Atlas of Breast Implant Ultrasound

Jae Hong Kim

Atlas of Breast Implant Ultrasound

Springer

Jae Hong Kim
Breast Center
The W Clinic
Seoul, Korea (Republic of)

ISBN 978-981-16-8281-0 ISBN 978-981-16-8282-7 (eBook)
https://doi.org/10.1007/978-981-16-8282-7

This Springer imprint is published by the registered company Springer Nature Singapore Pte Ltd.
The registered company address is: 152 Beach Road, #21-01/04 Gateway East, Singapore 189721, Singapore

Preface

Currently, an implant-based augmentation mammaplasty is the most popular plastic surgery in women worldwide. Moreover, breast cancer is the most common malignancy in women. Therefore, there has been an increase in the number of women who undergo breast reconstruction after mastectomy. According to the 2018 statistics in Korea, breast cancer occurred in approximately 26,000 women. It is also estimated that approximately 20,000 women receive an implant-based augmentation mammaplasty every year. In particular, women receiving total mastectomy have been covered by the national health insurance since 2015. This is closely associated with a continual increase in the number of women receiving an implant-based augmentation mammaplasty for reconstructive purposes. Breast is a symbol of feminity; women desire to have a beautiful breast, where breast health is an essential factor that cannot be overlooked. Women receiving an implant-based augmentation mammaplasty are vulnerable to diverse types of complications as there has been a dramatic increase in the use of a breast implant, for which an early detection of post-implantation complications is mandatory for assurance of patient health and safety.

Recently, breast implant-associated anaplastic large cell lymphoma (BIA-ALCL) has been reported worldwide; three cases of BIA-ALCL have also been described in three Korean women receiving a textured implant. This warns healthcare professionals of the importance of an early diagnosis and treatment of complications that may affect women receiving a breast implant. I have performed a meticulous observation of women receiving a breast implant with the use of a high-resolution ultrasound over the decade. I am now writing this book to share my knowledge and experience with other healthcare professionals. With images and video presentations in association with surgical procedures, readers of this book will comprehend overall aspects of an evidence-based approach to an early detection of post-implantation complications.

In my experience, breast ultrasound is *not only* an evidence-based imaging modality in making a diagnosis of complications in women receiving a breast implant at the earliest opportunities possible *but also* a useful tool for identifying a specific type of an implant like shell type, shape type, and the corresponding manufacturer. This book will provide a guidance to practitioners who are involved in an implant-based augmentation mammaplasty.

Seoul, Korea (Republic of) Jae Hong Kim

Acknowledgment

I dedicate this book to my family, especially wife, Ji Ha Kim, and my daughter, Min Seo Kim, with love and gratitude.

I am greatly thankful to Drs. Nam Sun Paik, Woo Chul Noh, Eun Kyu Kim, Hyun Ah Kim, Min Ki Sung, Hai Lin Park, Heung Kyu Park, and Young Bum Yoo for their helpful advice.

I also express gratitude to my colleagues, Drs. Min Soo Kim, Angela Soen Lee, and Hye Jin Kim, and the members of the Korean Society of Breast Implant Research for their critical reading of this book.

Finally, I send my gratitude to all the staffs of my clinic: Mrs. Go Eun Bi Seo, Yeo Jin, Lee, and Hui Xu for their great help.

Contents

1 Current Status and Future Implications of Ultrasound in the Context of Implant-Based Breast Aesthetic and Reconstructive Surgery 1
1.1 Overview 1
1.2 Diagnostic Imaging Studies in Patients Receiving a Breast Implant 2
1.3 The Emerging Value of Ultrasound as a Novel Diagnostic Modality 2
1.4 Comparison of HRUS and MRI 2
References 3

2 An Evidence-Based Approach to an Implant-Based Mammaplasty 5
2.1 Overview 5
2.2 Treatment Protocol 5
2.2.1 Preoperative Simulation of Postoperative Outcomes 5
2.2.2 Surgical Procedures 5
2.2.3 An Evidence-Based Radiologic Protocol for the Early Detection of Complications of an Implant-Based Breast Surgery 7
2.3 Clinical Cases 8
2.3.1 Case 1 8
2.3.2 Case 2 9
2.3.3 Case 3 9
2.3.4 Case 4 10
2.3.5 Case 5 10
2.3.6 Case 6 10
2.3.7 Case 7 12
2.3.8 Case 8 12
2.3.9 Case 9 12
2.3.10 Case 10 12
2.3.11 Case 11 12
2.3.12 Case 12 14
2.3.13 Case 13 14
2.3.14 Case 14 14
2.3.15 Case 15 16
2.3.16 Case 16 16

2.3.17 Case 17. 16
2.3.18 Case 18. 18
2.3.19 Case 19. 41
References. 45

3 Role of Ultrasound in the Implant-Based Aesthetic and Reconstructive Mammaplasty 47
3.1 Overview 47
3.2 Role of Ultrasound in the Context of an Implant-Based Aesthetic and Reconstructive Mammaplasty. 47
3.2.1 Characteristics of a Breast Implant 47
3.2.2 Ultrasound-Guided Assessment of a Breast Implant . . 47
3.2.3 Ultrasound-Guided Diagnosis of Postoperative Complications 48
3.2.4 Ultrasound as a Screening Tool for Patients Who Are Suspected of Having Breast Implant-Associated Anaplastic Large Cell Lymphoma (BIA-ALCL). 49
3.2.5 Ultrasound as a Component of a Multi-Disciplinary Algorithm-Based Approach to an Early Detection of Complications of an Implant-Based Augmentation Mammaplasty. 49
References. 53

4 Distinguishing Various Types of Breast Implant Using High-Resolution Ultrasonography 55
4.1 Location of a Breast Implant 55
4.2 Constituents of a Breast Implant 55
4.3 Surface Topography of a Breast Implant 56
4.4 Shape and Manufacturer of a Breast Implant 60

5 Usefulness of High-Resolution Ultrasound in Detecting Complications of an Implant-Based Mammaplasty 89
5.1 Overview 89
5.2 Folding. 89
5.3 Periprosthetic Fluid Collection 90
5.4 Rupture. 92
5.4.1 Saline Implant Rupture 92
5.4.2 Silicone Implant Rupture. 94
5.5 Thickened Capsule and Capsular Contracture. 101
5.6 Upside-Down (USD) Rotation. 110
References. 122

6 Breast Implant-Associated Anaplastic Large Cell Lymphoma. 123
6.1 Overview 123
6.2 A Vicious Circle of Crisis of a Breast Implant 123
6.3 Association Between the Onset of BIA-ALCL and a Textured Implant. 124
6.4 Approaches to Risk Management for an Early Detection of BIA-ALCL. 124

6.5 Conflict of Interest (COI) in Plastic Surgery and Its Possible Involvement in Crisis of Stakeholders in an Implant-Based Augmentation Mammaplasty . . . 125
References . . . 126

7 Usefulness of High-Resolution Ultrasound (HRUS) in Planning Revision or Reoperation for Patients Receiving an Implant-Based Augmentation Mammaplasty . . . 129
7.1 Overview . . . 129
7.2 Preoperative Considerations Based on HRUS for Reoperation . . . 129
7.3 An Algorithm-Based Approach to HRUS-Assisted Reoperation . . . 131
7.3.1 Location of a Pocket . . . 131
7.3.2 Surface Topography of the Shell of a Breast Implant . . . 131
7.3.3 Status of a Capsule . . . 131
7.3.4 Implant-Related Complications . . . 138
7.3.5 Previous Surgical Approaches . . . 148
References . . . 148

8 Clinical Presentation . . . 151
8.1 Overview . . . 151
8.2 Illustrative Cases . . . 151
8.2.1 Case 1 . . . 151
8.2.2 Case 2 . . . 151
8.2.3 Case 3 . . . 156
8.2.4 Case 4 . . . 156
8.2.5 Case 5 . . . 156
8.2.6 Case 6 . . . 164
8.2.7 Case 7 . . . 164
8.2.8 Case 8 . . . 166
8.2.9 Case 9 . . . 166
8.2.10 Case 10 . . . 166
8.2.11 Case 11 . . . 168
8.2.12 Case 12 . . . 175
8.2.13 Case 13 . . . 183
8.2.14 Case 14 . . . 186
8.2.15 Case 15 . . . 189
8.2.16 Case 16 . . . 191
8.2.17 Case 17 . . . 191
8.2.18 Case 18 . . . 193
8.2.19 Case 19 . . . 197
8.2.20 Case 20 . . . 197
8.2.21 Case 21 . . . 197
8.2.22 Case 22 . . . 200
8.2.23 Case 23 . . . 208
8.2.24 Case 24 . . . 214
8.2.25 Case 25 . . . 214

8.2.26 Case 26. 216
8.2.27 Case 27. 216
8.2.28 Case 28. 224
8.2.29 Case 29. 224
8.2.30 Case 30. 227
8.2.31 Case 31. 232
8.2.32 Case 32. 232
8.2.33 Case 33. 238
8.2.34 Case 34. 238
8.2.35 Case 35. 244
8.2.36 Case 36. 244
8.2.37 Case 37. 248
8.2.38 Case 38. 248
8.2.39 Case 39. 250
8.2.40 Case 40. 254
8.2.41 Case 41. 257
8.2.42 Case 42. 257
8.2.43 Case 43. 257
8.2.44 Case 44. 257
8.2.45 Case 45. 266
8.2.46 Case 46. 266
8.2.47 Case 47. 266
8.2.48 Case 48. 275
8.2.49 Case 49. 277
8.2.50 Case 50. 277
8.2.51 Case 51. 281
8.2.52 Case 52. 285
References. 288

9 Conclusions 289
References. 291

Current Status and Future Implications of Ultrasound in the Context of Implant-Based Breast Aesthetic and Reconstructive Surgery

1

1.1 Overview

Breast is a symbol of feminity that serves as a key factor of quality of life [1]. Implant-based augmentation mammaplasty is performed for the purposes of enlarging a normal breast and reconstructing an absent or abnormal breast [2, 3]. It remains as one of the most popular procedures in the setting of aesthetic and reconstructive plastic surgery. In the USA in 2018, a total of 313,000 procedures were performed. Moreover, it has also been reported that a total of 1,862,506 procedures were performed worldwide [4].

Still, controversial opinions exist regarding the safety of silicone gel-filled breast implants. This deserves special attention [5]. In more detail, there has been an extensive debate on the safety of breast implants, classified as a type III medical device, since they were first introduced in the 1960s; their use in cosmetic surgery was transiently prohibited by the US Food and Drug Administration (FDA) between 1992 and 2006, but it was approved by the FDA in 2006 on condition that it would be under a long-term follow-up, further analyzed after explanted and released with more detailed labeling [6, 7]. Nevertheless, a causal relationship of silicone gel-filled breast implants with postoperative complications, such as cancer, autoimmune diseases, and connective tissue diseases, has not been established, as described by a systematic review and meta-analyses of previously published studies in this series [7, 8].

Concerns for possible health risks after augmentation mammaplasty arose from earlier case reports about women exhibiting connective tissue disease after receiving breast implants or silicone injections [9, 10]. Such a key public health issue should be answered with scientific efforts rather than anti-scientific and irrational methods; it should be handled with evidence-based scientific grounds [11].

On the other hand, there are also some concerns that local complications may occur following the use of silicone gel-filled breast implants; its major drawbacks include capsular contracture (CC) and a loss of the implant integrity [12, 13]. Thus, safety concerns have shifted from systemic adverse effects to local complications that are closely associated with the primary safety profile of silicone gel-filled breast implants, as described in a report published by the Institute of Medicine of the National Academy of Science [14]. Potential postoperative complications include CC, implant malposition, breast deformation and asymmetry, wound and skin problems, infection, hematoma and hemorrhage, implant rupture, seroma, abscess, silicone granuloma, and implant extrusion [15–19]. But the incidence, severity, and long-term sequelae of these local complications have been studied only in a limited scope [20–24]. Moreover, differences in study design and methodology have made it difficult to directly compare the results between the studies in this series [25].

J. H. Kim, *Atlas of Breast Implant Ultrasound*, https://doi.org/10.1007/978-981-16-8282-7_1

1.2 Diagnostic Imaging Studies in Patients Receiving a Breast Implant

Patients receiving a breast implant should be evaluated with diagnostic imaging studies for several reasons: these include (1) regular screening mammography, (2) additional imaging for Breast Imaging. Reporting and Data System (BI-RADS) 0, 3, 4, and 5 lesions, (3) interventional biopsy, (4) certain types of complications of an implant-based augmentation mammaplasty (e.g., impaired immune response, connective tissue disorders, or BIA-ALCL), and (5) leakage or rupture of a breast implant [26–28].

Surgeons often encounter challenges arising from a breast implant; they should identify and distinguish shell types of a breast implant, make a diagnosis of implant failure or other complications of an implant-based augmentation mammaplasty, and perform a regular follow-up [29]. It has been reported that patients receiving a breast implant are vulnerable to mortality from malignant conditions [30]. This suggests that diagnostic imaging studies have their own merits and demerits in detecting complications of an implant-based augmentation mammaplasty [31]. It can therefore be concluded that novel imaging studies should apply to the diagnosis of complications of an implant-based augmentation mammaplasty.

1.3 The Emerging Value of Ultrasound as a Novel Diagnostic Modality

Since the US FDA approval of a silicone gel-filled breast implant, dated November of 2006, it has been recommended that patients receiving a breast implant are evaluated with magnetic resonance imaging (MRI) scans at three years post-operatively and at a 2-year interval thereafter [32]. Thus, efforts have been made to detect complications of an implant-based augmentation mammaplasty, such as capsular contracture and rupture imaging studies [33]. Since then, the use of MRI has been considered a gold standard for the non-invasive assessment of a breast implant [34]. In addition to its disadvantages including high cost *as well as* inconvenience, however, its sensitivity and specificity for detecting implant failure have been reported to show discrepancies between the radiologists [35–37]. Further, it remains questionable whether an MRI can also be used to detect implant failure in asymptomatic patients receiving the fourth and fifth generation of device [38].

A US has also been used to detect implant failure, although it has been established as an alternative to an MRI [35, 39–45]. With technological advancements, its specifications have been much improved. As a non-invasive, cost-effective diagnostic modality for patients receiving a breast implant, it deserves special attention [46].

1.4 Comparison of HRUS and MRI

HRUS has many advantages in identifying various breast implant types and measurement of thickened capsule and complications like upside-down rotation.

The biggest advantage of HRUS are the ability to diagnose side effects and excellence in distinguishing side effects.

So, HRUS is an effective diagnostic image modality than MRI (Table 1.1).

Table 1.1 Comparison between HRUS and MRI

	MRI	HRUS
Identify implant information Shell type Shape type Manufacturer Constituent	Impossible	Possible (sometimes even there are ruptures)
Rupture	Possible	Possible
Periprosthetic fluid collection	Possible	Possible
Upside-down rotation	Impossible	Possible
Thickened capsule	Possible	Possible (>0.4 mm)
Radiation exposure	Yes	No
Time	40 minutes	<10 minutes
Radiologic result	Days	Immediate

References

1. Webb C, Jacox N, Temple-Oberle C. The making of breasts: navigating the symbolism of breasts in women facing cancer. Plast Surg (Oakv). 2019;27(1):49–53.
2. Champaneria MC, Wong WW, Hill ME, Gupta SC. The evolution of breast reconstruction: a historical perspective. World J Surg. 2012;36(4):730–42.
3. Rizki H, Nkonde C, Ching RC, Kumiponjera D, Malata CM. Plastic surgical management of the contralateral breast in post-mastectomy breast reconstruction. Int J Surg. 2013;11(9):767–72.
4. Oh JS, Jeong JH, Myung Y, et al. BellaGel breast implant: 6-year results of a prospective cohort study. Arch Plast Surg. 2020;47(3):235–41.
5. Hillard C, Fowler JD, Barta R, Cunningham B. Silicone breast implant rupture: a review. Gland Surg. 2017 Apr;6(2):163–8.
6. Tanne JH. FDA approves silicone breast implants 14 years after their withdrawal. BMJ. 2006 Dec 2;333(7579):1139.
7. Balk EM, Earley A, Avendano EA, Raman G. Long-term health outcomes in women with silicone gel breast implants: a systematic review. Ann Intern Med. 2016 Feb 2;164(3):164–75.
8. Janowsky EC, Kupper LL, Hulka BS. Meta-analyses of the relation between silicone breast implants and the risk of connective-tissue diseases. N Engl J Med. 2000 Mar 16;342(11):781–90.
9. van Nunen SA, Gatenby PA, Basten A. Post-mammoplasty connective tissue disease. Arthritis Rheum. 1982 Jun;25(6):694–7.
10. Kumagai Y, Shiokawa Y, Medsger TA Jr, Rodnan GP. Clinical spectrum of connective tissue disease after cosmetic surgery. Observations on eighteen patients and a review of the Japanese literature. Arthritis Rheum. 1984 Jan;27(1):1–12.
11. Angell M. Shattuck Lecture--evaluating the health risks of breast implants: the interplay of medical science, the law, and public opinion. N Engl J Med. 1996 Jun 6;334(23):1513–8.
12. Steiert AE, Boyce M, Sorg H. Capsular contracture by silicone breast implants: possible causes, biocompatibility, and prophylactic strategies. Med Devices (Auckl). 2013 Dec 2;6:211–8.
13. Berry MG, Davies DM. Breast augmentation: Part I--A review of the silicone prosthesis. J Plast Reconstr Aesthet Surg. 2010 Nov;63(11):1761–8.
14. Kulmala I, McLaughlin JK, Pakkanen M, Lassila K, Hölmich LR, Lipworth L, Boice JD Jr, Raitanen J, Luoto R. Local complications after cosmetic breast implant surgery in Finland. Ann Plast Surg. 2004 Nov;53(5):413–9.
15. Quirós MC, Bolaños MC, Fassero JJ. Six-year prospective outcomes of primary breast augmentation with Nano surface implants. Aesthet Surg J. 2019 Apr 8;39(5):495–508.
16. Nava MB, Rancati A, Angrigiani C, Catanuto G, Rocco N. How to prevent complications in breast augmentation. Gland Surg. 2017 Apr;6(2):210–7.
17. Duteille F, Rouif M, Laurent S, Cannon M. Five-year safety data for Eurosilicone's round and anatomical silicone gel breast implants. Plast Reconstr Surg Glob Open. 2014 May 7;2(4):e138.
18. Mazzocchi M, Dessy LA, Corrias F, Scuderi N. A clinical study of late seroma in breast implantation surgery. Aesthet Plast Surg. 2012 Feb;36(1):97–104.
19. Wong T, Lo LW, Fung PY, Lai HY, She HL, Ng WK, Kwok KM, Lee CM. Magnetic resonance imaging of breast augmentation: a pictorial review. Insights Imaging. 2016 Jun;7(3):399–410.
20. Hall-Findlay EJ. Breast implant complication review: double capsules and late seromas. Plast Reconstr Surg. 2011 Jan;127(1):56–66.
21. Baek WY, Lew DH, Lee DW. A retrospective analysis of ruptured breast implants. Arch Plast Surg. 2014 Nov;41(6):734–9.
22. Alderman A, Pusic A, Murphy DK. Prospective analysis of primary breast augmentation on body image using the BREAST-Q: results from a Nationwide study. Plast Reconstr Surg. 2016 Jun;137(6):954e–60e.
23. Maxwell GP, Van Natta BW, Bengtson BP, Murphy DK. Ten-year results from the Natrelle 410 anatomi-

cal form-stable silicone breast implant core study. Aesthet Surg J. 2015 Feb;35(2):145–55.
24. Headon H, Kasem A, Mokbel K. Capsular contracture after breast augmentation: an update for clinical practice. Arch Plast Surg. 2015 Sep;42(5):532–43.
25. Fryzek JP, Signorello LB, Hakelius L, Lipworth L, McLaughlin JK, Blot WJ, Nyren O. Local complications and subsequent symptom reporting among women with cosmetic breast implants. Plast Reconstr Surg. 2001 Jan;107(1):214–21.
26. Muir Gray JA. Breast implants: evidence based patient choice and litigation. BMJ. 1999;318:414.
27. Balzer BL, Weiss SW. Do biomaterials cause implant associated mesenchymal tumors of the breast. Analysis of eight new cases and review of the literature. Hum Pathol. 2009;40:1564–70.
28. Di Benedetto G, Cecchini S, Grassetti L, Baldassarre S, Valeri G, Leva L, Giuseppetti GM, Bertani A. Comparative study of breast implant rupture using mammography, sonography, and magnetic resonance imaging: correlation with surgical findings. Breast J. 2008;14:532–7.
29. Stöblen F, Rezai M, Kümmel S. Imaging in patients with breast implants-results of the first international breast (implant) conference 2009. Insights Imaging. 2010;1(2):93–7.
30. Koot VCM, Peeters PHM, Granath F, Grobbee DE, Nyren O. Total and cause specific mortality among Swedish women with cosmetic breast implants: prospective study. BMJ. 2003;326:527–8.
31. Handel N. The effect of silicone implants on the diagnosis, prognosis, and treatment of breast cancer. Plast Reconstr Surg. 2007;120(7 Suppl 1):81S–93S.
32. Sung JY, Jeong JP, Moon DS, et al. Short-term safety of augmentation Mammaplasty using the BellaGel implants in Korean women. Plast Reconstr Surg Glob Open. 2019;7(12):e2566.
33. Juanpere S, Perez E, Huc O, Motos N, Pont J, Pedraza S. Imaging of breast implants-a pictorial review. Insights Imaging. 2011;2(6):653–70.
34. Wong T, Lo LW, Fung PY, et al. Magnetic resonance imaging of breast augmentation: a pictorial review. Insights Imaging. 2016;7(3):399–410.
35. Goodman CM, Cohen V, Thornby J, Netscher D. The life span of silicone gel breast implants and a comparison of mammography, ultrasonography, and magnetic resonance imaging in detecting implant rupture: a metaanalysis. Ann Plast Surg. 1998;41:577–85.
36. Collis N, Litherland J, Enion D, Sharpe DT. Magnetic resonance imaging and explantation investigation of long-term silicone gel implant integrity. Plast Reconstr Surg. 2007;120:1401–6.
37. Song JW, Kim HM, Bellfi LT, Chung KC. The effect of study design biases on the diagnostic accuracy of magnetic resonance imaging for detecting silicone gel breast implant ruptures: a meta-analysis. Plast Reconstr Surg. 2011;127:1029–44.
38. Bengtson BP, Eaves FF 3rd. High-resolution ultrasound in the detection of silicone gel breast implant shell failure: background, in vitro studies, and early clinical results. Aesthet Surg J. 2012;32(2):157–74.
39. Ahn CY. Comparative silicone gel breast implant evaluation using mammography, sonography, and magnetic resonance imaging: experience with 59 implants. Plast Reconstr Surg. 1994;94:620–7.
40. Di Benedetto G, Cecchini S, Grassetti L, et al. Comparative study of breast implant rupture using mammography, sonography, and magnetic resonance imaging: correlation with surgical findings. Breast J. 2008;14:532–7.
41. Ikeda DM, Borofsky HB, Herfkens RJ, et al. Silicone gel breast implant rupture: Pitfalls of magnetic resonance imaging and relative efficacies of magnetic resonance, mammography and ultrasound. Plast Reconst Surg. 1999;104:2054–62.
42. Rohrich RJ, Adams WP Jr, Beran SJ, et al. An analysis of silicone gel-filled breast implants: diagnosis and failure rates. Plast Reconstr Surg. 1998;102:2304–8.
43. Chung KC, Wilkins EG, Beil RJ Jr, et al. Diagnosis of silicone gel breast implant rupture by ultrasonography. Plast Reconstr Surg. 1996;97:104–9.
44. Caskey CI, Berg WA, Anderson ND, et al. Breast implant rupture: diagnosis with US. Radiology. 1994;190:819–23.
45. Venta LA, Salomon CG, Flisak ME, et al. Sonographic signs of breast implant rupture. AJR Am J Roentgenol. 1996;166:1413–9.
46. Chung KC, Malay S, Shauver MJ, Kim HM. Economic analysis of screening strategies for rupture of silicone gel breast implants. Plast Reconstr Surg. 2012;130(1):225–37.

2 An Evidence-Based Approach to an Implant-Based Mammaplasty

2.1 Overview

An implant has been used for aesthetic and reconstructive mammaplasty (Fig. 2.1).

An implant-based augmentation mammaplasty is commonly performed based on what surgeons learned in training, but it may be altered by anecdotal evidence with regard to complications and personal experiences [1–3]. Surgical approaches and implants vary, for which a considerable amount of clinical data has been published to provide an evidence-based approach to an implant-based augmentation mammaplasty [4, 5]. An evidence-based implant-based augmentation mammaplasty has been previously described [6–8].

2.2 Treatment Protocol

2.2.1 Preoperative Simulation of Postoperative Outcomes

Preoperatively, the Divina™ 3-dimensional Scanner (Establishment Labs Holdings Inc., Alajuela, Costa Rica) is used to allow the patients to view possible results of an implant-based augmentation mammaplasty (Fig. 2.2). It *not only* helps a surgeon obtain anthropometric measurements of the breast *but also* visualizes its preoperative characteristics. Thus, it stimulates possible results through an analysis of data and information about diverse types of a silicone gel-filled breast implant for the purposes of helping a patient select optimal types of a breast implant and thereby yielding satisfactory outcomes.

2.2.2 Surgical Procedures

Surgical procedures are performed in compliance with the American Society of Plastic Surgery (ASPS) recommendations, as previously described [9]. Periareolar, inframammary fold, and axillary incisions are made under general anesthesia and intravenous sedation for the purposes of preventing visible scarring (Fig. 2.3). Selection of surgical incision is based on desired outcomes, types of breast implants, the degree of augmentation, the anatomical characteristics of patients, and patient-surgeon preference.

Based on the Ranquist formula, the distance extending from the nipple to the inframammary fold, the size of breast implant, and the scope of dissection are determined. After the dissection, each breast is irrigated using a 100 mL of normal saline mixed with H_2O_2 solution at a ratio of 1:1, followed by the use of betadine 100 cc. Then, a breast implant is immersed in a normal saline mixed with ceftezole 1 vial and gentamicin 1 ample and then inserted in a pocket either under

Supplementary Information The online version contains supplementary material available at [https://doi.org/10.1007/978-981-16-8282-7_2].

J. H. Kim, *Atlas of Breast Implant Ultrasound*, https://doi.org/10.1007/978-981-16-8282-7_2

the pectoralis major muscle (a submuscular placement) or in the retromammary space above it (subglandular/submammary placement).

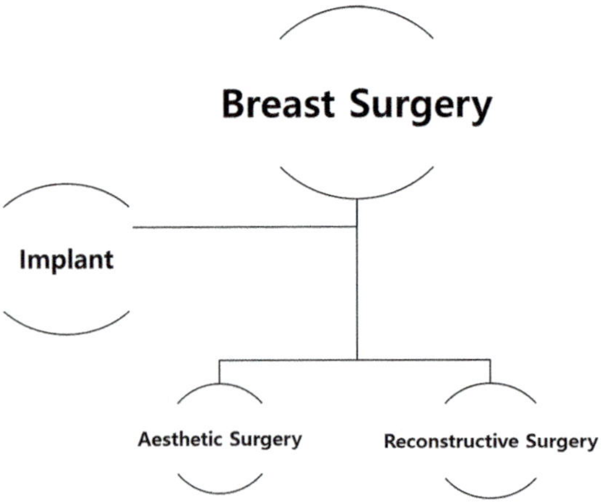

Fig. 2.1 Breast implant surgery

There are two types of breast implant position, subpectoral and subglandular pocket (Fig. 2.4). Subpectoral pocket means that breast implant is positioned under the pectoralis major muscle.

Methods for inserting and positioning a breast implant in the pocket are dependent on its types, the degree of augmentation, characteristics of a patient's body, and surgeons' recommendations. Thus, a dual-plane I/II augmentation is performed on a case-by-case basis.

Dual plane I, II, II is determined by dissection range and height of P. major muscle during operation for aesthetic result (Fig. 2.5). Best aesthetic result is achieved by appropriate N-IMF distance.

Intraoperatively, the patients are intravenously given ceftezole 1.0 g. Incisions are closed using layered sutures in the breast tissue. In addition, skin adhesive or surgical tape is used to close the skin. Postoperatively, the patients are given cefa-

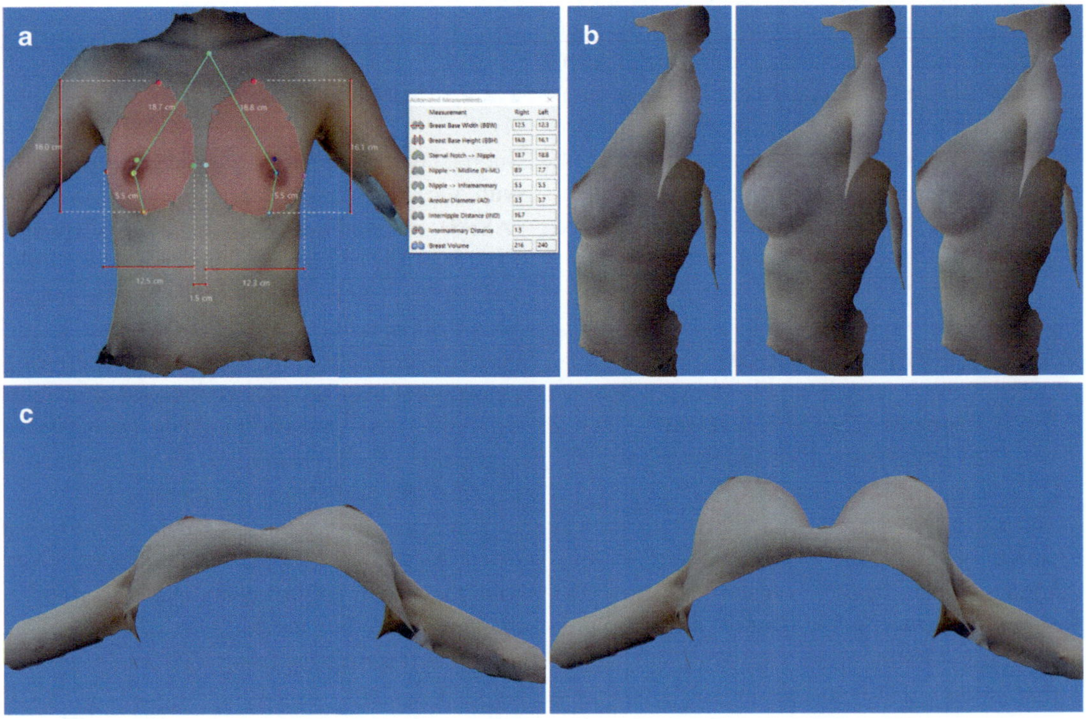

Fig. 2.2 Preoperative anthropometric measurement by 3D simulation. (**a**) Measurement of Breast base width, Breast base height, Sternal notch- > nipple, Nipple- > midline, Nipple- > inframammary fold, Areolar diameter, Internal distance, Intermammary distance, Breast volume. (**b**) Before and after simulation. (**c**) Correction of projection asymmetry

clor, non-steroidal anti-inflammatory drugs (NSAIDs), and antacid 3 times daily for a week. Moreover, they are also recommended to take montelukast sodium 10 mg (Lucast tab.; Wooridul Pharmaceutical Ltd., Seoul, Korea) for a month for the prevention of capsular contracture (CC) and to wear a compressive garment for 3 months. Furthermore, they are also recommended to use an upper or lower band, if necessary, and most of them use an upper one for 1–2 months. Postoperative course is meticulously monitored during a regular follow-up at 1, 2, 3, and 4 weeks; 3, 6, 9, and 12 months; and thereafter [9].

I use the Delmar breast endoscope set for trans-axillary approach (Fig. 2.6). Delmar set has advantages not only in primary augmentation surgery, but also in capsulectomy in revisional surgery (Video 2.2).

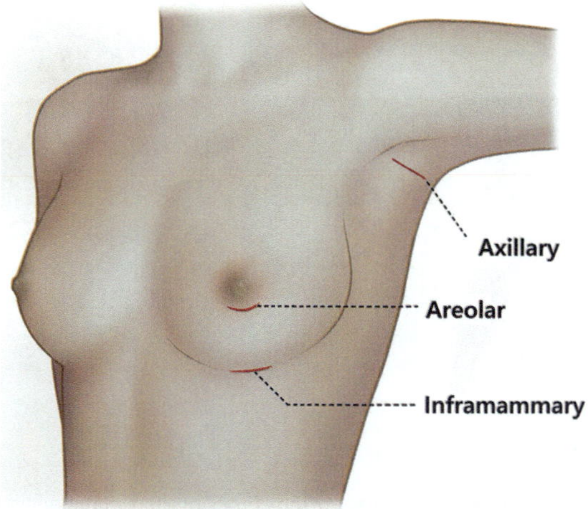

Fig. 2.3 Various types of incision in augmentation mammaplasty

2.2.3 An Evidence-Based Radiologic Protocol for the Early Detection of Complications of an Implant-Based Breast Surgery

Early detection of postoperative complications is achieved by breast ultrasound at 3 months, 6 months (if necessary), and every year postoperatively which is performed routinely in every patient with Aplio i600 (Canon Medical Systems, Otawara, Tochigi, Japan) system with a 7–18-MHz linear transducer, as previously described [10] (Fig. 2.7).

High-resolution ultrasound is used for checking breast parenchyma, implant (shell), and periprosthetic capsule (Fig. 2.8).

Normal ultrasonography after implant-based mammaplasty shows flattened shell and no rupture sign and thickened capsule (Video 2.1).

Fig. 2.4 Position of breast implant pocket

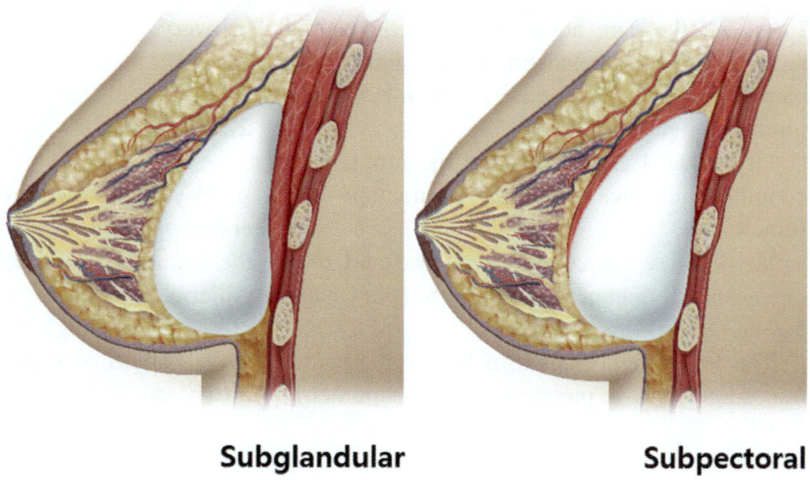

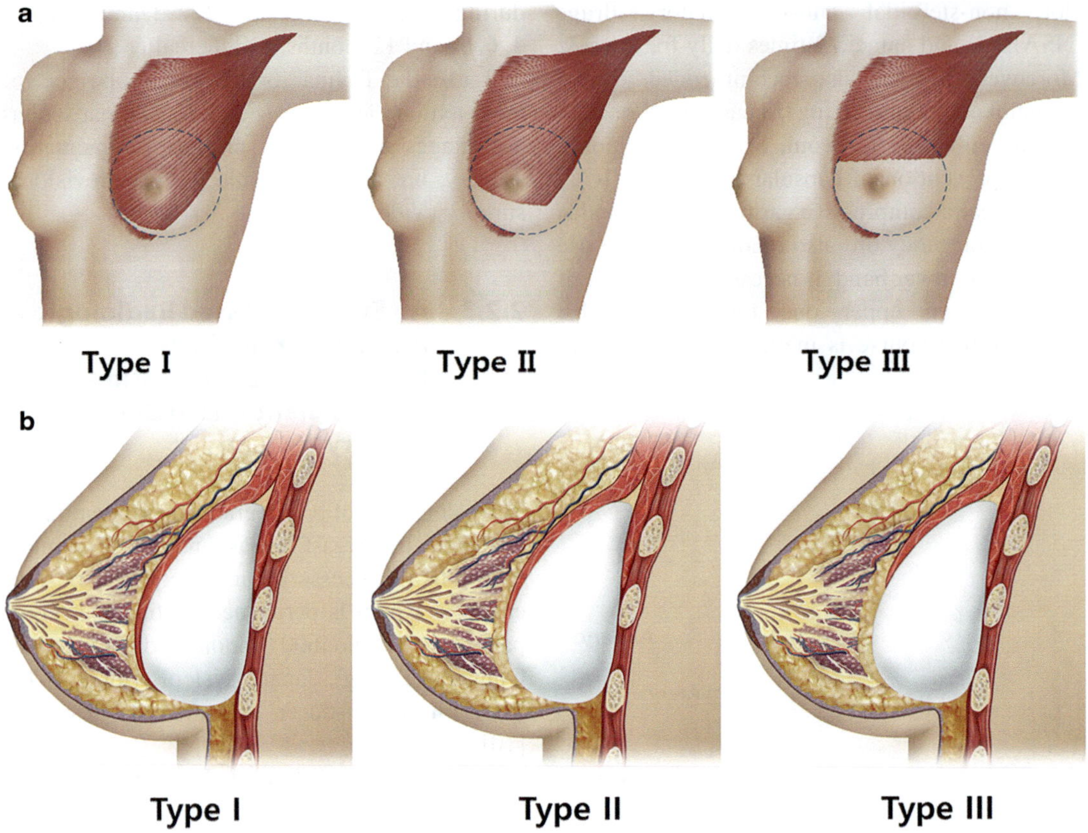

Fig. 2.5 (**a**, **b**): dividing and separating of P. major muscle from breast parenchyma. Various types of dual-plane operation technique

2.3 Clinical Cases

I can get the data about normal sequence of recovery of periprosthetic tissue and breast parenchyma through high-resolution ultrasonography.

Of course, I can understand the progress of complications like capsular contracture and rupture.

I will show the complicated case and their diagnosis and treatment and the results in Chaps. 5, 7 and 8.

The following 19 cases of breast augmentation surgery show preoperative anthropometric measurement, pre/post-operative gross finding, and ultrasonographic image and normal recovery.

2.3.1 Case 1

A 23-year-old woman received a trans-axillary endoscopic augmentation mammaplasty using the Naturgel™ (Groupe Sebbin SAS, Boissy-l' Aillerie, France), for which the patient did have placement of a high-profile device (LS 71285 cc) in the subpectoral pocket on both sides of the breast using preoperative anthropometric data

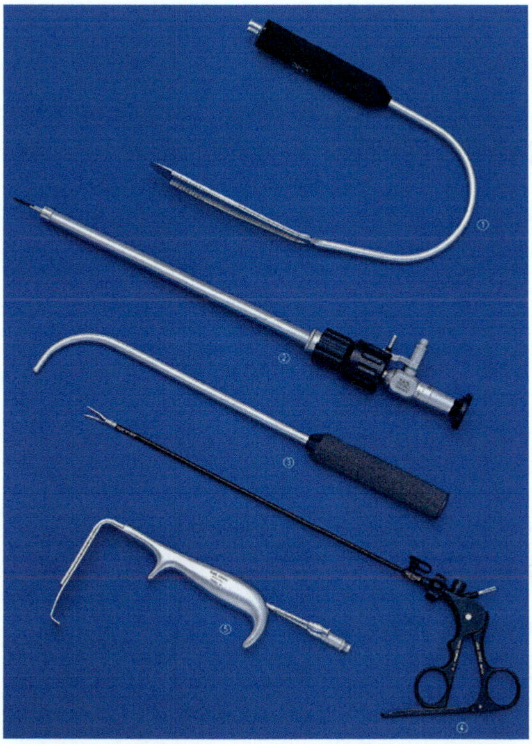

Fig. 2.6 Instrument of breast endoscopic surgery: Delmar set, Karl Storz

(Fig. 2.9). And preoperative front and lateral view & post-operative front and lateral view, postoperative ultrasonographic finding was checked during routine follow-up (Fig. 2.9).

2.3.2 Case 2

A 28-year-old woman received a trans-axillary endoscopic augmentation mammaplasty using the BellaGel SmoothFine (HansBiomed Co. Ltd., Seoul, Korea), for which the patient did have placement of a high-profile device (300 cc) in the subpectoral pocket on both sides of the breast using preoperative anthropometric data (Fig. 2.10). And pre & post-operative view, post-operative ultrasonographic finding was checked during routine follow-up (Fig. 2.10).

2.3.3 Case 3

A 39-year-old woman received a trans-axillary endoscopic augmentation mammaplasty using the

Fig. 2.7 Postoperative ultrasonographic finding after the breast implant-based mammaplasty

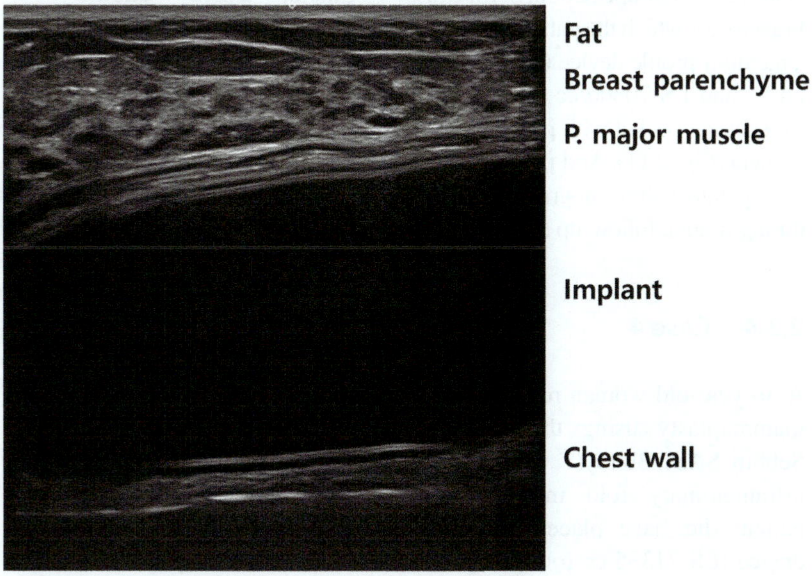

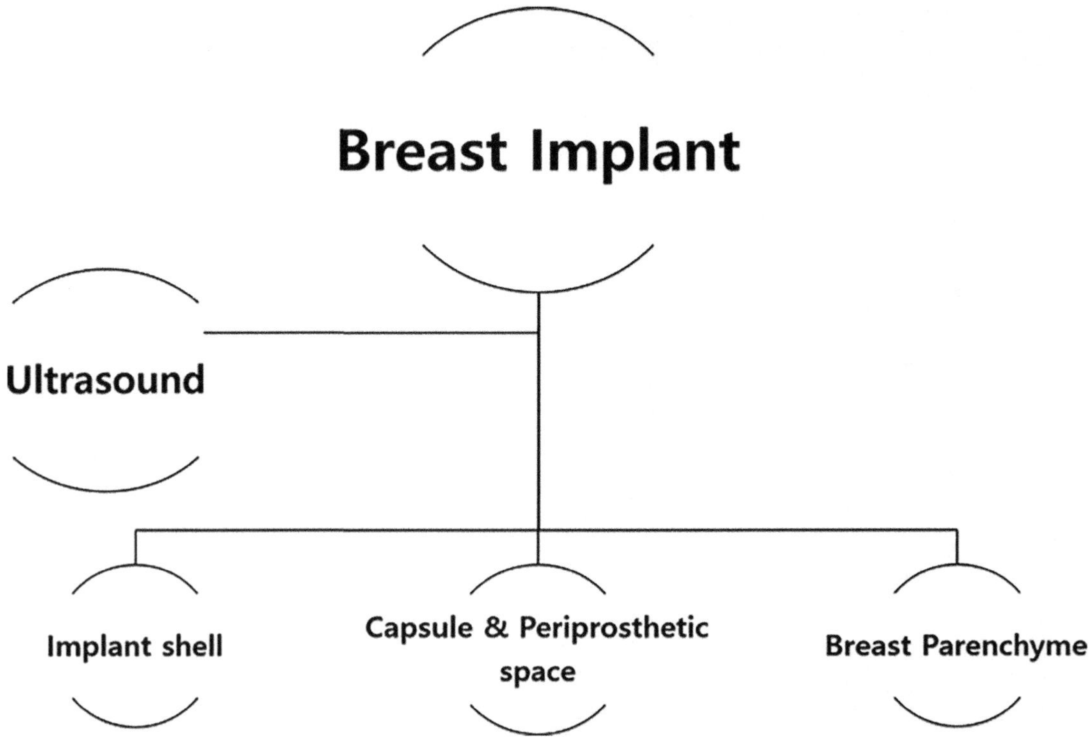

Fig. 2.8 Checkpoints of high-resolution ultrasound in patient received implant mammaplasty

Naturgel™ (Groupe Sebbin SAS, Boissy-l' Aillerie, France), for which the patient did have placement of a medium-profile device (LS70 330 cc for the right breast and LS 70300 cc for the left breast) in the subpectoral pocket with preoperative anthropometric data (Fig. 2.11). And pre & post-operative view, postoperative ultrasonographic finding was checked during routine follow-up (Fig. 2.11).

2.3.4 Case 4

A 36-year-old woman received an augmentation mammaplasty using the Naturgel™ (Groupe Sebbin SAS, Boissy-l' Aillerie, France) via an inframammary fold incision, for which the patient did have placement of a high-profile device (LS 71335 cc for the right breast and LS 71365 cc for the left breast) in the subpectoral pocket with preoperative anthropometric data (Fig. 2.12). And pre & post-operative view, postoperative ultrasonographic finding was checked during routine follow-up (Fig. 2.12).

2.3.5 Case 5

A 35-year-old woman received a trans-axillary endoscopic augmentation mammaplasty using the Naturgel™ (Groupe Sebbin SAS, Boissy-l' Aillerie, France) for which the patient did have placement of a high-profile device (LS 71395 cc for the right breast and LS 71365 cc for the left breast) in the subpectoral pocket with preoperative anthropometric data (Fig. 2.13). And pre & post-operative view, postoperative ultrasonographic finding was checked during routine follow-up (Fig. 2.13).

2.3.6 Case 6

A 44-year-old woman received a trans-axillary endoscopic augmentation mammaplasty using the Naturgel™ (Groupe Sebbin SAS, Boissy-l' Aillerie, France) for which the patient did have placement of a medium-profile device (LS 71305 cc for the right breast and LS 71285 cc for

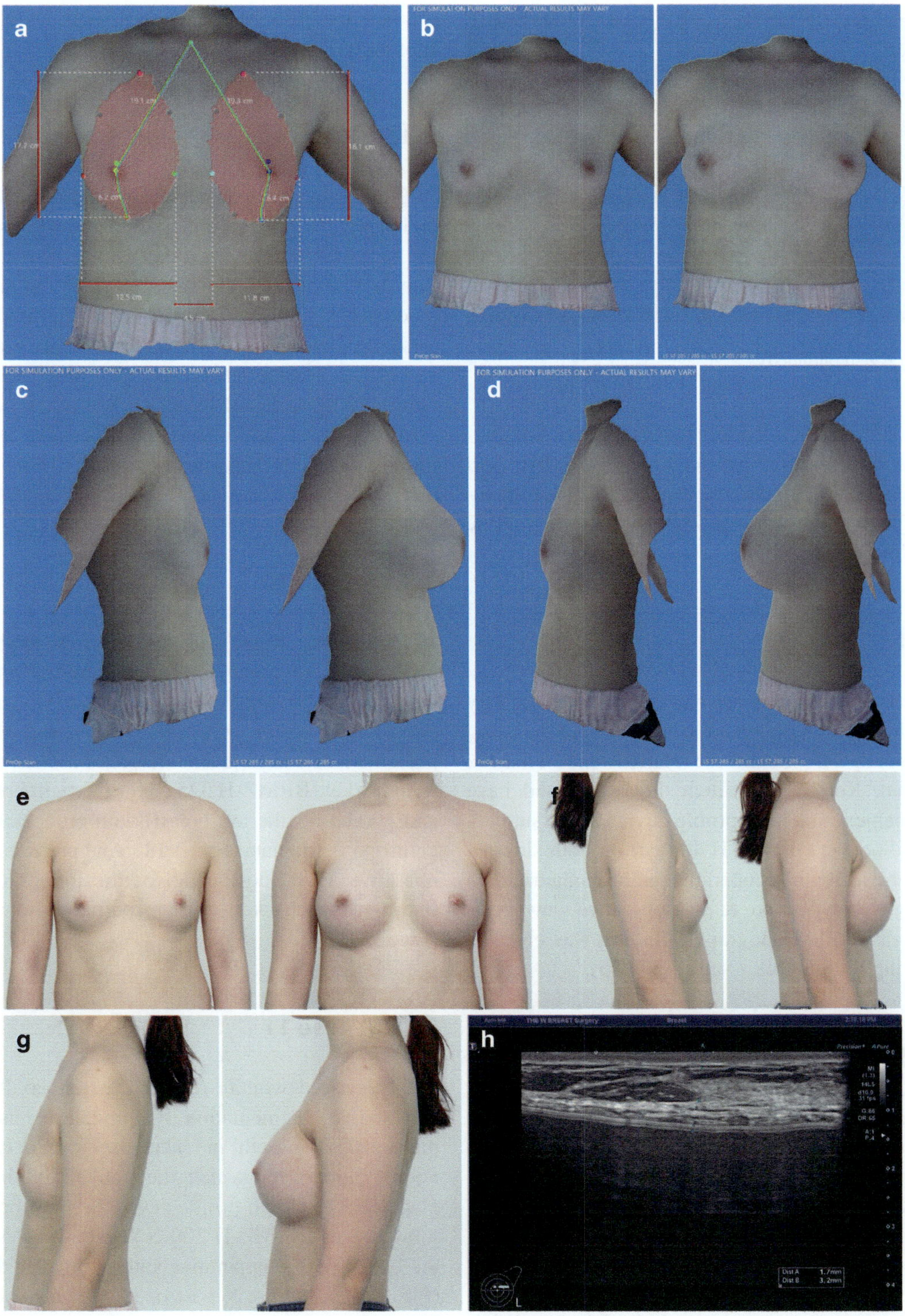

Fig. 2.9 (**a**) Preoperative anthropometric data by 3D simulation. (**b**) Front view of before and after 3D simulation. (**c**) Right side view of before and after 3D simulation. (**d**) Left side view of before and after 3D simulation. (**e**) Preoperative and postoperative front view. (**f**) Preoperative and postoperative right side view. (**g**) Preoperative and postoperative left side view. (**h**) Left ultrasound image shows normal device placed in the subpectoral pocket on 52 weeks postoperatively. (**i**) Right ultrasound image shows normal device placed in the subpectoral pocket on 52 weeks postoperatively

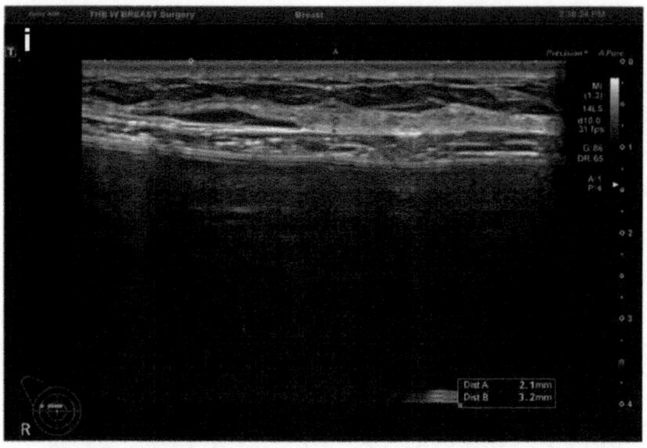

Fig. 2.9 (continued)

the left breast) in the subpectoral pocket with preoperative anthropometric data (Fig. 2.14). And pre & post-operative view, postoperative ultrasonographic finding was checked during routine follow-up (Fig. 2.14).

2.3.7 Case 7

A 26-year-old woman received a trans-axillary endoscopic augmentation mammaplasty using the BellaGel SmoothFine (HansBiomed Co. Ltd., Seoul, Korea), for which the patient did have placement of a high-profile device in the subpectoral pocket (BRMZ-H 400 cc) on both sides of the breast with preoperative anthropometric data (Fig. 2.15). And pre & post-operative view, postoperative ultrasonographic finding was checked during routine follow-up (Fig. 2.15).

2.3.8 Case 8

A 34-year-old woman received a trans-axillary endoscopic augmentation mammaplasty using the Motiva Ergonomix™Round SilkSurface (Establishment Labs Holdings Inc., Alajuela, Costa Rica), for which the patient did have placement of a high-profile device in the subpectoral pocket (ERSF 335 cc) on both sides of the breast with preoperative anthropometric data (Fig. 2.16). And pre & post-operative view, postoperative ultrasonographic finding was checked during routine follow-up (Fig. 2.16).

2.3.9 Case 9

A 28-year-old woman received a trans-axillary endoscopic augmentation mammaplasty using the BellaGel SmoothFine (HansBiomed Co. Ltd., Seoul, Korea), for which the patient did have placement of a high-profile device in the subpectoral pocket (BRMZ-H 275 cc for the right breast and 325 cc for the left breast) with preoperative anthropometric data (Fig. 2.17). And pre & post-operative view, postoperative ultrasonographic finding was checked during routine follow-up (Fig. 2.17)..

2.3.10 Case 10

A 28-year-old woman received a trans-axillary endoscopic augmentation mammaplasty using the BellaGel SmoothFine (HansBiomed Co. Ltd., Seoul, Korea), for which the patient did have placement of a high-profile device in the subpectoral pocket (BRMZ-H 325 cc for the right breast and 300 cc for the left breast) with preoperative anthropometric data (Fig. 2.18). And pre & post-operative view, postoperative ultrasonographic finding was checked during routine follow-up (Fig. 2.18).

2.3.11 Case 11

A 31-year-old woman received a trans-axillary endoscopic augmentation mammaplasty using the BellaGel SmoothFine (HansBiomed Co. Ltd., Seoul, Korea) for which the patient did have placement of a high-profile device in the subpectoral pocket (BRMZ-H 300 cc) on both sides of the breast with preoperative anthropometric data (Fig. 2.19). And pre & post-operative view, postoperative ultrasonographic finding was checked during routine follow-up (Fig. 2.19).

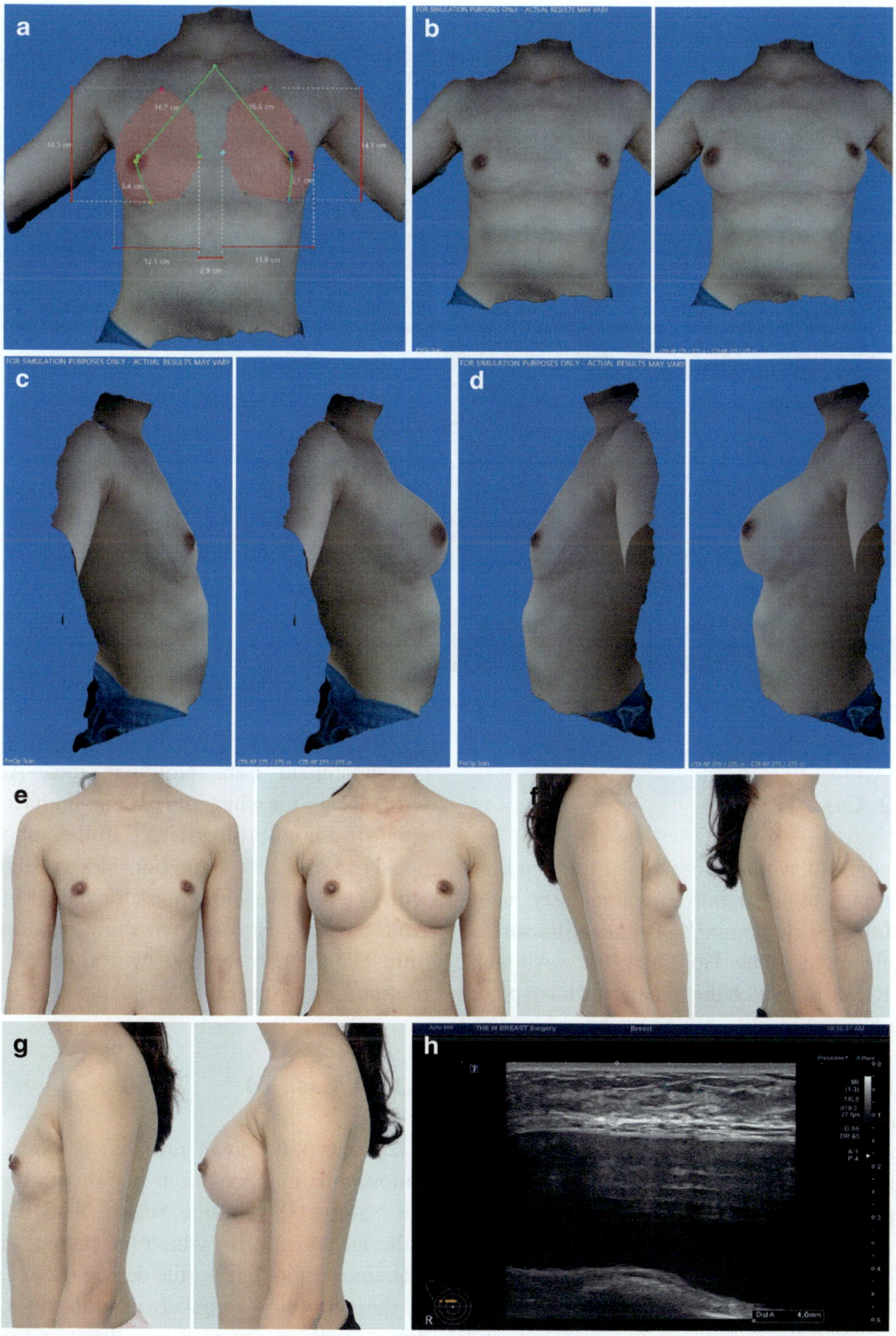

Fig. 2.10 (**a**) Preoperative anthropometric data by 3D simulation. (**b**) Front view of before and after 3D simulation. (**c**) Right side view of before and after 3D simulation. (**d**) Left side view of before and after 3D simulation. (**e**) Preoperative and postoperative front view. (**f**) Preoperative and postoperative right side view. (**g**) Preoperative and postoperative left side view. (**h**) Left ultrasound image shows normal device placed in the subpectoral pocket on 12 weeks postoperatively. (**i**) Right ultrasound image shows normal device placed in the subpectoral pocket on 12 weeks postoperatively. (**j**) Left ultrasound image shows normal device placed in the subpectoral pocket on 122 weeks postoperatively. (**k**) Right ultrasound image shows normal device placed in the subpectoral pocket on 122 weeks postoperatively

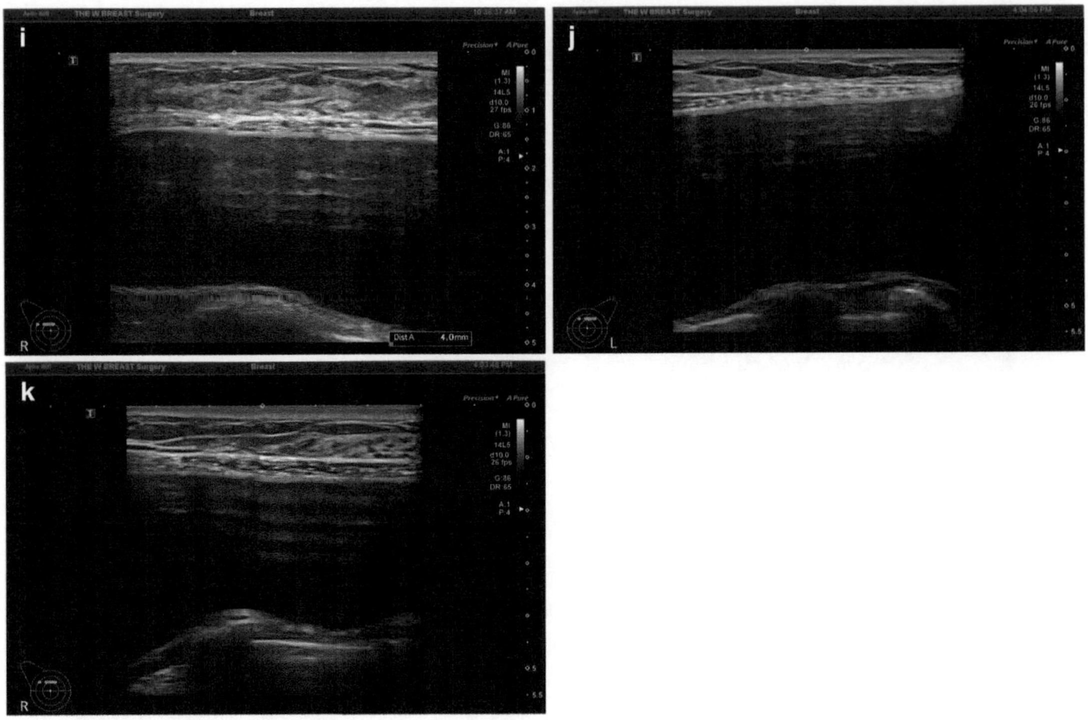

Fig. 2.10 (continued)

2.3.12 Case 12

A 27-year-old woman received a trans-axillary endoscopic augmentation mammaplasty using the Motiva Ergonomix™ Round SilkSurface (Establishment Labs Holdings Inc., Alajuela, Costa Rica), for which the patient did have placement of a high-profile device in the subpectoral pocket (ERSF 355 cc for the right breast and ERSD 300 cc for the left breast) with preoperative anthropometric data (Fig. 2.20). And pre & post-operative view, postoperative ultrasonographic finding was checked during routine follow-up (Fig. 2.20).

2.3.13 Case 13

A 41-year-old woman received a trans-axillary endoscopic augmentation mammaplasty using the Motiva Ergonomix™ Round SilkSurface (Establishment Labs Holdings Inc., Alajuela, Costa Rica), for which the patient did have placement of a high-profile device in the subpectoral pocket (ERSF 335 cc) on both sides of the breast with preoperative anthropometric data (Fig. 2.21). And pre & post-operative view, postoperative ultrasonographic finding was checked during routine follow-up (Fig. 2.21).

2.3.14 Case 14

A 28-year-old woman received a trans-axillary endoscopic augmentation mammaplasty using the Naturgel™ (Groupe Sebbin SAS, Boissy-l' Aillerie, France), for which the patient did have placement of a high-profile device (LS 71305 cc) in the subpectoral pocket on both sides of the breast with preoperative anthropometric data (Fig. 2.22). And pre & post-operative view, post-operative ultrasonographic finding was checked during routine follow-up (Fig. 2.22).

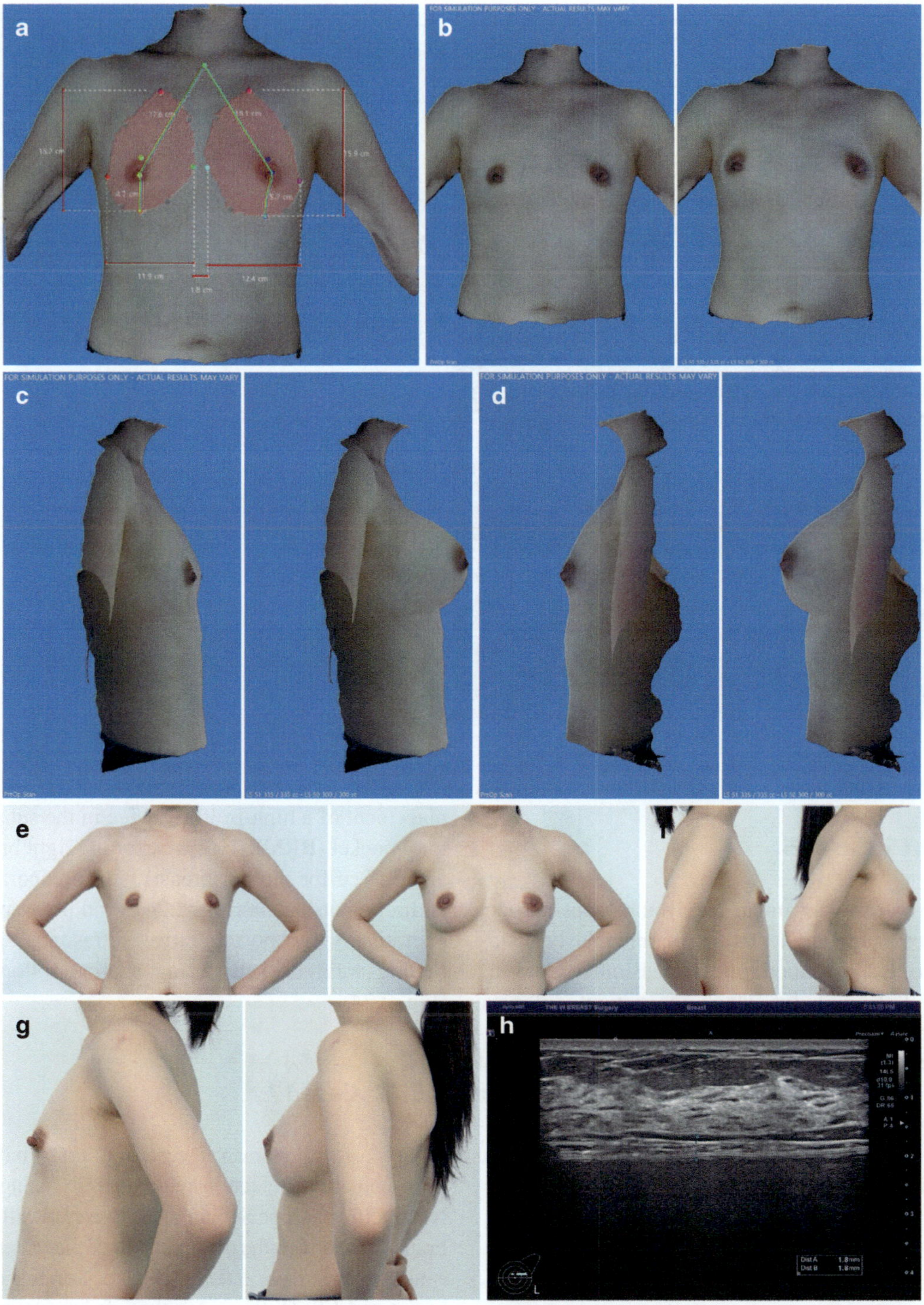

Fig. 2.11 (**a**) Preoperative anthropometric data by 3D simulation. (**b**) Front view of before and after 3D simulation. (**c**) Right side view of before and after 3D simulation. (**d**) Left side view of before and after 3D simulation. (**e**) Preoperative and postoperative front view. (**f**) Preoperative and postoperative right side view. (**g**) Preoperative and postoperative left side view. (**h**) Left ultrasound image shows normal device placed in the subpectoral pocket on 55 weeks postoperatively. (**i**) Right ultrasound image shows normal device placed in the subpectoral pocket on 55 weeks postoperatively. (**j**) Left ultrasound image shows normal device placed in the subpectoral pocket on 181 weeks postoperatively. (**k**) Right ultrasound image shows normal device placed in the subpectoral pocket on 181 weeks postoperatively

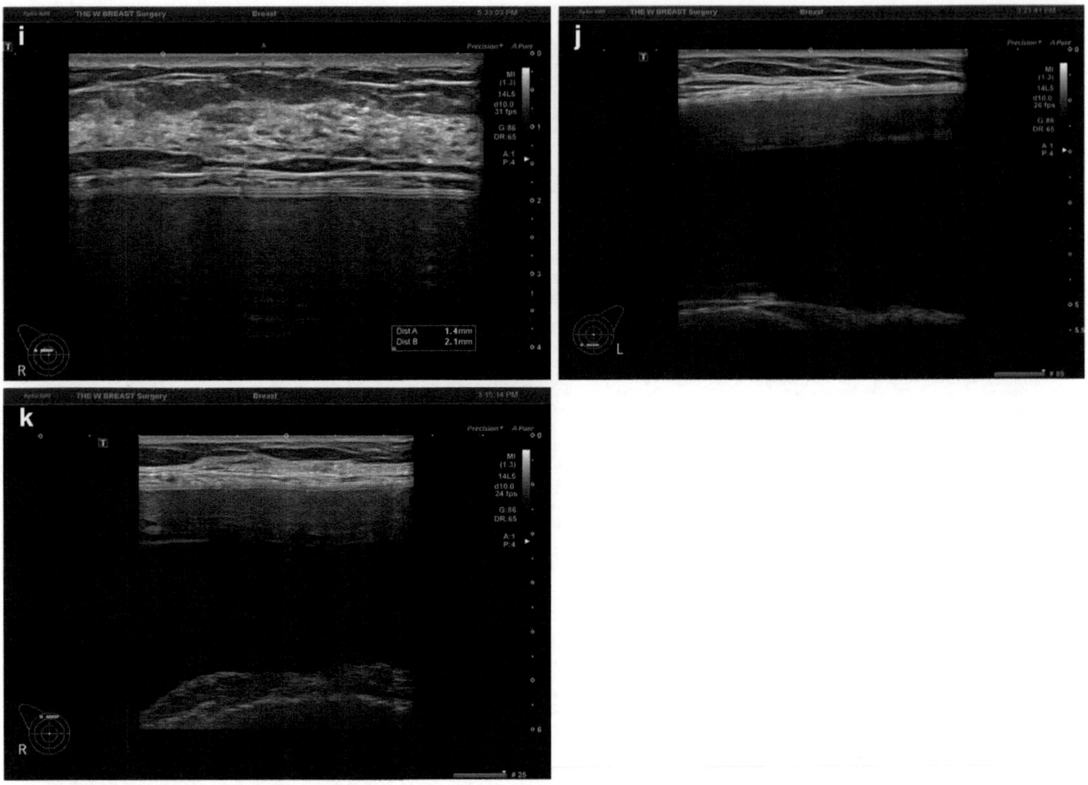

Fig. 2.11 (continued)

2.3.15 Case 15

A 31-year-old woman received a trans-axillary endoscopic augmentation mammaplasty using the BellaGel SmoothFine (HansBiomed Co. Ltd., Seoul, Korea), for which the patient did have placement of a high-profile device in the subpectoral pocket (BRMZ-H 300 cc) on both sides of the breast with preoperative anthropometric data (Fig. 2.23). And pre & post-operative view, postoperative ultrasonographic finding was checked during routine follow-up (Fig. 2.23).

2.3.16 Case 16

A 29-year-old woman received a trans-axillary endoscopic augmentation mammaplasty using the BellaGel SmoothFine (HansBiomed Co. Ltd., Seoul, Korea), for which the patient did have placement of a high-profile device in the subpectoral pocket (BRMZ-H 350 cc for the right breast and 325 cc for the left breast) with preoperative anthropometric data (Fig. 2.24). And pre & post-operative view, postoperative ultrasonographic finding was checked during routine follow-up (Fig. 2.24).

2.3.17 Case 17

A 30-year-old woman received a trans-axillary endoscopic augmentation mammaplasty using the Naturgel™ (Groupe Sebbin SAS, Boissy-l' Aillerie, France), for which the patient did have placement of a high-profile device (LS 71335 cc for the right breast and LS 71305 cc for the left breast) in the subpectoral pocket with preoperative anthropometric data (Fig. 2.25). And pre & post-operative view, postoperative ultrasonographic finding was checked during routine follow-up (Fig. 2.25).

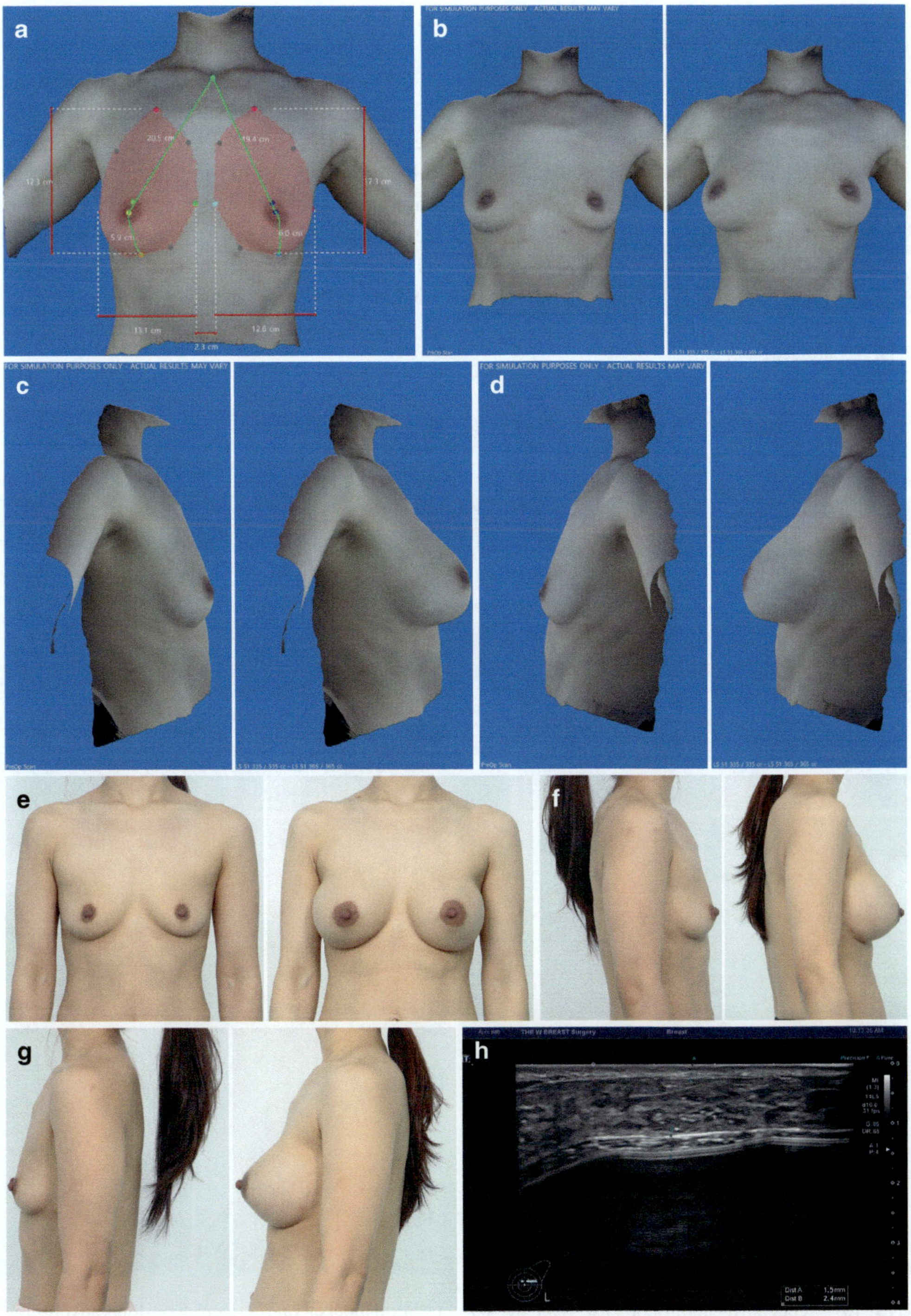

Fig. 2.12 (**a**) Preoperative anthropometric data by 3D simulation. (**b**) Front view of before and after 3D simulation. (**c**) Right side view of before and after 3D simulation. (**d**) Left side view of before and after 3D simulation. (**e**) Preoperative and postoperative front view. (**f**) Preoperative and postoperative right side view. (**g**) Preoperative and postoperative left side view. (**h**) Left ultrasound image shows normal device placed in the subpectoral pocket on 52 weeks postoperatively. (**i**) Right ultrasound image shows normal device placed in the subpectoral pocket on 52 weeks postoperatively

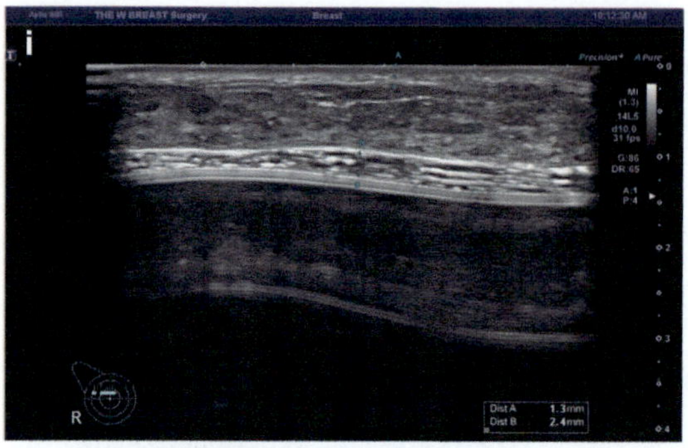

Fig. 2.12 (continued)

2.3.18 Case 18

A 33-year-old woman received an augmentation mammaplasty using the Naturgel™ (Groupe Sebbin SAS, Boissy-l' Aillerie, France) via an inframammary fold incision, for which the patient did have placement of a high-profile device (LS 71265 cc for the right breast and LS 71245 cc for the left breast) in the subpectoral pocket with preoperative anthropometric data (Fig. 2.26). And pre & post-operative view, post-

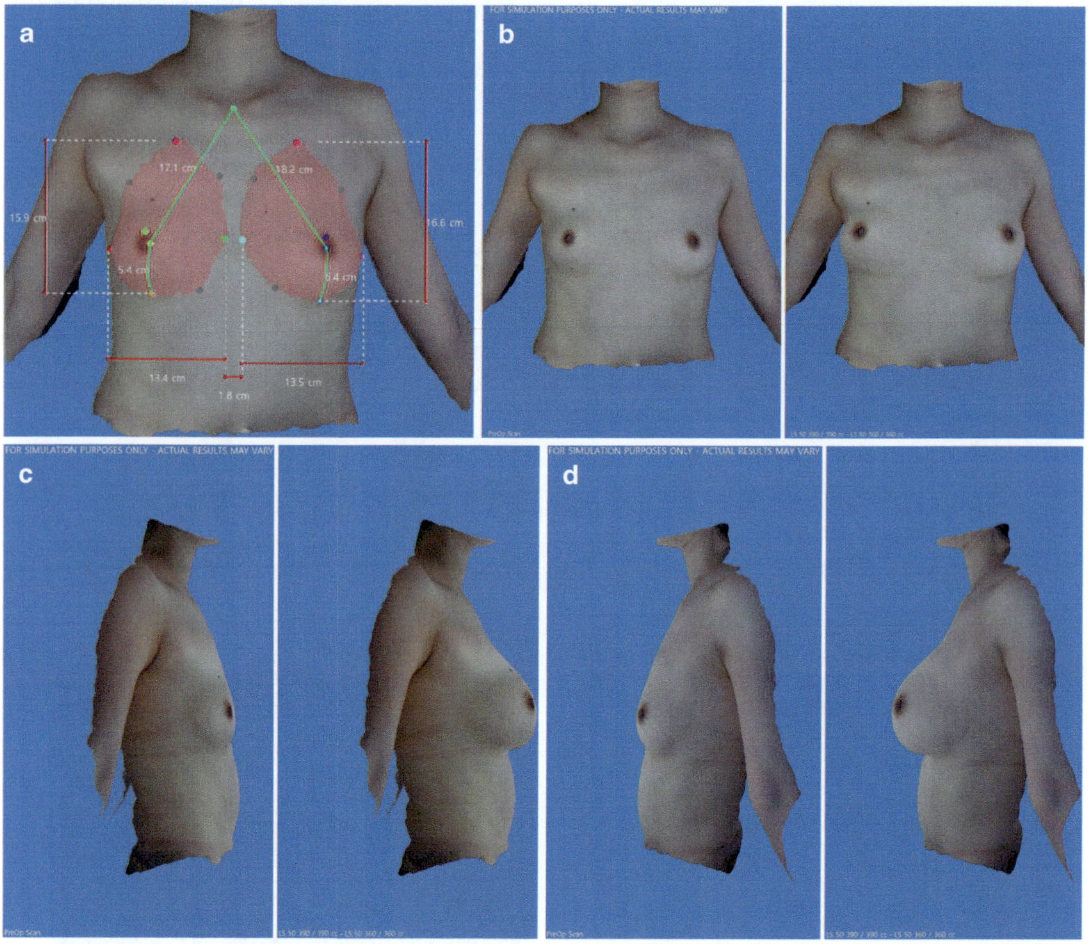

Fig. 2.13 (**a**) Preoperative anthropometric data by 3D simulation. (**b**) Front view of before and after 3D simulation. (**c**) Right side view of before and after 3D simulation. (**d**) Left side view of before and after 3D simulation. (**e**) Preoperative and postoperative front view. (**f**) Preoperative and postoperative right side view. (**g**) Preoperative and postoperative left side view. (**h**) Left ultrasound image shows normal device placed in the subpectoral pocket on 12 weeks postoperatively. (**i**) Right ultrasound image shows normal device placed in the subpectoral pocket on 12 weeks postoperatively. (**j**) Left ultrasound image shows normal device in the subpectoral pocket on 122 weeks postoperatively. (**k**) Right ultrasound image shows normal device in the subpectoral pocket on 122 weeks postoperatively

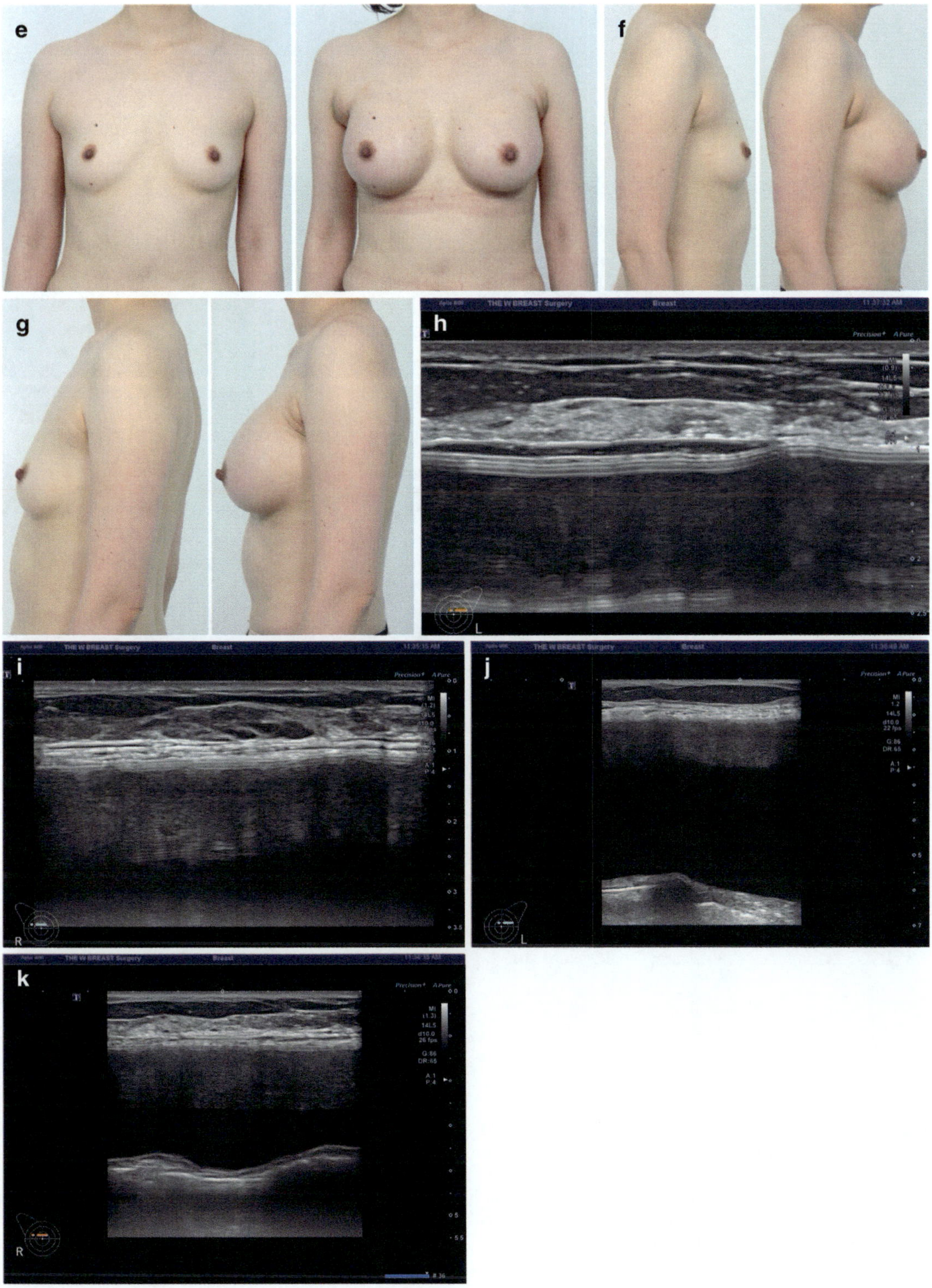

Fig. 2.13 (continued)

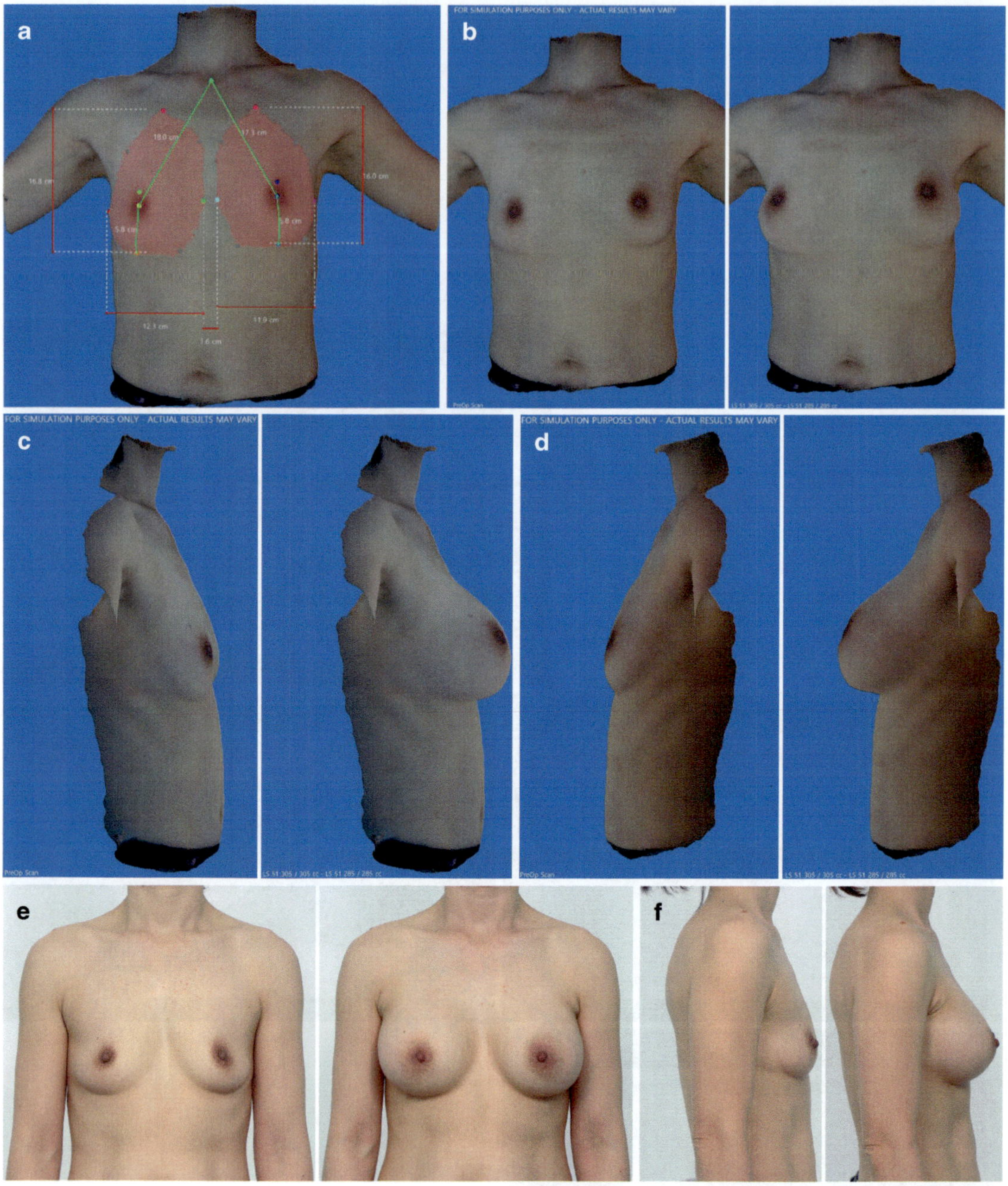

Fig. 2.14 (**a**) Preoperative anthropometric data by 3D simulation. (**b**) Front view of before and after 3D simulation. (**c**) Right side view of before and after 3D simulation. (**d**) Left side view of before and after 3D simulation. (**e**) Preoperative and postoperative front view. (**f**) Preoperative and postoperative right side view. (**g**) Preoperative and postoperative left side view. (**h**) Left ultrasound image shows normal device placed in the subpectoral pocket on 12 weeks postoperatively. (**i**) Right ultrasound image shows normal device placed in the subpectoral pocket on 12 weeks postoperatively

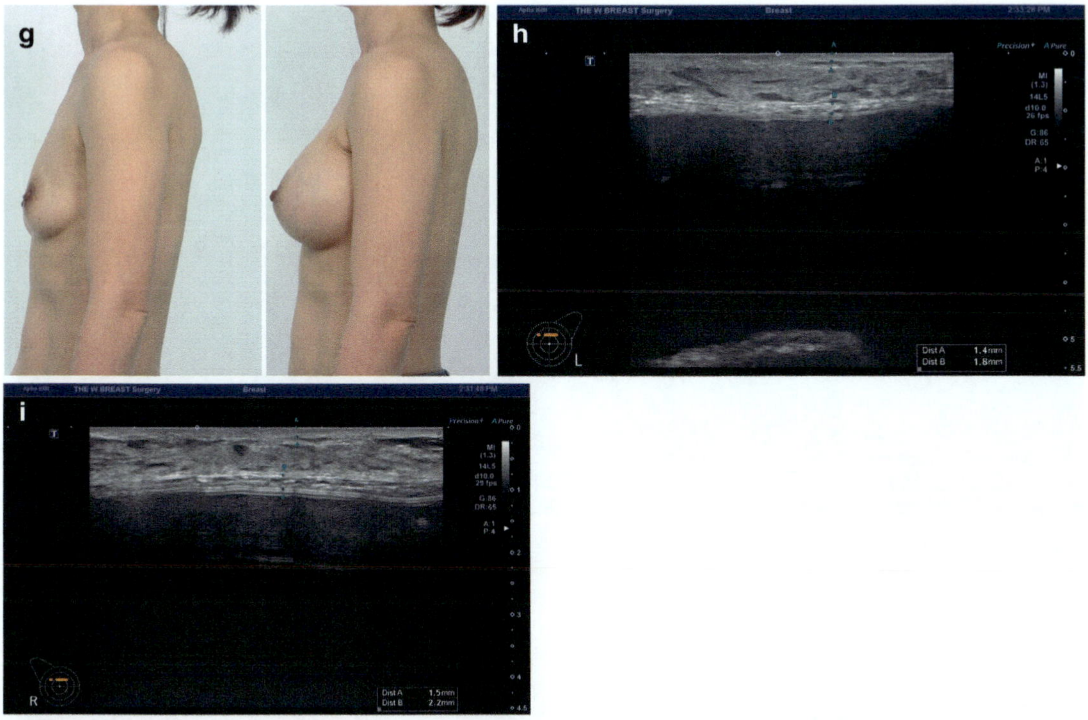

Fig. 2.14 (continued)

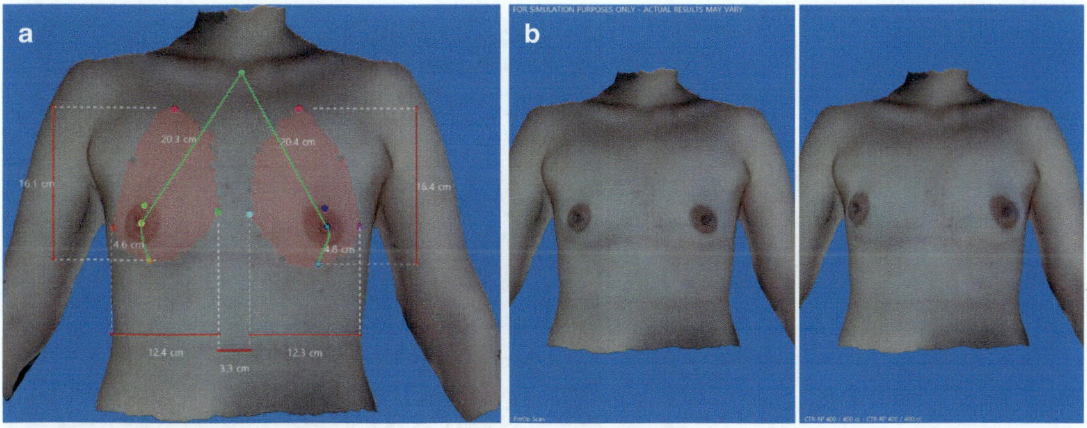

Fig. 2.15 (**a**) Preoperative anthropometric data by 3D simulation. (**b**) Front view of before and after 3D simulation. (**c**) Right side view of before and after 3D simulation. (**d**) Left side view of before and after 3D simulation. (**e**) Preoperative and postoperative front view. (**f**) Preoperative and postoperative right side view. (**g**) Preoperative and postoperative left side view. (**h**) Left ultrasound image shows normal device placed in the subpectoral pocket on 12 weeks postoperatively. (**i**) Right ultrasound image shows normal device placed in the subpectoral pocket on 12 weeks postoperatively

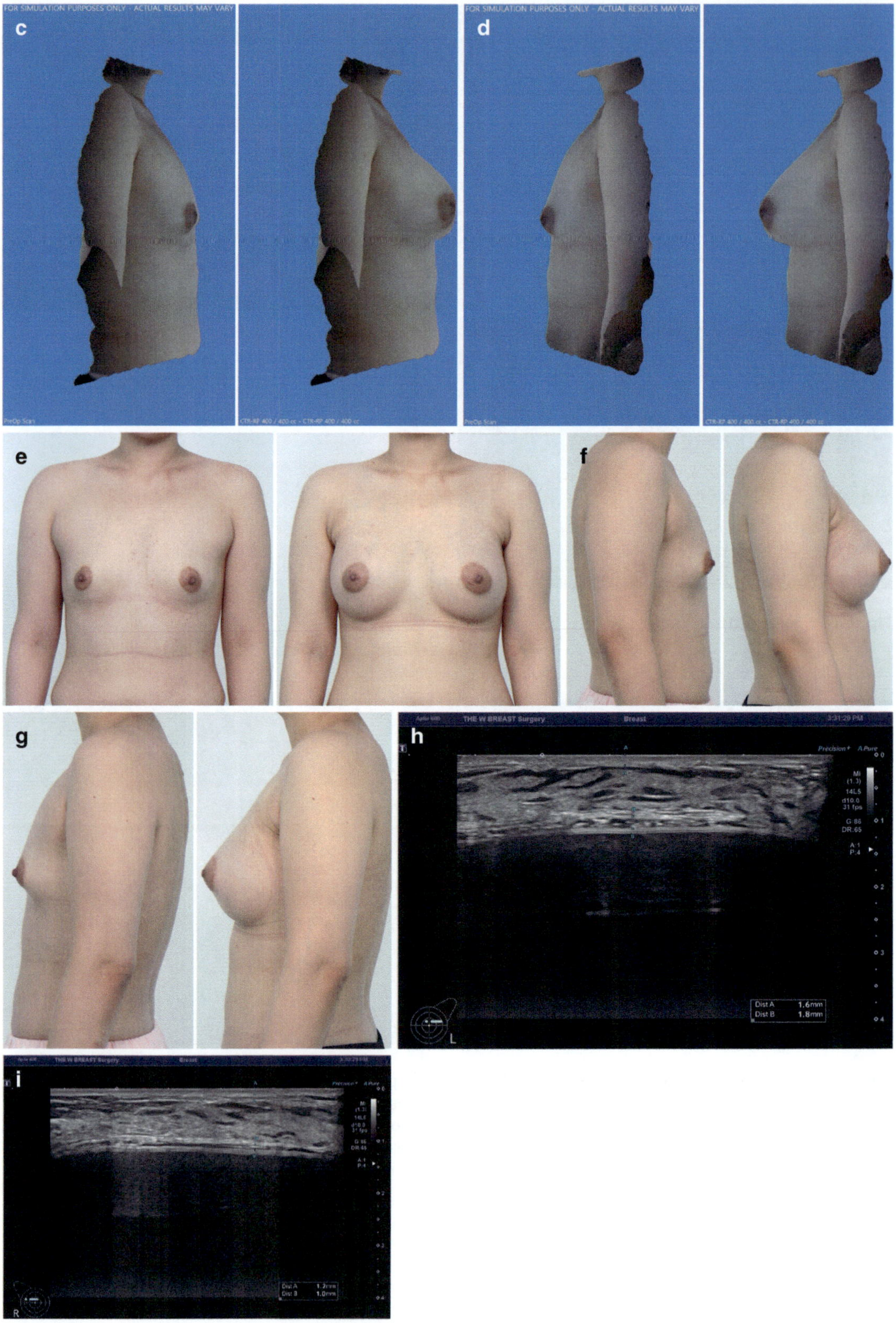

Fig. 2.15 (continued)

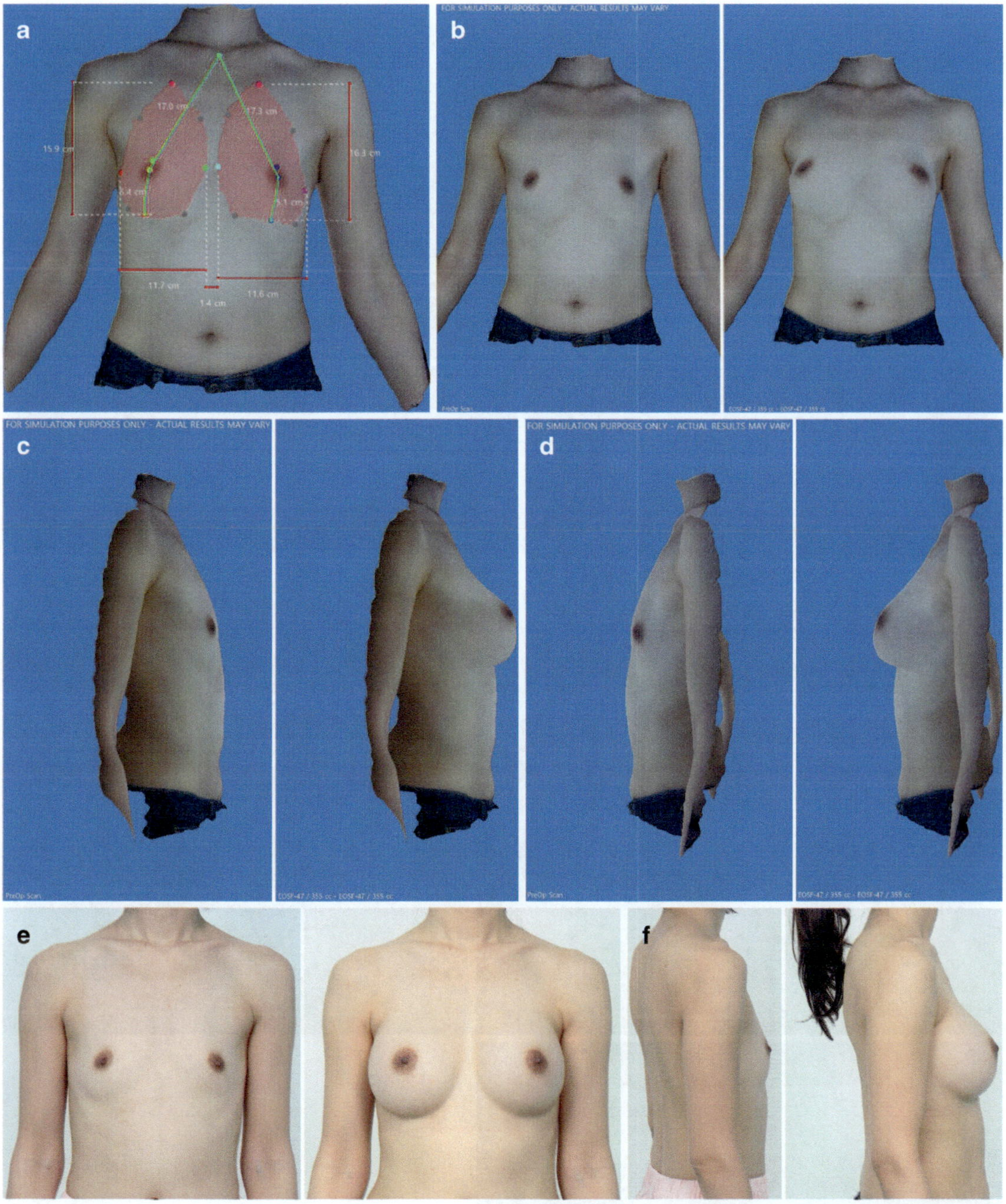

Fig. 2.16 (**a**) Preoperative anthropometric data by 3D simulation. (**b**) Front view of before and after 3D simulation. (**c**) Right side view of before and after 3D simulation. (**d**) Left side view of before and after 3D simulation. (**e**) Preoperative and postoperative front view. (**f**) Preoperative and postoperative right side view. (**g**) Preoperative and postoperative left side view. (**h**) Left ultrasound image shows normal device placed in the subpectoral pocket on 60 weeks postoperatively. (**i**) Right ultrasound image shows normal device placed in the subpectoral pocket on 60 weeks postoperatively. (**j**) Left ultrasound image shows normal device placed in the subpectoral pocket on 120 weeks postoperatively. (**k**) Right ultrasound image shows normal device placed in the subpectoral pocket on 120 weeks postoperatively. (**l**) Left ultrasound image shows normal device placed in the subpectoral pocket on 156 weeks postoperatively. (**m**) Right ultrasound image shows normal device placed in the subpectoral pocket on 156 weeks postoperatively

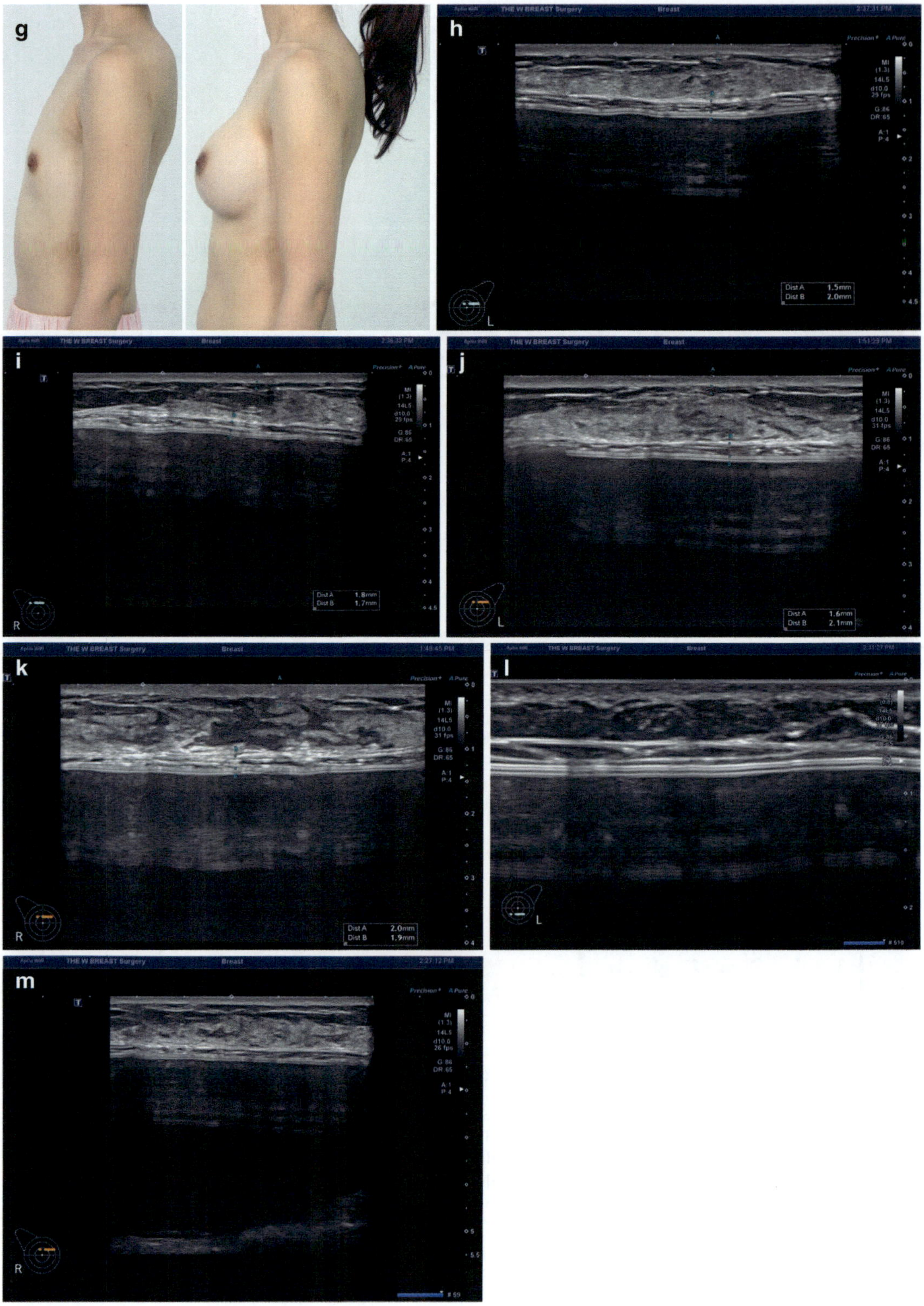

Fig. 2.16 (continued)

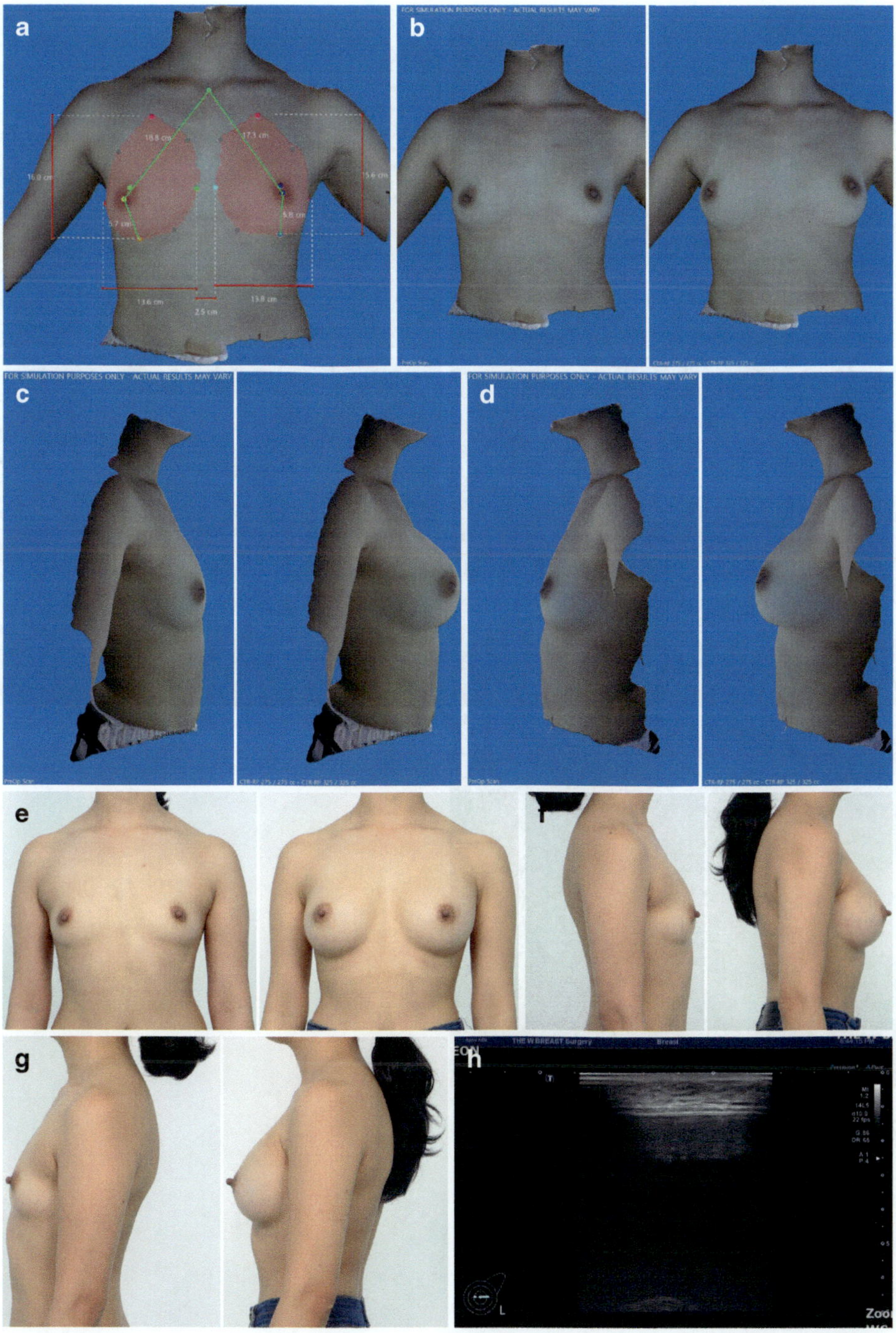

Fig. 2.17 (**a**) Preoperative anthropometric data by 3D simulation. (**b**) Front view of before and after 3D simulation. (**c**) Right side view of before and after 3D simulation. (**d**) Left side view of before and after 3D simulation. (**e**) Preoperative and postoperative front view. (**f**) Preoperative and postoperative right side view. (**g**) Preoperative and postoperative left side view.(**h**) Left ultrasound image shows normal device placed in the subpectoral pocket on 12 weeks postoperatively. (**i**) Right ultrasound image shows normal device placed in the subpectoral pocket on 12 weeks postoperatively. (**j**) Left ultrasound image shows normal device placed in the subpectoral pocket on 52 weeks postoperatively. (**k**) Right ultrasound image shows normal device placed in the subpectoral pocket on 52 weeks postoperatively. (**l**) Left ultrasound image shows normal device placed in the subpectoral pocket on 119 weeks postoperatively. (**m**) Right ultrasound image shows normal device placed in the subpectoral pocket on 119 weeks postoperatively

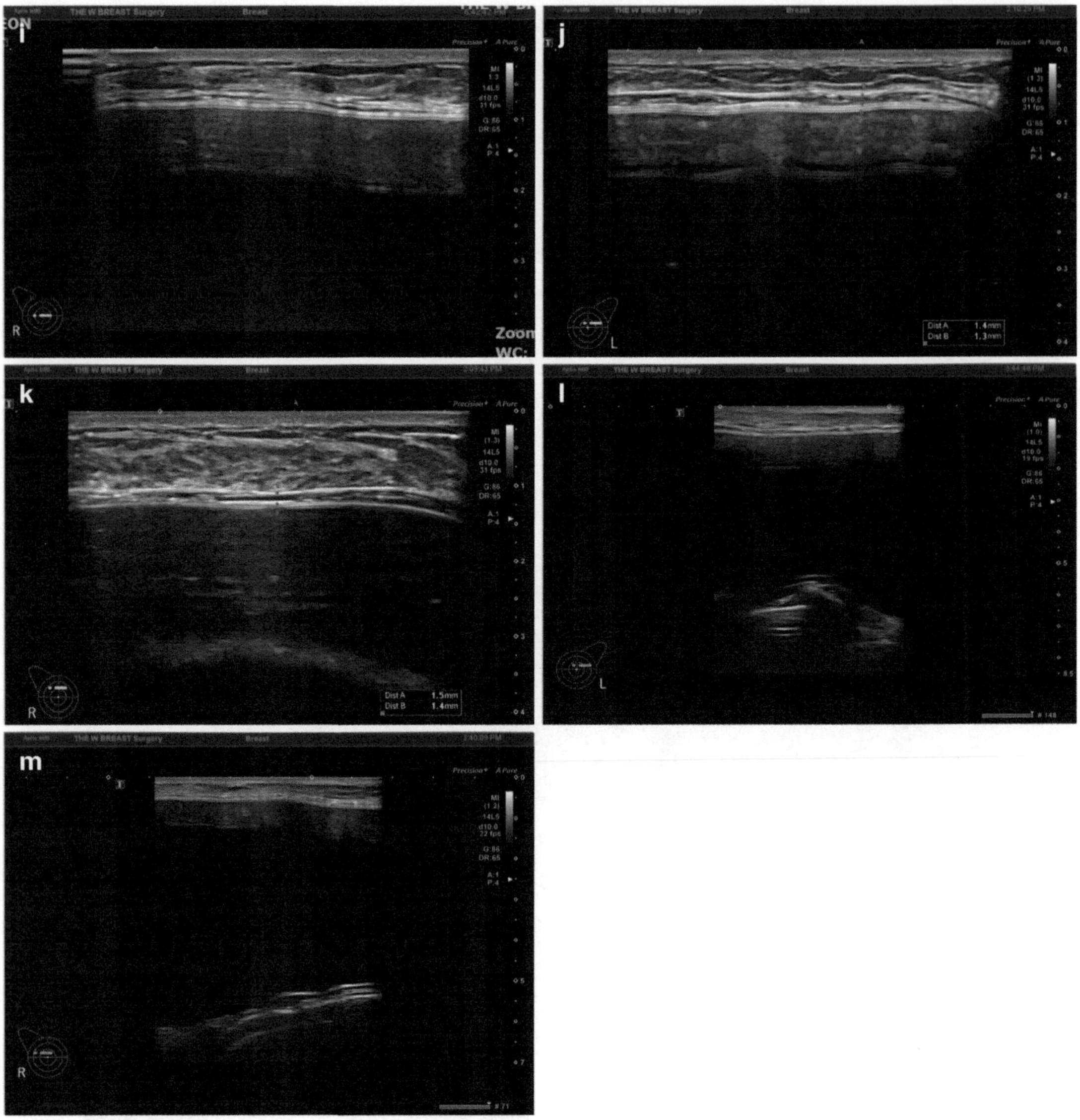

Fig. 2.17 (continued)

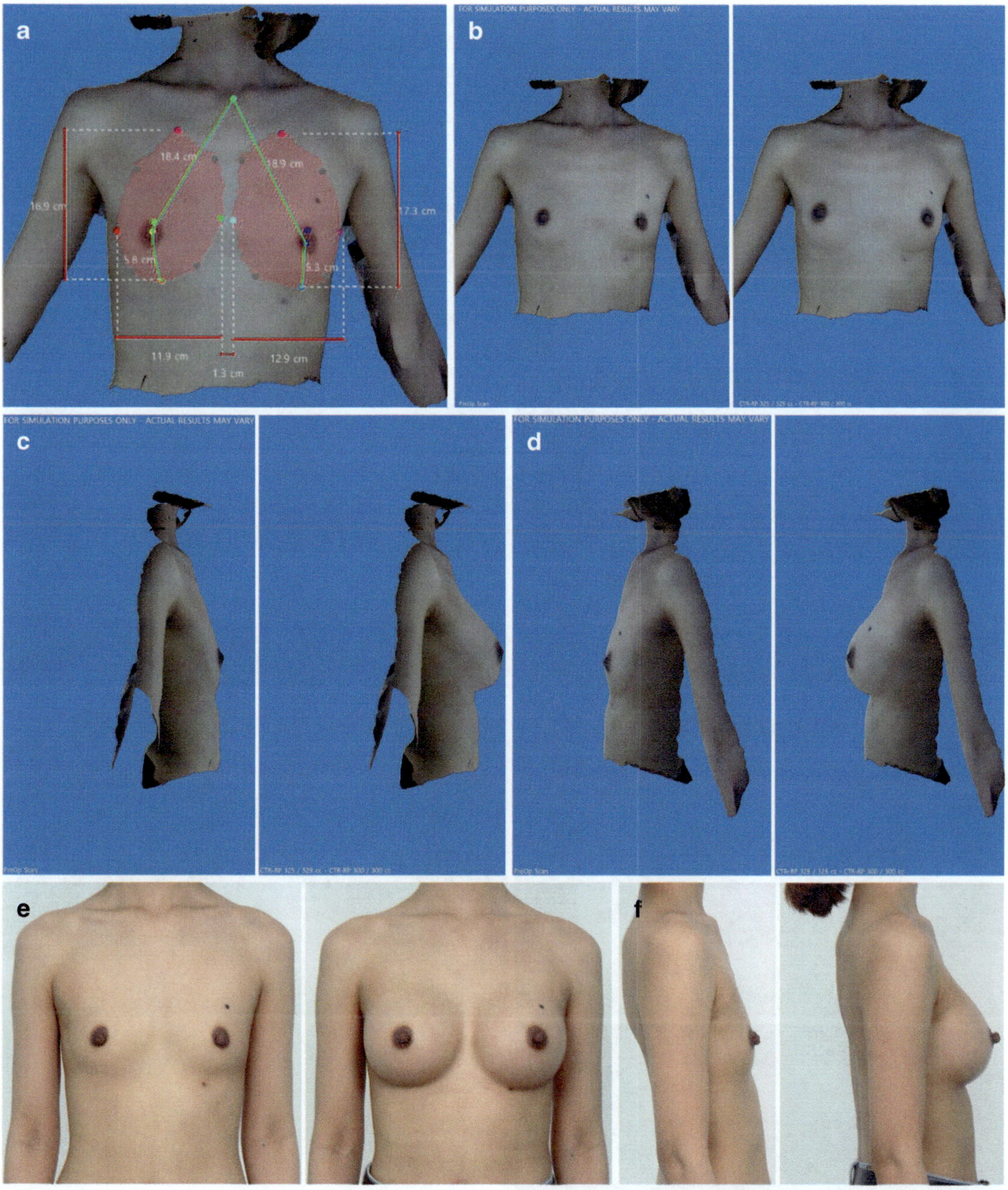

Fig. 2.18 (**a**) Preoperative anthropometric data by 3D simulation. (**b**) Front view of before and after 3D simulation. (**c**) Right side view of before and after 3D simulation. (**d**) Left side view of before and after 3D simulation. (**e**) Preoperative and postoperative front view. (**f**) Preoperative and postoperative right side view. (**g**) Preoperative and postoperative left side view. (**h**) Left ultrasound image shows normal device placed in the subpectoral pocket on 12 weeks postoperatively. (**i**) Right ultrasound image shows normal device placed in the subpectoral pocket on 12 weeks postoperatively. (**j**) Left ultrasound image shows normal device placed in the subpectoral pocket on 52 weeks postoperatively. (**k**) Right ultrasound image shows normal device placed in the subpectoral pocket on 52 weeks postoperatively. (**l**) Left ultrasound image shows normal device placed in the subpectoral pocket on 113 weeks postoperatively. (**m**) Right ultrasound image shows normal device placed in the subpectoral pocket on 113 weeks postoperatively

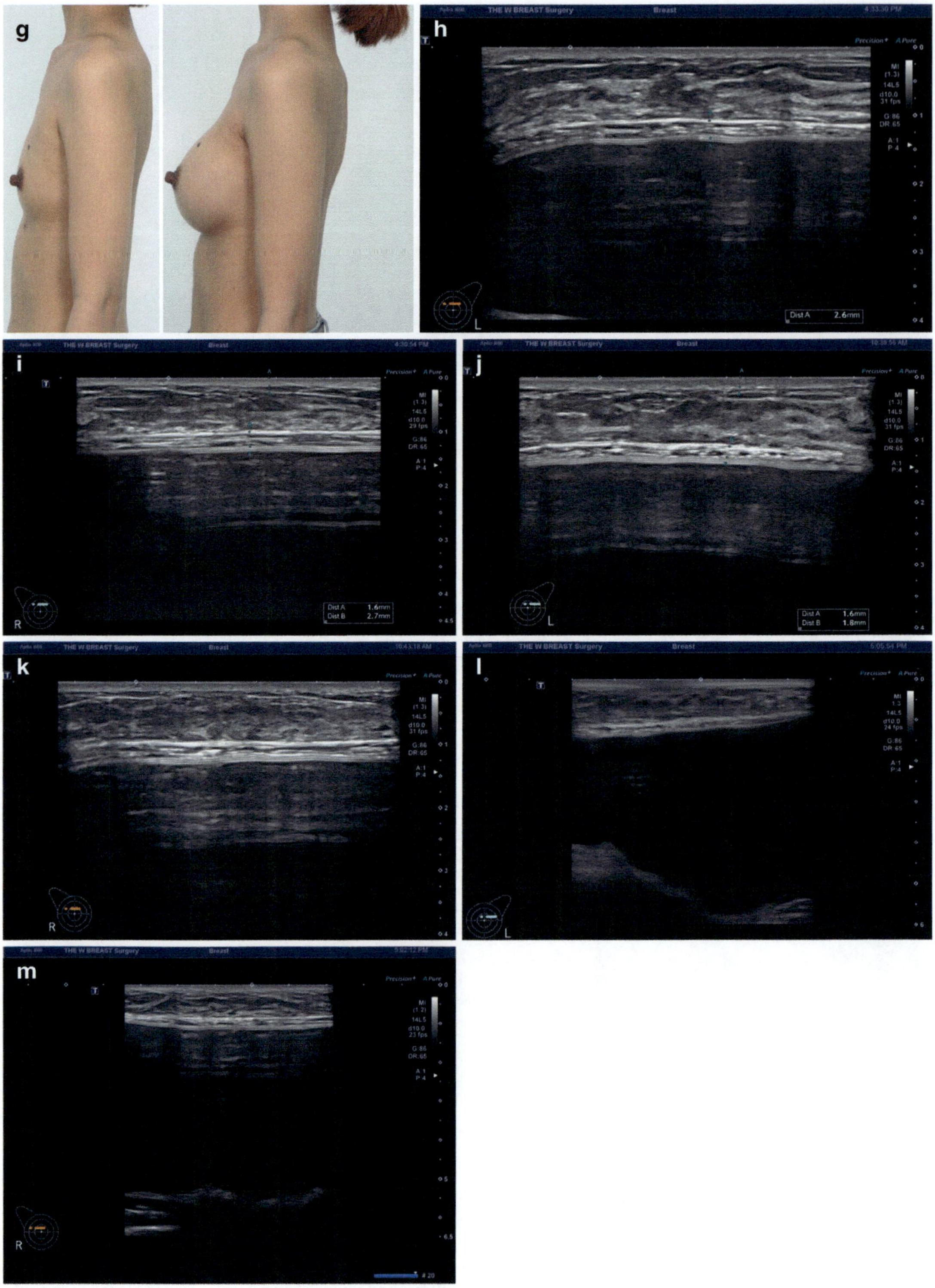

Fig. 2.18 (continued)

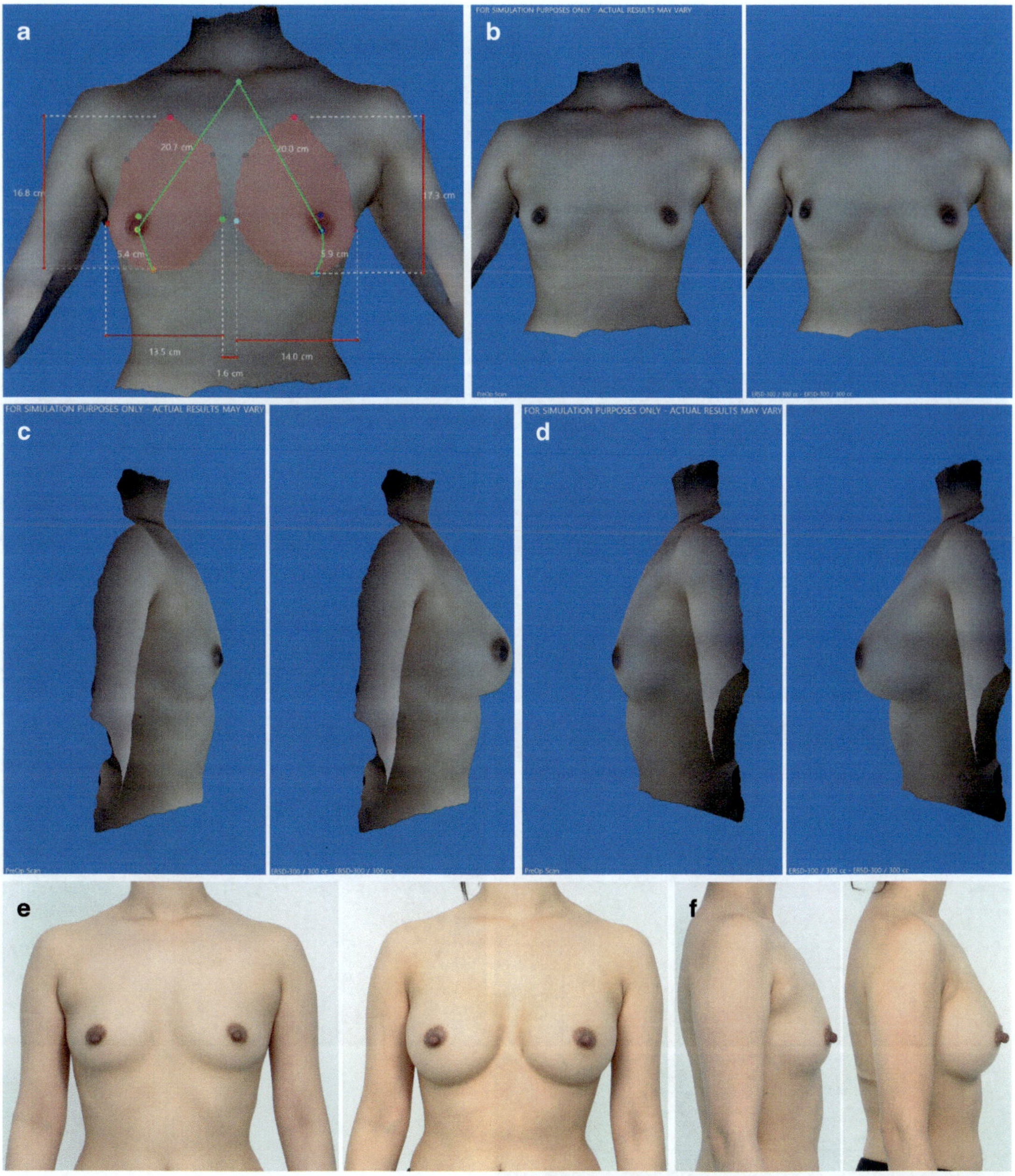

Fig. 2.19 (**a**) Preoperative anthropometric data by 3D simulation. (**b**) Front view of before and after 3D simulation. (**c**) Right side view of before and after 3D simulation. (**d**) Left side view of before and after 3D simulation. (**e**) Preoperative and postoperative front view. (**f**) Preoperative and postoperative right side view. (**g**) Preoperative and postoperative left side view. (**h**) Left ultrasound image shows normal device placed in the subpectoral pocket on 12 weeks postoperatively. (**i**) Right ultrasound image shows normal device placed in the subpectoral pocket on 12 weeks postoperatively. (**j**) Left ultrasound image shows normal device placed in the subpectoral pocket on 52 weeks postoperatively. (**k**) Right ultrasound image shows normal device placed in the subpectoral pocket on 52 weeks postoperatively. (**l**) Left ultrasound image shows normal device placed in the subpectoral pocket on 108 weeks postoperatively. (**m**) Right ultrasound image shows normal device placed in the subpectoral pocket on 108 weeks postoperatively

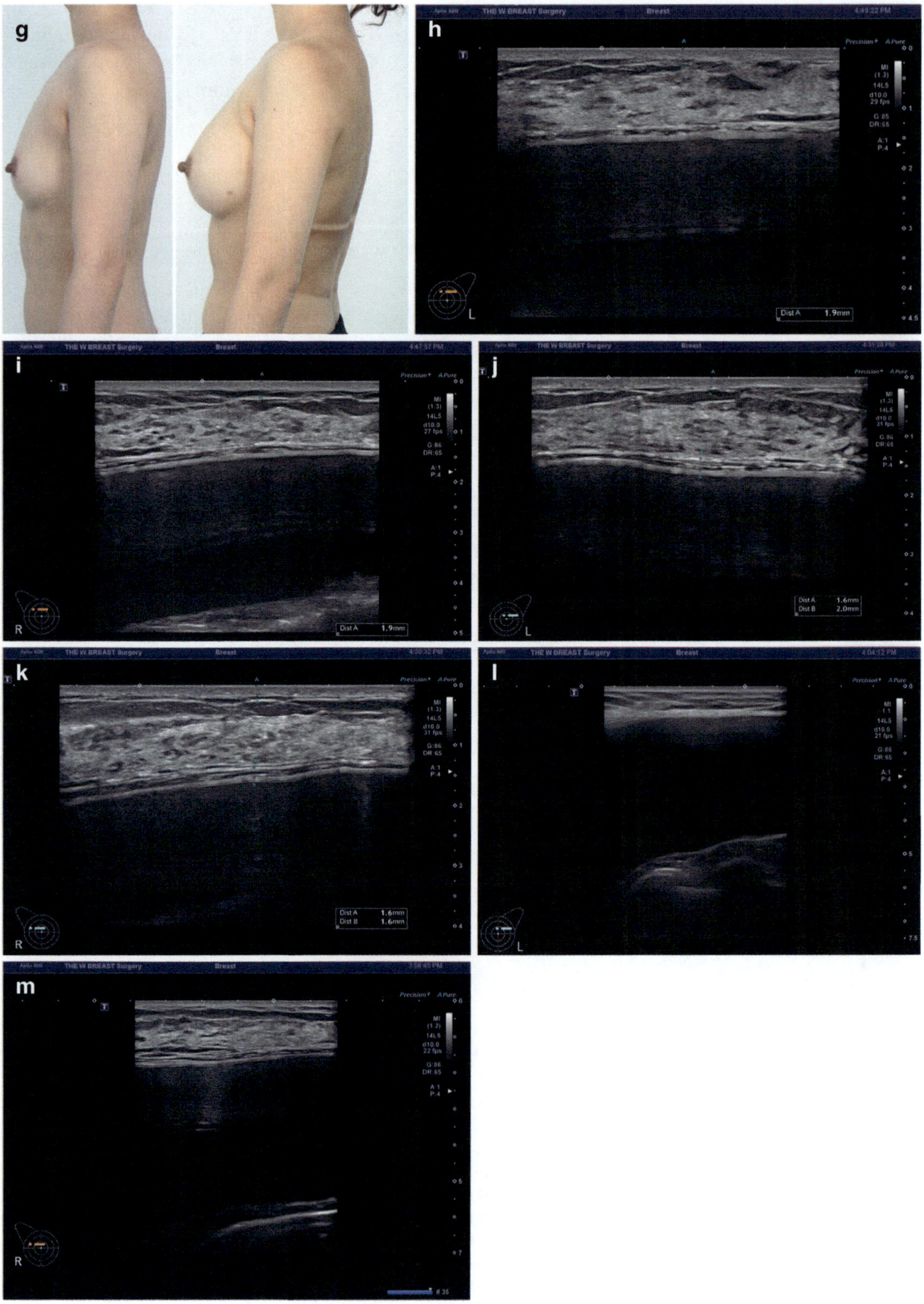

Fig. 2.19 (continued)

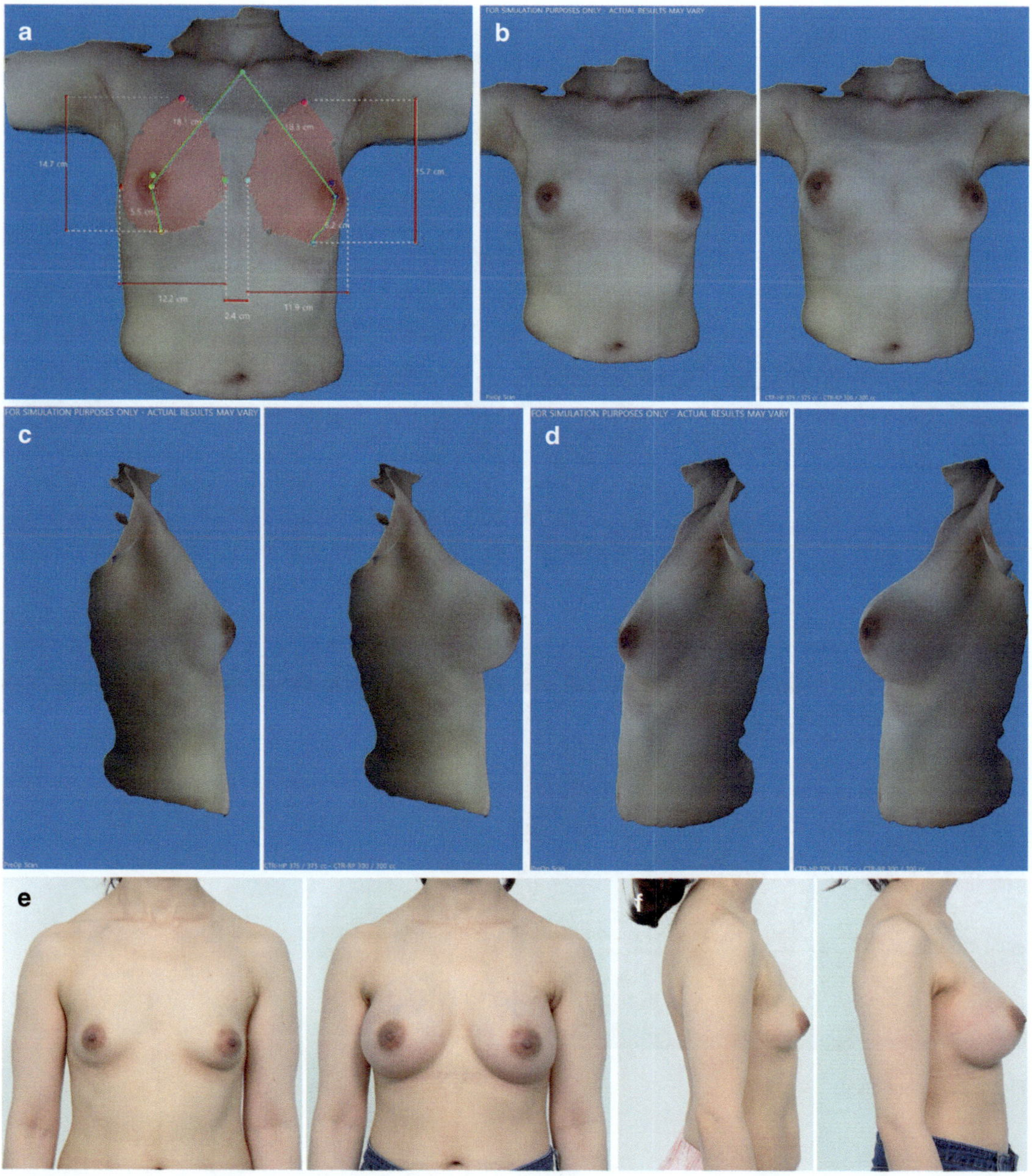

Fig. 2.20 (**a**) Preoperative anthropometric data by 3D simulation. (**b**) Front view of before and after 3D simulation. (**c**) Right side view of before and after 3D simulation. (**d**) Left side view of before and after 3D simulation. (**e**) Preoperative and postoperative front view. (**f**) Preoperative and postoperative right side view. (**g**) Preoperative and postoperative left side view. (**h**) Left ultrasound image shows normal device placed in the subpectoral pocket on 12 weeks postoperatively. (**i**) Right ultrasound image shows normal device placed in the subpectoral pocket on 12 weeks postoperatively. (**j**) Left ultrasound image shows normal device placed in the subpectoral pocket on 54 weeks postoperatively. (**k**) Right ultrasound image shows normal device placed in the subpectoral pocket on 54 weeks postoperatively

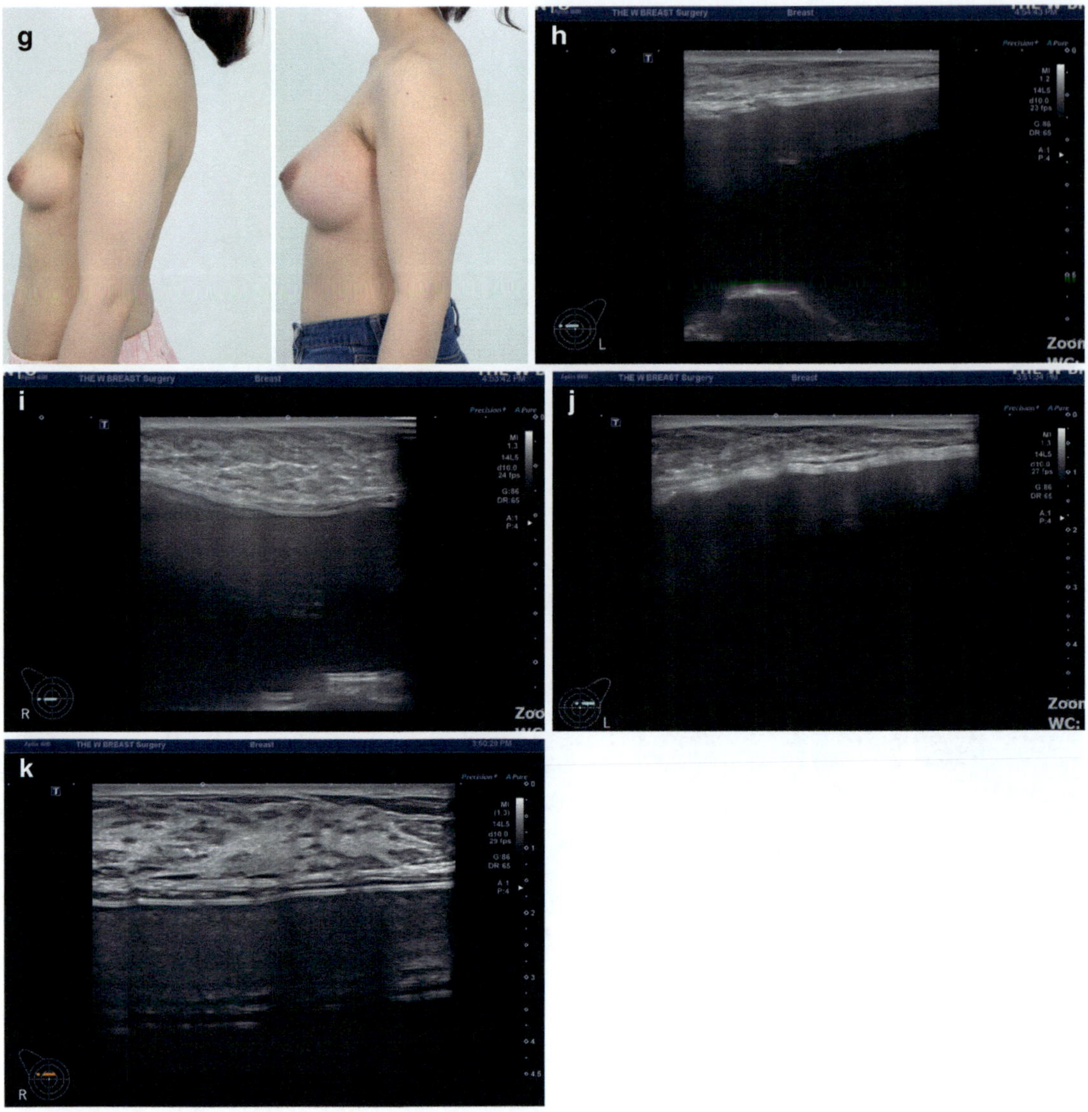

Fig. 2.20 (continued)

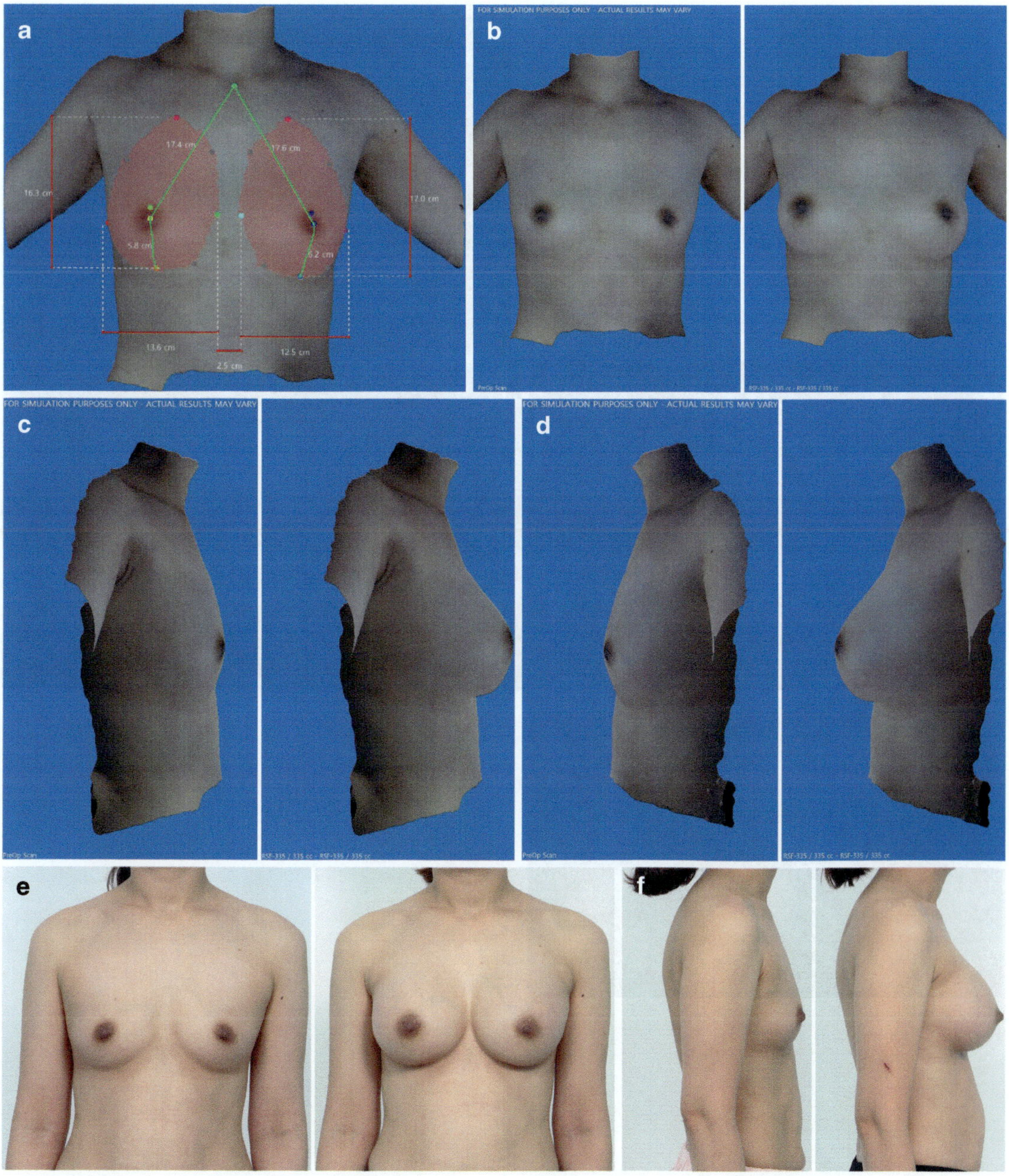

Fig. 2.21 (**a**) Preoperative anthropometric data by 3D simulation. (b) Front view of before and after 3D simulation. (**c**) Right side view of before and after 3D simulation. (**d**) Left side view of before and after 3D simulation. (**e**) Preoperative and postoperative front view. (**f**) Preoperative and postoperative right side view. (**g**) Preoperative and postoperative left side view. (**h**) Left ultrasound image shows normal device placed in the subpectoral pocket with benign mass on 12 weeks postoperatively. (**i**) Right ultrasound image shows normal device placed in the subpectoral pocket with benign mass on 12 weeks postoperatively. (**j**) Left ultrasound image shows normal device placed in the subpectoral pocket with benign mass on 54 weeks postoperatively. (**k**) Right ultrasound image shows normal device placed in the subpectoral pocket with benign mass on 54 weeks postoperatively

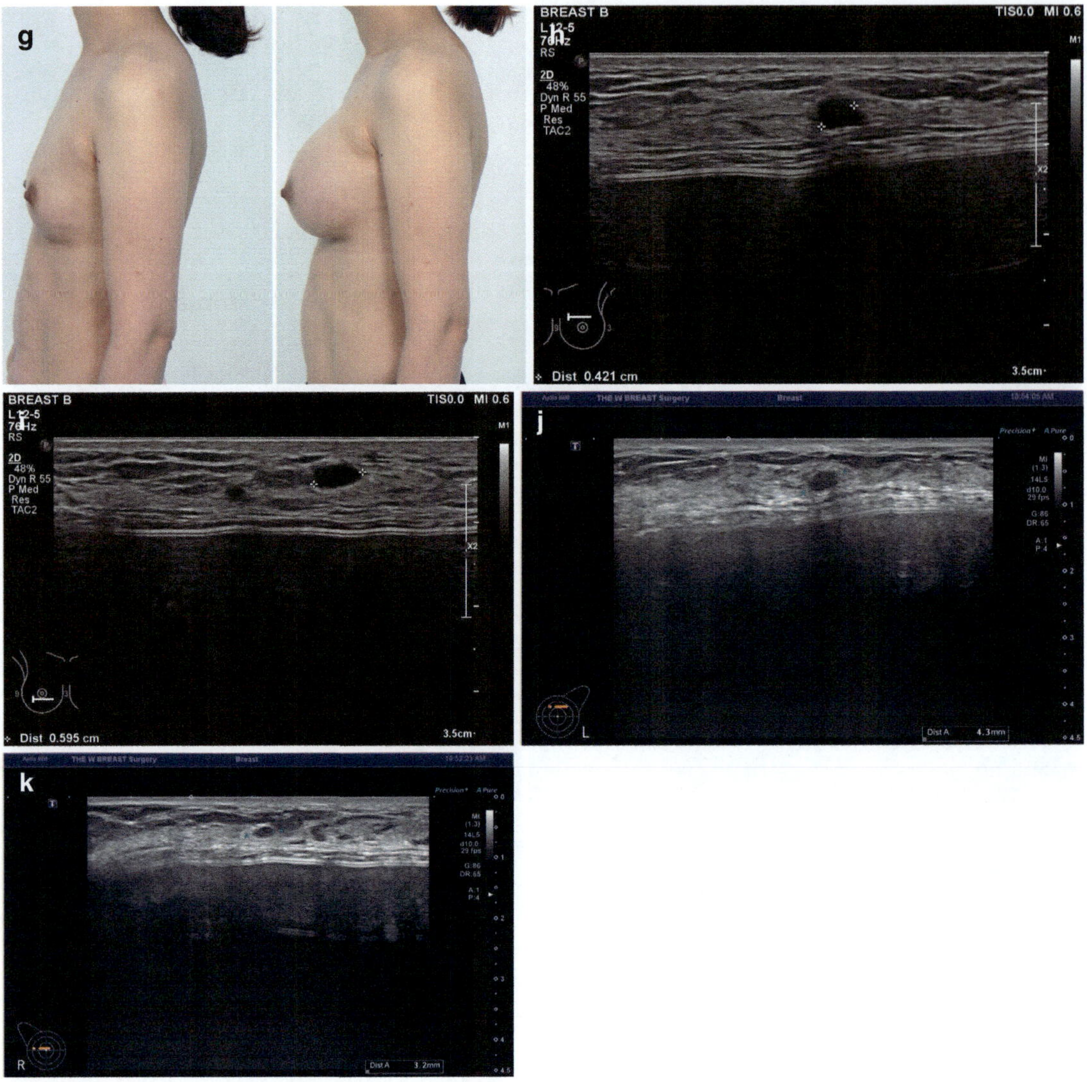

Fig. 2.21 (continued)

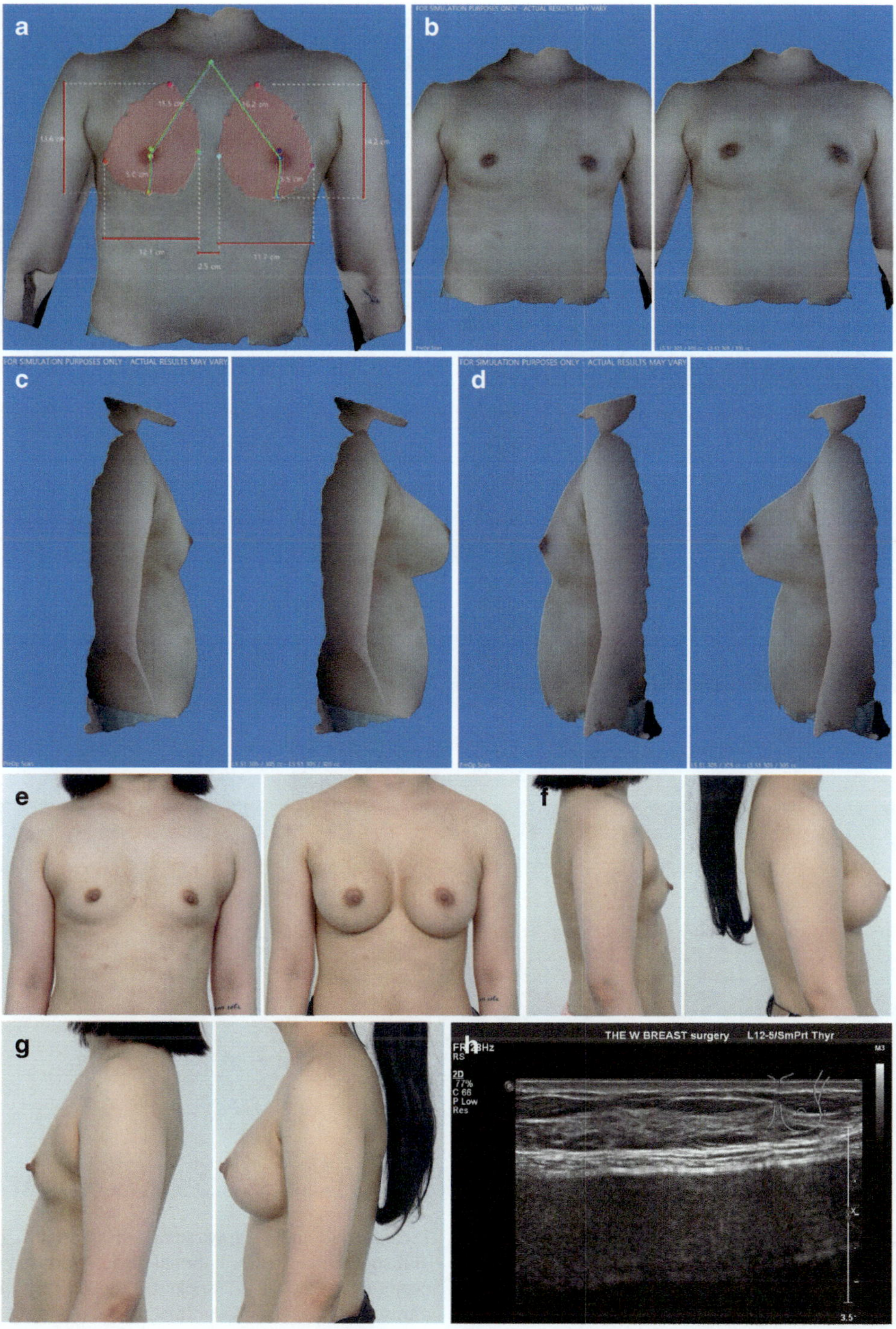

Fig. 2.22 (**a**) Preoperative anthropometric data by 3D simulation. (**b**) Front view of before and after 3D simulation. (**c**) Right side view of before and after 3D simulation. (**d**) Left side view of before and after 3D simulation. (**e**) Preoperative and postoperative front view. (**f**) Preoperative and postoperative right side view. (**g**) Preoperative and postoperative left side view. (**h**) Left ultrasound image shows normal device placed in the subpectoral pocket on 12 weeks postoperatively. (**i**) Right ultrasound image shows normal device placed in the subpectoral pocket on 12 weeks postoperatively. (**j**) Left ultrasound image shows normal device placed in the subpectoral pocket on 55 weeks postoperatively. (**k**) Right ultrasound image shows normal device placed in the subpectoral pocket with benign mass on 55 weeks postoperatively

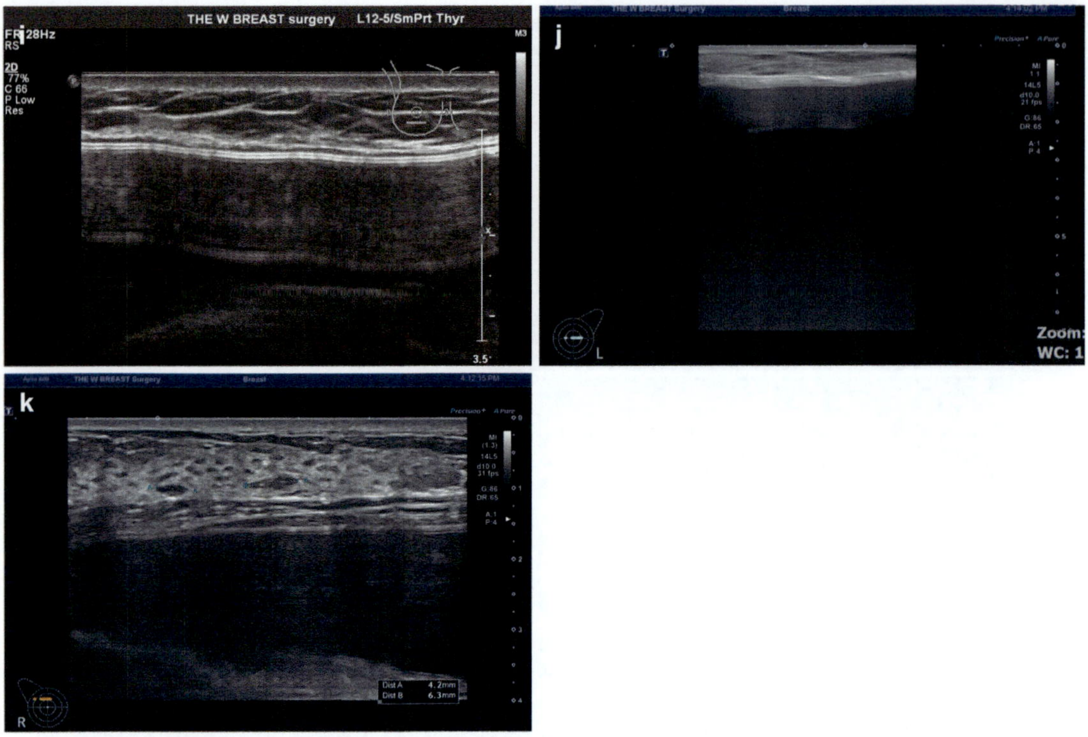

Fig. 2.22 (continued)

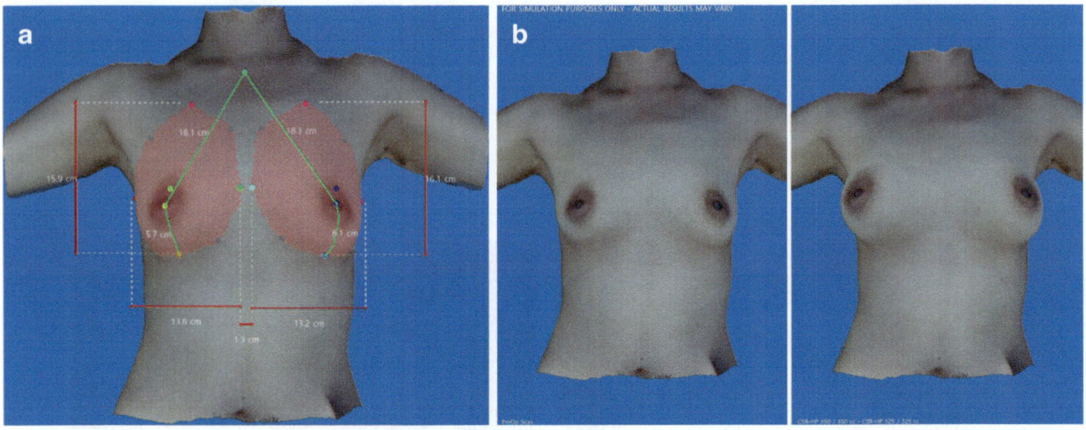

Fig. 2.23 (**a**) Preoperative anthropometric data by 3D simulation. (**b**) Front view of before and after 3D simulation. (**c**) Right side view of before and after 3D simulation. (**d**) Left side view of before and after 3D simulation. (**e**) Preoperative and postoperative front view. (**f**) Preoperative and postoperative right side view. (**g**) Preoperative and postoperative left side view. (**h**) Left ultrasound image shows normal device placed in the subpectoral pocket on 12 weeks postoperatively. (**i**) Right ultrasound image shows normal device placed in the subpectoral pocket on 12 weeks postoperatively

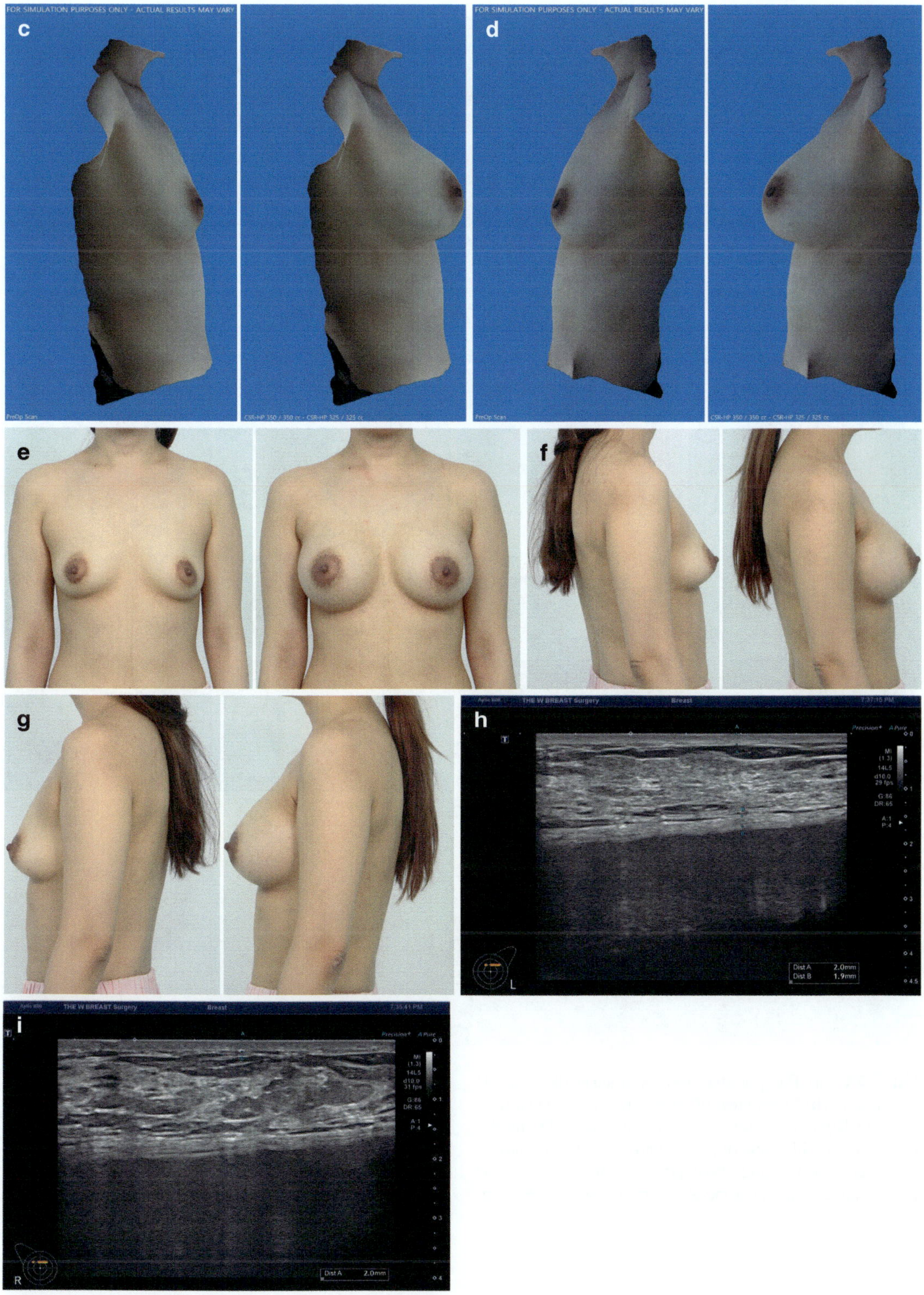

Fig. 2.23 (continued)

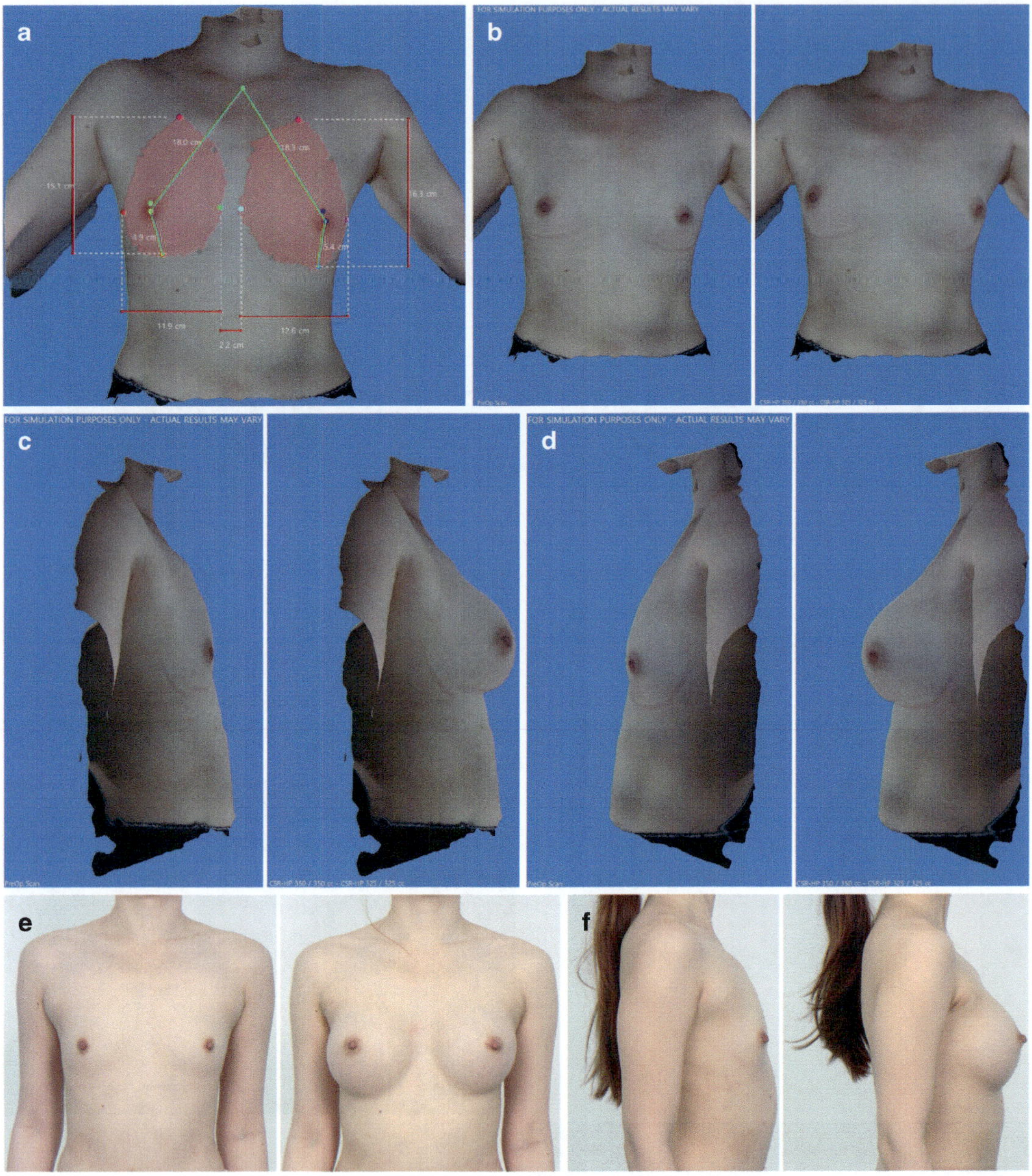

Fig. 2.24 (**a**) Preoperative anthropometric data by 3D simulation. (**b**) Front view of before and after 3D simulation. (**c**) Right side view of before and after 3D simulation. (**d**) Left side view of before and after 3D simulation. (**e**) Preoperative and postoperative front view. (**f**) Preoperative and postoperative right side view. (**g**) Preoperative and postoperative left side view. (**h**) Left ultrasound image shows normal device placed in the subpectoral pocket on 12 weeks postoperatively. (**i**) Right ultrasound image shows normal device placed in the subpectoral pocket on 12 weeks postoperatively

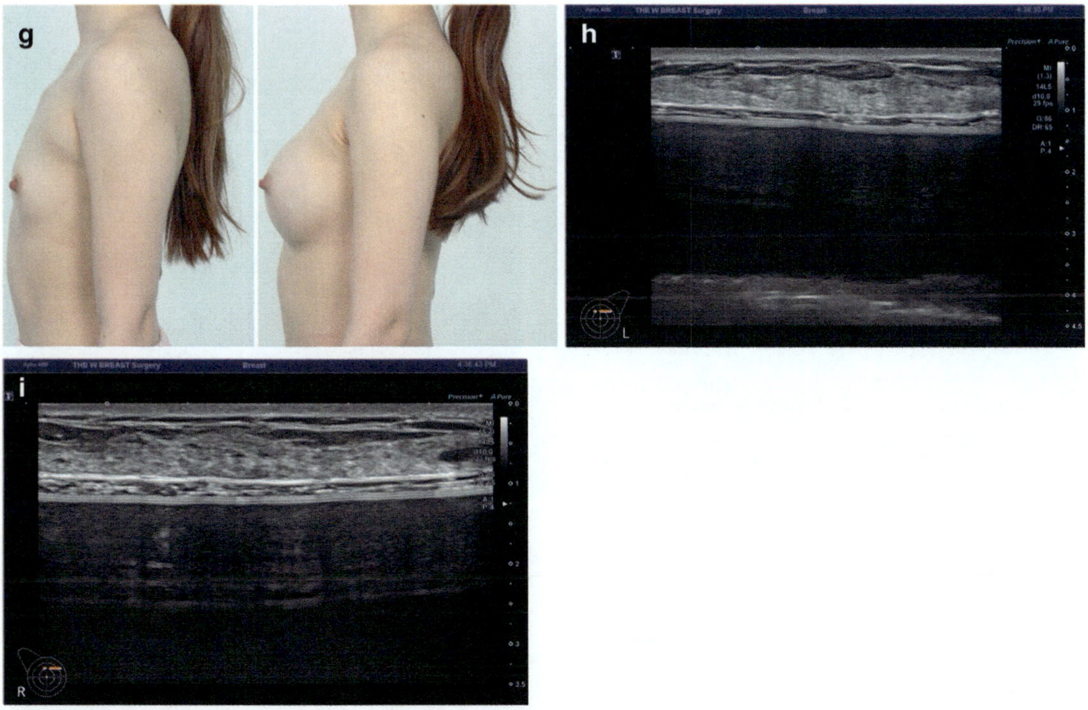

Fig. 2.24 (continued)

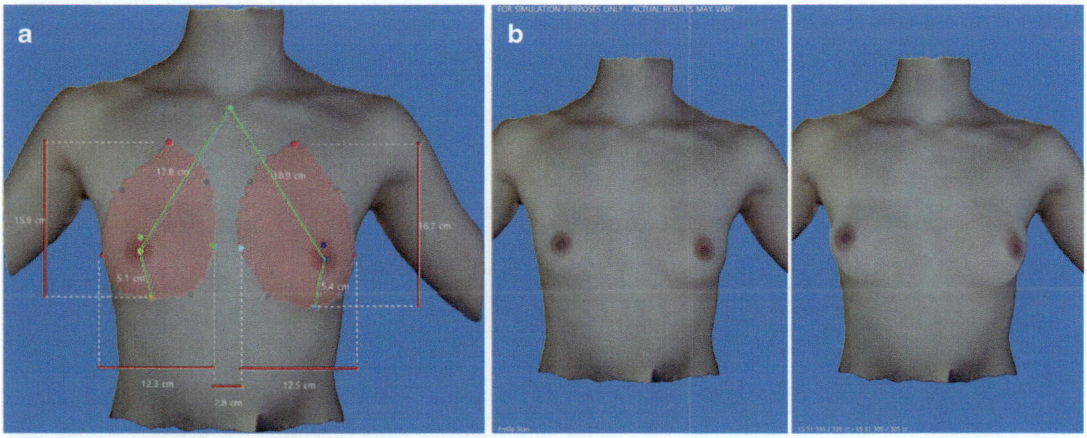

Fig. 2.25 (**a**) Preoperative anthropometric data by 3D simulation. (**b**) Front view of before and after 3D simulation. (**c**) Right side view of before and after 3D simulation. (**d**) Left side view of before and after 3D simulation. (**e**) Preoperative and postoperative front view. (**f**) Preoperative and postoperative right side view. (**g**) Preoperative and postoperative left side view. (**h**) Left ultrasound image shows normal device placed in the subpectoral pocket on 12 weeks postoperatively. (**i**) Right ultrasound image shows normal device placed in the subpectoral pocket on 12 weeks postoperatively. (**j**) Left ultrasound image shows normal device placed in the subpectoral pocket on 54 weeks postoperatively. (**k**) Right ultrasound image shows normal device placed in the subpectoral pocket on 54 weeks postoperatively. (**l**) Left ultrasound image shows normal device placed in the subpectoral pocket on 120 weeks postoperatively. (**m**) Right ultrasound image shows normal device placed in the subpectoral pocket on 120 weeks postoperatively

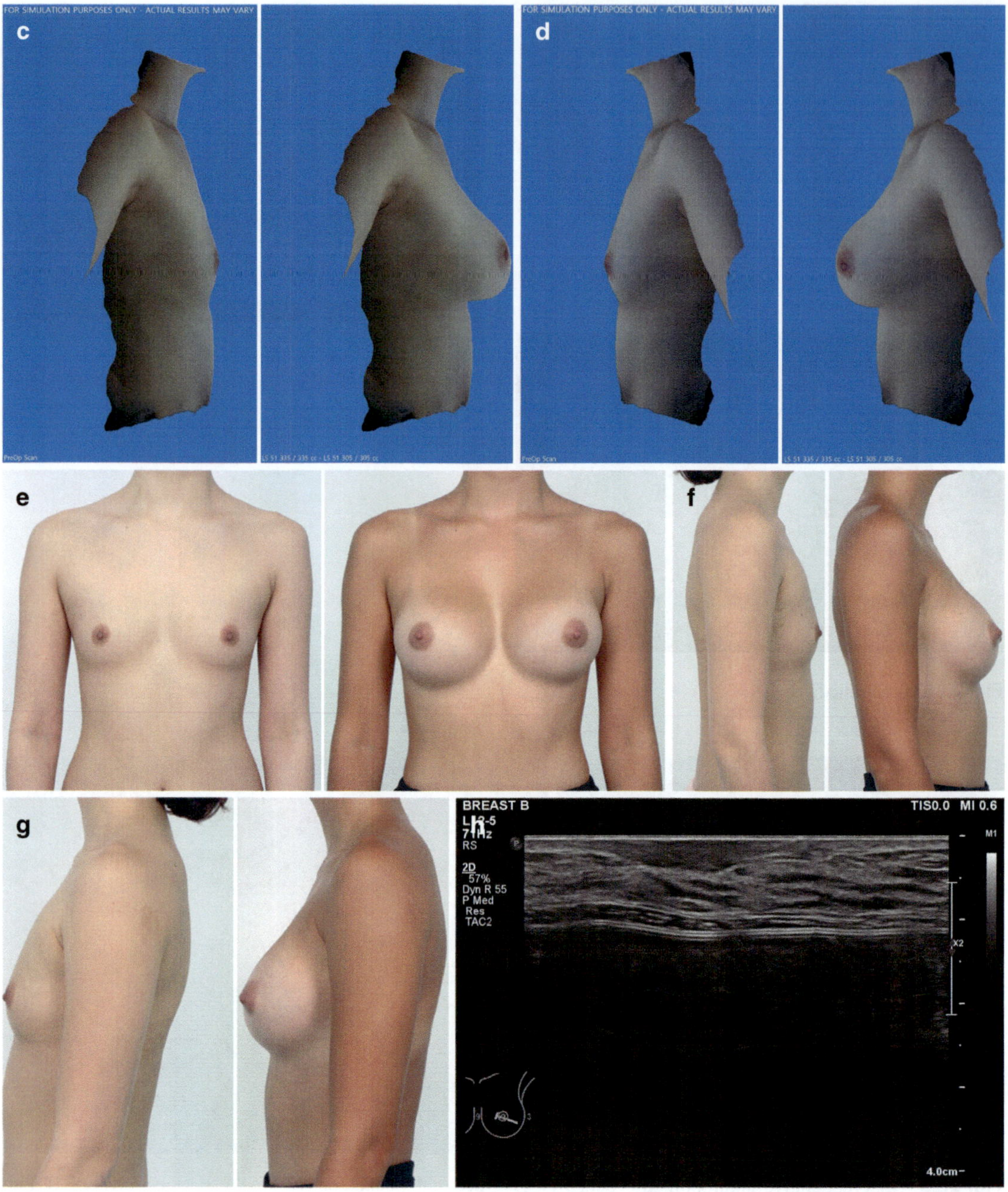

Fig. 2.25 (continued)

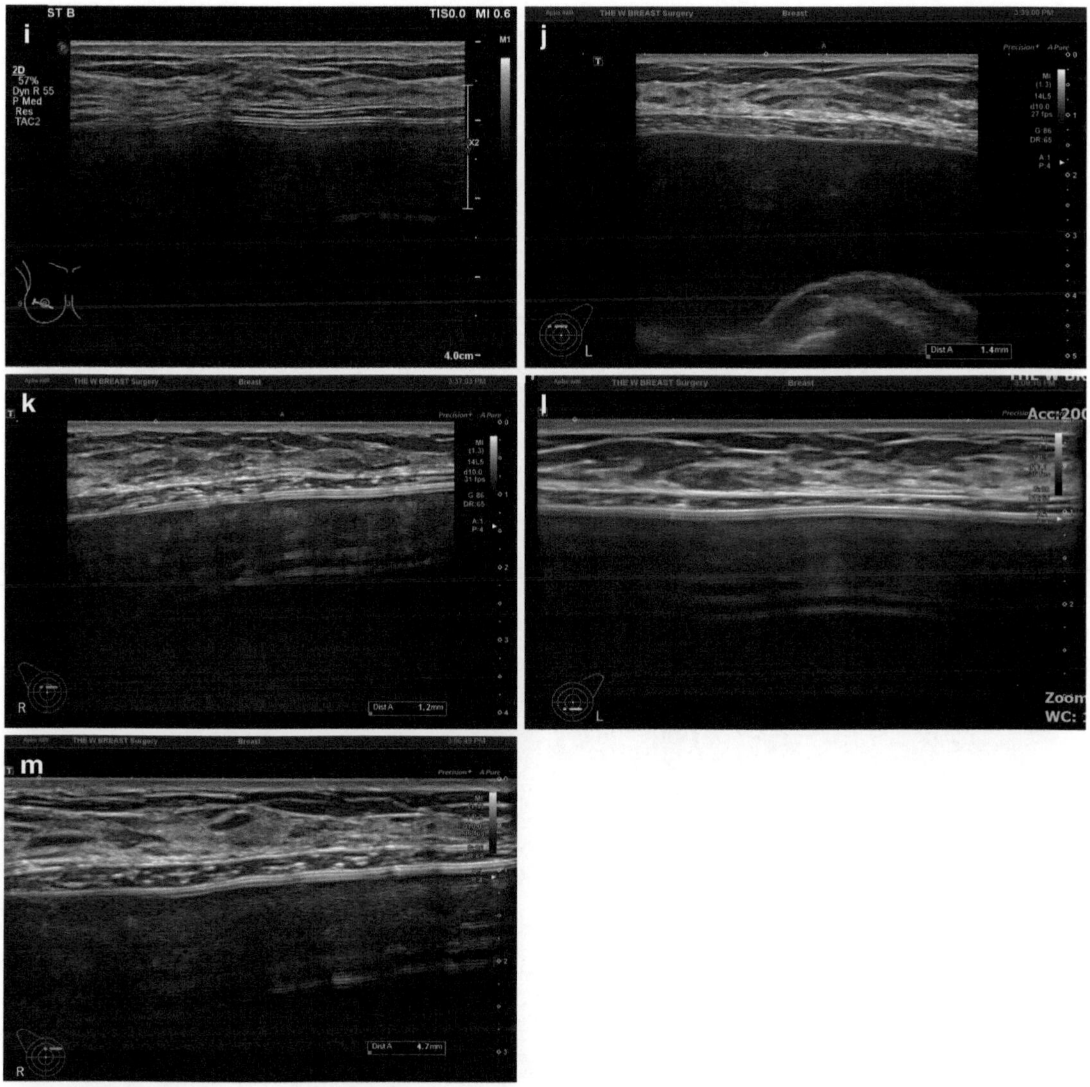

Fig. 2.25 (continued)

operative ultrasonographic finding was checked during routine follow-up (Fig. 2.26).

2.3.19 Case 19

A 28-year-old woman received an augmentation mammaplasty using the Naturgel™ (Groupe Sebbin SAS, Boissy-l' Aillerie, France) via an inframammary fold incision, for which the patient did have placement of a high-profile device (LS 71335 cc) in the subpectoral pocket on both sides of the breast with preoperative anthropometric data (Fig. 2.27). And pre & post-operative view, postoperative ultrasonographic finding was checked during routine follow-up (Fig. 2.27).

If surgeon is familiar with ultrasonography, he or she can understand the course of recovery sequelae.

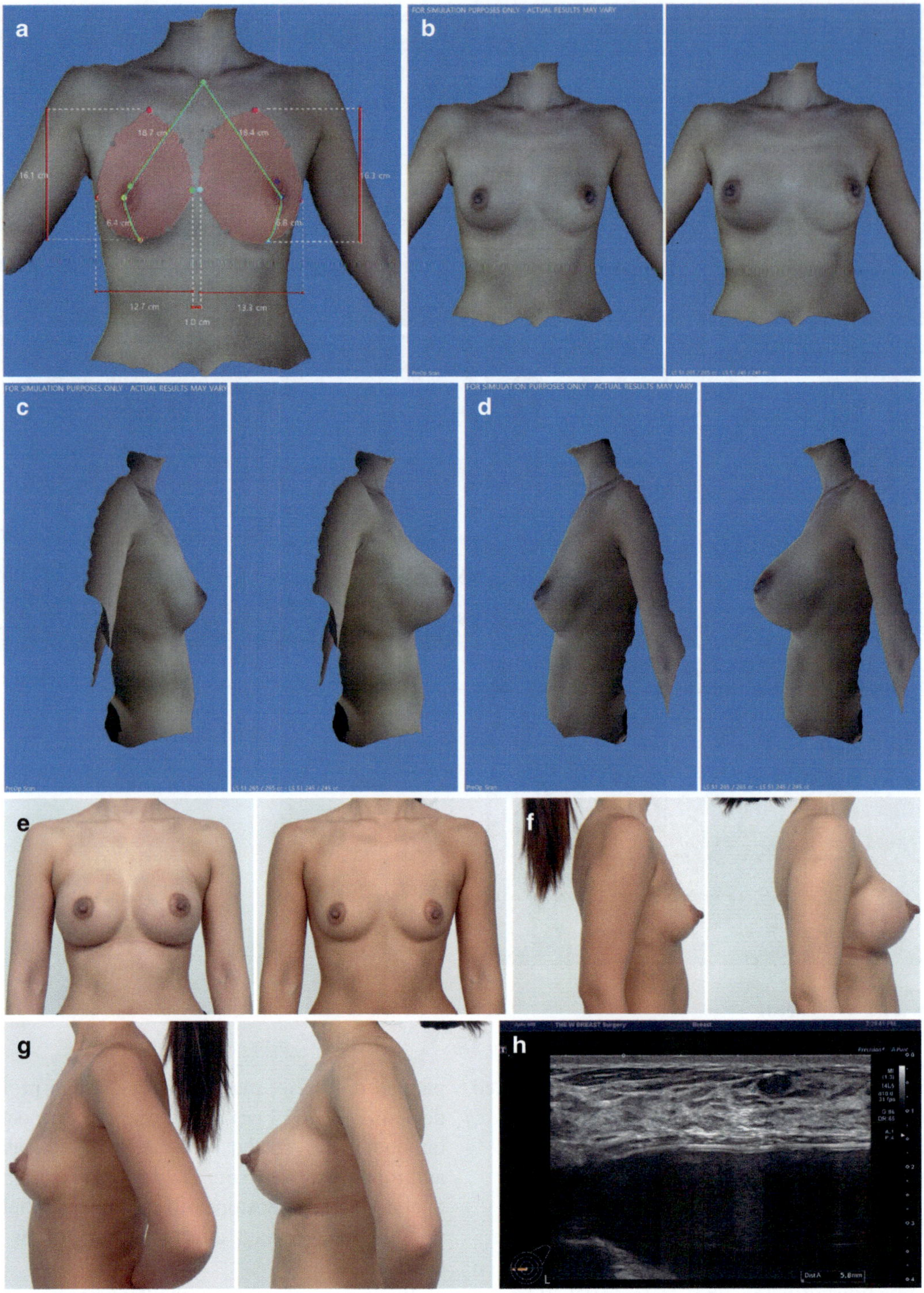

Fig. 2.26 (**a**) Preoperative anthropometric data by 3D simulation. (**b**) Front view of before and after 3D simulation. (**c**) Right side view of before and after 3D simulation. (**d**) Left side view of before and after 3D simulation. (**e**) Preoperative and postoperative front view. (**f**) Preoperative and postoperative right side view. (**g**) Preoperative and postoperative left side view. (**h**) Left ultrasound image shows normal device placed in the subpectoral pocket with benign mass on 12 weeks postoperatively. (**i**) Right ultrasound image shows normal device placed in the subpectoral pocket on 12 weeks postoperatively

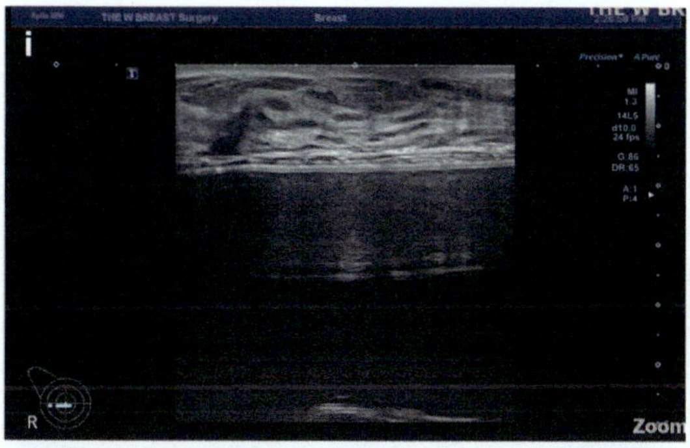

Fig. 2.26 (continued)

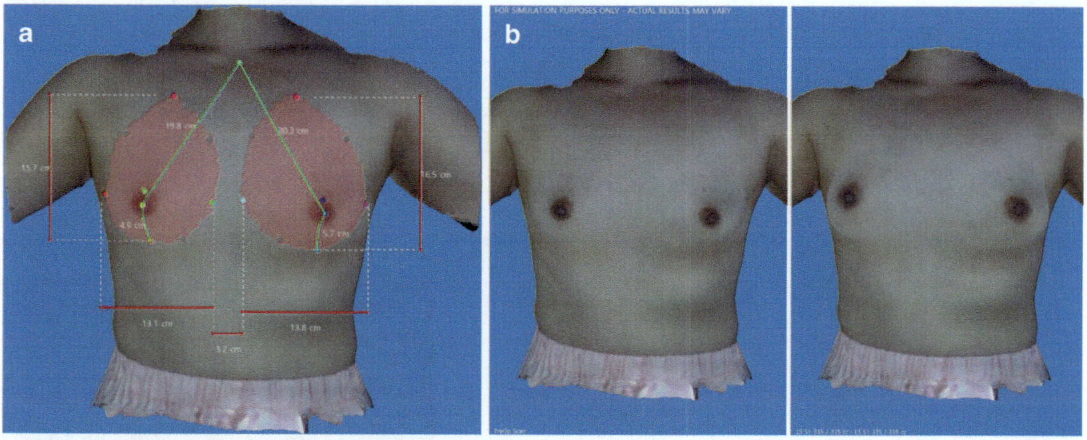

Fig. 2.27 (**a**) Preoperative anthropometric data by 3D simulation. (**b**) Front view of before and after 3D simulation. (**c**) Right side view of before and after 3D simulation. (**d**) Left side view of before and after 3D simulation. (**e**) Preoperative and postoperative front view. (**f**) Preoperative and postoperative right side view. (**g**) Preoperative and postoperative left side view. (**h**) Left ultrasound image shows normal device placed in the subpectoral pocket on 12 weeks postoperatively. (**i**) Right ultrasound image shows normal device placed in the subpectoral pocket on 12 weeks postoperatively. (**j**) Left ultrasound image shows normal device placed in the subpectoral pocket on 56 weeks postoperatively. (**k**) Right ultrasound image shows normal device placed in the subpectoral pocket on 56 weeks postoperatively. (**l**) Left ultrasound image shows normal device on 126 weeks postoperatively. (**m**) Right ultrasound image shows normal device on 126 weeks postoperatively. (**n**) Left ultrasound image shows normal device on 180 weeks postoperatively. (**o**) Right ultrasound image shows normal device on 180 weeks postoperatively

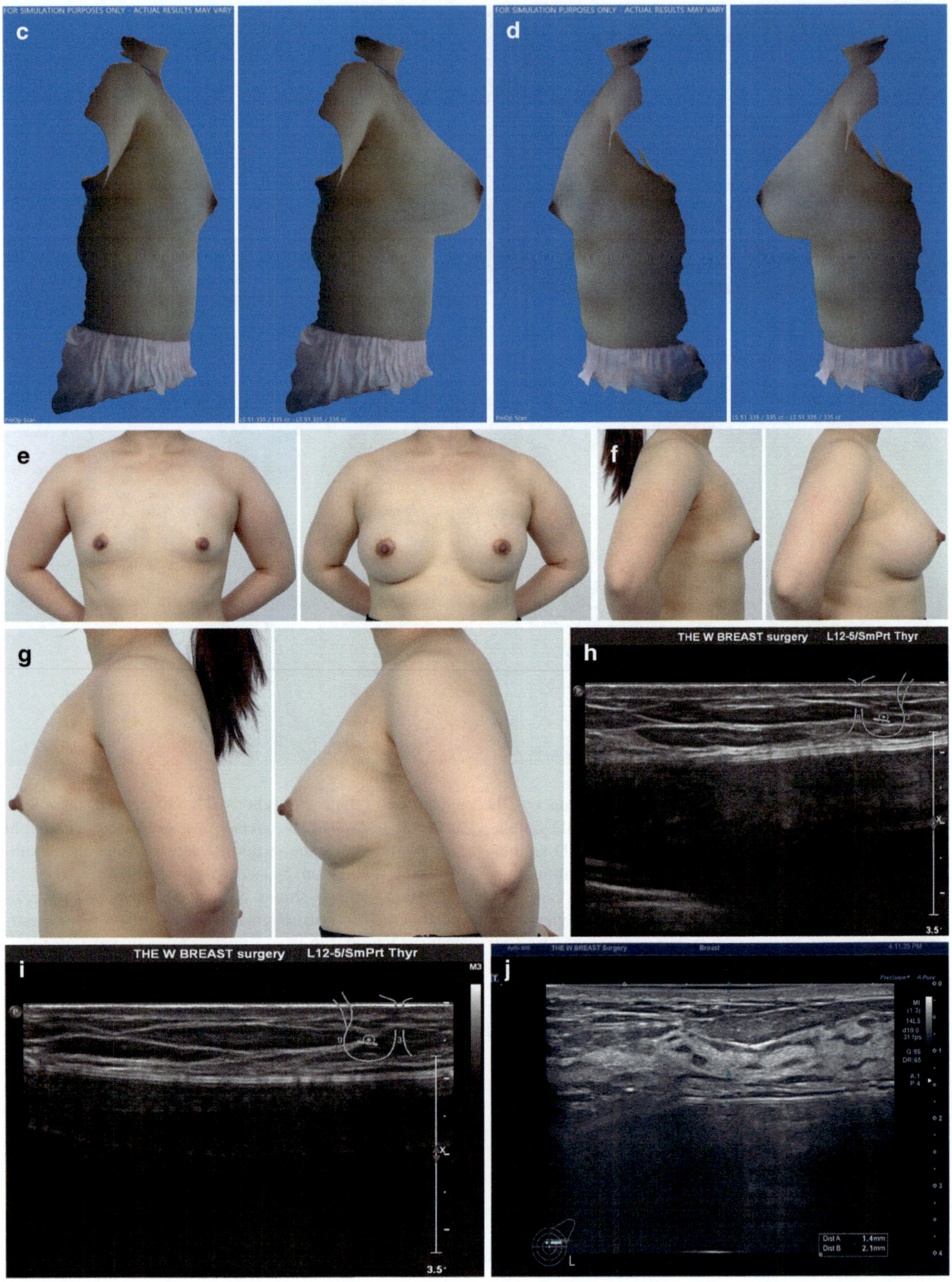

Fig. 2.27 (continued)

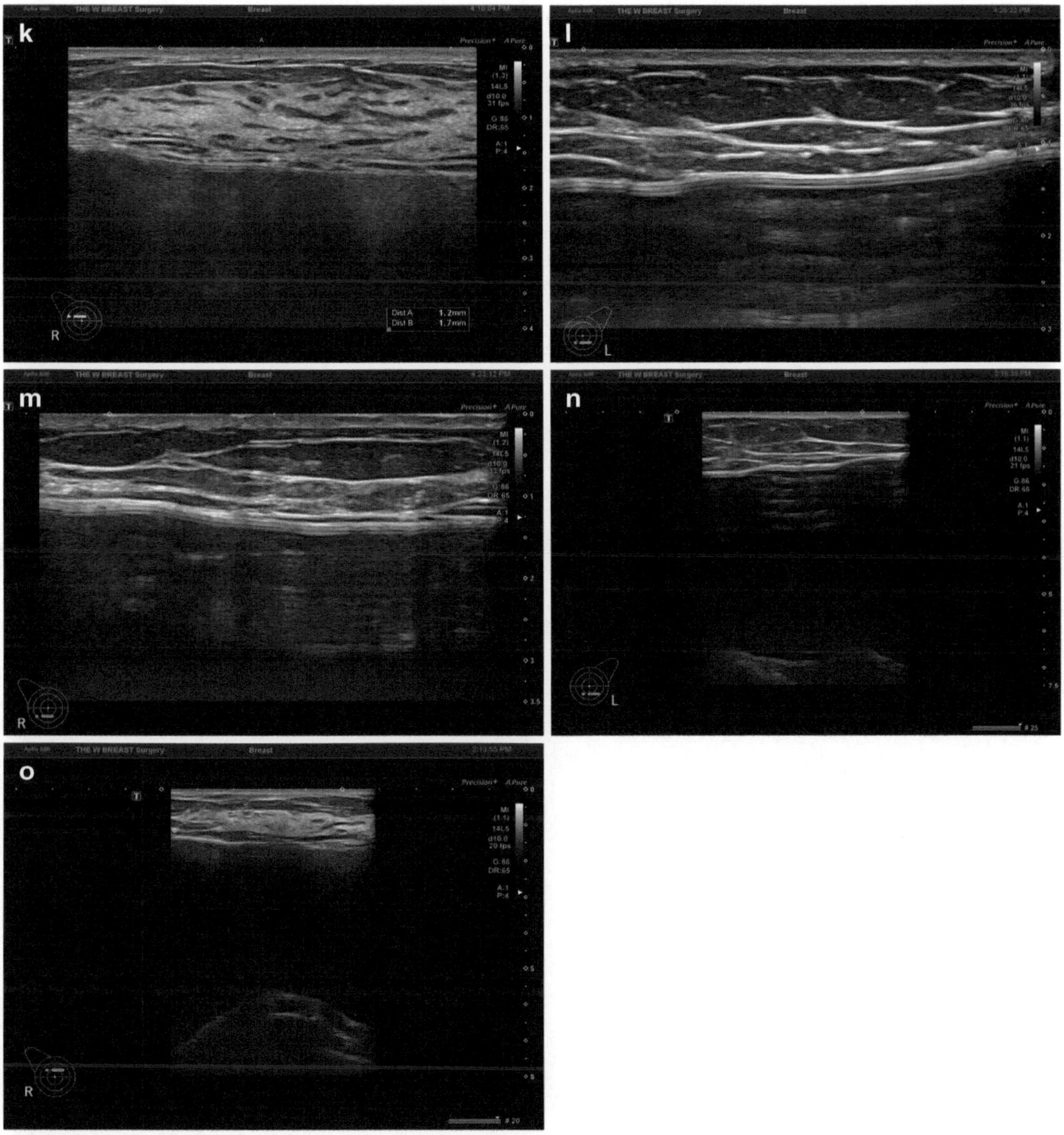

Fig. 2.27 (continued)

References

1. Heidekrueger PI, Sinno S, Hidalgo DA, Colombo M, Broer PN. Current trends in breast augmentation: an international analysis. Aesthet Surg J. 2018;38(2):133–48.
2. Jacobson JM, Gatti ME, Schaffner AD, Hill LM, Spear SL. Effect of incision choice on outcomes in primary breast augmentation. Aesthet Surg J. 2012;32(4):456–62.
3. Deva AK, Cuss A, Magnusson M, Cooter R. The "Game of implants": a perspective on the crisis-prone history of breast implants. Aesthet Surg J. 2019;39(Suppl_1):S55–65.
4. Tebbetts JB. A system for breast implant selection based on patient tissue characteristics and implant-soft tissue dynamics. Plast Reconstr Surg. 2002;109(4):1396–415.
5. Montemurro P, Hedén P, Behr B, Wallner C. Controllable factors to reduce the rate of complications in primary breast augmentation: a review

of the literature [published online ahead of print, 2020 May 1]. Aesthetic Plast Surg. 2020; https://doi.org/10.1007/s00266-020-01726-x.
6. Thorne CH. An evidence-based approach to augmentation mammaplasty. Plast Reconstr Surg. 2010;126:2184–8.
7. Lista F, Ahmad J. Evidence-based medicine: augmentation mammaplasty. Plast Reconstr Surg. 2013;132:1684–96.
8. Schwartz MR. Evidence-based medicine: breast augmentation. Plast Reconstr Surg. 2017;140:109e–19e.
9. Sung JY, Jeong JP, Moon DS, et al. Short-term safety of augmentation Mammaplasty using the BellaGel implants in Korean women. Plast Reconstr Surg Glob Open. 2019;7(12):e2566.
10. Park AY, Seo BK, Cho KR, Woo OH. The utility of MicroPure™ ultrasound technique in assessing grouped microcalcifications without a mass on mammography. J Breast Cancer. 2016;19:83–6.

3 Role of Ultrasound in the Implant-Based Aesthetic and Reconstructive Mammaplasty

3.1 Overview

To date, ultrasound has played a role in examining the integrity and rotation of a breast implant [1–9]. Moreover, its role has been expanded to manage patients who are suspected of having breast implant-associated anaplastic large cell lymphoma *as well as* to evaluate a breast mass [10, 11]. For the appropriate management of a patient receiving an implant-based augmentation mammaplasty, surgeons should perform an ultrasound-guided assessment of two matters:

(1) information about a breast implant (e.g., location, constituents, shell, shape, and manufacturer) and (2) possible occurrence of implant-related complications (e.g., folding with or without detachment, periprosthetic fluid collection, thickened capsule, rupture, capsular mass, malrotation of an anatomical device, upside-down rotation, and foreign body reactions) (Fig. 3.1).

3.2 Role of Ultrasound in the Context of an Implant-Based Aesthetic and Reconstructive Mammaplasty

3.2.1 Characteristics of a Breast Implant

A breast implant is equipped with a single or double lumen with saline or silicone. The single lumen breast implant is commonly encountered in a clinical setting even if it is a saline- or silicone gel-filled breast implant. All the devices are equipped with implants which have an external silicone shell.

After placement, a breast implant is characterized by the formation of a thin fibrous capsule around it, considered a normal physiological phenomenon in response to foreign body.

3.2.2 Ultrasound-Guided Assessment of a Breast Implant

Patients receiving a breast implant should be evaluated for the breast implant position, content, and periprosthetic tissue and axilla on ultrasound. On ultrasound, a silicone gel-filled breast implant is characterized by anechoic findings surrounded by a linear echogenic envelope. Moreover, its interior side may be characterized by low-level echoes.

Supplementary Information The online version contains supplementary material available at [https://doi.org/10.1007/978-981-16-8282-7_3].

J. H. Kim, *Atlas of Breast Implant Ultrasound*, https://doi.org/10.1007/978-981-16-8282-7_3

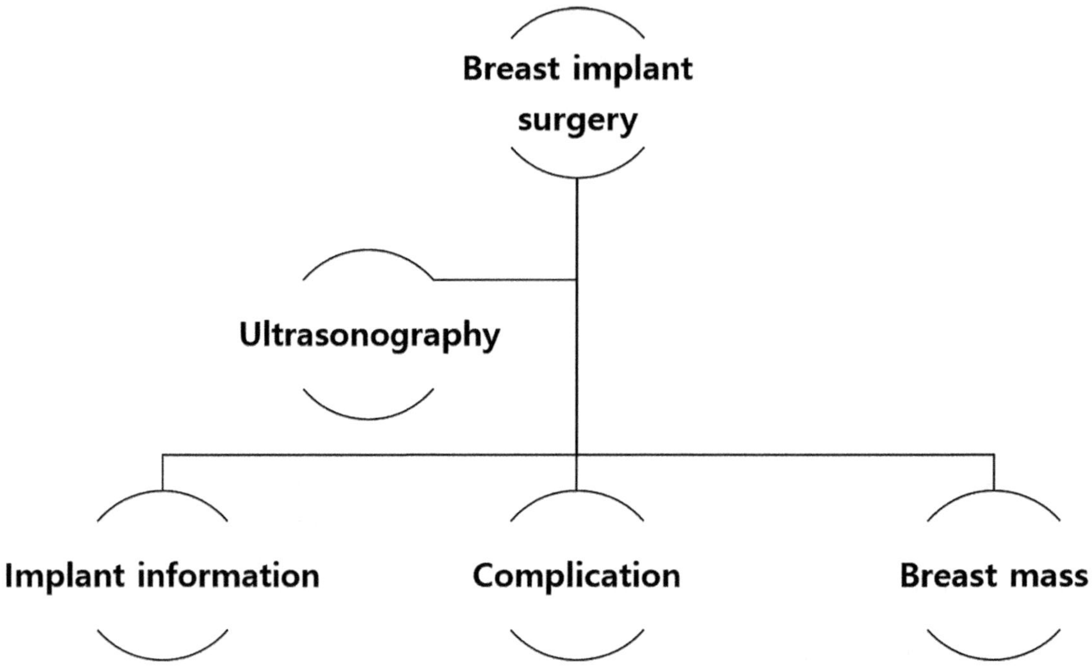

Fig. 3.1 Role of ultrasonography after breast implant surgery

The shell of a silicone gel-filled breast implant may be observed as a single echogenic line or parallel echogenic lines. Moreover, the fibrous capsule is observed as two parallel echogenic lines that are superficial to the surface of a silicone gel-filled breast implant. Normal undulations of the envelope may be observed as wavy echogenic lines irrespective of the presence of minimal intervening fluid.

3.2.3 Ultrasound-Guided Diagnosis of Postoperative Complications

Early complications of an implant-based augmentation mammaplasty include infection and hematoma. Delayed complications include thickened capsule, rupture. As described earlier, in 2006, the US Food and Drug Administration (FDA) mandated the use of a magnetic resonance imaging (MRI) in women receiving a silicone gel-filled breast implant at 3 years postoperatively and at a 2-year interval thereafter [2]. But this causes an economic burden for them. A cost-effective imaging study should therefore be employed to make an early diagnosis of complications of an implant-based augmentation.

In Europe, ultrasound is a more preferred imaging modality in the initial assessment of implant rupture as compared with MRI that has been established as a gold standard strategy [3, 7]. According to a review of literatures, an agreement rate of 87% between ultrasound and MRI has been reported, accompanied by a close association between ultrasound images and findings at explantation.

Moreover, surgeons' use of ultrasound in assessing the status of a breast implant has been advocated [1]. Further, ultrasound has been reported to be a useful modality in postoperatively assessing the rotation of a shaped breast implant seen in 42% of patients receiving an implant-based augmentation mammaplasty [9].

3.2.4 Ultrasound as a Screening Tool for Patients Who Are Suspected of Having Breast Implant-Associated Anaplastic Large Cell Lymphoma (BIA-ALCL)

Usefulness of ultrasound in screening BIA-ALCL has been advocated in the literature; Adrada et al. performed a review of imaging studies in 44 cases of BIA-ALCL, thus reporting that ultrasound showed a sensitivity of 84% and a specificity of 75% in detecting an effusion. These values were higher as compared with the sensitivity and specificity of computed tomography, MRI (82% and 33%), and positron emission computed tomography (38% and 83%) [12]. Ultrasound may be therefore recommended as the first line of screening for BIA-ALCL.

Initially, breast ultrasound is performed to assess periprosthetic fluid collection, mass, or regional adenopathy [14–16]. According to a retrospective study conducted by Adrada et al., breast ultrasound showed a sensitivity of 84% and a specificity of 75% in detecting a periprosthetic fluid collection. These authors also reported that it showed a sensitivity of 46% and a specificity of 100% in detecting a mass [17]. A periprosthetic fluid should be aspirated and then sent for culture and Gram stain, cell block cytology, immunohistochemistry, and flow cytometry [15, 16]. A minimum volume of 20 mL is needed, but a 50–100 mL of the fluid sample should be collected to avoid a risk of false-negative or intermediate results [14]. A pathologist should consider the possibility of BIA-ALCL for the purposes of performing appropriate tests including comprehensive flow cytometric markers.

3.2.5 Ultrasound as a Component of a Multi-Disciplinary Algorithm-Based Approach to an Early Detection of Complications of an Implant-Based Augmentation Mammaplasty

Kim et al. analyzed medical examination data that was collected from a total of 2,037 women ($n = 2{,}037$) between August 12 and December 31, 2021. They were evaluated for whether they were in healthy conditions. Moreover, their baseline characteristics were also examined; these include age, sex, height (cm), weight (kg), duration since surgery (years), possession of a breast implant card, the site of surgical incision, side of symptoms, and reasons for outpatient visit. Furthermore, the patients were also evaluated for their subjective awareness of the manufacturer, surface, and shape of the breast implant.

Potential complications include malrotation, folding, seroma, capsule thickening, upside-down rotation, rupture, capsule mass, and breast mass (Fig. 3.2). According to these

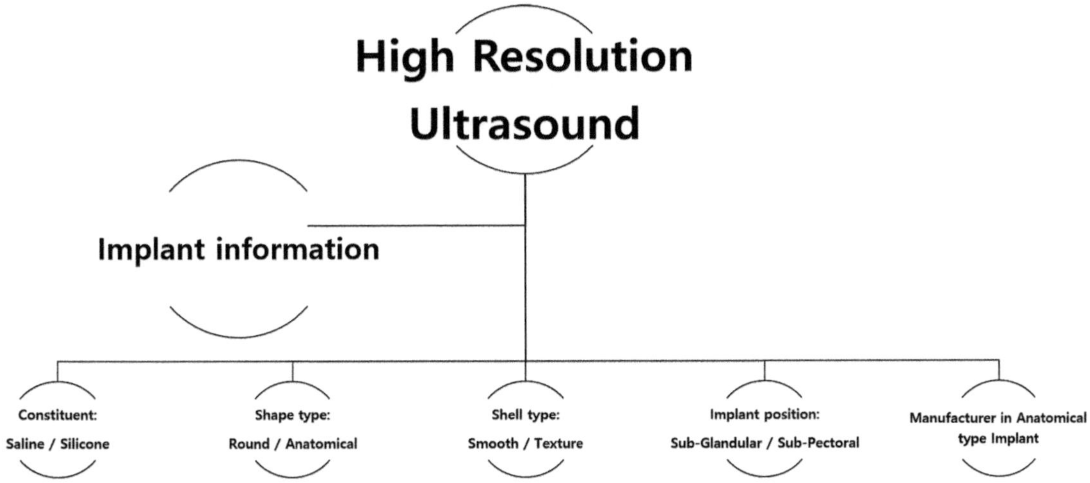

Fig. 3.2 Checkpoint of breast implant ultrasonography for breast implant information

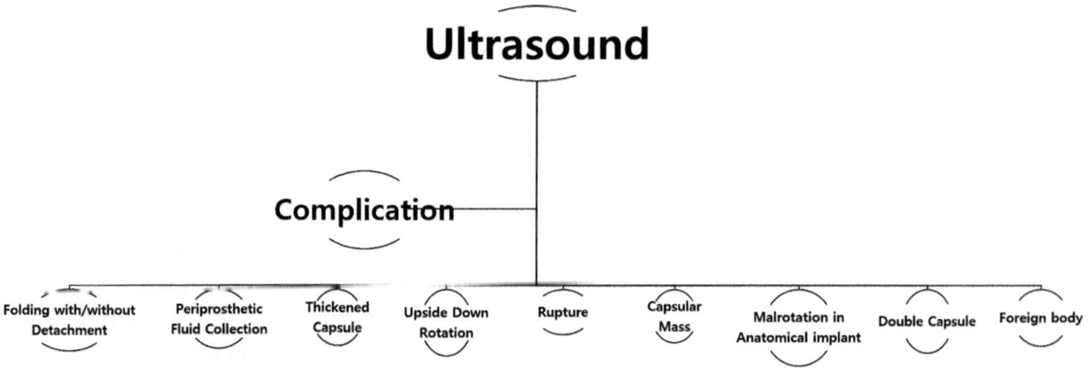

Fig. 3.3 Checklist of breast implant-related complications after breast implant surgery

authors, a majority of the patients had a past history of receiving textured implants. Based on these findings, Kim et al. proposed that such patients be further evaluated for a risk of BIA-ALCL through a multi-disciplinary algorithm-based approach to an early detection of complications of an implant-based augmentation mammaplasty [13].

There is a nine-point checklist for diagnosis of breast implant-related complications (Fig. 3.3).

1. Folding with or without detachment.
2. Periprosthetic fluid collection.
3. Thickened capsule.
4. Double capsule.
5. Rupture (intracapsular and extracapsular rupture with or without LN silicone invasion).
6. Capsular mass.
7. Malrotation in anatomical type implant.
8. Upside-down rotation.
9. Foreign body.

Usually, there will be minimally 12 photos and 12 video for patients who have breast implant for the meticulous follow-up using ultrasonography. And also physician records more photos for problematic site (Figs. 3.4 and 3.5), (Videos 3.1, 3.2, 3.3, 3.4, 3.5 and 3.6).

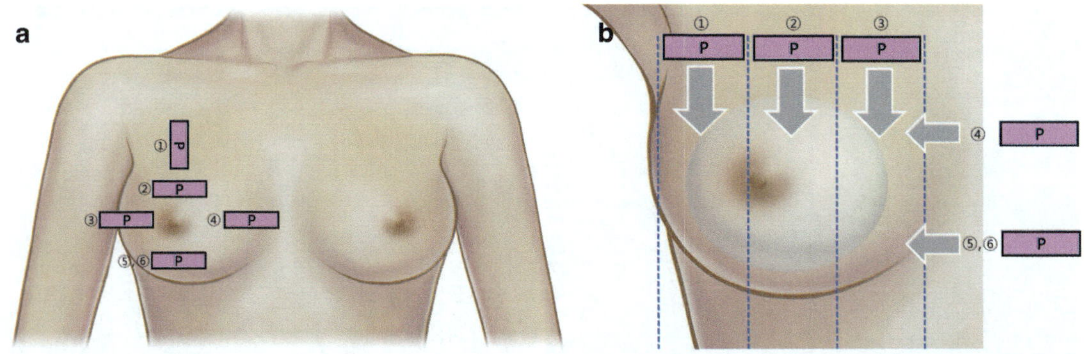

Fig. 3.4 (**a**, **b**) Breast implant specified ultrasonography. (**a**) 6 photos for one breast: each point has a role. ① Point: Best position for checking breast implant pocket. ② Point: Checkpoint for upper part of breast implant and periprosthetic space. ③ Point: Checkpoint for lateral part of breast implant and periprosthetic space. ④ Point: Checkpoint for medial part of breast implant and periprosthetic space. ⑤ Point: Checkpoint for inferior part of breast implant and periprosthetic space. ① Point: Best position for identifying the breast implant shell type. (**b**) 6 videos for one breast. Video: For checking lateral part of breast implant and periprosthetic space. ① Video: For checking central part of breast implant and periprosthetic space. ② Video: For checking medial part of breast implant and periprosthetic space. ③ Video: For checking upper part of breast implant and periprosthetic space. ④ Video: For checking lower part of breast implant and periprosthetic space. ⑤ Video: For checking shell of breast implant

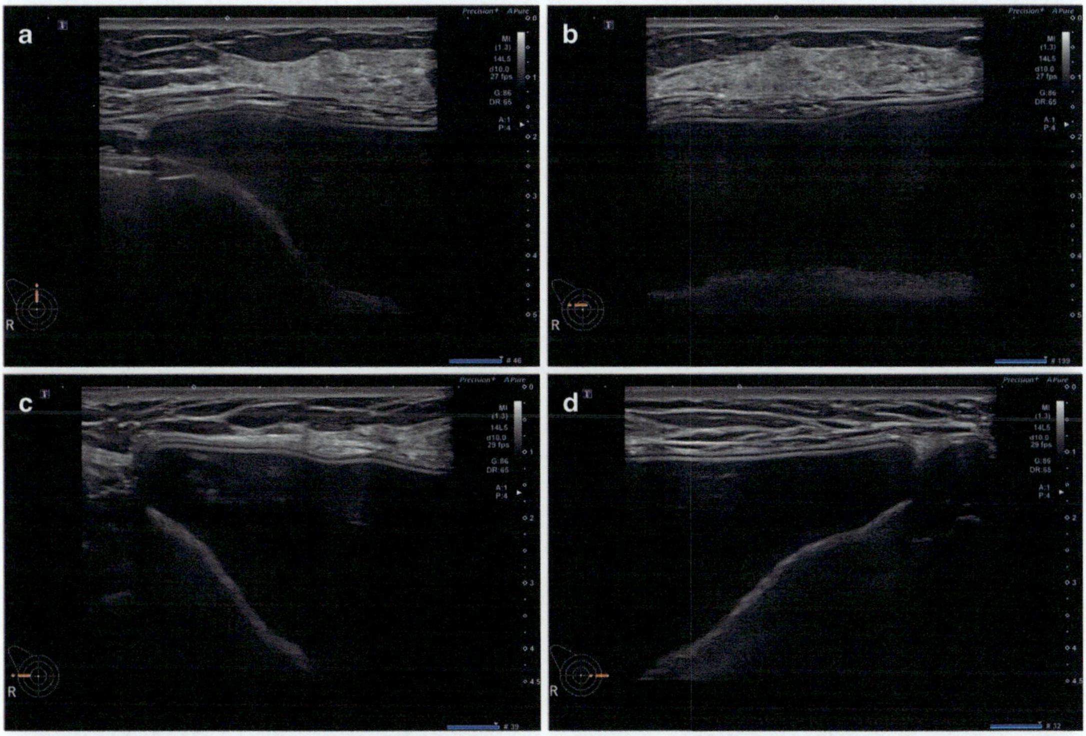

Fig. 3.5 Example of two different shell types breast implant ultrasonography. (**a–f**) Textured shell type breast implant. (**g–l**) Smooth shell type breast implant. (**a**): ① point. (**b**): ② point. (**c**): ③ point. (**d**): ④ point. (**e**): ⑤ point. (**f**): ⑥ point. (**g**): ① point. (**h**): ② point. I: ③ point. (**j**): ④ point. (**k**): ⑤ point. (**l**): ⑥ point

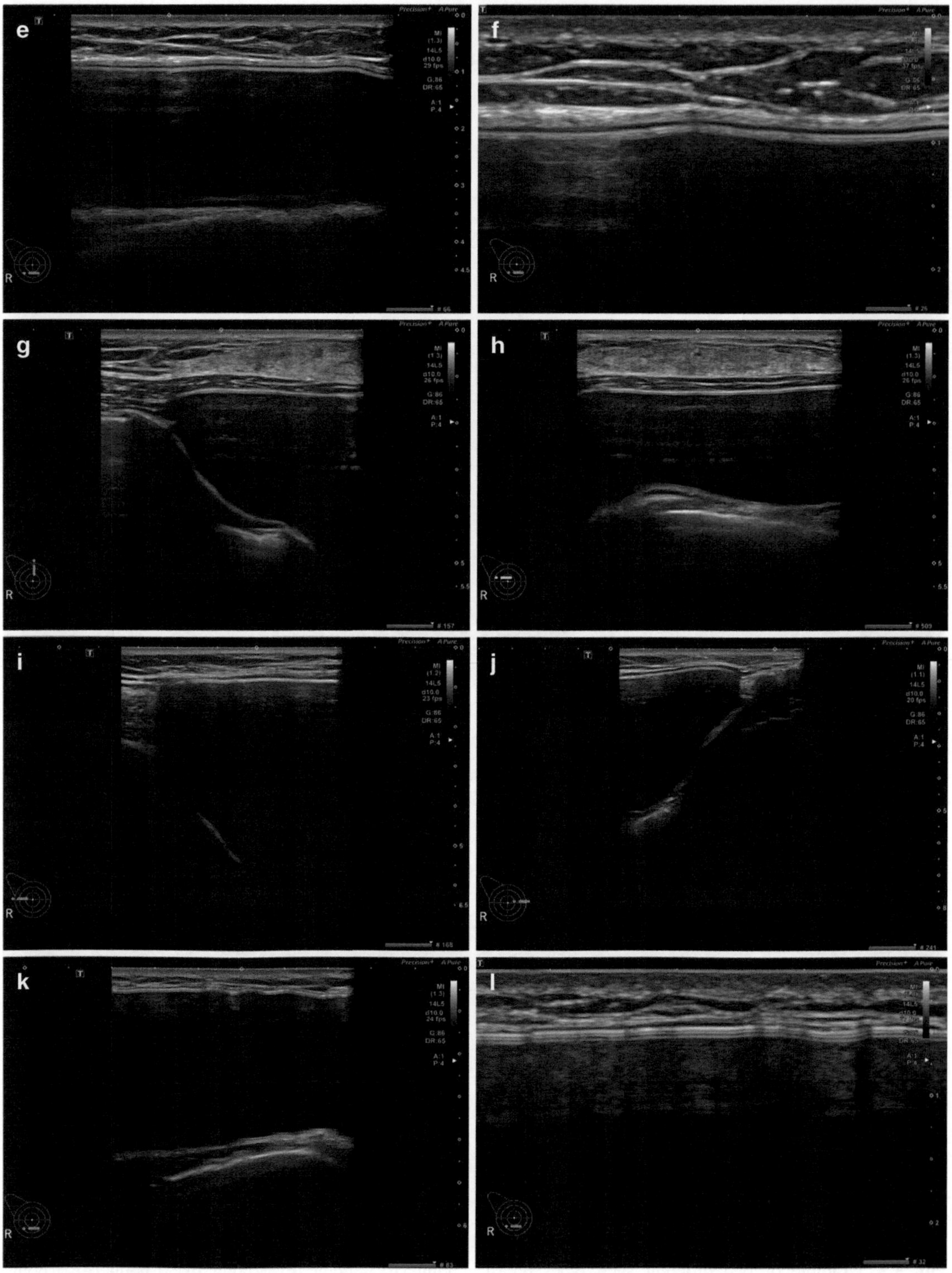

Fig. 3.5 (continued)

References

1. Bengtson BP, Eaves FF 3rd. High-resolution ultrasound in the detection of silicone gel breast implant shell failure: background, in vitro studies, and early clinical results. Aesthet Surg J. 2012;32:157–74.
2. Chung KC, Malay S, Shauver MJ, et al. Economic analysis of screening strategies for rupture of silicone gel breast implants. Plast Reconstr Surg. 2012;130:225–37.
3. Rietjens M, Villa G, Toesca A, et al. Appropriate use of magnetic resonance imaging and ultrasound to detect early silicone gel breast implant rupture in postmastectomy reconstruction. Plast Reconstr Surg. 2014;134:13e–20e.
4. Nahabedian MY. Discussion: appropriate use of magnetic resonance imaging and ultrasound to detect early silicone gel breast implant rupture in postmastectomy reconstruction. Plast Reconstr Surg. 2014;134:21e–3e.
5. Stachs A, Dieterich M, Hartmann S, et al. Diagnosis of ruptured breast implants through high-resolution ultrasound combined with real-time elastography. Aesthet Surg J. 2015;35:410–8.
6. Mennie JC, Quaba O, Smith M, et al. Diagnosing PIP breast implant failure: a prospective analysis of clinical and ultrasound accuracy. J Plast Reconstr Aesthet Surg. 2015;68:540–5.
7. Sisti A, Tassinari J, Milonia L, et al. Comparison of Allergan, Mentor, and Sientra contoured cohesive gel breast implants: a single surgeon's 10-year experience. Plast Reconstr Surg. 2016;138:548e–9e.
8. Stivala A, Rem K, Leuzzi S, et al. Efficacy of ultrasound, mammography and magnetic resonance imaging in detecting breast implant rupture: a retrospective study of 175 reconstructive and aesthetic sub-pectoral breast augmentation cases. J Plast Reconstr Aesthet Surg. 2017;70:1520–6.
9. Sieber DA, Stark RY, Chase S, et al. Clinical evaluation of shaped gel breast implant rotation using high-resolution ultrasound. Aesthet Surg J. 2017;37:290–6.
10. Clemens MW, Brody GS, Mahabir RC, et al. How to diagnose and treat breast implant-associated anaplastic large cell lymphoma. Plast Reconstr Surg. 2018;141:586e–99e.
11. Shida M, Chiba A, Ohashi M, et al. Ultrasound diagnosis and treatment of breast lumps after breast augmentation with autologous fat grafting. Plast Reconstr Surg Glob Open. 2017;5:e1603.
12. Adrada BE, Miranda RN, Rauch GM, et al. Breast implant-associated anaplastic large cell lymphoma: sensitivity, specificity, and findings of imaging studies in 44 patients. Breast Cancer Res Treat. 2014;147:1–14.
13. Kim JH, Paik NS, Nam SY, Cho Y, Park HK. The emerging crisis of stakeholders in implant-based augmentation Mammaplasty in Korea. J Korean Med Sci. 2020;35(15):e103.
14. Mehta-Shah N, Clemens MW, Horwitz SM. How I treat breast implant-associated anaplastic large cell lymphoma. Blood. 2018;132:1889–98.
15. O'Neill AC, Zhong T, Hofer SOP. Implications of breast implant associated anaplastic large cell lymphoma (BIA-ALCL) for breast cancer reconstruction: an update for surgical oncologists. Ann Surg Oncol. 2017;24:3174–9.
16. Clemens MW, Horwitz SM. NCCN consensus guidelines for the diagnosis and management of breast implant-associated anaplastic large cell lymphoma. Aesthet Surg J. 2017;37:285–9.
17. Adrada BE, Miranda RN, Rauch GM, et al. Breast implant-associated anaplastic large cell lymphoma: sensitivity, specificity, and findings of imaging studies in 44 patients. Breast Cancer Res Treat. 2014;147:1–14.

4 Distinguishing Various Types of Breast Implant Using High-Resolution Ultrasonography

High-resolution ultrasound (HRUS) should be used to evaluate some essential factors for a patient receiving an implant-based aesthetic or reconstructive mammaplasty; these include location, constituents, surface topography of the shell, shape, and manufacturer of the breast implant (Fig. 4.1).

4.1 Location of a Breast Implant

A breast implant can be placed either above or below the muscle, and its accurate location can be identified (Fig. 4.2, Videos 4.11 and 4.12). The easiest way to identify its location is to examine the upper quadrant of the breast on its 12 o'clock position. That is, an ultrasound probe is vertically positioned on the border of a breast implant on its 12 o'clock position (Fig. 4.3). The following sonographic finding shows the placement of a breast implant above the pectoralis major muscle (Fig. 4.4); this can be further understood on video (Videos 4.9 and 4.10). A breast implant might be partly placed below the muscle in patients receiving multiple surgeries or those who did not achieve a complete dissection of the tissue. Otherwise, a breast implant could be correctly placed above or below the muscle. The location of a breast implant is an essential factor that is closely associated with a soft feel of the breast. Once identified, it is a helpful information for making a plan for revisional surgery or reoperation.

4.2 Constituents of a Breast Implant

A breast implant can be classified into a saline-filled or silicone gel-filled device. But there are also other types of breast implant that can be equipped with a double lumen. Step-off sign is a clue to characterization of constituents of a breast implant placed in a pocket. This may be supported by an inlet of a saline-filled breast implant (Fig. 4.5), (Video 4.2). Sometimes there is no inlet in the superior part of a saline-filled breast implant. In patients receiving a breast implant in an upside-down position, it is important to cautiously differentiate between an inlet and a patch of a saline-filled breast implant, considering that the shell of a saline-filled breast implant is also available as either a smooth or textured surface. This suggests that there is no correlation between the surface topography and constituents of a saline-filled breast implant. Definite sign of saline breast implant even in dual chamber is no step-off sign (Videos 4.1, 4.3 and 4.4).

Step-off sign is a definite indicator of a difference in the velocity of ultrasound wave between a saline-filled and silicone gel-filled breast implant. Step-off sign can be identified through

Supplementary Information The online version contains supplementary material available at (https://doi.org/10.1007/978-981-16-8282-7_4).

J. H. Kim, *Atlas of Breast Implant Ultrasound*, https://doi.org/10.1007/978-981-16-8282-7_4

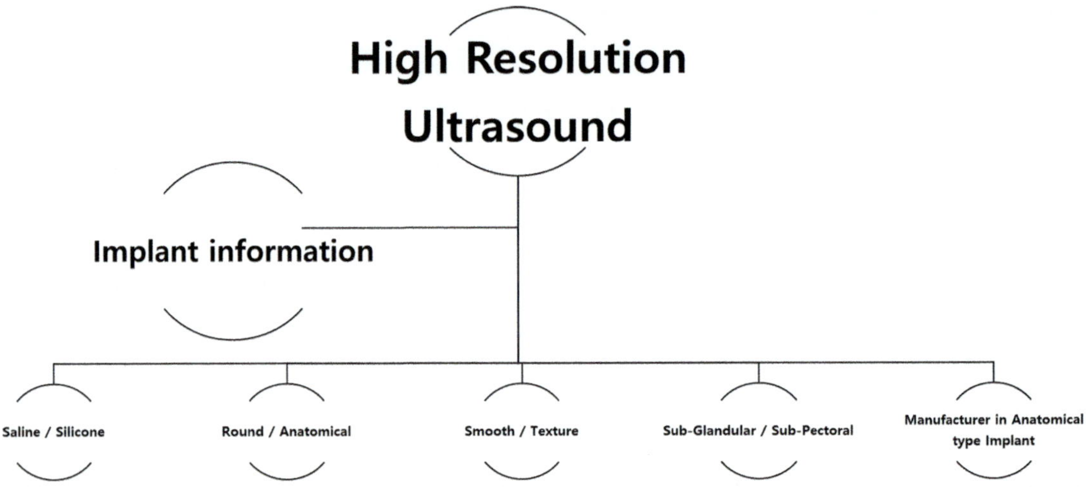

Fig. 4.1 Checkpoint of breast implant-related information using ultrasonography

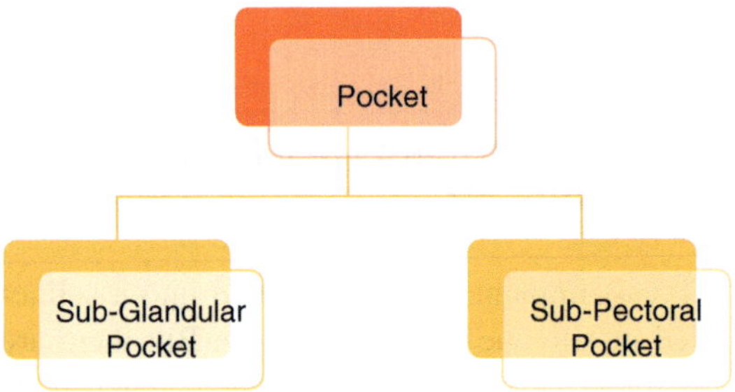

Fig. 4.2 Position of breast implant

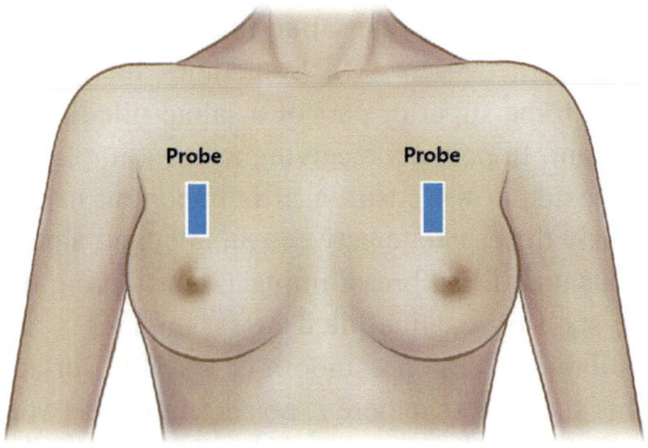

Fig. 4.3 Best site for identifying implant pocket position

application of an ultrasound probe to the border of a breast implant with compression (Fig. 4.6), (Video 4.2). The continuous line between chest wall and inferior border of breast implant is broken when there is step-off sign. A continuity between the base of a breast implant and the chest wall suggests a lack of step-off sign, based on which the presence of a saline-filled breast implant can be identified. By contrast, a discontinuity between the base of a silicone gel-filled breast implant and the chest wall suggests step-off sign. A lack of step-off sign is indicative of a saline-filled breast implant.

4.3 Surface Topography of a Breast Implant

Identification of the surface topography of a breast implant is helpful for not only examining whether the corresponding device has a causal relationship with the onset of breast implant-associated anaplastic lymphoma (BIA-ALCL) but also making a plan for reoperation.

In patients who are suspected of having BIA-ALCL, a clinical course should be meticulously monitored in association with a macro-textured device. Thus, such patients cannot be overlooked.

In this regard, patients receiving a smooth device are free from a risk of BIA-ALCL. Unfortunately, most of the patients were not aware of a breast implant they received, some of whom even lost a warranty card. Identification of the surface topography of a breast implant is therefore helpful for these patients.

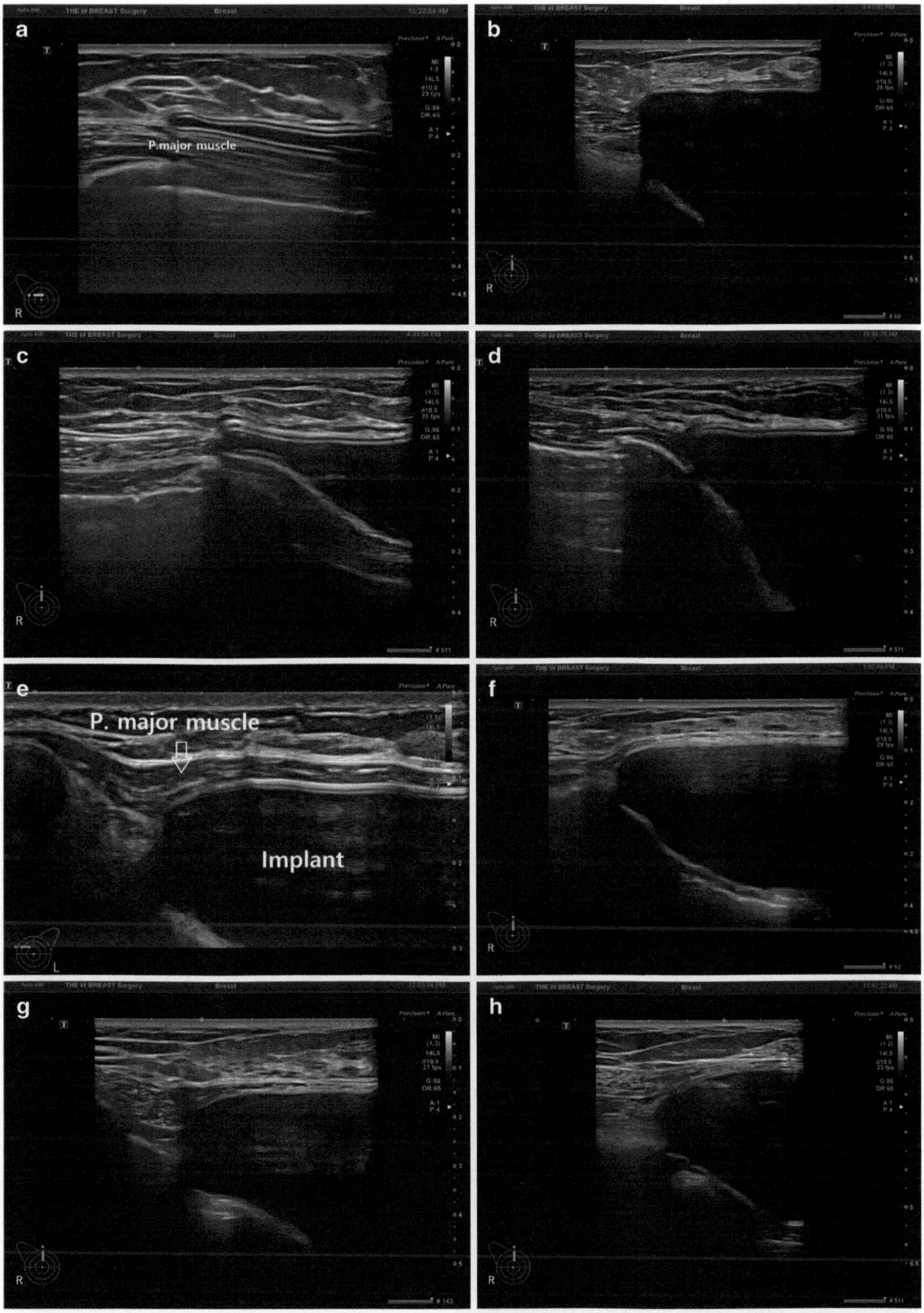

Fig. 4.4 Ultrasonographic images of subglandular and subpectoral implant pocket. (**a–d**) Breast implant in subglandular pocket. (**e–o**) Breast implant in subpectoral pocket

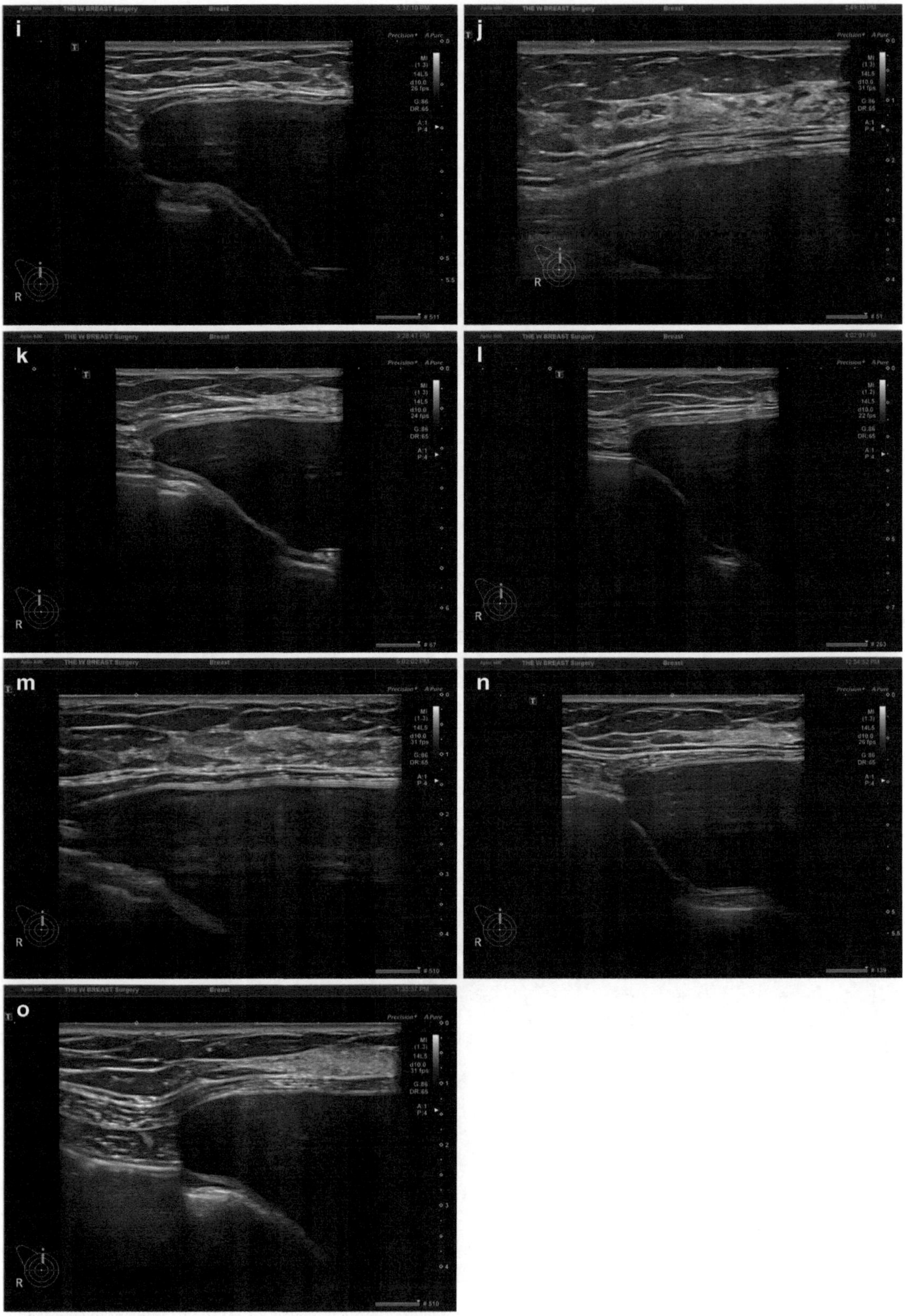

Fig. 4.4 (continued)

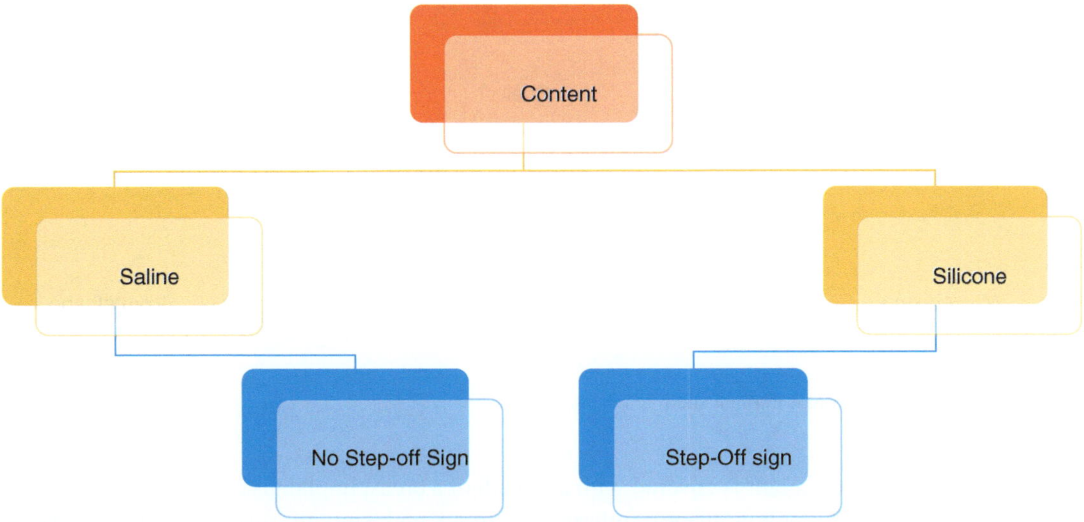

Fig. 4.5 Distinguishing sign saline and silicone breast implant by ultrasonography

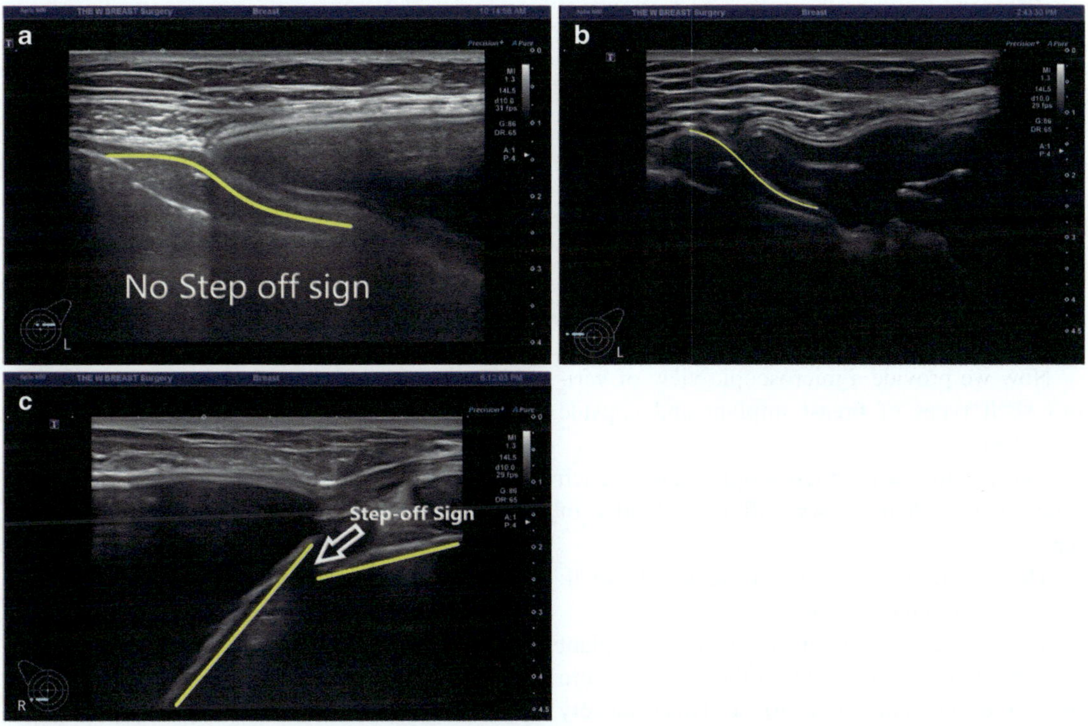

Fig. 4.6 Step-off sign and no step-off sign in ultrasonography. (**a**) No step-off sign in single-lumen saline implant. (**b**) No step-off sign in double-lumen saline implant. (**c**) Step-off sign in silicone implant

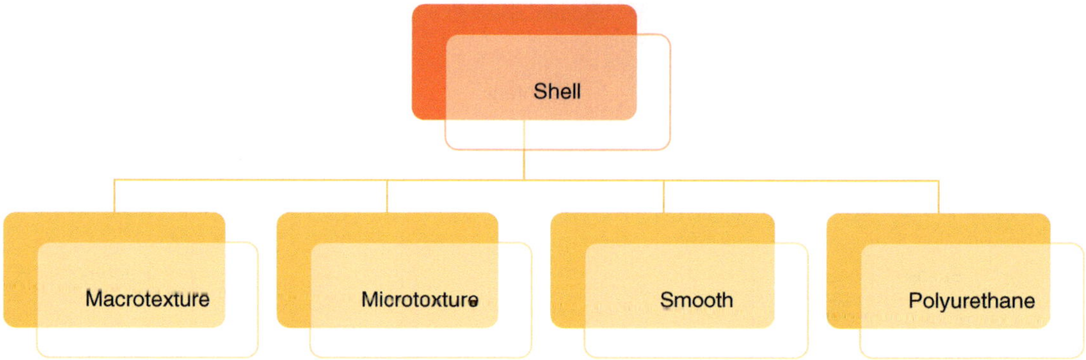

Fig. 4.7 Various types of breast implant shell

The shell of a breast implant is covered with a macro-textured (include polyurethane), micro-textured, or smooth surface, each of which can be observed on ultrasound as follows (Figs. 4.7 and 4.8): HRUS is useful in making a definite differentiation of a macro-textured breast implant from a micro-textured or smooth device.

There are three shell types: macro-texture (including polyurethane), micro-texture, smooth (Fig. 4.8), (Videos 4.5, 4.6 and 4.7).

In sonography, shell type can be divided two types: macro-texture (including polyurethane), smooth Micro-texture and smooth shell type is almost same features in ultrasonography. HRUS cannot distinguish the difference.

Now we provide a microscopic view of various shell types of breast implant and capsule (Fig. 4.9).

And the following microscopic view of each type of the shell shows different depths of texturing.

There are two types of textured shell: Embossing or engraving type.

The surface topography of a breast implant can be differentiated based on the depth of pore that is present on the shell surface. This is closely associated with the manufacturing process of each manufacturer. There is a broad spectrum of the depth; even the micro-textured breast implant had a depth of 5–50 μm. On HRUS, a micro-textured breast implant and a smooth device share almost similar surface topography (Fig. 4.10). It is therefore difficult to differentiate between the two devices. For this reason, the shell of a breast implant is classified into a macro-textured and smooth surface unless otherwise noted.

4.4 Shape and Manufacturer of a Breast Implant

The shape of a breast implant can be classified into a round and anatomical shape (Fig. 4.11). An anatomical breast implant was developed because its shape was considered appropriate for aesthetic or reconstructive purposes. But it is vulnerable to malrotation, and no objective studies have demonstrated its advantages. Because it is equipped with a textured surface, it has a causal relationship with the onset of BIA-ALCL.

The following photograph shows an anatomical breast implant placed in the left breast and a round device in the right breast.

Identification of an anatomical breast implant can be made based on the orientation mark that is unique to the manufacturer. The OM was devised to place a breast implant to correct directions, and it is observed as a dot or a line in the superior and inferior part of a breast implant. The following table summarizes the OM that is unique to the manufacturer of an anatomical breast implant. Values in the parenthesis denote its numbers (Table 4.1).

It is worthwhile to note that the length, width, and height of the line vary depending on the manufacturer. A closer look at it would therefore be helpful for identifying the manufacturer. The

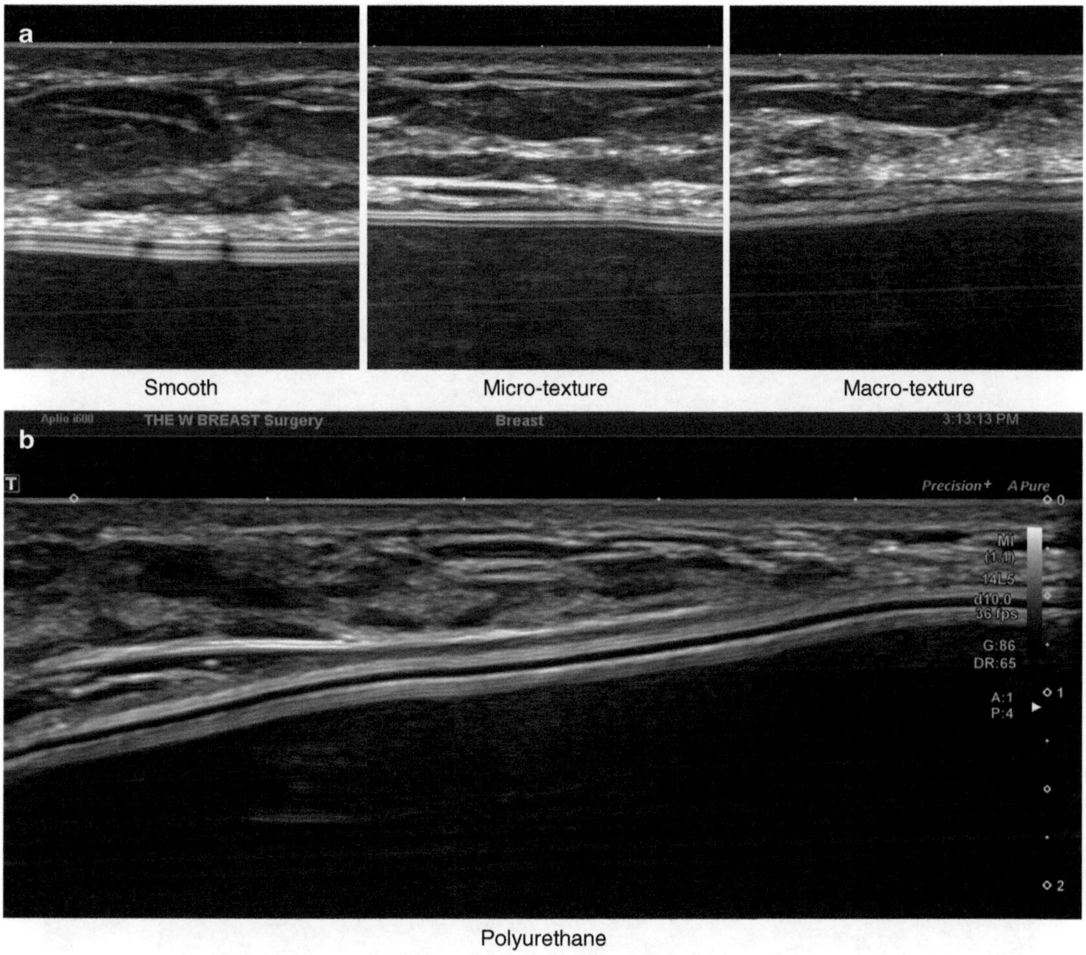

Fig. 4.8 Various shell types of breast implant in ultrasonography. (**a**) Smooth, micro-texture, macro-textured shell type breast implant in HRUS image. (**b**) Polyurethane shell type breast implant in HRUS image

direction of the superior OM may serve as an indicator of malrotation. Grossly, the Sebbin and the Mentor share very similar OM with each other. It is somewhat difficult to identify an anatomical breast implant manufactured by the Silimed. This is because its superior OM is not visible even on HRUS. Therefore, an anatomical breast implant manufactured by the Silimed should be identified based on the characteristic features of its textured surface. Thus, it can be identified based on a dot that is present on the base of a breast implant.

The time point of clinical release of an anatomical breast implant is also a useful information for identification of the corresponding manufacturer. For example, the Polytech anatomical breast implant was first approved for clinical use in Korea in 2012. This information will be helpful for the type of a breast implant depending on the period during which a patient received an implant-based augmentation mammaplasty. Gross findings of an anatomical breast implant are shown below. (Mentor, Allergan, Silimed, Sebbin, Polytech, Eurosilicone, Hansbiomed) (Figs. 4.12, 4.13, 4.14, 4.15, 4.16, 4.17 and 4.18), (Videos 4.33, 4.34, 4.35, 4.36, 4.37, 4.38, 4.39 and 4.40).

Briefly, the OM is unique to an anatomical breast implant. But there are no anatomical breast implants branded as the Motiva because the Motiva Ergonomix Round SilkSurface was solely imported to Korea. To identify the manufacturer

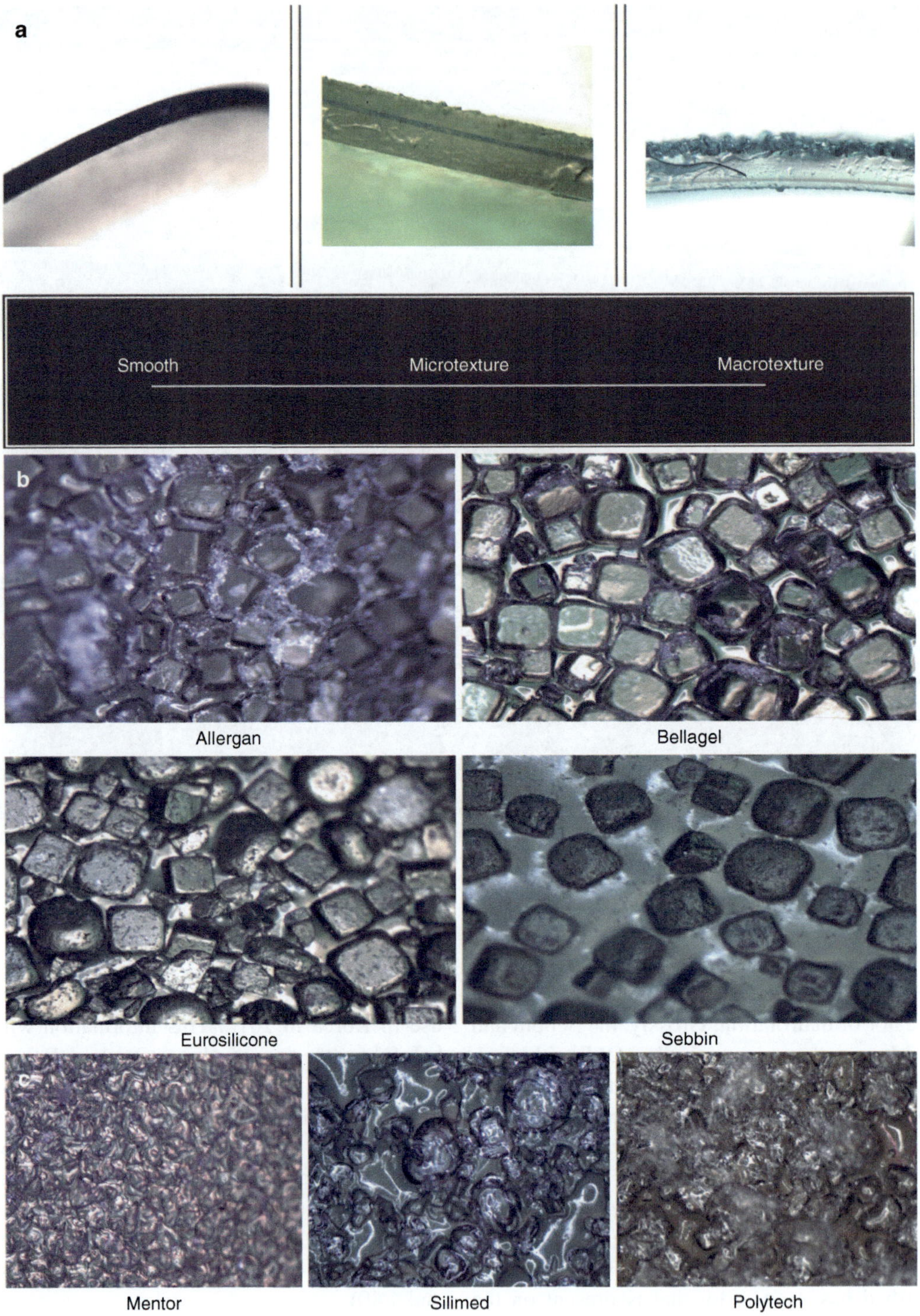

Fig. 4.9 Three different breast implant shell images and microscopic view of capsule in microscopy. (**a**) Microscopic view of three different shell types. (**b**) Microscopic view of embossing shell type breast implant. (**c**) Microscopic view of engraving shell type breast implant. (**d**) Microscopic view of polyurethane shell. (**e**) Microscopic view of capsule that had contained macro-textured shell type breast implant that shows many undulations. (**f**) Microscopic view of capsule that had contained smooth shell type breast implant that shows smooth inner line

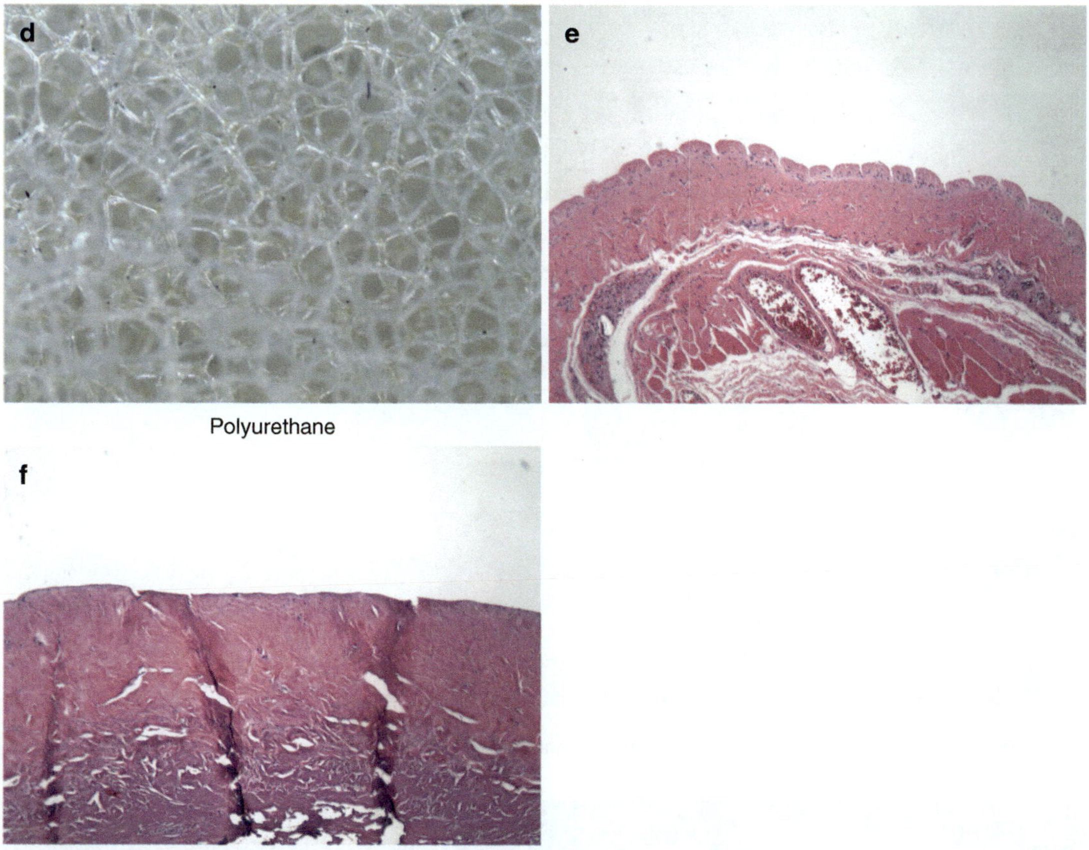

Fig. 4.9 (continued)

of an anatomical breast implant based on the presence of OM, a breast implant should be examined using an ultrasound probe from the superior to inferior directions (Videos 4.8, 4.15, 4.18, 4.21, 4.23, 4.24, 4.27, 4.29, 4.30 and 4.32). This is followed by examination of the border of a breast implant in a circle at an angle of 360°. Subsequently, specific findings on the shell are observed (Figs. 4.19, 4.20, 4.21, 4.22, 4.23, 4.24, 4.25 and 4.26). An ultrasound probe should be rotated when there are any notable findings, based on which it can be determined whether the OM has a shape of line or dot. It is necessary to examine the shell of a breast implant manufactured by the Silimed at a higher magnification. Moreover, it is also necessary to adjust the depth of probing, which is essential for examining the inferior part of a device. Thus, the manufacturer of a breast implant can be completely identified (Fig. 4.21).

It is common to see patients who do not know what type of breast implants she has.

So far, you can see the ultrasonographic clue for identifying the various manufacturers by OM.

From now on, you can see the gross photos and ultrasonographic images of round texture or smooth shell type breast implant by various manufacturers.

In the case of round shape type breast implant, since there is no mark that specifies the manufacturer, in theory, it is impossible to determine the manufacturer, but the manufacturer can be identified if there is an RFID chip, upside-down rotation, specific shell type in some manufacturer (Fig. 4.27).

And we can get the information by upside-down rotation because posterior patch is manufacturer specific. This will be discussed next in Chap. 5.

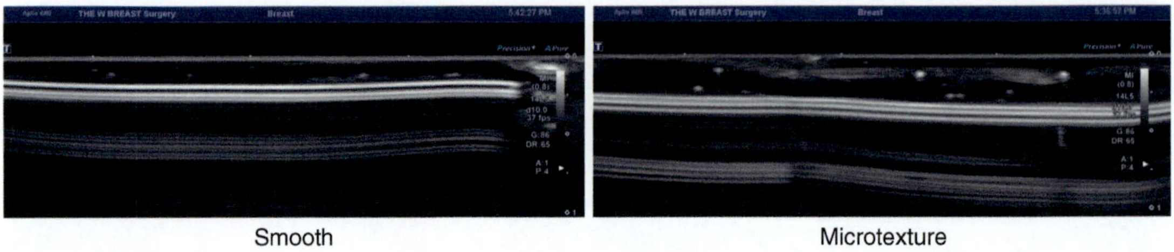

Fig. 4.10 Smooth and micro-textured shell looks almost identical in HRUS

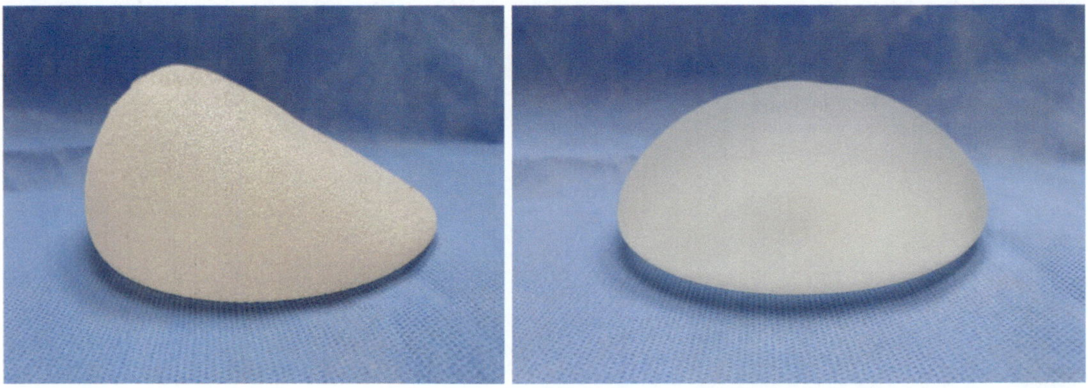

Fig. 4.11 Two different shape types of breast implant: anatomical type and round type

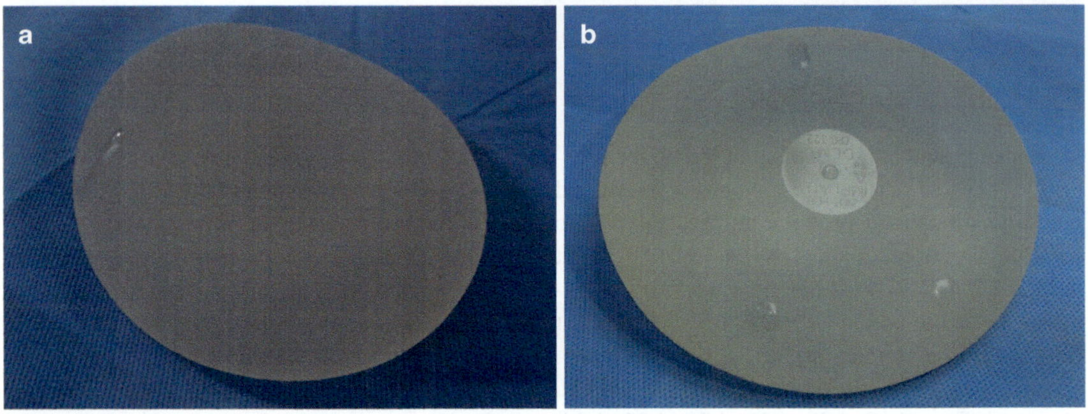

Fig. 4.12 Orientation mark of Mentor anatomical shape type breast implant. (**a**) Anterior view. (**b**) Posterior view

Table 4.1 Various types of orientation mark

	Anterior orientation mark		Posterior orientation mark	
Manufacturer	Line	Dot	Line	Dot
Allergan	None	Yes (3)	None	Yes (4)
Mentor	Yes (1), Short	None	Yes (1)	Yes (2)
Silimed	Yes (1), Long	None	None	Yes (4)
Sebbin	Yes (1), Short	None	Yes (1)	Yes (2)
Polytech	Yes (1), Long	None	None	Yes (2)
Hansbiomed	Yes (1), Short	None	None	Yes (5)
Eurosilicone	None	Yes (2)	None	Yes (5)

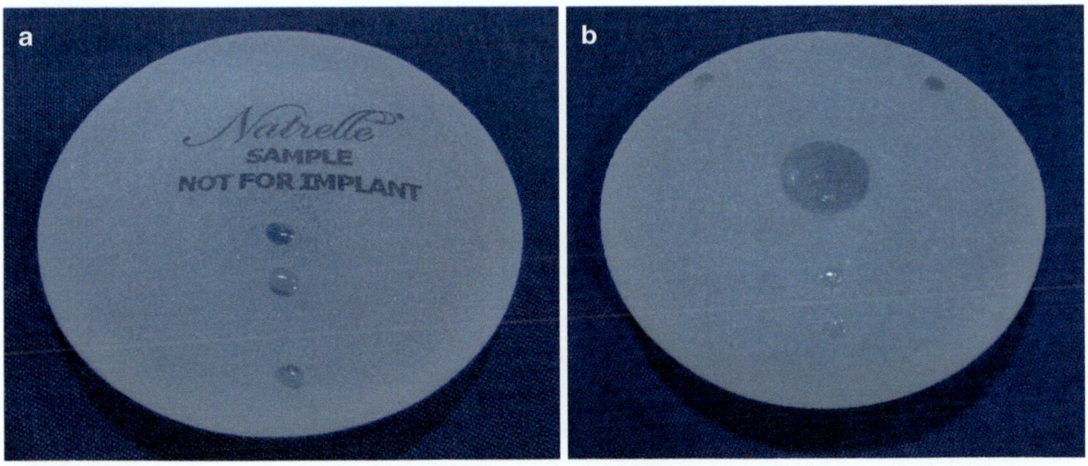

Fig. 4.13 Orientation mark of Allergan anatomical shape type breast implant. (**a**) Anterior view. (**b**) Posterior view

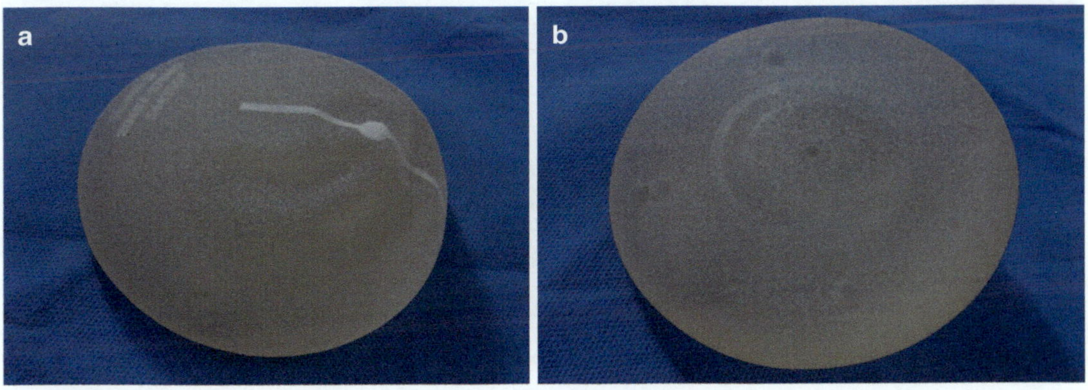

Fig. 4.14 Orientation mark of Polytech anatomical shape type breast implant. (**a**) Anterior view. (**b**) Posterior view

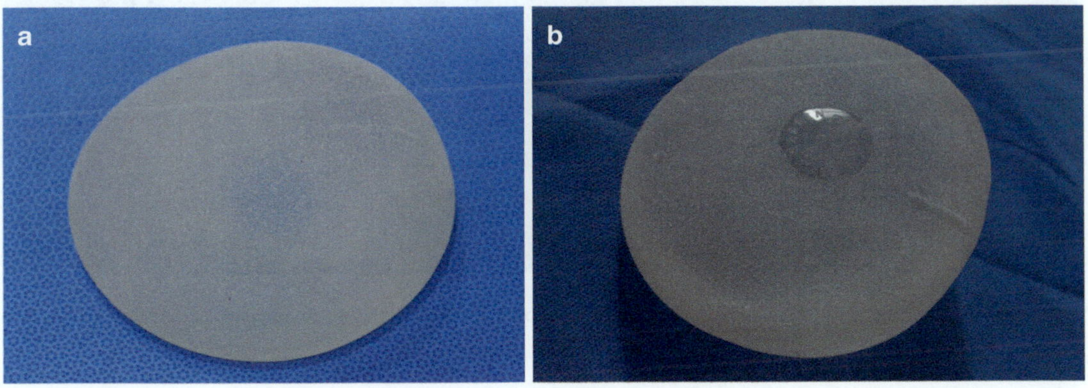

Fig. 4.15 Orientation mark of Sebbin anatomical shape type breast implant. (**a**) Anterior view. (**b**) Posterior view

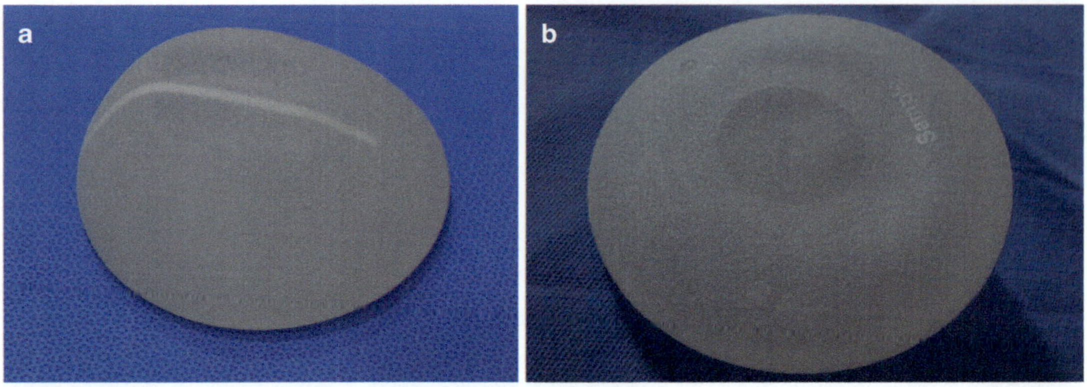

Fig. 4.16 Orientation mark of Silimed anatomical shape type breast implant. (**a**) Anterior view. (**b**) Posterior view

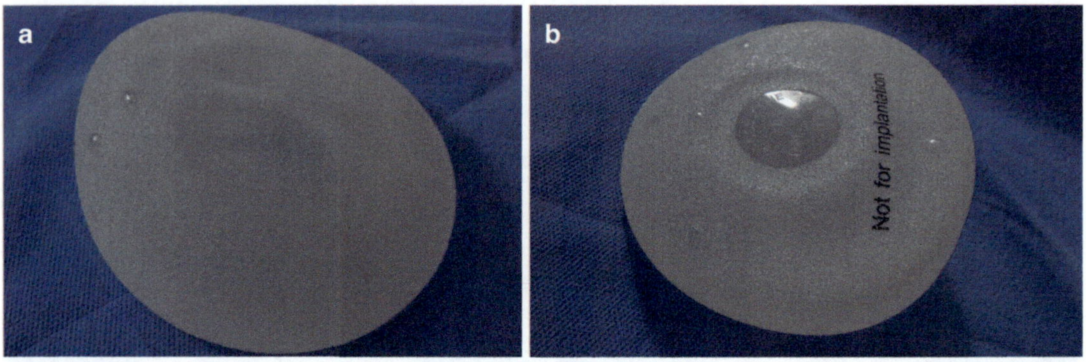

Fig. 4.17 Orientation mark of Eurosilicone anatomical shape type breast implant. (**a**) Anterior view. (**b**) Posterior view

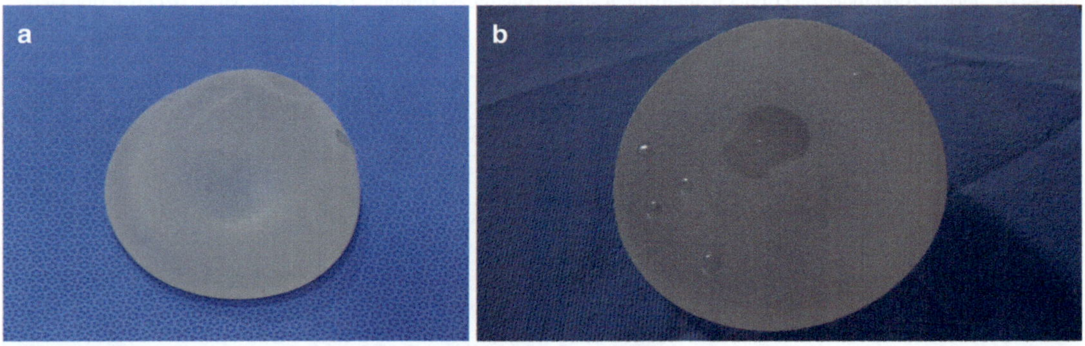

Fig. 4.18 Orientation mark of Hansbiomed Bellagel anatomical shape type breast implant. (**a**) Anterior view. (**b**) Posterior view

From now, gross and ultrasonographic view of various round type breast implants is shown.

There are round texture and smooth type of Mentor, Allergan, Silimed, Sebbin, Hansbiomed, Polytech, Eurosilicone, Motiva (Figs. 4.28, 4.29, 4.30, 4.31, 4.32, 4.33, 4.34, 4.35, 4.36 and 4.37), (Videos 4.13, 4.14, 4.16, 4.17, 4.19, 4.20, 4.22, 4.25, 4.26, 4.28 and 4.31).

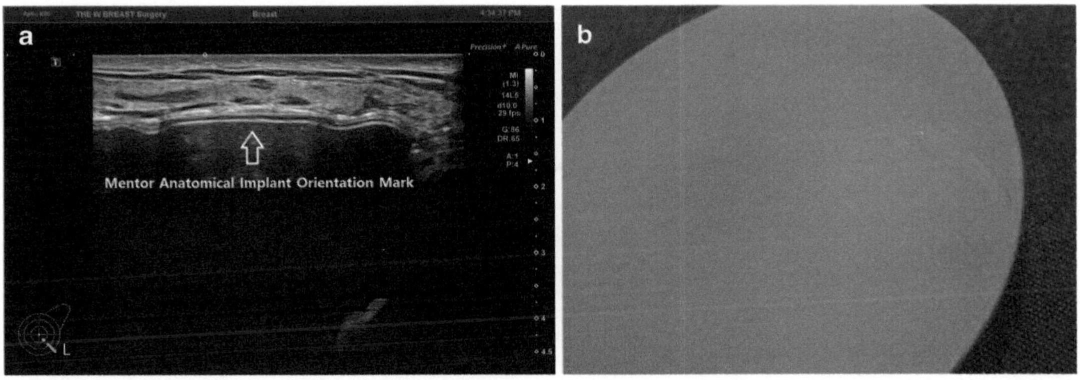

Fig. 4.19 Mentor anatomical type. The OM of Sebbin, Hansbiomed, Mentor is similar, but there is definite difference in shape, height, and length, so it can be distinguished in HRUS. (**a**) Ultrasonographic image of OM (3 cm Linear type at anterior shell). (**b**) Gross finding of OM of Mentor anatomical type implant

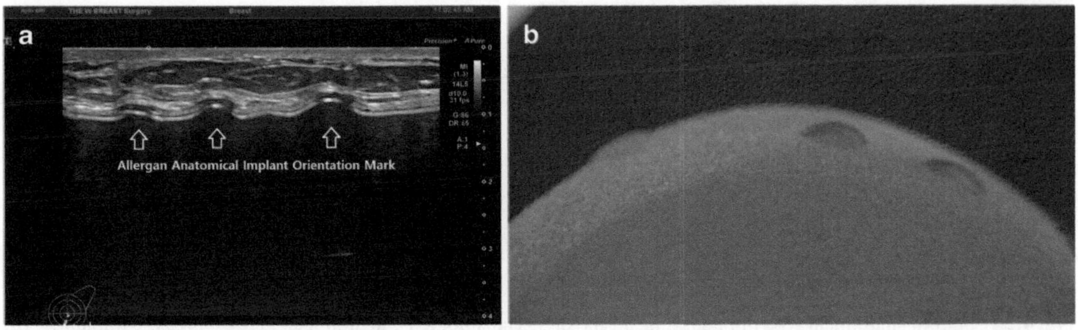

Fig. 4.20 Allergan anatomical type. Three dots is anterior shell, sometimes two dots type of OM is seen. (**a**) Ultrasonographic image of three orientation dot. (**b**) Gross finding of OM of Allergan anatomical type implant

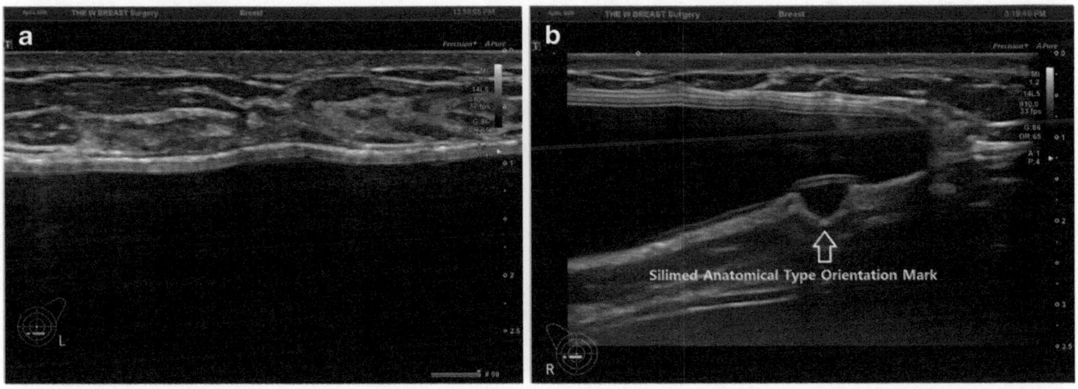

Fig. 4.21 Silimed anatomical type implant (2 stage). For the identification of Silimed anatomical type, it is necessary to identify Silimed specified texture shell type. After identification of Silimed textured shell type, then looking for OM in posterior shell layer is necessary. There is no difference between anatomical type and round textured shell type of Silimed implant in anterior shell, only posterior dot is seen in ultrasonography, for the identification of Silimed anatomical type implant, operator should check posterior shell of implant if Silimed textured shell is checked in anterior shell image. (**a**) Identification of Silimed macro-texture shell type. (**b**) Ultrasonographic image of OM. (**c**) Gross image of posterior OM of Silimed anatomical breast implant

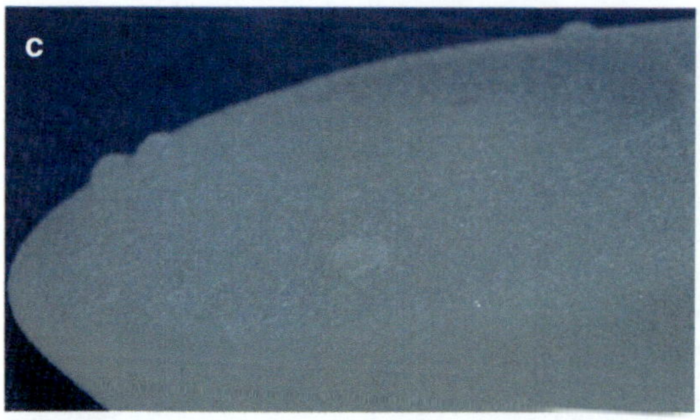

Fig. 4.21 (continued)

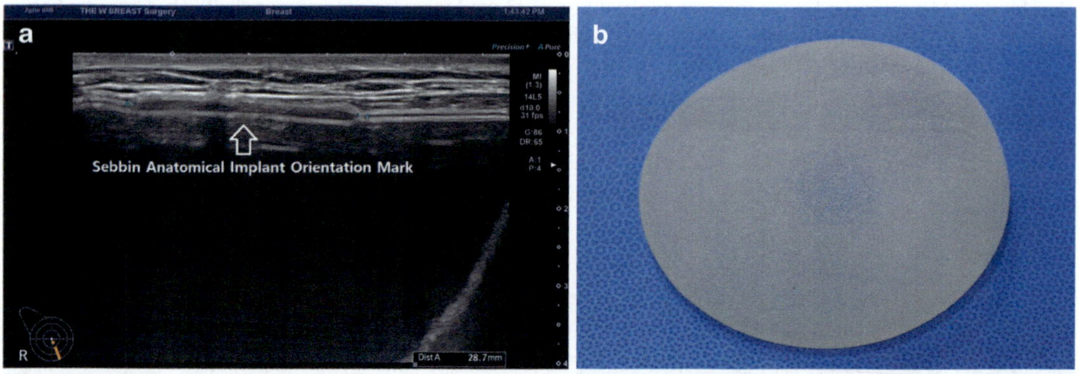

Fig. 4.22 Sebbin anatomical type implant. Linear type of OM is checked by HRUS. Sebbin OM is distinguished from shape and textured shell image from Mentor, Hansbiomed anatomical type breast implant. (**a**) Ultrasonographic image of OM. (**b**) Gross image of OM in anterior shell of Sebbin anatomical type breast implant

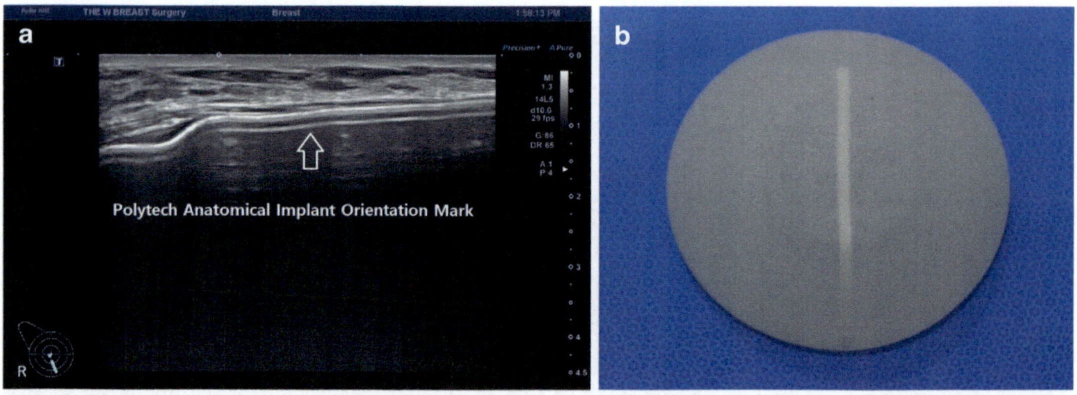

Fig. 4.23 Polytech anatomical type implant. There is a long line below textured shell. It is very easy to confirm Polytech anatomical type breast implant. See the video (**a**) Ultrasonographic image of OM. (**b**) Gross image of OM in anterior shell of Polytech anatomical type breast implant

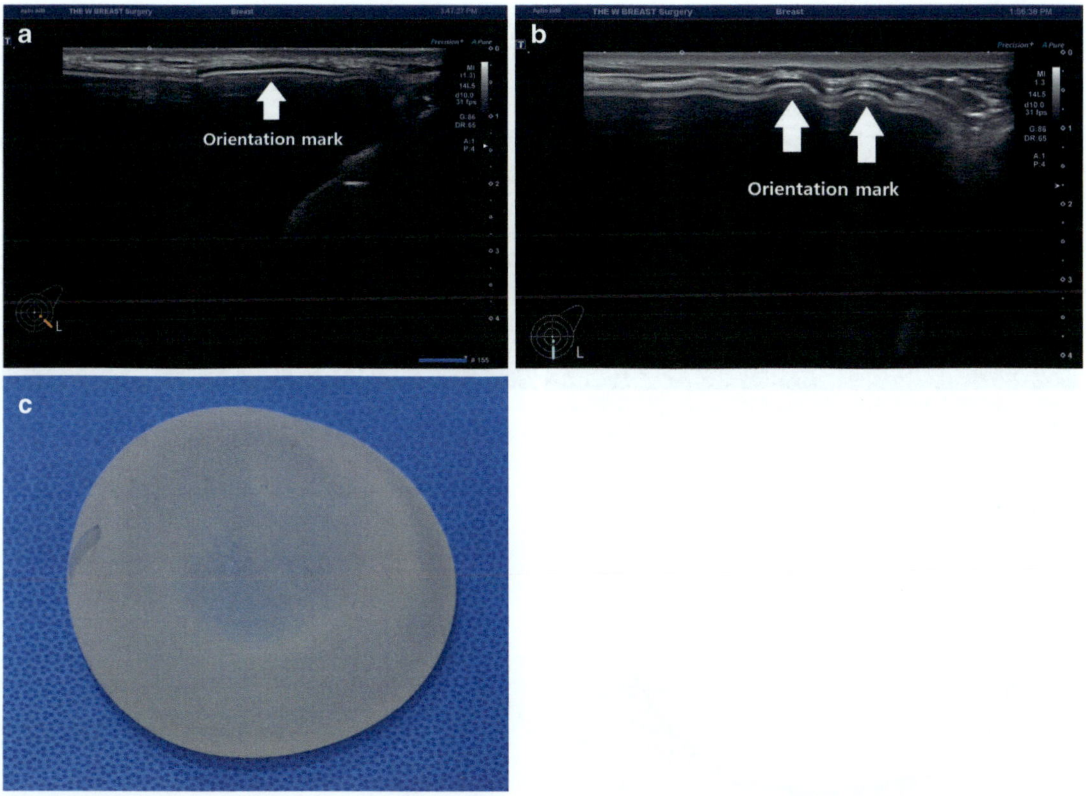

Fig. 4.24 Hansbiomed “Bellagel” anatomical type implant. There is linear type OM that can be distinguished from Sebbin and Mentor anatomical type by HRUS. (**a**) Ultrasonographic image of OM. (**b**) Ultrasonographic image of OM (Old two dot version of OM of Bellagel anatomical implant). (**c**) Gross image of Bellagel anatomical type implant

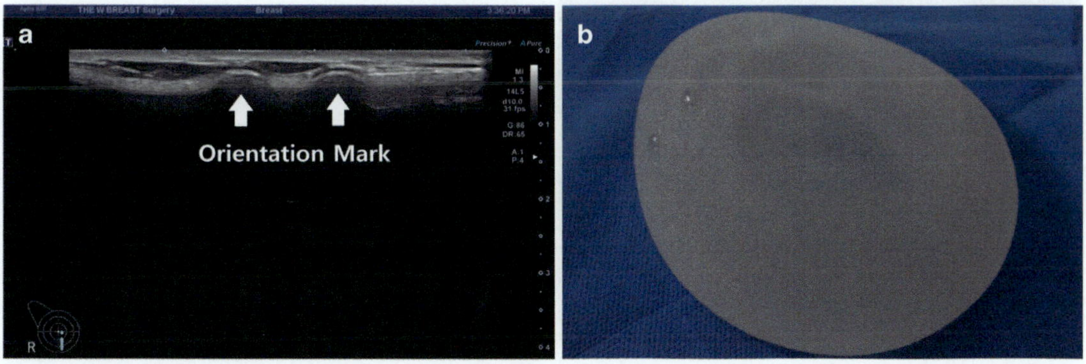

Fig. 4.25 Eurosilicone anatomical type implant. Eurosilicone anatomical OM is similar with Hansbiomed anatomical type. (**a**) Ultrasonographic image of OM. (**b**) Gross image of Eurosilicone anatomical type breast implant

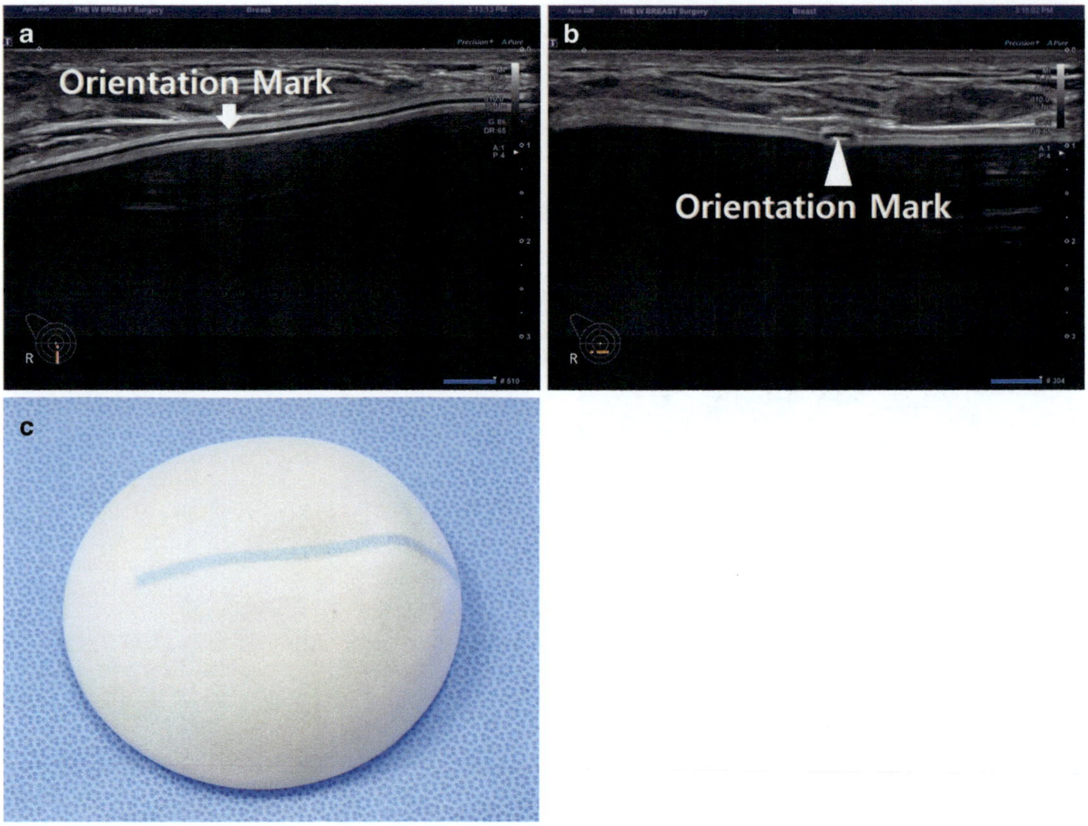

Fig. 4.26 Polytech polyurethane anatomical implant. (**a**) Ultrasonographic image of OM (Sagittal view). (**b**) Ultrasonographic image of OM (coronal view). (**c**) Gross image of polyurethane breast implant

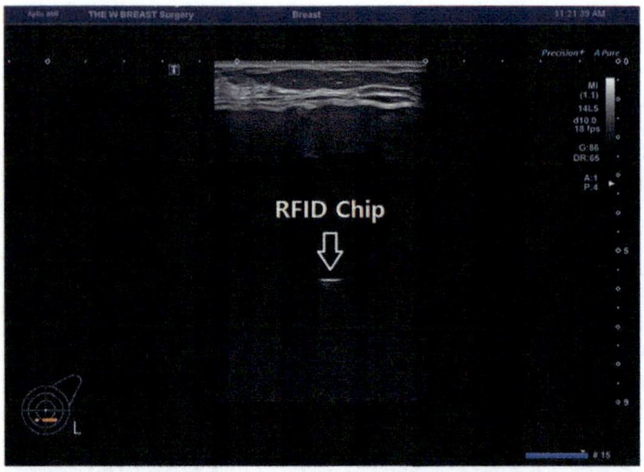

Fig. 4.27 RFID chip is seen in the bottom of implant

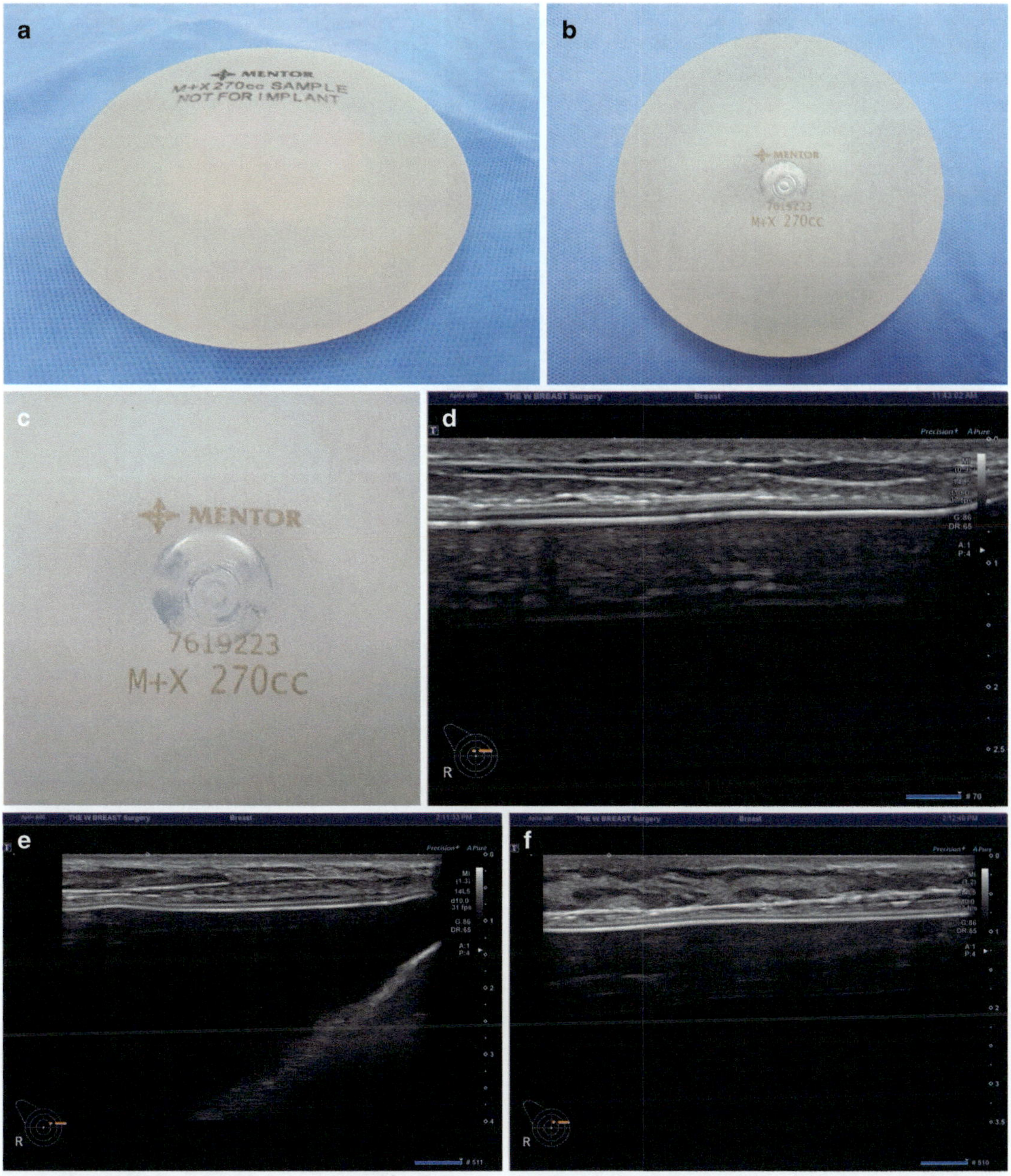

Fig. 4.28 Mentor round texture and smooth type breast implant. (**a**) Anterior view of round textured shell type breast implant. (**b**) Posterior view of round textured shell type breast implant. (**c**) Gross view of posterior patch. (**d–g**) Ultrasonographic image of Mentor textured shell. (**h**) Anterior view of round smooth shell type breast implant. (**i**) Posterior view of round smooth shell type breast implant. (**j**) Gross view of posterior patch. (**k–t**) Ultrasonographic image of smooth shell of Mentor

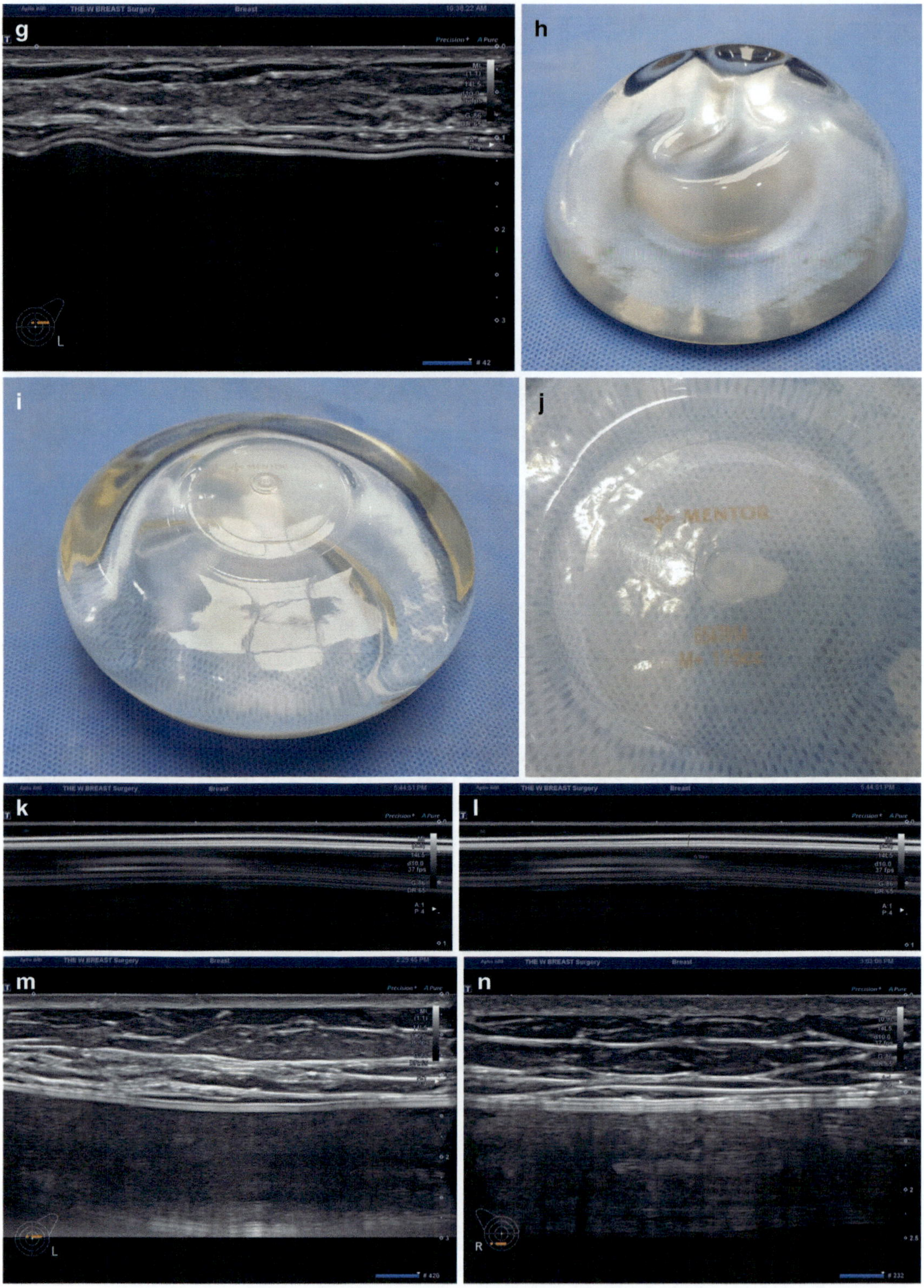

Fig. 4.28 (continued)

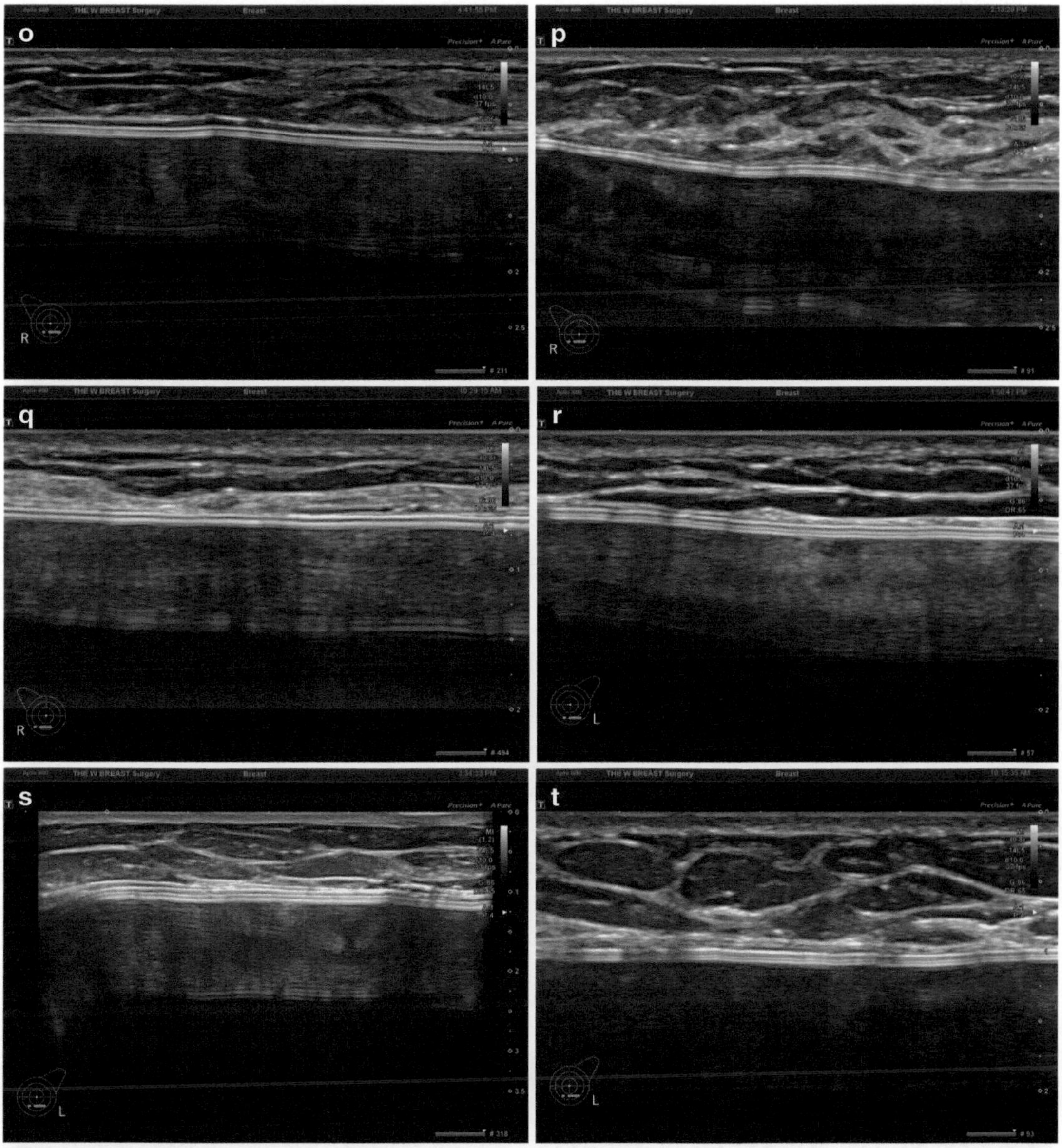

Fig. 4.28 (continued)

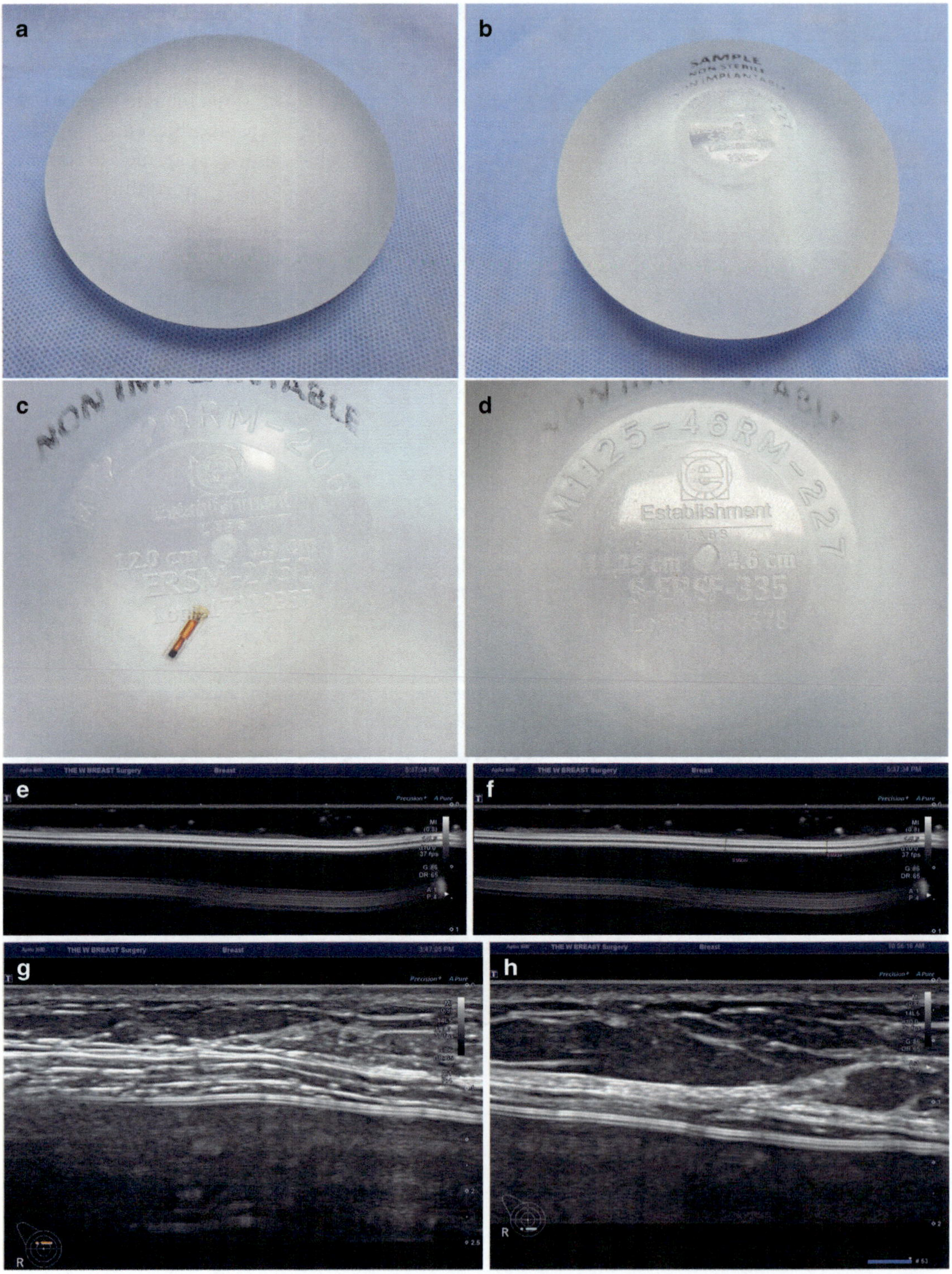

Fig. 4.29 Motiva round micro-textured implant gross with/without RFID chip. (**a**) Gross finding of anterior view. (**b**) Gross finding of posterior view. (**c**) RFID chip of posterior patch. (**d**) No RFID chip of posterior patch. (**e–q**) Ultrasonographic image of Motiva Ergonomix Round. SilkSurface breast implant. (**r**) Ultrasonographic image of RFID chip (This is the clue for identifying the manufacturer)

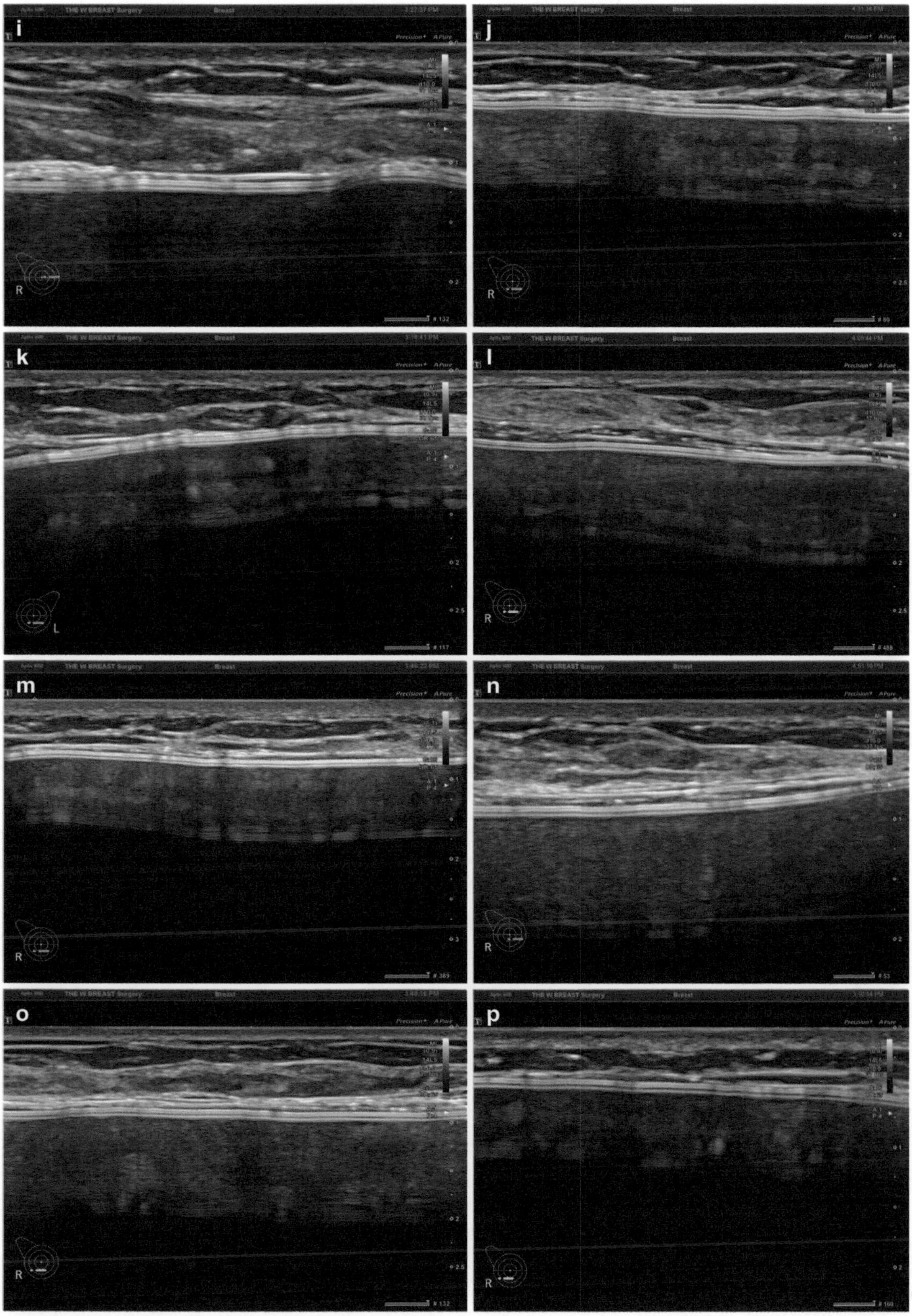

Fig. 4.29 (continued)

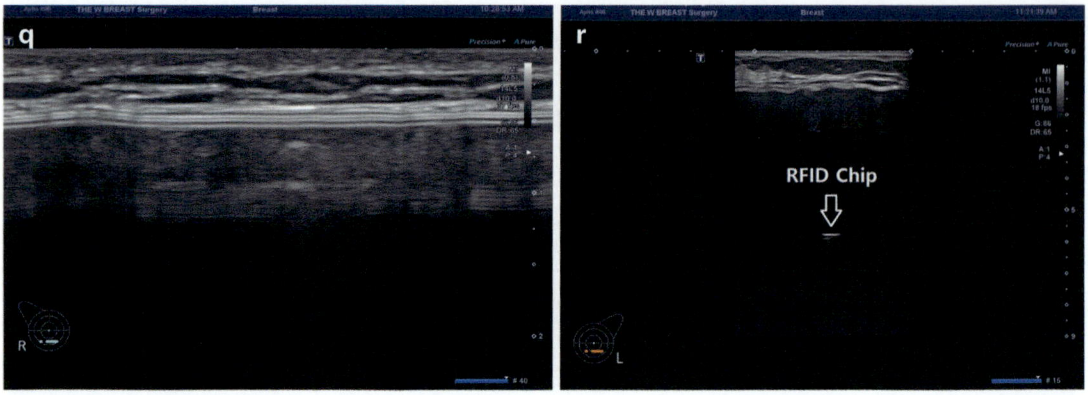

Fig. 4.29 (continued)

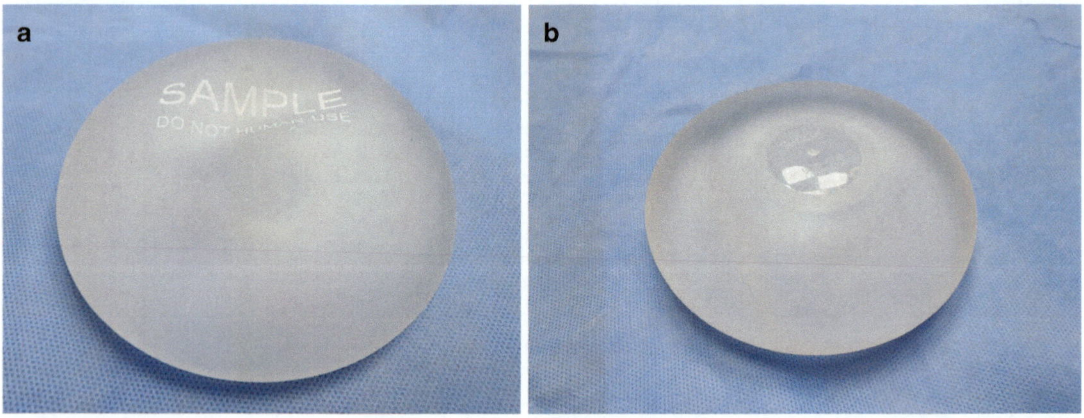

Fig. 4.30 Hansbiomed Bellagel round micro-textured shell type breast implant. (**a**) Anterior view of round micro-texture shell type breast implant. (**b**) Posterior view of round micro-texture shell type breast implant. (**c**) Posterior patch of Bellagel micro-texture breast implant. (**d**, **e**) Ultrasonographic image of Bellagel micro-texture shell. (**f**) Ultrasonographic image of Bellagel micro-texture shell. (**g**) Ultrasonographic image shows different shell layers of Bellagel micro-texture shell. (**h–l**) Different shell layers in same patient of Bellagel micro-texture shell. (High-resolution ultrasonography shows the shell layer modification)

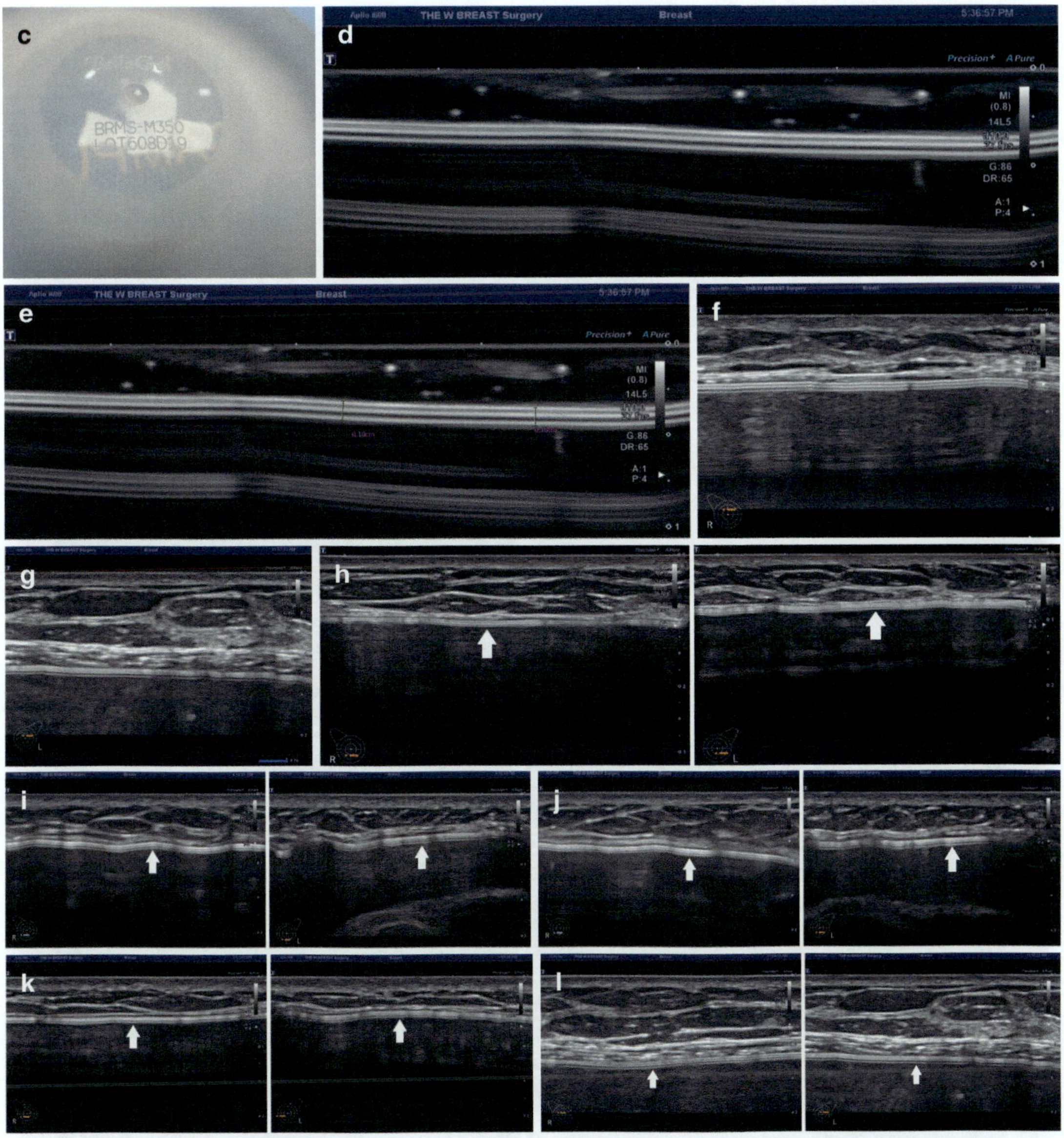

Fig. 4.30 (continued)

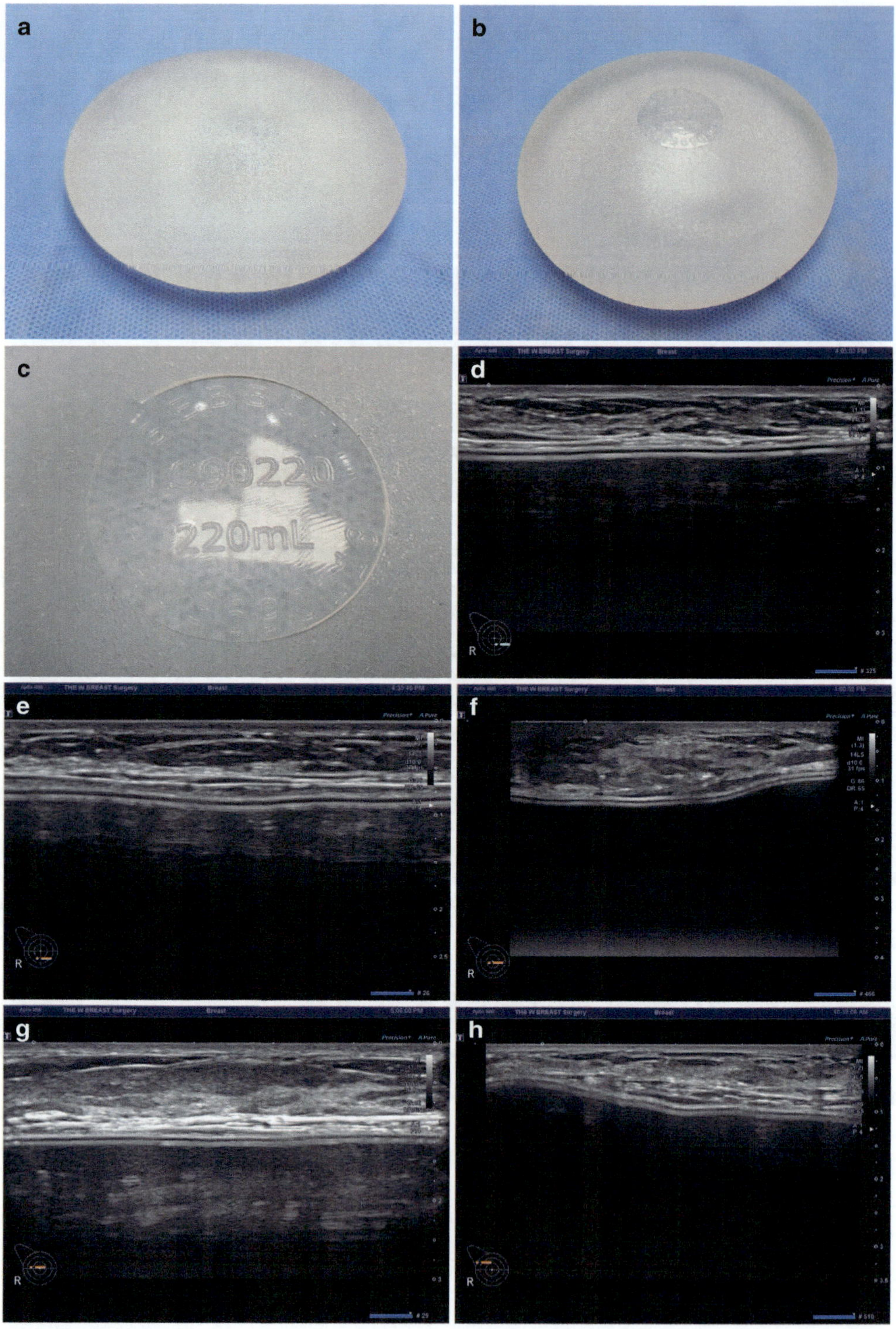

Fig. 4.31 Sebbin round macro-textured shell type breast implant. (**a**) Gross image of anterior view of Sebbin round texture implant. (**b**) Gross image of posterior view of Sebbin round texture implant. (**c**) Gross image of posterior patch. (**d–h**) Ultrasonographic image of Sebbin macro-textured shell type breast implant

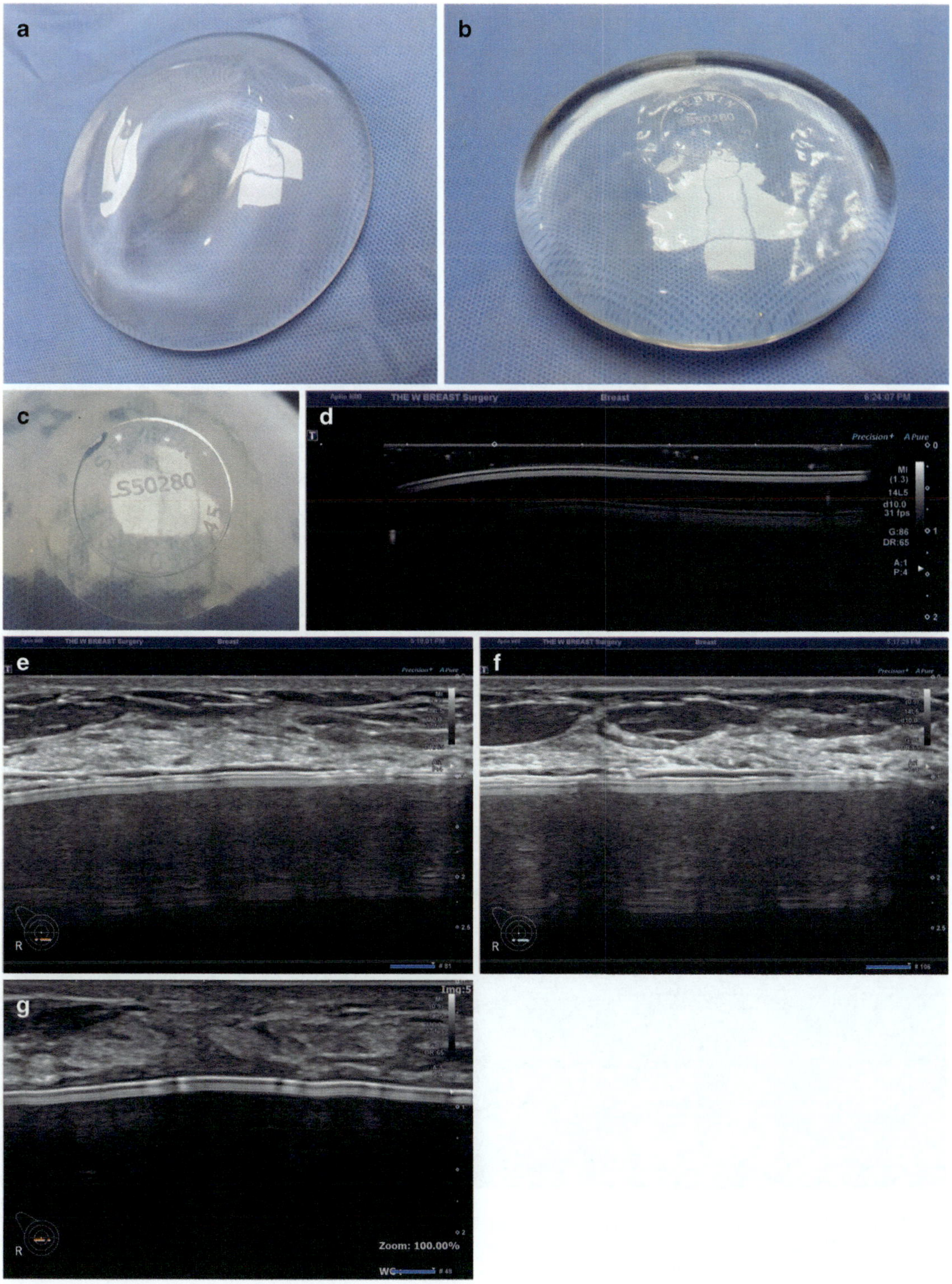

Fig. 4.32 Sebbin round smooth shell type breast implant. (**a**) Gross image of anterior view of Sebbin round smooth shell type implant. (**b**) Gross image of posterior view of Sebbin round smooth shell type implant. (**c**) Gross image of posterior patch. (**d–g**) Ultrasonographic image of Sebbin smooth shell type breast implant

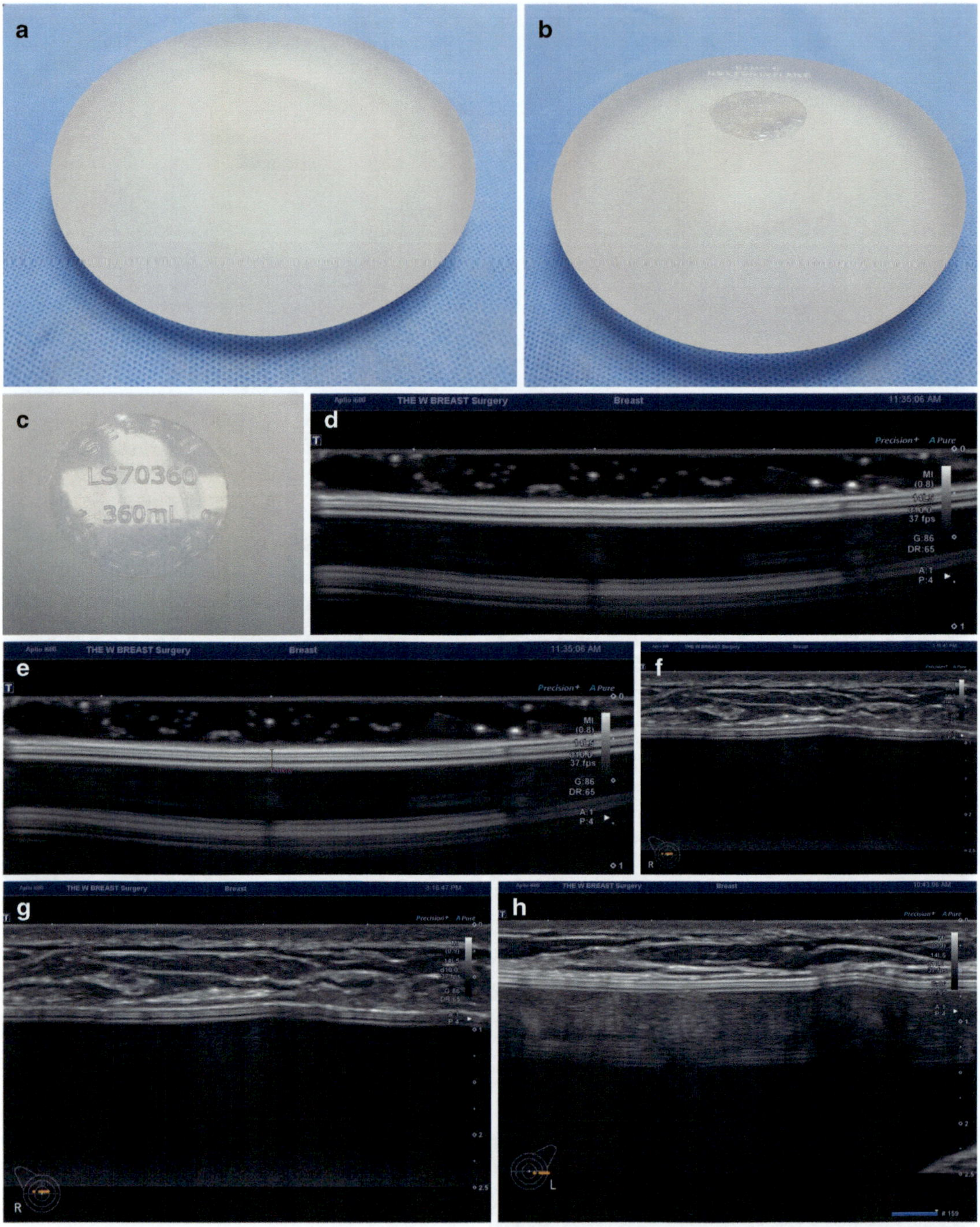

Fig. 4.33 Sebbin round micro-textured shell type breast implant. (**a**) Gross image of anterior view of Sebbin micro-texture implant. (**b**) Gross image of posterior view of Sebbin micro-texture implant. (**c**) Gross image of posterior patch. (**d–m**) Ultrasonographic image of Sebbin micro-textured shell type breast implant

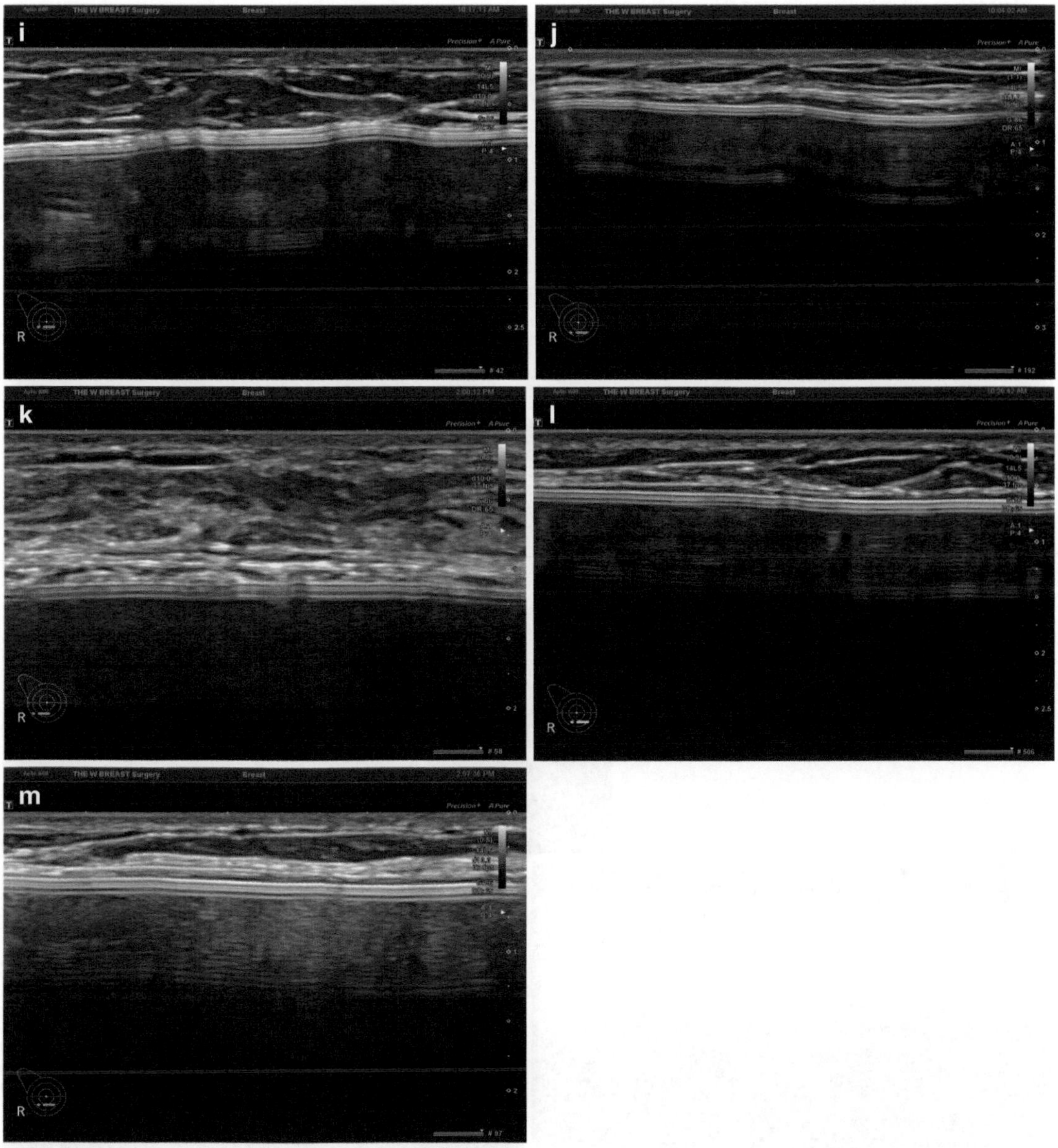

Fig. 4.33 (continued)

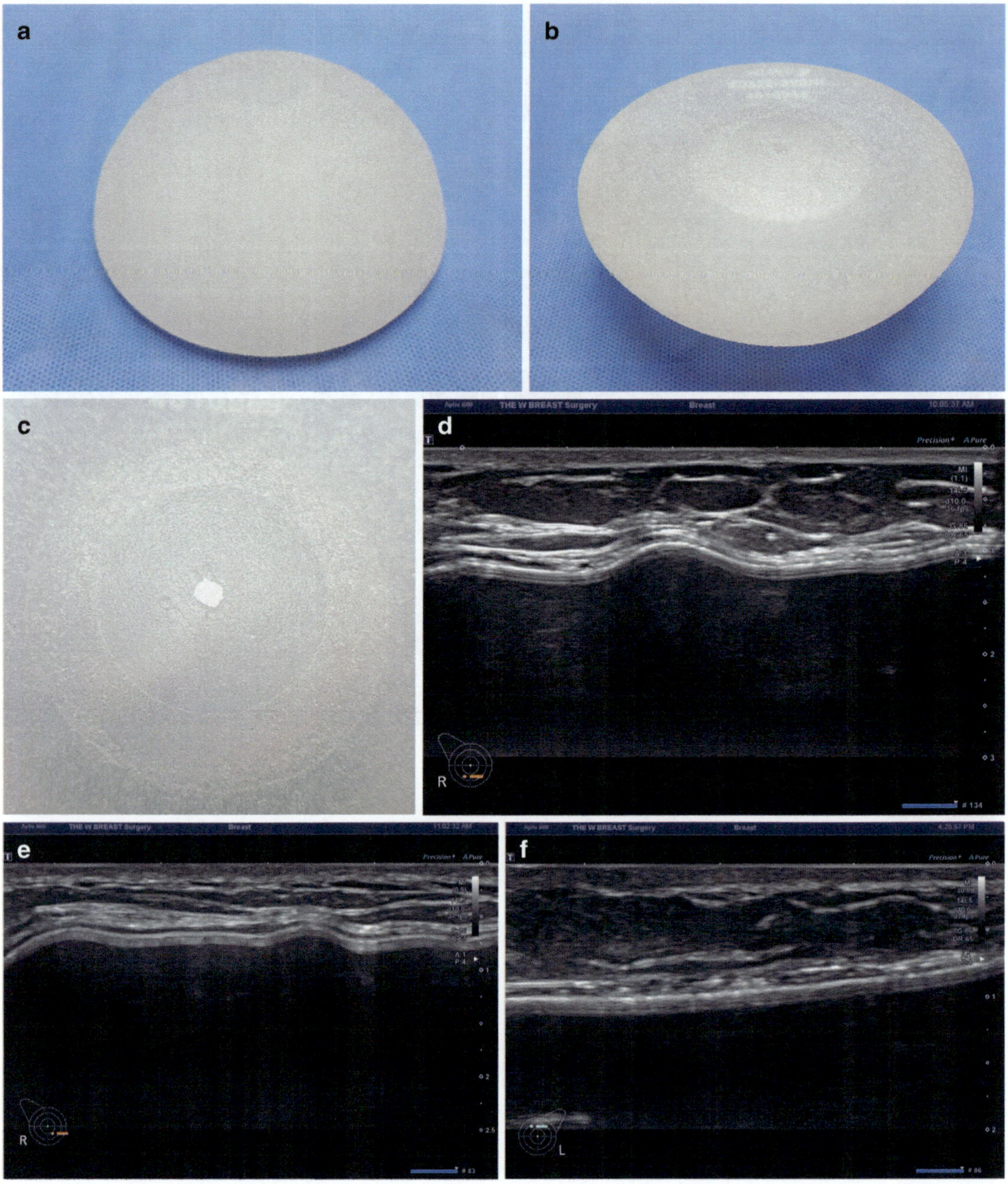

Fig. 4.34 Silimed round macro-textured shell type breast implant. (**a**) Gross image of anterior view of Silimed macro-texture implant. (**b**) Gross image of posterior view of Silimed macro-texture implant. (**c**) Gross image of posterior patch. (**d–i**) Ultrasonographic image of Silimed macro-textured shell type breast implant

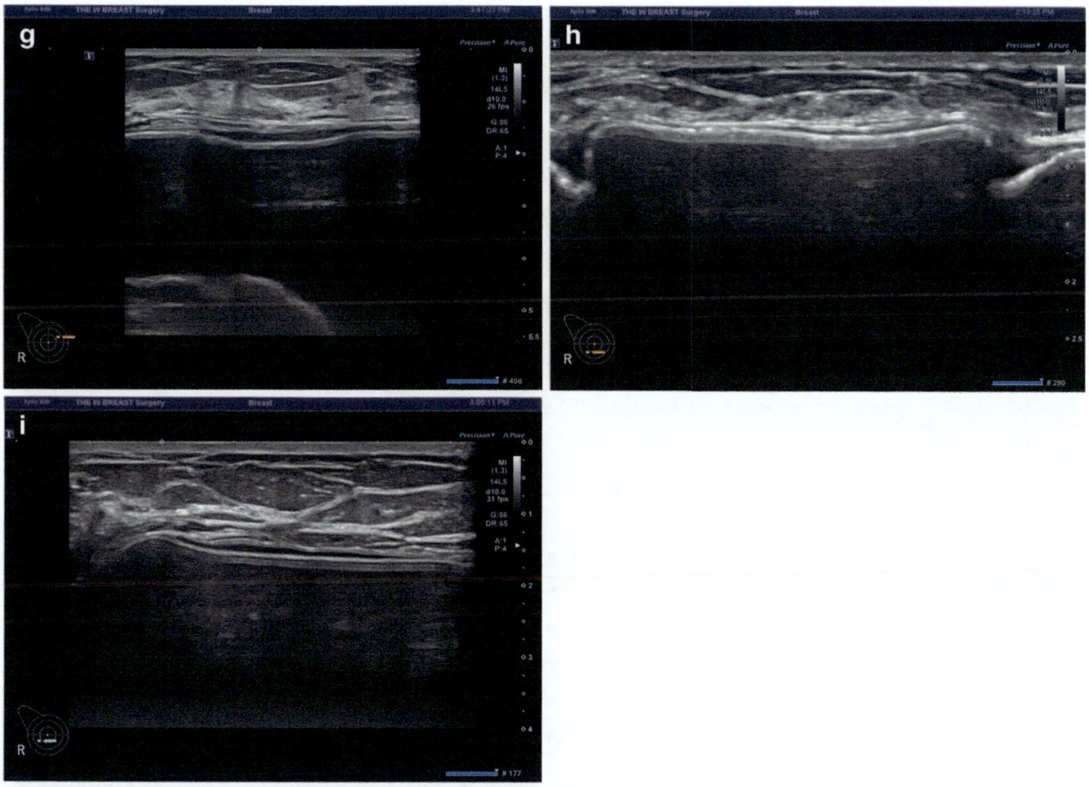

Fig. 4.34 (continued)

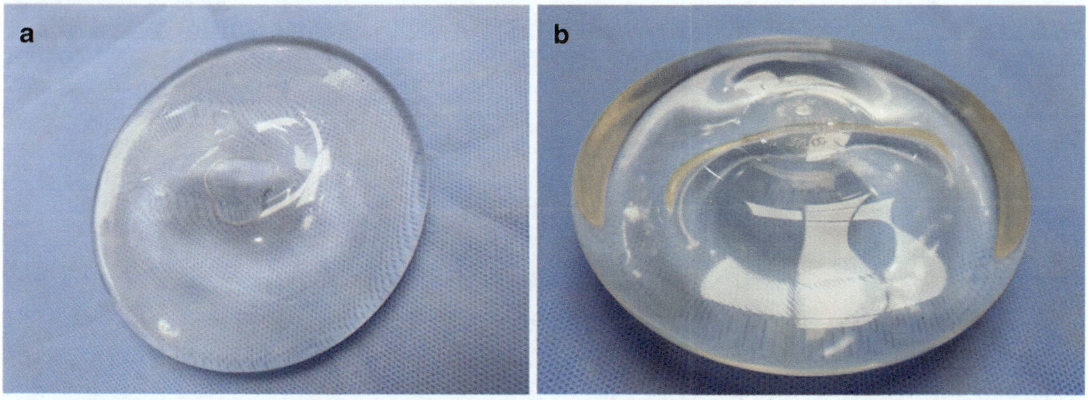

Fig. 4.35 Allergan round smooth shell type breast implant. (**a**) Gross image of anterior view of Allergan round smooth shell type implant. (**b**) Gross image of posterior view of Allergan round smooth shell type implant. (**c**) Gross image of posterior patch. (**d–l**) Ultrasonographic image of Allergan smooth shell type breast implant

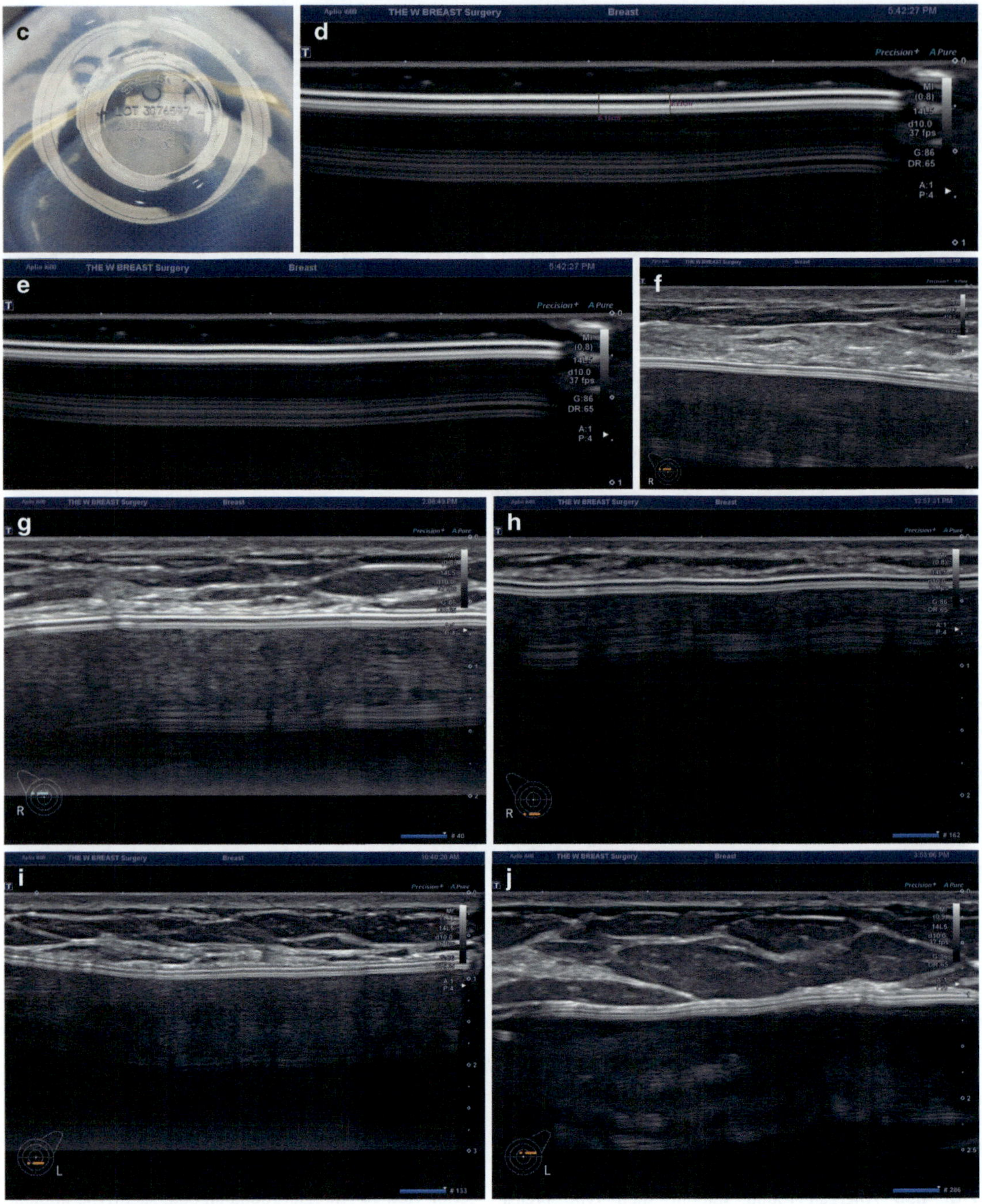

Fig. 4.35 (continued)

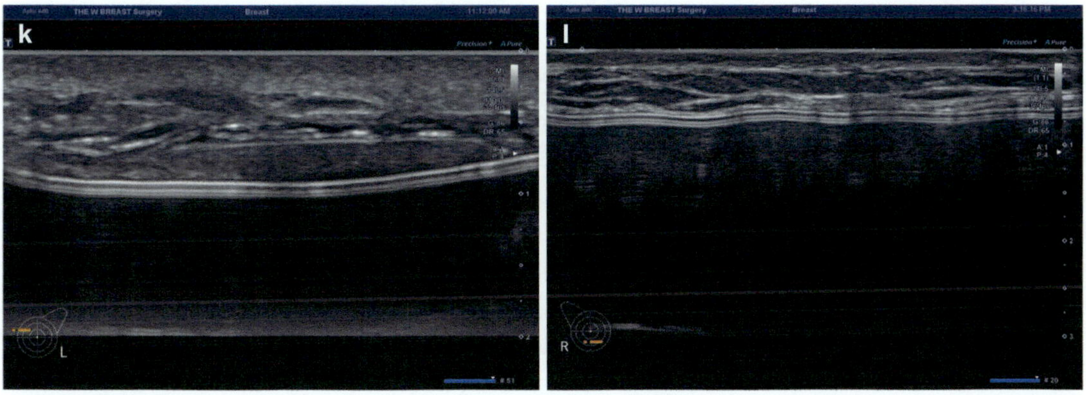

Fig. 4.35 (continued)

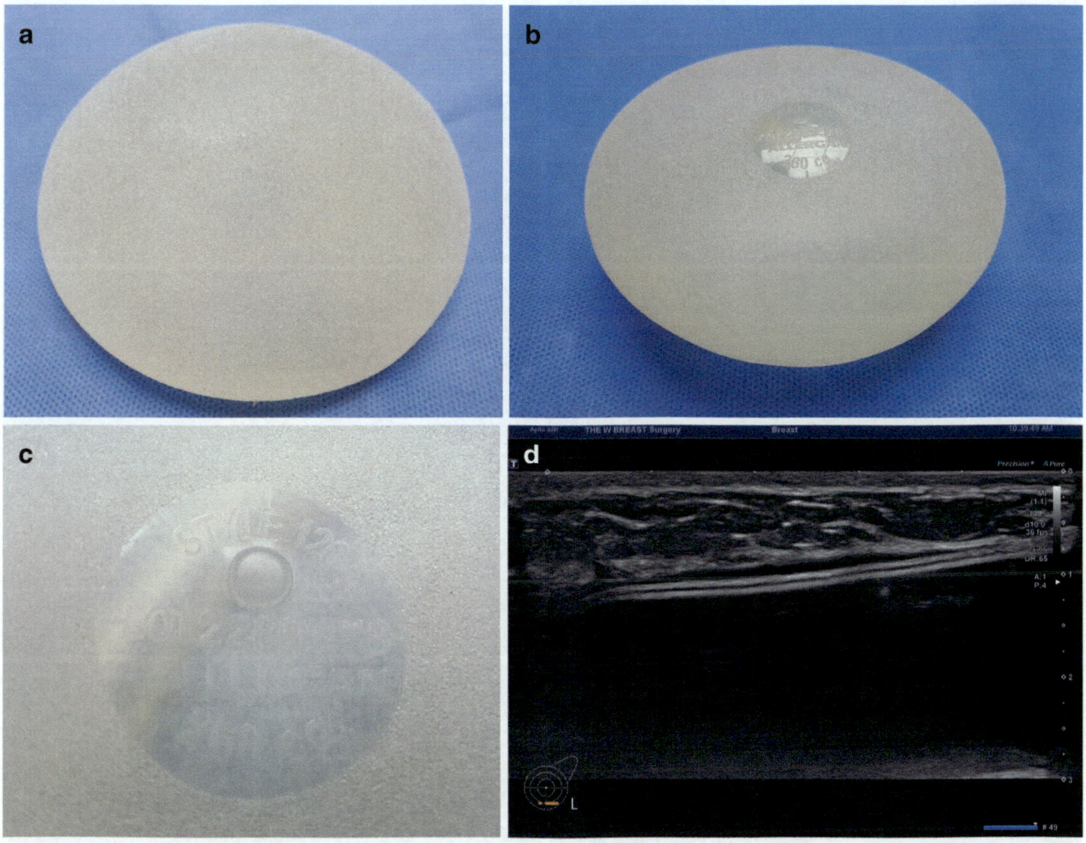

Fig. 4.36 Allergan round macro-textured shell type breast implant. (**a**) Gross image of anterior view of Allergan macro-texture implant. (**b**) Gross image of posterior view of Allergan macro-texture implant. (**c**) Gross image of posterior patch. (**d–l**) Ultrasonographic image of Allergan macro-textured shell type breast implant

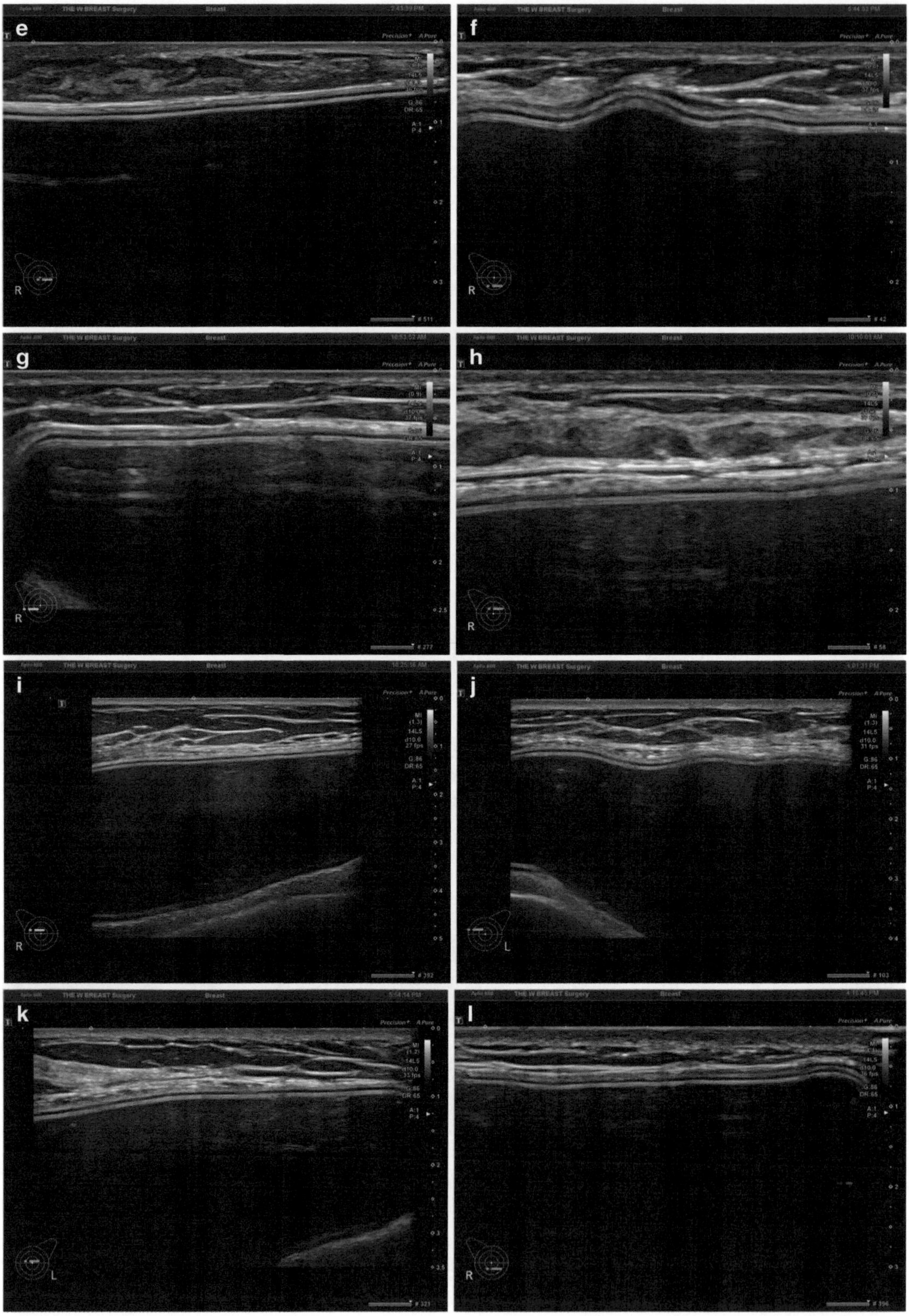

Fig. 4.36 (continued)

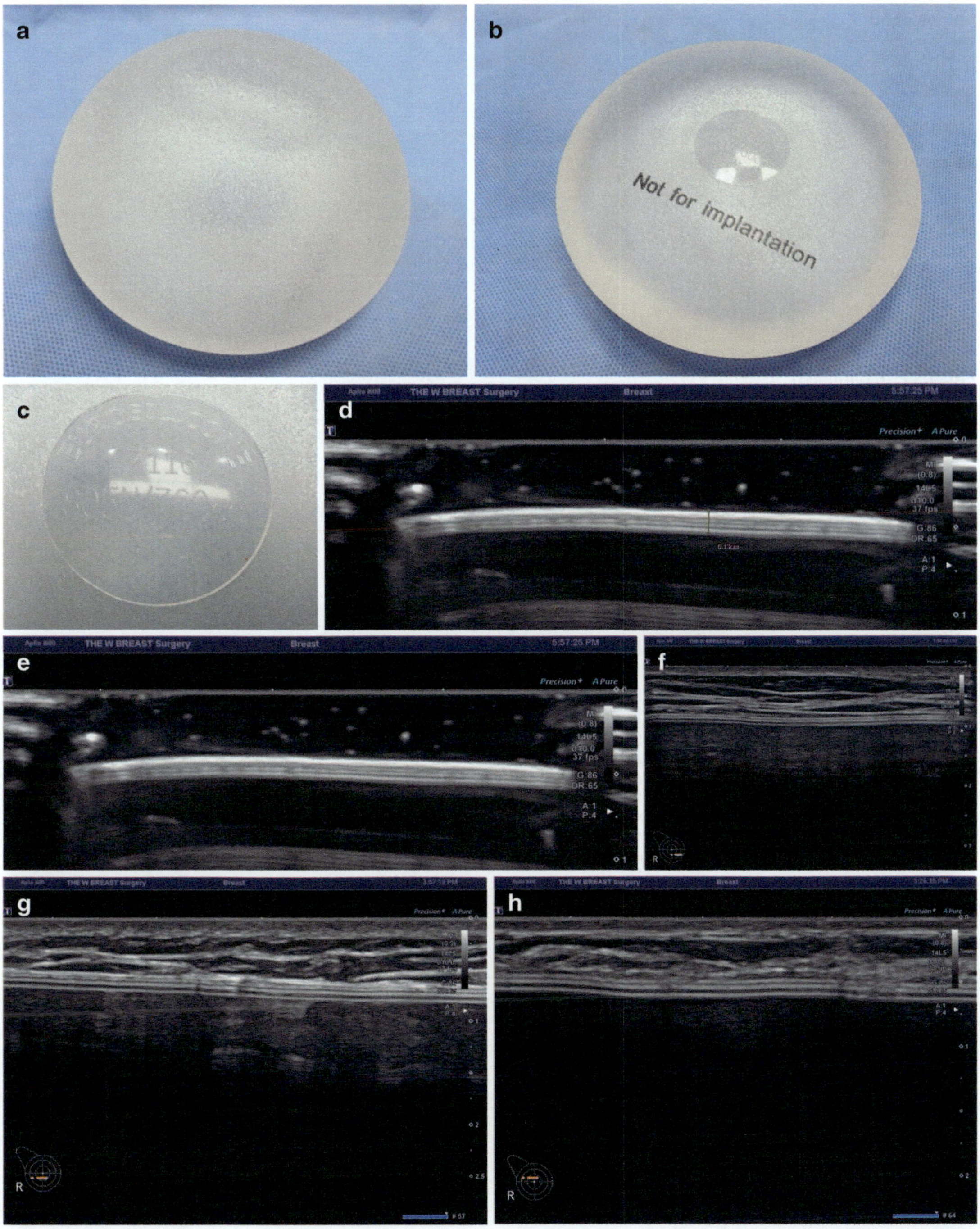

Fig. 4.37 Eurosilicone round micro-textured shell type breast implant. (**a**) Gross image of anterior view of Eurosilicone micro-texture implant. (**b**) Gross image of posterior view of Eurosilicone micro-texture implant. (**c**) Gross image of posterior patch. (**d–i**) Ultrasonographic image of Eurosilicone micro-textured shell type breast implant

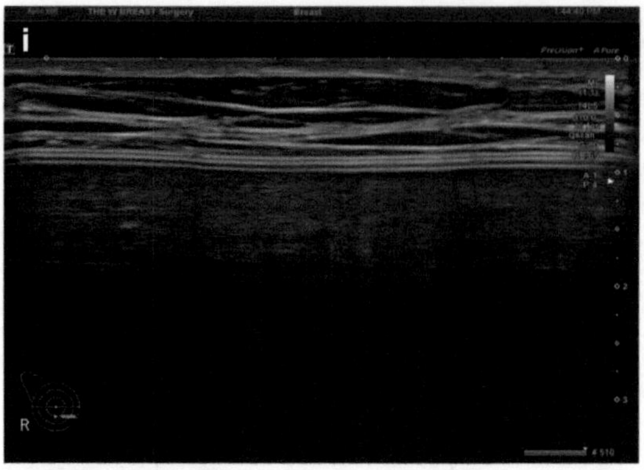

Fig. 4.37 (continued)

5 Usefulness of High-Resolution Ultrasound in Detecting Complications of an Implant-Based Mammaplasty

5.1 Overview

When a breast implant is inserted in a human's body, it may cause diverse complications (Fig. 5.1). An early diagnosis of them is essential for ensuring the safety of a patient.

For the past 15 years, I have performed aesthetic or reconstructive implant-based mammaplasty. During this period, I have made all efforts to meticulously monitor the patient's postoperative course. I have therefore found that most of the postoperative complications could not be diagnosed on physical examination and they should be accurately diagnosed on ultrasound in association with signs and symptoms that are suggestive of them. Thus, I have regularly performed a breast ultrasound for patients receiving an implant-based augmentation mammaplasty after 3 months postoperatively, thus making all efforts to diagnose postoperative complications at the earliest opportunities possible. Here, I provide numerous images and videos which I have accumulated until now.

The current book is advantageous in simultaneously examining radiological, pathological, and plastic surgical findings, thus contributing to evaluating a patient's findings based on clinical findings and imaging characteristics. The following complications are closely associated with a patient's discomfort, particularly including pain *as well as* the shape and feel of breast.

Supplementary Information The online version contains supplementary material available at (https://doi.org/10.1007/978-981-16-8282-7_5.)

5.2 Folding

Folding is a very common sonographic finding after breast implant augmentation. It is not a serious complication in almost any case (Fig. 5.2), (Video 5.1). But folding may cause pain, foreign body sensation or palpation of a breast implant which a patient can exhibit at the outpatient clinic.

Its occurrence is associated with a relatively smaller size of pocket; it may occur as a result of capsular contracture (CC) and under-dissection. It is commonly manifested on ultrasound as shown below (Figs. 5.3 and 5.4).

An ultrasound-guided monitoring of a patient's clinical course is useful in determining the scope of dissection at surgery. This is because an excessive mobility of the device due to over-dissection requires a reduction in the scope of dissection. From this context, the scope of dissection should be re-considered in a patient who commonly presents with a folding of the device due to under-dissection even in the absence of CC. This would be helpful for preventing a surgeon from repeatedly making mistakes.

The severity of a patient's symptoms may vary depending on the scope of folding and the depth of groove. For example, there would be no discomfort without TC, deep groove, and thin

J. H. Kim, *Atlas of Breast Implant Ultrasound*, https://doi.org/10.1007/978-981-16-8282-7_5

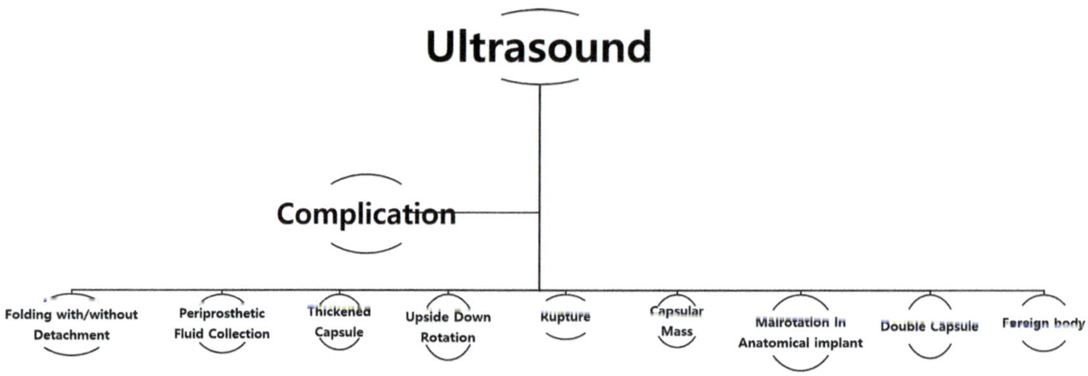

Fig. 5.1 Complications of an implant-based augmentation mammaplasty

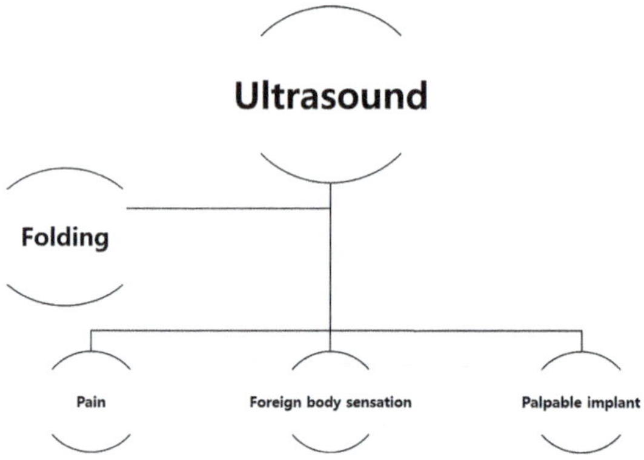

Fig. 5.2 Symptom of implant shell folding

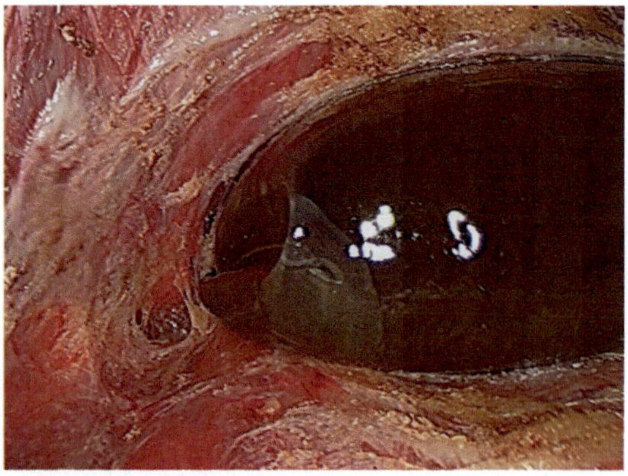

Fig. 5.3 An intraoperative finding of folding with thickened capsule

subcutaneous tissue. But palpation of a breast implant or pain would be present if there is more than one of these. Folding of a breast implant might also lead to the disruption of shell, which may also cause rupture of the device. Therefore, an ultrasound-guided examination at a follow-up should be performed to determine the optimal scope and degree of folding.

Some cases of folding may be accompanied by the detachment of the affected site. A relatively longer, wider detachment may be associated with a patient's foreign body sensation.

The following sonographic finding is folding with or without detachment (Figs. 5.5 and 5.6), (Videos 5.2 and 5.3).

5.3 Periprosthetic Fluid Collection

Periprosthetic fluid collection can be classified into normal and abnormal cases depending on the time point of its onset, volume, hematoma, and seroma (Fig. 5.7). If abnormal fluid collection is found in ultrasonography, ultrasound-guided aspiration should be performed followed by cytology and culture for the appropriate management.

Seroma can occur after a prosthesis is inserted in a human body. Most of which is absorbed after three months postoperatively or left minimally. So, there is no or minimal fluid collection in periprosthetic space (Fig. 5.8), (Video 5.4).

This can be confirmed based on ultrasound findings obtained at 1 or 3 months, which has been verified from a total of more than 700 patients receiving primary or secondary implant-based augmentation mammaplasty. Normally a small amount of seroma (<10 cc) on the medial side of the breast can be present persistently.

In a patient who grossly had a swelling or did have a widespread presence of seroma around a breast implant rather than a minimal periprosthetic fluid collection on ultrasound, aspiration should be performed (Fig. 5.9). Thus, additional examination should be performed and the appropriate treatment should be planned accordingly.

The following sonographic image shows large amount of delayed seroma formed around a breast implant (Fig. 5.10). Physician should distinguish between seroma and rupture.

As shown above, an ultrasound-guided aspiration should be performed to avoid damages to a breast implant in a patient with a large amount of periprosthetic fluid collection. In a patient who is suspected of having an infection based on the color and smell of the specimen, empirical antibiotics is prescribed with cytology and culture test.

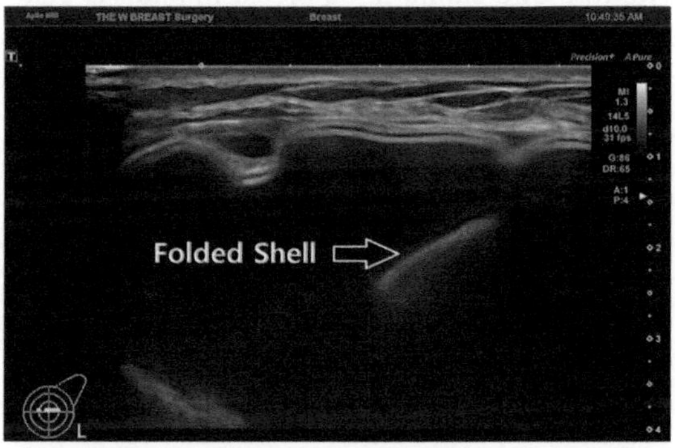

Fig. 5.4 Sonographic finding of folding

If necessary, however, antibiotics can be changed based on cytology and culture.

In my experience, CC is inevitable following condition even if there were appropriate management of infectious seroma which is immediate postoperative onset. If a patient has such condition, surgeon may consider explantation or second stage reoperation option. Explantation should be performed in severe infectious conditions or refractory to antibiotics therapy.

The following sonographic image shows a case of non-infectious seroma occurring after drinking alcohol at 6 months postoperatively. This case was treated with several sessions of ultrasound-guided aspiration (Fig. 5.11).

A sudden appearance of seroma with textured breast implant should be considered serious if it disappeared postoperatively, for which a rule-out diagnosis of breast implant-associated anaplastic large cell lymphoma (BIA-ALCL) and infection should be made on ultrasound-guided aspiration. This should be followed by cytology, culture, and CD30-positive immunohistochemistry.

Delayed seroma should also be considered serious because a patient receiving a macrotextured breast implant is vulnerable to BIA-ALCL. An early detection of delayed seroma would therefore be essential. It would also be mandatory to examine whether it is of infectious origin. Even a patient with non-infectious delayed seroma would be at increased risk of developing capsular thickening over time. Such patient should be meticulously followed up using ultrasound with appropriate treatment, by which the

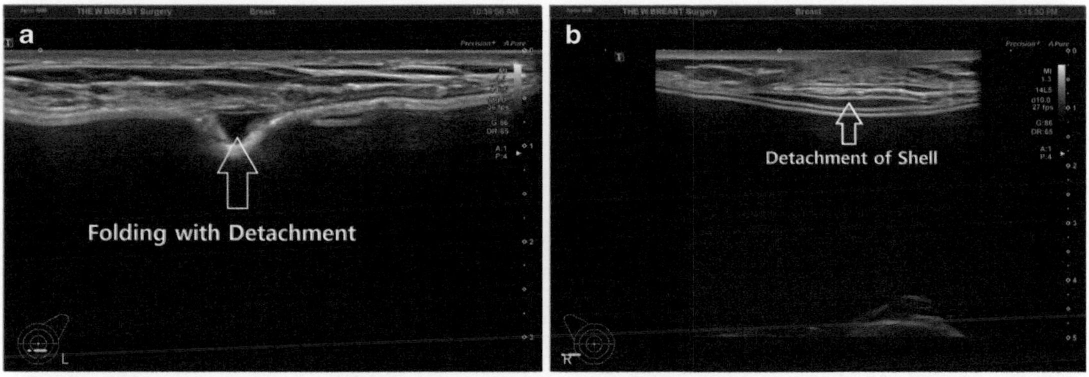

Fig. 5.5 Folding with detachment. (**a**) Transverse view of detachment. (**b**) Longitudinal view of detachment

possible absorption of seroma and changes in the capsule thickness should be evaluated. This would be helpful for planning for more active treatments for patients who may be vulnerable to possible complications.

A tentative diagnosis of hematoma can be made based on ultrasound findings after a history taking and clinical examination (e.g., bruise). Then, the appropriate treatment should be planned based on the severity of swelling and the scope of hematoma.

The following sonographic images show hematoma-related cases (Fig. 5.12).

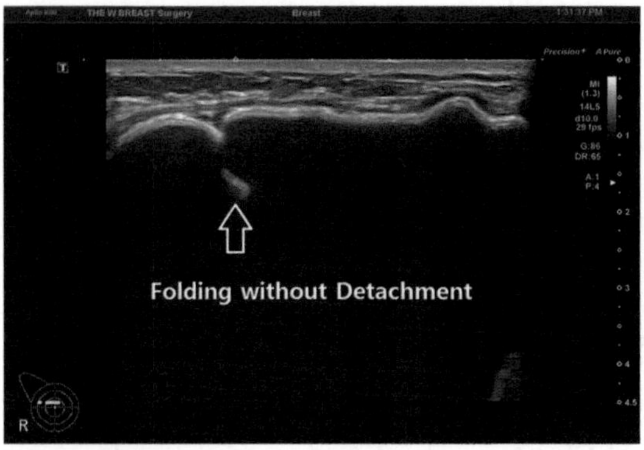

Fig. 5.6 Sonographic finding of folding without detachment

5.4 Rupture

Rupture is a major complication after breast implant surgery which is a cause of reoperation. Rupture occurs in both saline and silicone implants (Fig. 5.13). The ultrasonographic finding is different in both ruptures (Video 5.5). There are various diagnostic image modalities for detecting implant rupture.

Ultrasonography is the most cost-effective and useful diagnostic modality for detecting implant failure.

But sufficient level of expertise would be mandatory to make an accurate diagnosis of rupture on ultrasound. This is because it is important to make a differential diagnosis of rupture from periprosthetic fluid collection, thickened capsule, and folding with or without detachment.

5.4.1 Saline Implant Rupture

Rupture of a saline-filled breast implant is characterized by a flattened shell after disappearance of saline filler in a single lumen (Videos 5.6, 5.7, 5.8, 5.9 and 5.10).

Stepladder sign is a typical clue to diagnosis of rupture of a saline-filled breast implant, which may also be compared with the contralateral breast [1, 2].

Fig. 5.7 Periprosthetic fluid

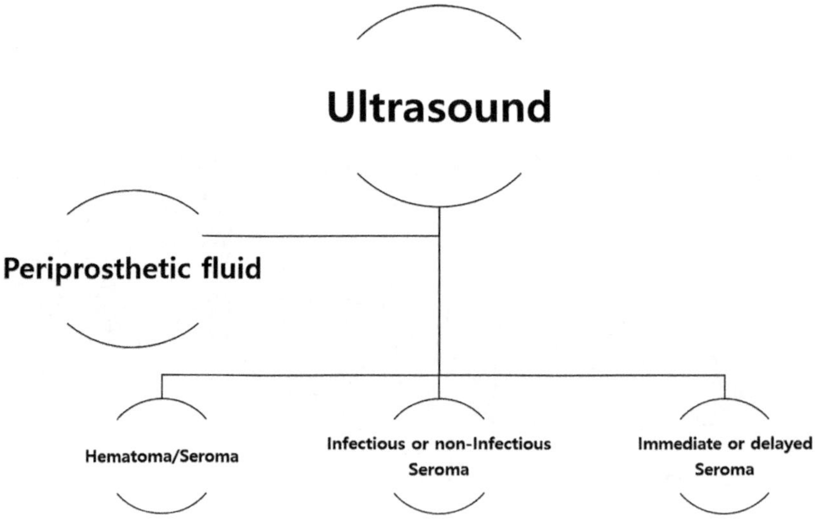

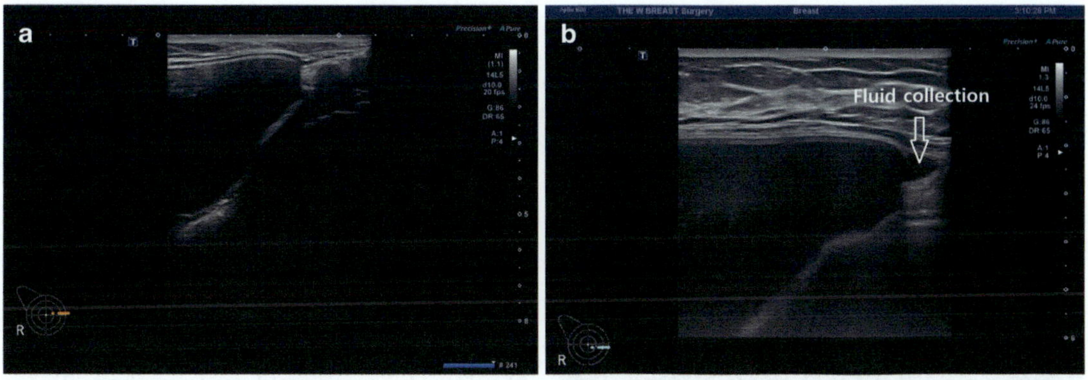

Fig. 5.8 Normal US finding in postoperatively 12 weeks. (**a**) No medial fluid collection. (**b**) Minimal fluid collection

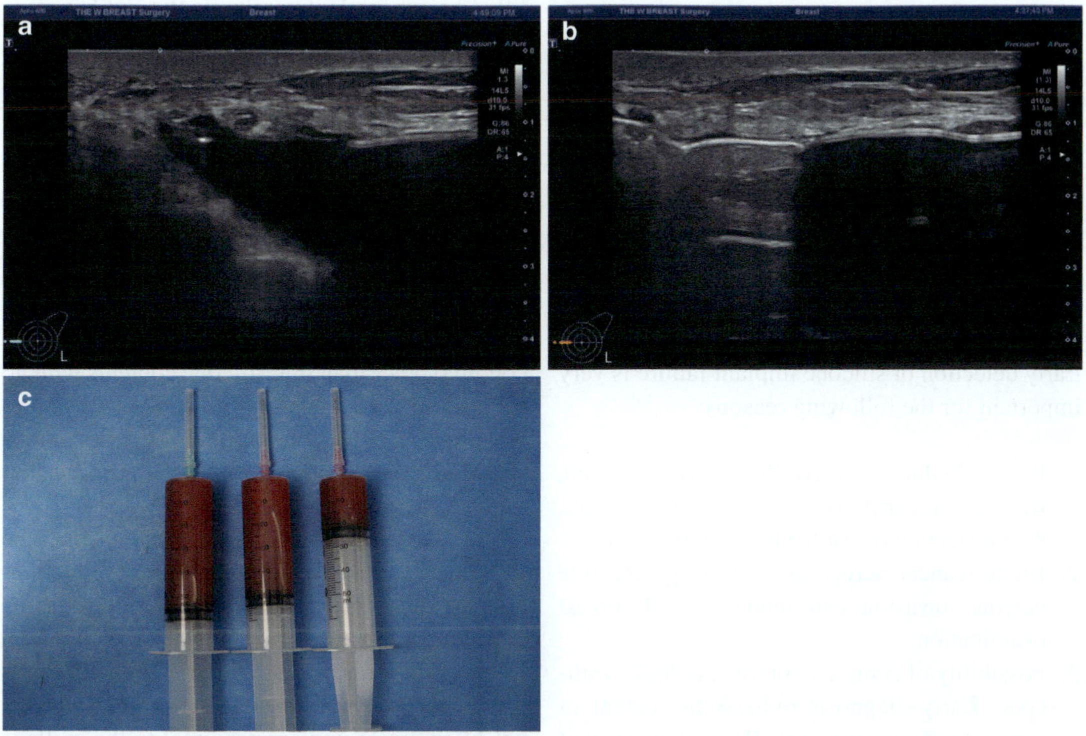

Fig. 5.9 Fluid collection after reoperation d/t capsular contracture. (**a**) Sonographic image during US-guided needle aspiration for the left medial fluid collection. (**b**) Sonographic image after aspiration with intact breast implant. (**c**) Aspirated seroma for cytology and culture

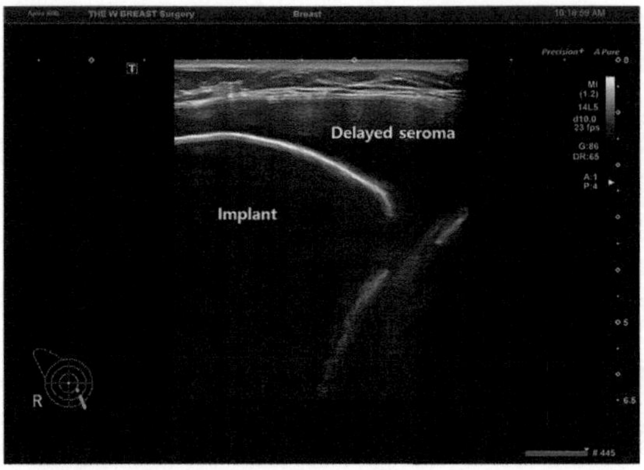

Fig. 5.10 Delayed seroma in periprosthetic space after breast augmentation

Rupture of a saline-filled breast implant can be easily detected on ultrasound with history taking and physical examination.

The following sonographic image shows the characteristics of rupture of a saline-filled breast implant (Fig. 5.14).

5.4.2 Silicone Implant Rupture

Early detection of silicone implant failure is very important for the following reasons:

1. Breast feeding: If early diagnosis is missed, free silicone can progress extracapsular rupture, then ipsilateral breast feeding is interfered.
2. Breast cancer screening: Extracapsular free silicone invasion can interfere with breast examination.
3. Possibility of complete removal of leaked silicone: Early diagnosis reduces the extent of surgery and recovery time. Radical removal of free silicone cannot be achieved in extracapsular rupture with or without LN silicone invasion.

Surgeon cannot prevent failure of implant, but early detection of rupture using any diagnostic modality can minimize hazard of free silicone.

Silicone implant rupture can be classified by scope and type (Fig. 5.15).

Depending on the infiltration of silicone contents into the tissue after it is leaked from a ruptured breast implant, rupture of the device can also be classified into intracapsular rupture and extracapsular rupture; the latter is further divided based on the infiltration of silicone contents into the ipsilateral axillary lymph node [3].

Rupture of a breast implant can be classified into major rupture, grossly characterized by a shell tear (Fig. 5.16), and minor rupture, characterized by a gel bleed despite a lack of gross finding of shell tear [3–5].

Major rupture of a silicone gel-filled breast implant can be diagnosed based on the shell and silicone leakage (free silicone) [3, 6, 7]. A gel bleed can be confirmed based on a free silicone without shell tear [3–5].

An extracapsular rupture of a silicone gel-filled breast implant can be confirmed based on the concurrent presence of posterior acoustic shadowing (reverberating echoes with loss of detail posterior to the echogenic area, which has been variably described as snowstorm, echodense noise, echodense shadowing, or echogenic confusion) and diagnosed when there is a concurrent presence of extracapsular mass or LN invasion [4, 5, 8–12].

Unless there are notable findings (Snowstorm sign (+), LN silicone invasion, extracapsular siliconoma) other than free silicone contents with no snowstorm sign, extra-capsular silicone granuloma and LN silicone infiltration), the corresponding cases are diagnosed as an intracapsular rupture of a breast implant.

An infiltration of silicone contents into the ipsilateral axillary lymph node is a clue to diagnosis of an extracapsular rupture of a silicone gel-filled breast implant [13–15]. This is not seen in cases of intracapsular rupture. A widespread presence of an extracapsular rupture of a silicone gel-filled breast implant proximal to the axilla is commonly seen with the involvement of axillary lymph node in a patient with a long-standing presence of rupture [13, 14, 16].

Signs of silicone implant rupture in ultrasonography are as follows:

1. Tear of shell.
2. Hyperechoic capsule d/t free silicone.
3. Gel fracture (change of integrity of implant).
4. Stepladder sign.
5. Free silicone presence.
6. Snowstorm appearance (seen in extracapsular rupture).

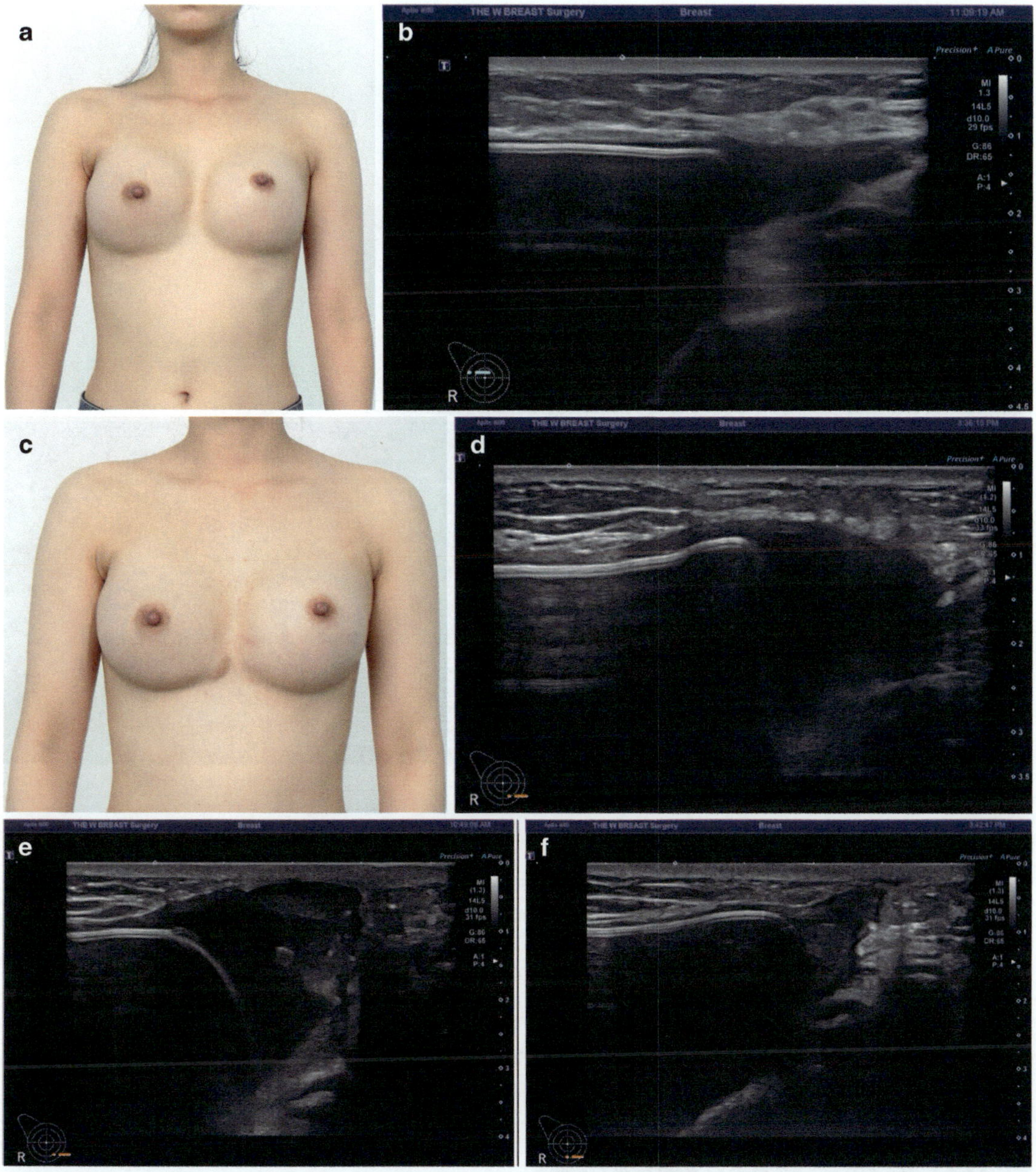

Fig. 5.11 Non-infectious seroma treatment using US-guided aspiration. (**a**) Gross finding of POD 13 weeks. (**b**) Ultrasonographic finding of the right medial small fluid collection. (**c**) Gross finding of POD 30 weeks. (**d**) Ultrasonographic image of LIQ area. (**e**) Ultrasonographic image of POD 35 weeks. (**f**) Ultrasonographic image of POD 47 weeks. (**g**) Ultrasonographic image of POD 50 weeks. (**h**) Gross finding of the right breast. (**i**) Ultrasonographic image of POD 55 weeks. (**j**) Ultrasonographic image of POD 74 weeks

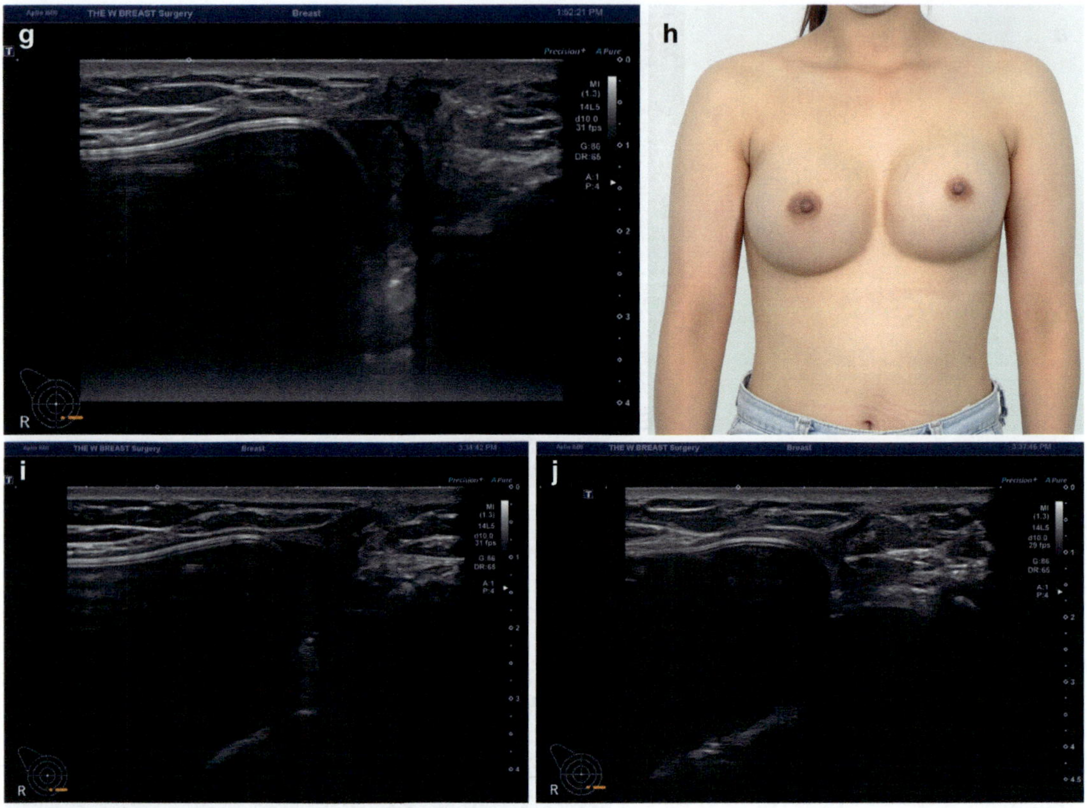

Fig. 5.11 (continued)

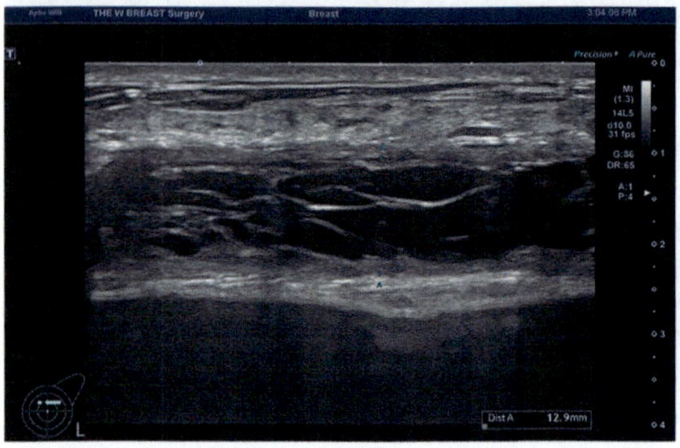

Fig. 5.12 Postoperative hematoma

5.4.2.1 Gel Bleed

There are some points to consider in detecting a rupture of a silicone gel-filled breast implant on ultrasound. Depending on the degree of rupture, rupture of a silicone gel-filled breast implant can be classified into major and minor ruptures.

Gel bleed called with minor rupture is checked free silicone without shell tearing.

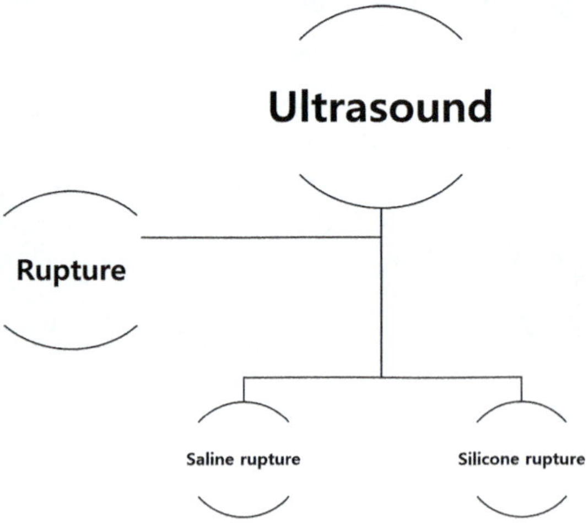

Fig. 5.13 Breast implant rupture

The following image shows minor rupture of a silicone gel-filled breast implant: High-resolution ultrasonography will make it possible for early detection of minor rupture (Fig. 5.17), (Videos

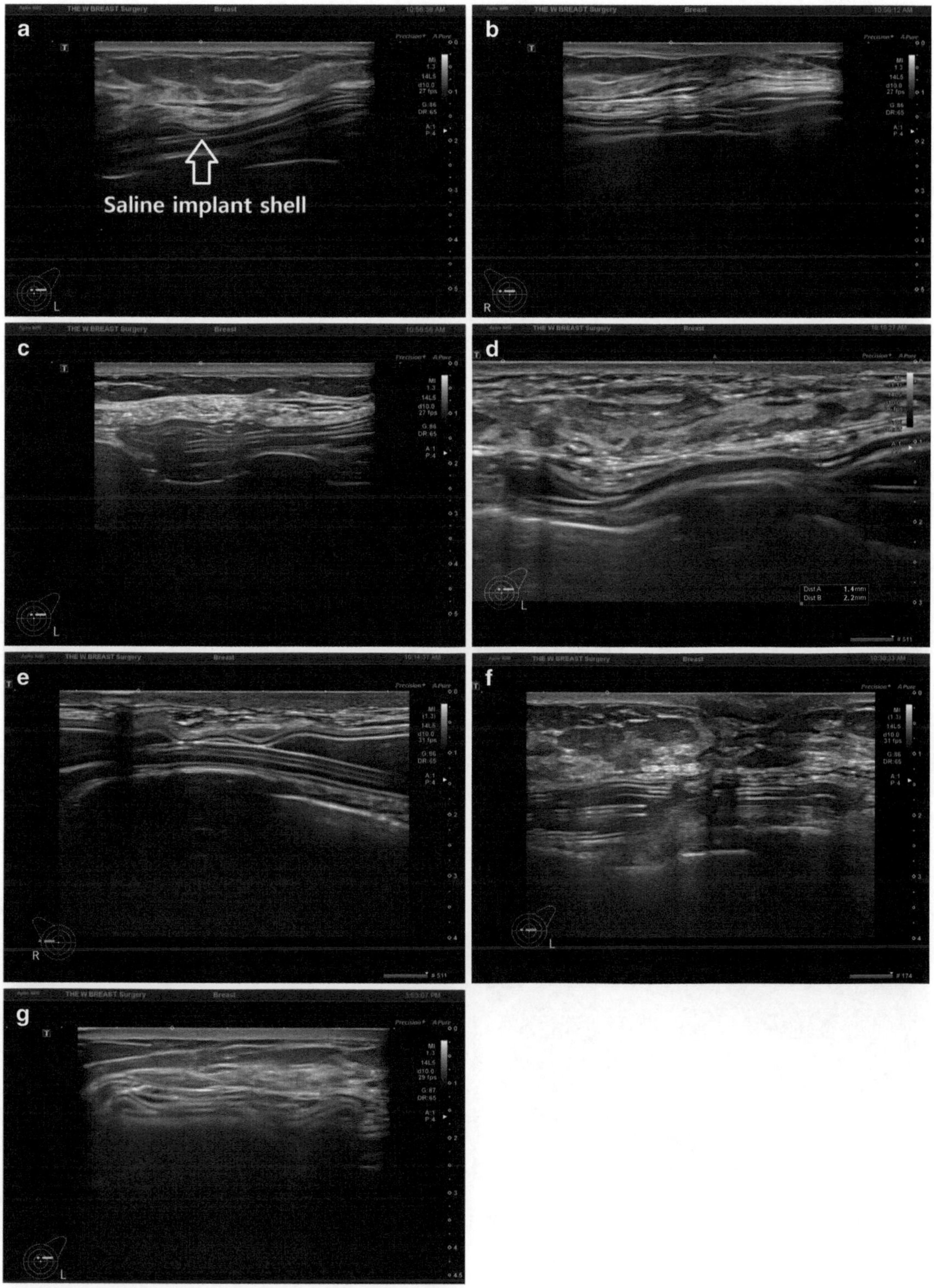

Fig. 5.14 Ultrasonographic image of saline implant rupture d/t shell tear or leakage. (**a**) White arrow indicates saline implant shell with no remnant saline. (**b–g**) Deflated saline breast implant with saline leakage

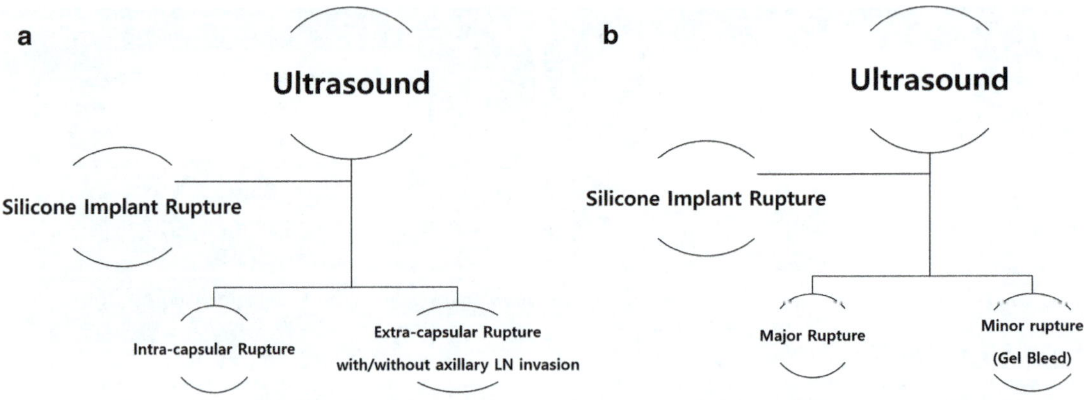

Fig. 5.15 Scope of silicone implant rupture by ultrasonography. (**a**) Classified by silicone invasion: Intracapsular rupture and extracapsular rupture. (**b**) Classified by shell tear: Major rupture (shows shell tear in gross finding) and minor rupture (no shell tear in gross finding, gel bleed)

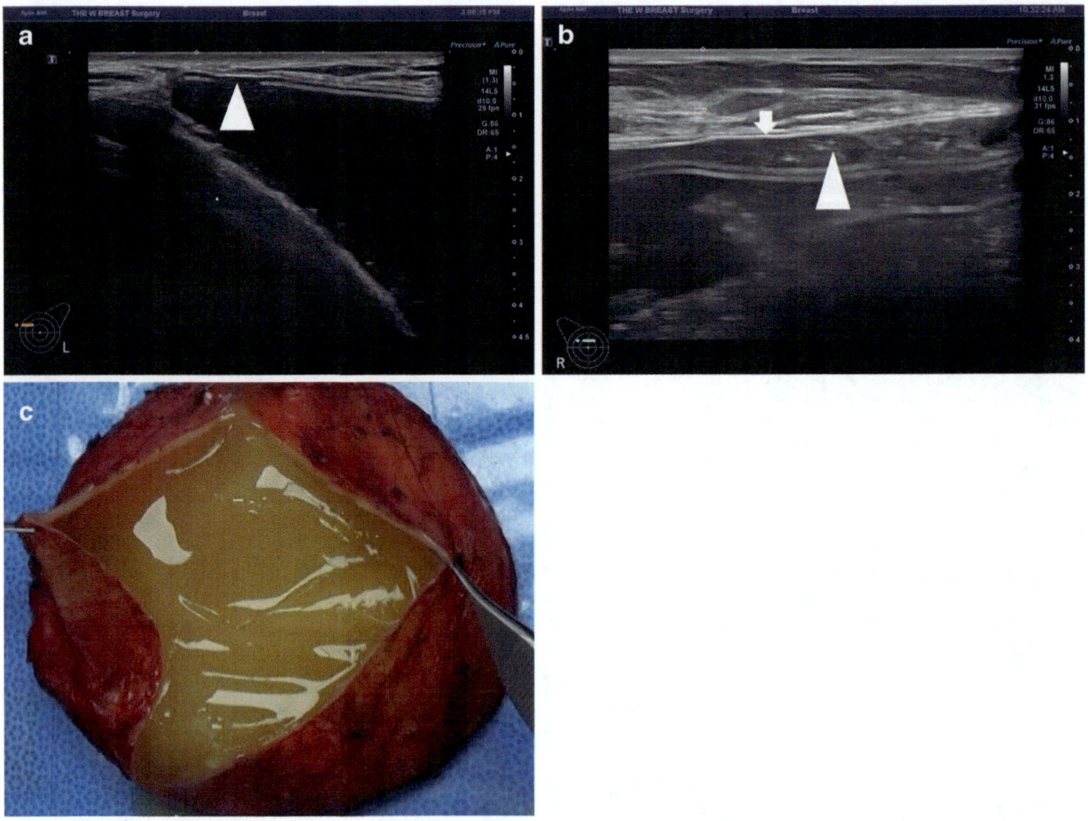

Fig. 5.16 The following sonographic image shows the characteristics of major rupture of a silicone gel-filled breast implant: (**a**) White triangle is the point of tear of shell. (**b**) White triangle is leaked silicone and white arrow is hyperechoic capsule. (**c**) Gross finding of ruptured breast implant

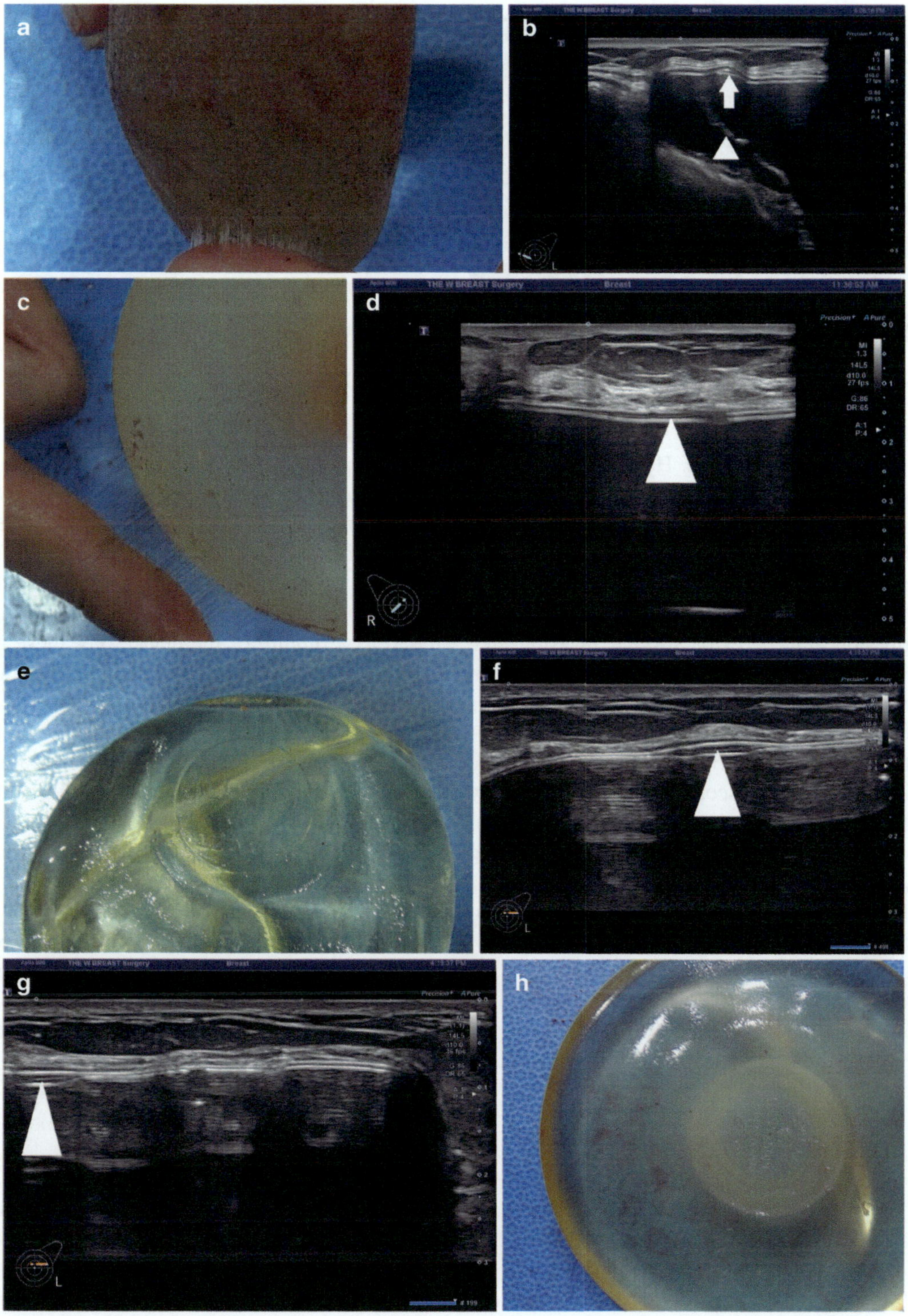

Fig. 5.17 Gross and ultrasonographic image of minor rupture (gel bleeding) which is lack of shell tear. (**a**, **b**): Case I. (**c**, **d**): Case II. (**e–g**): Case III. (**h**, **i**): Case IV. (**a**) Gross finding of gel bleed. (**b**) Ultrasonographic image of gel bleed (white arrow shows abnormal shell condition, white triangle shows gel fracture). (**c**) Gross finding of gel bleed. (**d**) Preoperative ultrasonographic diagnosis of gel bleed (white triangle). (**e**) Gross finding of gel bleed. (**f**) Preoperative diagnosis of gel bleed (white triangle). (**g**) Preoperative diagnosis of gel bleed (white triangle). (**h**) Gross finding of gel bleed. (**i**) Preoperative ultrasonographic diagnosis of gel bleed (white triangle)

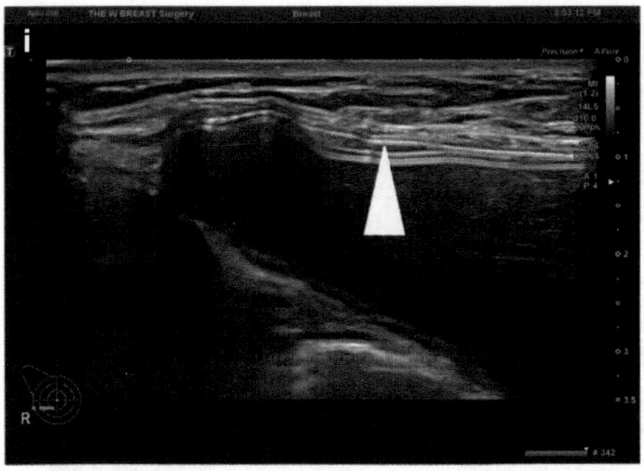

Fig. 5.17 (continued)

5.11, 5.12, 5.13 and 5.14). Hyperechoic capsule is also seen in gel bleed site.

5.4.2.2 Intracapsular Major Rupture

Intra-capsular rupture is diagnosed when there are no signs of extracapsular rupture like snowstorm appearance, extracapsular invasion like regional lymph node. Distinguishing between intracapsular rupture and extracapsular rupture is difficult in some cases. In that case target capsulectomy is a key for accurate diagnosis. Distinguishing the scope of rupture is very important for management of possible residual siliconoma that may interfere with breast feeding in young patients.

Ultrasonographic signs of intracapsular rupture are as follows:

1. Free silicone.
2. Shell tearing without free silicone.
3. Hyperechoic capsule in both minor rupture and major rupture.
4. Step-ladder sign.
5. Gel fracture.

The following sonographic images show various intracapsular silicone rupture (Fig. 5.18), (Videos 5.15 and 5.16).

Sonographic finding of hyperechoic capsule is seen.

5.4.2.3 Extracapsular Rupture with or without Lymph Node Invasion

An extracapsular rupture is diagnosed with capsular invasion of free silicone. Extracapsular mass and ipsilateral lymph node siliconoma are a definite sign of extracapsular rupture (Videos 5.17, 5.18, 5.19, 5.20, 5.21, 5.22, 5.23, 5.24, 5.25 and 5.26).

Extracapsular silicone invasion to breast parenchyma may disturb breast examination and complete removal of the leaked silicone cannot be achieved. It would therefore be mandatory to inform a patient of the presence of extracapsular rupture.

In a patient with an extracapsular rupture of a breast implant, there is a possibility that remnant lesions in breast and lymph node might be left because of leaked silicone contents on ultrasound even after explantation or implant change.

It is noteworthy because there is a possibility that a normal breast implant may be misdiagnosed as a rupture of the device. For these reasons, the scope and degree of silicone involvement should be checked and then recorded through an ultrasound-guided examination of the breast. This would contribute to avoiding unnecessary surgeries and thereby ensuring a patient's healthcare rights.

Ultrasonographic signs of extracapsular rupture are as follows:

1. Reverberating echoes with loss of detail posterior to the echogenic area, which has been variably described as snowstorm, echodense noise, echodense shadowing, or echogenic confusion.
2. Extracapsular granuloma.
3. Regional LN siliconoma.

The following sonographic image shows an extracapsular rupture of a silicone gel-filled breast implant (Fig. 5.19).

By definition, silicone lymphadenopathy is referred to as involvement of silicone in a lymph node; it is a rare complication of augmentation mammaplasty using a silicone gel-filled breast implant [16–18]. This poses a diagnostic dilemma for surgeons. Malignancy may be initially considered, but its possibility should be ruled out in a patient with a lump in the neck or axilla who had a past history of receiving augmentation mammaplasty using a silicone gel-filled breast implant [19]. To date, two different mechanisms underlying the migration of silicone to the tissue have been proposed; these include rupture or erosion of a silicone-containing surface or continued leakage through an intact surface [20, 21]. The migration of silicone to the tissue causes fibrosis and foreign body granulomatous reactions [22]. This may be followed by the transportation of silicone particles to regional lymph nodes via macrophages in the reticulo-endothelial system [23]. Consequently, foreign body reactions may cause local swelling of the involved lymph node. It has been documented that silicone lymphadenopathy primarily affects the axillary lymph node in a patient receiving augmentation mammaplasty using a silicone gel-filled breast implant [20, 24].

The following ultrasonographic image shows silicone invasion to lymph node (Fig. 5.20).

Axillary lymph node ultrasonography should be performed with or without rupture.

5.5 Thickened Capsule and Capsular Contracture

Known as one of the major causes of reoperation, CC is characterized by thickening and ingrowth of the capsule composed of collagen around a breast implant, resulting in alterations in the shape and location of the device, which may lead to pain and hardening sensation.

CC can be classified depending on the capsule thickness, the elasticity of the capsule, and the scope of thickened capsule; it is divided into mild and severe cases. In association with this, the Baker classification system was introduced to express its degree in 1978.

For the past several years, I have studied correlations between the Baker grades I-IV and capsule thickness measured on breast ultrasound.

Table 5.1 Thickness of capsule with Baker grade

Baker grade	The capsule thickness on breast ultrasound
I	<0.4 mm
II	0.4–0.8 mm
III	0.8–1.4 mm
IV	>1.4 mm

The following sonographic image shows a normal breast without CC (Fig. 5.21). It is characterized by a lack of notable TC between the inferior border of the pectoralis major muscle and the shell of a breast implant.

Capsular contracture is a result of extensive thickened capsule (Fig. 5.22), (Videos 5.27, 5.28, 5.29, 5.30, 5.31 and 5.32). We can easily see the folding of shell in Baker III, IV capsular contracture.

Fortunately many patients have thickened capsule but are asymptomatic d/t focal or partial TC range. In these patients, careful observation of changes in the thickness and range of TC is necessary with ultrasonography. Then early detection of Baker III, IV capsular contracture is possible.

By measuring TC, cut-off values for the Baker grades I-IV were estimated as follows:

Correlation between the Baker classification system and the capsule thickness on breast ultrasound.

According to "the value of capsule thickness on breast ultrasound as an indicator of the severity of capsular contracture and its correlation with the baker classification," the capsule thickness might be used as an indicator of the severity of CC alternative to the Baker classification system [2], (Table 5.1).

As mentioned earlier, not only the thickness of capsule, but also the extent of thickened capsule and the elasticity of the capsule are important in severity of symptoms.

According to a study about periprosthetic capsule, there was no consistency in the capsule thickness, as shown above in the ultrasonographic image of thickened capsule.

But the place where a patient complains of the greatest discomfort was the point that has most thickened capsule. If there was a TC, it was matched to a patient's symptoms.

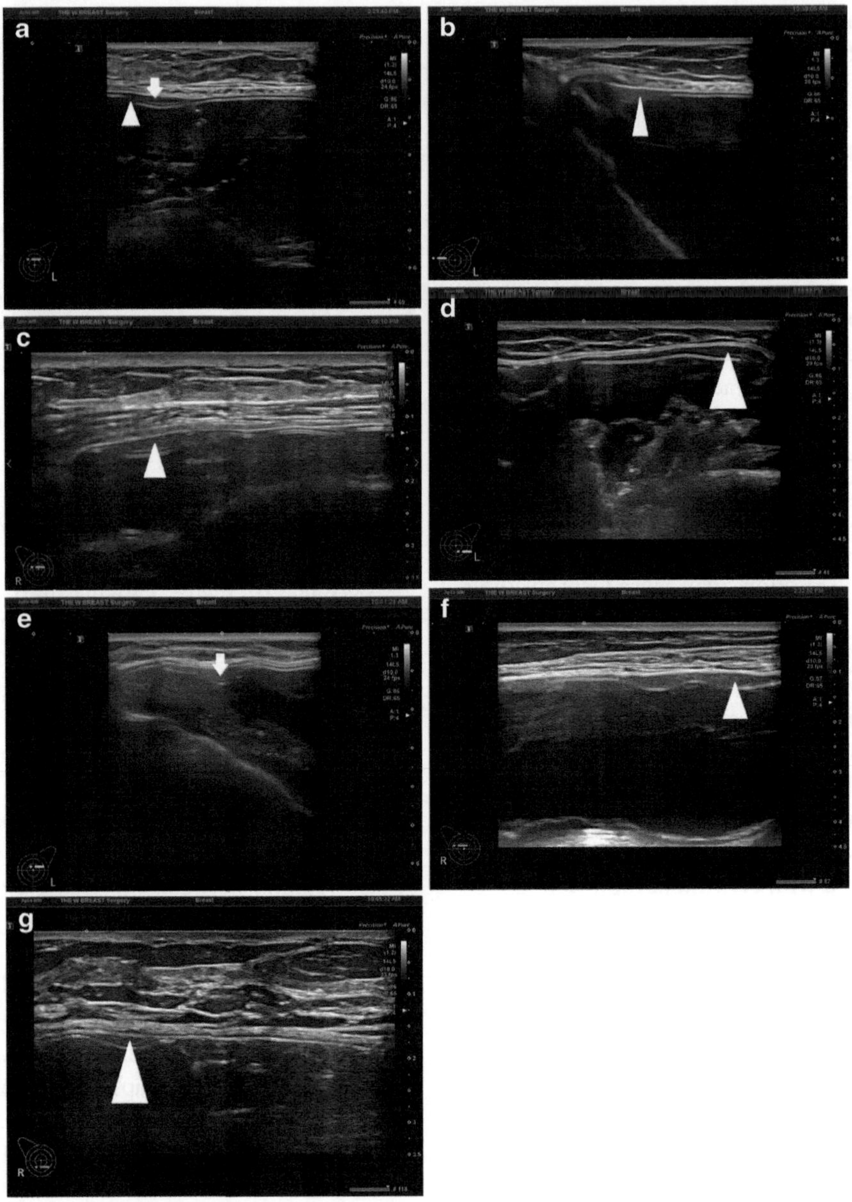

Fig. 5.18 Ultrasonographic finding of intracapsular silicone rupture. (**a**) White triangle is shell disruption, white arrow is free silicone. (**b**) White triangle is free silicone. (**c**) White triangle is free silicone. (**d**) White triangle is free silicone. (**e**) White arrow is free silicone. (**f**) White triangle is free silicone. (**g**) White triangle is free silicone. (**h**) White arrow is free silicone. (**i**) White triangle is free silicone. (**j**) White triangle is free silicone. (**k**) White arrow is free silicone. (**l**) White triangle is free silicone. (**m**) White triangle is free silicone. (**n**) White triangle is free silicone. (**o**) White triangle is free silicone. (**p**) White triangle is free silicone. (**q**) White triangle is free silicone. (**r**) White arrow is free silicone. (**s**) White arrow is free silicone. (**t**) White triangle is free silicone. (**u**) White arrow is free silicone. (**v**) White triangle is free silicone. (**w**) White triangle is free silicone. (**x**) White triangle is ruptured implant. (**y**) White triangle is free silicone. (**z1**) White triangle is free silicone, white arrow is hyperechoic capsule. (**z2**) White triangle is free silicone. (**z3**) White triangle is hyperechoic capsule d/t rupture. (**z4**) White triangle is free silicone and white arrow is hyperechoic capsule. (**z5**) White triangle is hyperechoic capsule d/t rupture. (**z6**) White triangle is free silicone and white arrow is hyperechoic capsule. (**z7**) White triangle is free silicone and white arrow is hyperechoic capsule. (**z8**) White triangle is free silicone and white arrow is hyperechoic capsule. (**z9**) White triangle is hyperechoic capsule d/t rupture. (**z10**) White triangle is free silicone and white arrow is hyperechoic capsule. (**z11**) White triangle is free silicone and white arrow is hyperechoic capsule. (**z12**) White triangle is free silicone and white arrow is hyperechoic capsule. (**z13**) White triangle is free silicone and white arrow is hyperechoic capsule. (**z14**) White triangle is hyperechoic capsule d/t rupture

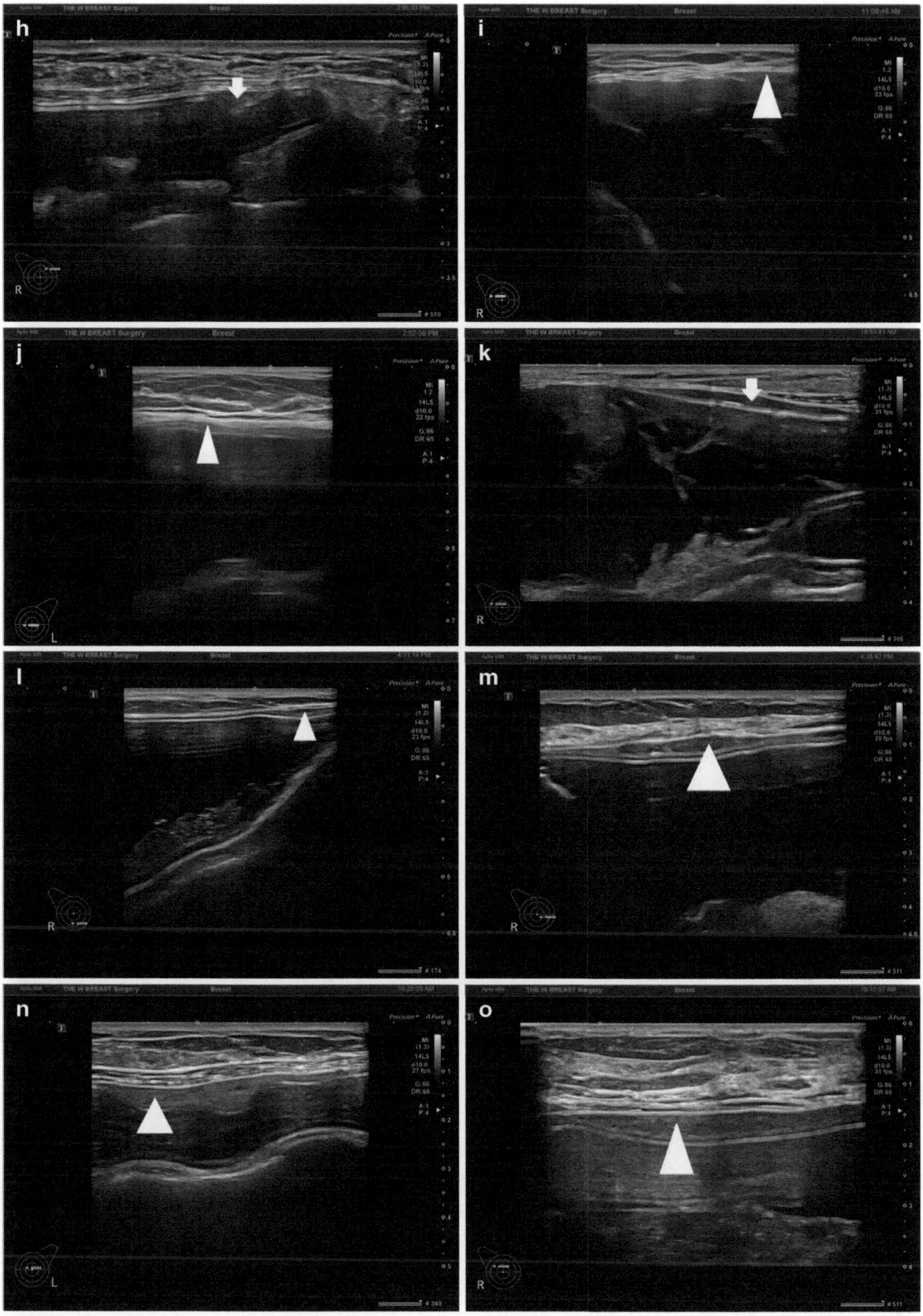

Fig. 5.18 (continued)

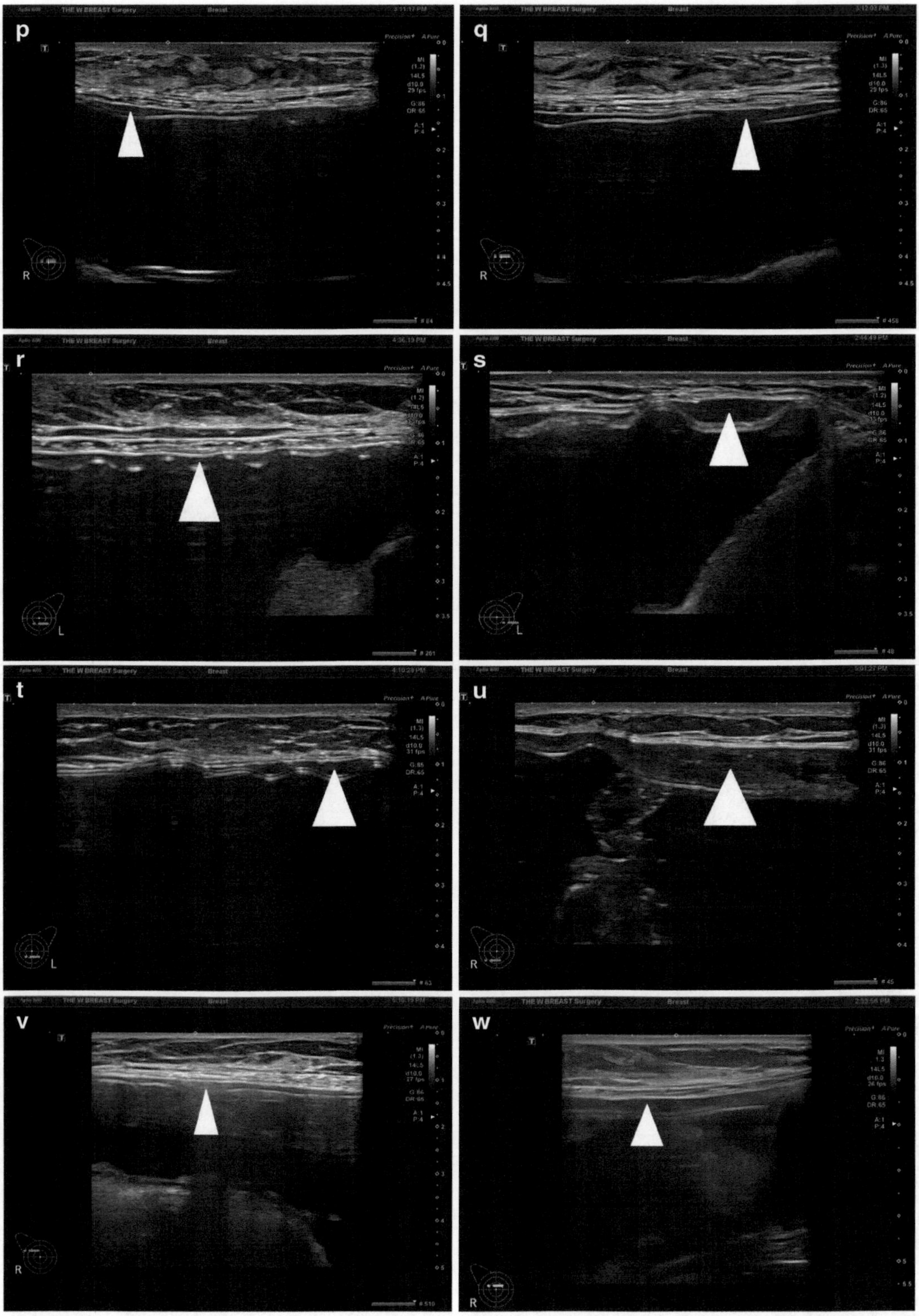

Fig. 5.18 (continued)

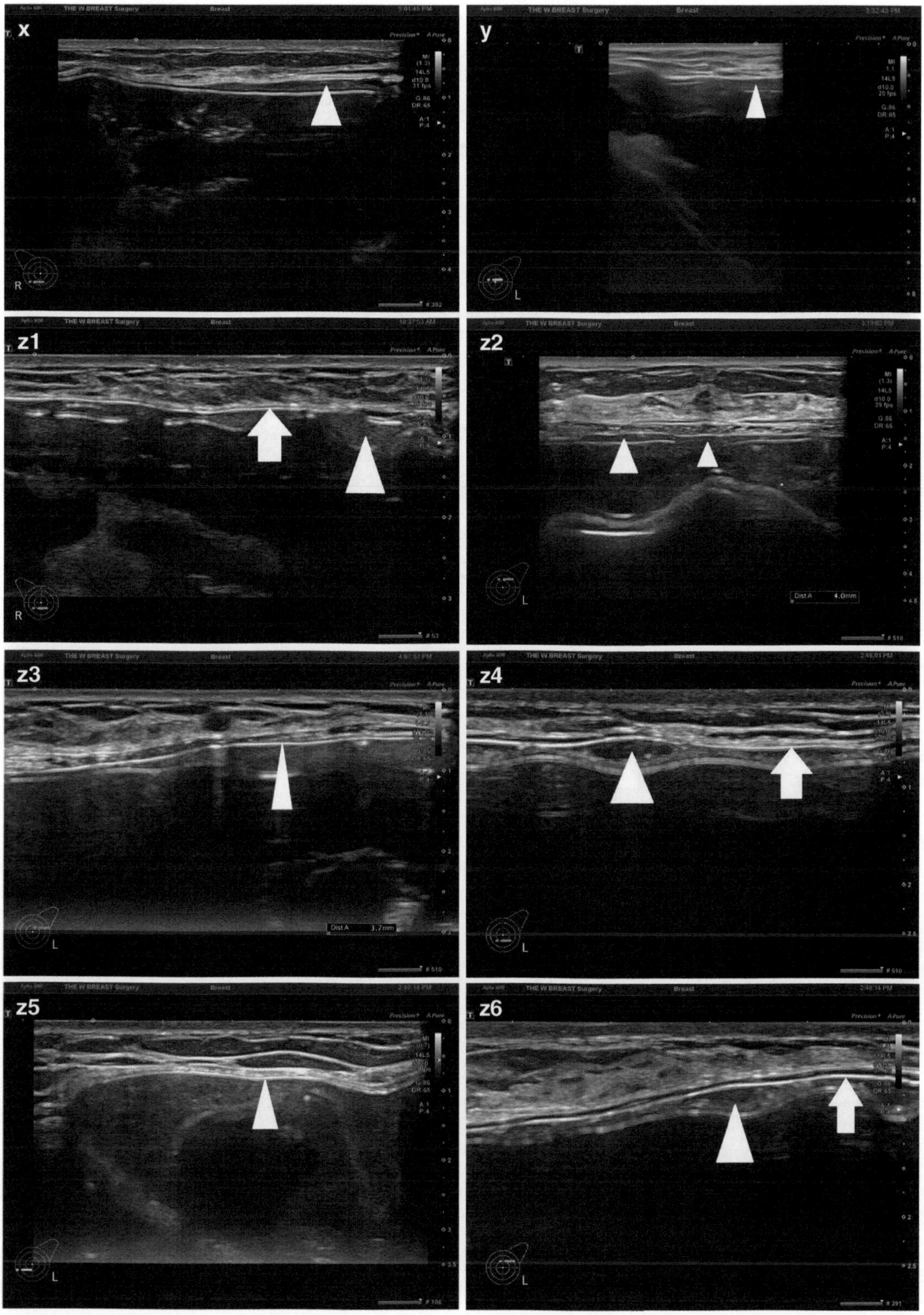

Fig. 5.18 (continued)

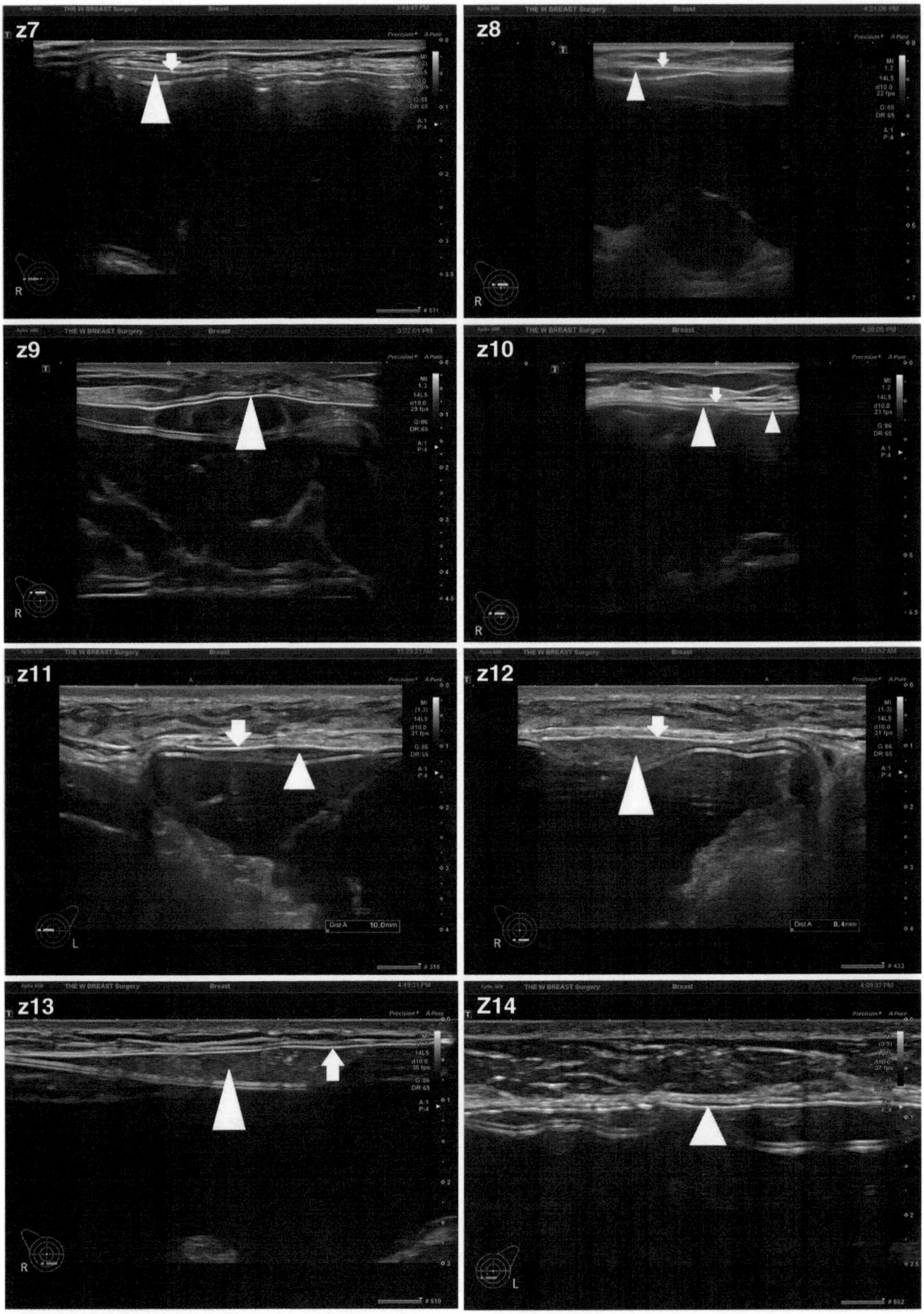

Fig. 5.18 (continued)

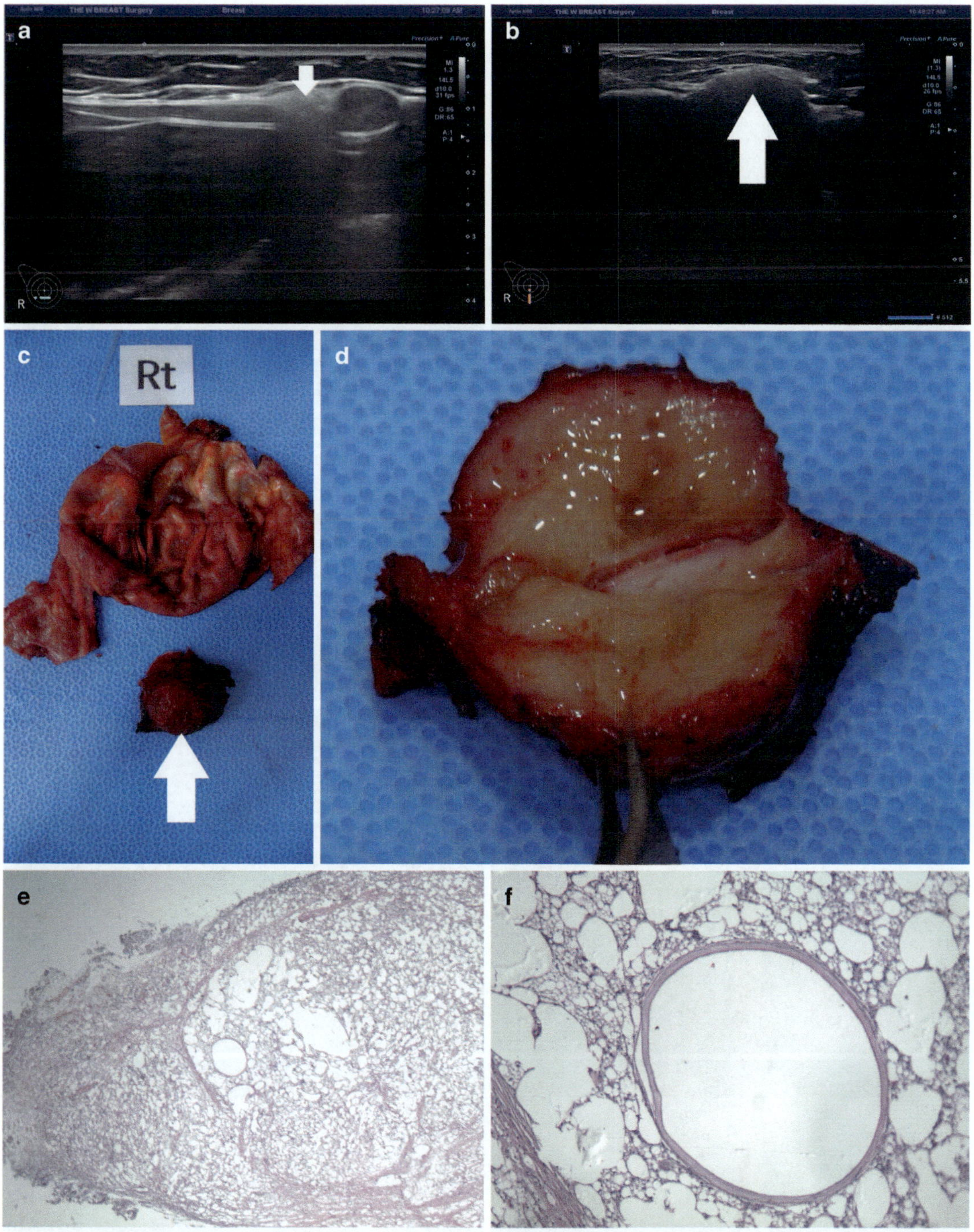

Fig. 5.19 Ultrasonographic finding of extracapsular rupture. (**a**) White arrow is extracapsular invasion of leaked silicone. It is impossible to assess the status of the inferior breast due to posterior acoustic shadowing in a patient with an extracapsular rupture of the device. (**b**) White arrow is preoperative ultrasonographic image of extracapsular mass. (**c**) Gross finding of capsule and extracapsular mass (white arrow). (**d**) Cross-sectional view of extracapsular mass. (**e, f**) Histopathologic image (H&E stain) (**g–o**) Snowstorm appearance in extra-capsular rupture in ultrasonography

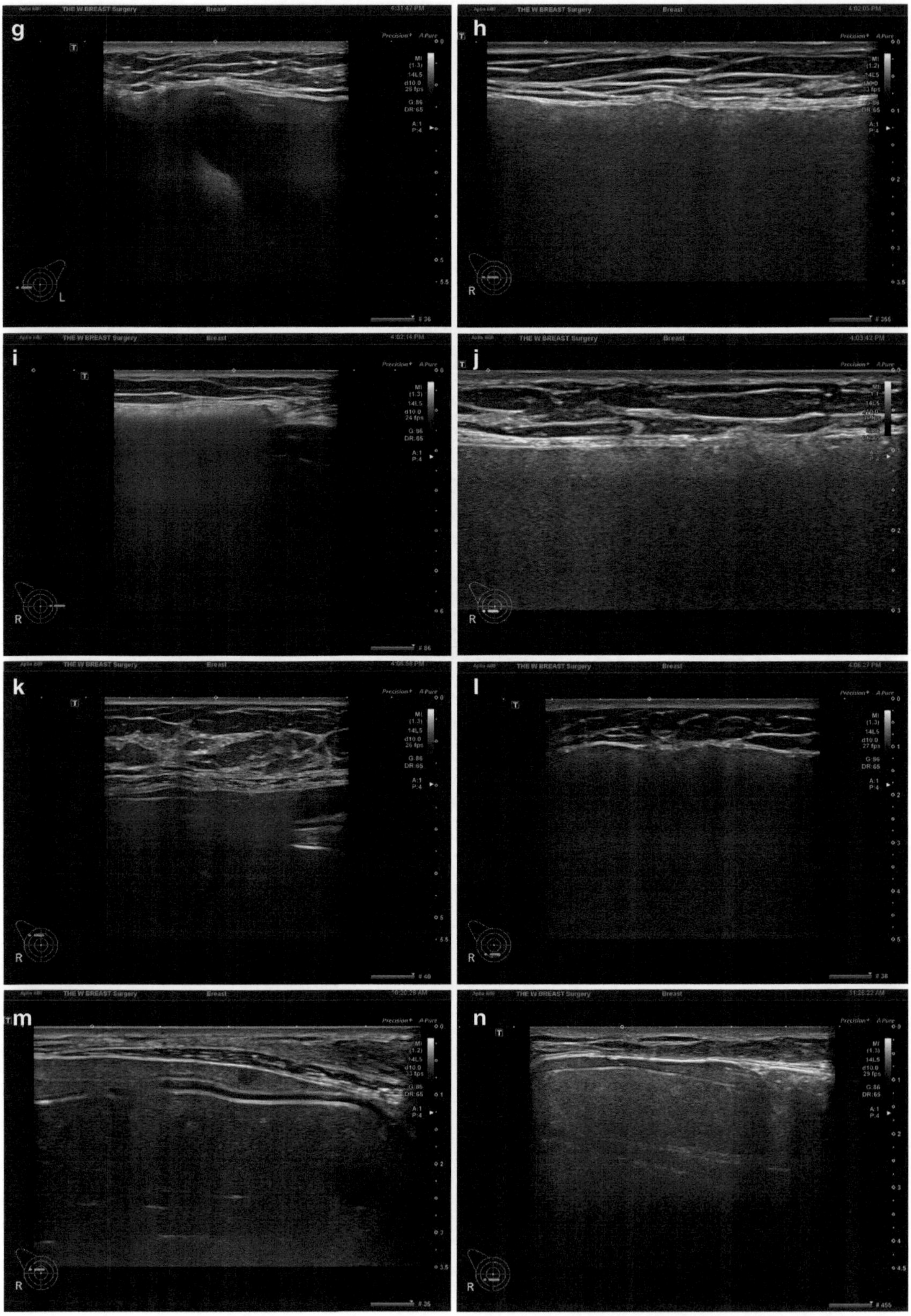

Fig. 5.19 (continued)

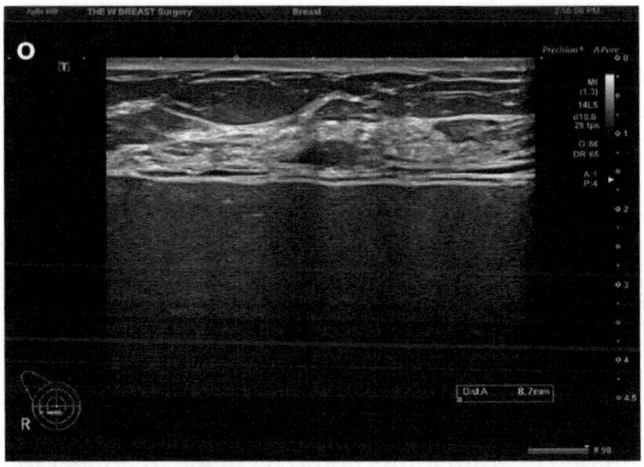

Fig. 5.19 (continued)

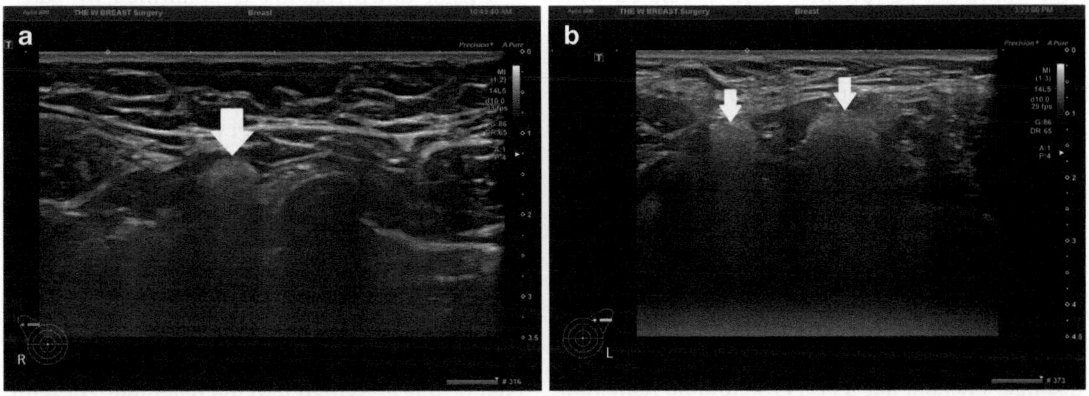

Fig. 5.20 (**a**, **b**) White arrow is preoperative ultrasonographic image of axillary lymph node silicone invasion

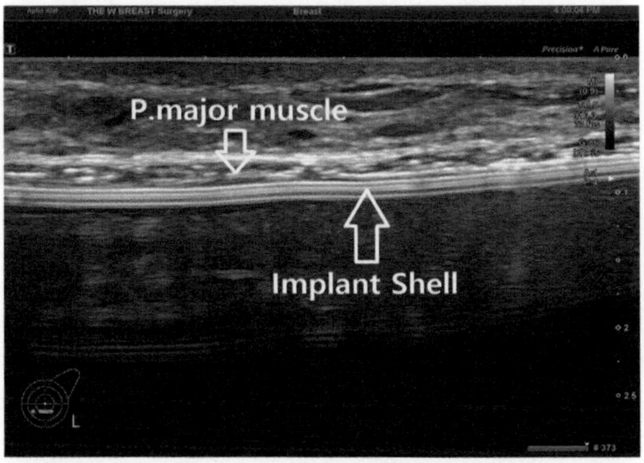

Fig. 5.21 Normal invisible capsule after breast implant-based mammaplasty. Micro-textured implant with invisible normal capsule thickness in subpectoral pocket

Even the same capsule thickness may cause a varying degree of discomfort depending on a patient, which may be related to the elasticity of the capsule.

The presence of early thickened capsule without symptom within 6 months after surgery is an important ultrasonographic indicator to monitor possibility of future capsular contracture deterioration.

5.6 Upside-Down (USD) Rotation

Without ultrasound, the presence of USD rotation would not be revealed. USD is related with pain, hardness d/t thick patch.

It is often observed that a breast implant is rotated in reverse directions *rather than* horizontal ones. It remains obscure, however, whether the device was placed in a wrong position or its location was changed later. This would not be clarified unless there are immediate postoperative data. It is also probable, however, that a textured breast implant or an anatomical device might have been placed in a wrong location at surgery. This should be cautioned by surgeons, who should examine whether a patient has a USD rotation by palpating a process or patch of the device.

I experienced 20 cases of USD rotation on ultrasound in patients who had been surgically treated at other hospitals. Of these, 90% (18/20) had a textured breast implant. Moreover, there were some patients receiving an anatomical device; even some patients had an anatomical device placed in an upside-down position in both breasts.

A patient with USD rotation may be vulnerable to alterations in the shape and may present with pain due to a thick patch on the base of a device. This suggests that USD rotation is a complication that deserves special attention.

Of note, a patch is unique to a manufacturer of a breast implant; it serves as a clue to the identification of the manufacturer as an orientation mark does. Similarly, the patch can also be used to identify the manufacturer of a round device.

More continuous efforts based on ultrasound-guided examination should be made to collect the data about a patch of all the breast implants that are commercially available in Korea.

Upside-down rotation is confirmed by patch. Sometimes it is necessary to distinguish between the saline injection port of the saline implant and the patch, so you need to be careful. The following images are various shapes of patch by manufacturers and ultrasonographic findings (Fig. 5.23), (Videos 5.33, 5.34, 5.35, 5.36, 5.37, 5.38, 5.39, 5.40 and 5.41). If the physician knows all shapes of patch by various manufacturers, it is easy to confirm the manufacturer.

As shown above, there is a variability in the shape of patch depending on the manufacturer. That is, it is classified into the patch with or without an embossing dot.

The video shows a complete difference in the shape between the patches, which may serve as a clue to identification of a manufacturer of a breast implant placed in an up-side down position (Videos 5.33, 5.34, 5.35, 5.36, 5.37, 5.38, 5.39, 5.40 and 5.41). Moreover, orientation mark on the base serves as another clue.

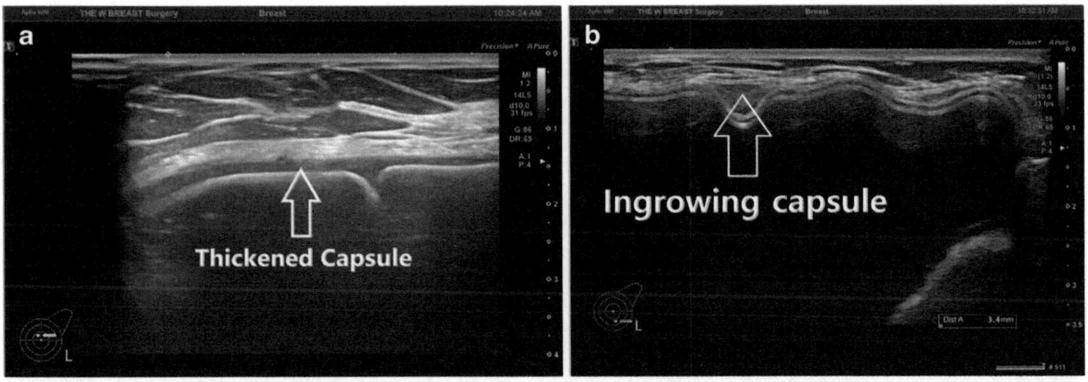

Fig. 5.22 The following sonographic image shows a thickened capsule. (**a**) Thickened capsule is seen with textured breast implant in subpectoral pocket. (**b**) Ultrasonographic image of ingrowing thick capsule with textured breast implant. (**c**) Ultrasonographic image of periprosthetic thickened capsule. (**d**) Ultrasonographic image of ingrowing thickened capsule. (**e**) Ultrasonographic image of TC with detachment. (**f**) White arrow is thickened capsule with textured type breast implant. (**g**) White triangle is thickened capsule with textured type breast implant. (**h**) White triangle is thickened capsule with textured type breast implant. (**i**) White arrow is thickened capsule with textured type breast implant. (**J**) White arrow is thickened capsule with textured type breast implant. (**k**) White arrow is thickened capsule with textured type breast implant. (**l**) White triangle is thickened capsule with textured type breast implant. (**m**) White arrow is thickened capsule with textured type breast implant. (**n**) White triangle is thickened capsule with textured type breast implant. (**o**) White triangle is thickened capsule with textured type breast implant. (**p**) White triangle is thickened capsule with textured type breast implant. (**q**) White triangle is thickened capsule with textured type breast implant. (**r**) White triangle is thickened capsule with textured type breast implant. (**s**) White triangle is thickened capsule with textured type breast implant. (**t**) White triangle is thickened capsule with smooth type breast implant. (**u**) White triangle is thickened capsule with textured type breast implant. (**v**) White triangle and arrow are thickened capsule with textured type breast implant. (**w**) White triangle is thickened capsule with textured type breast implant. (**x**) White triangle is thickened capsule with smooth type breast implant. (**y**) White triangle is thickened capsule with textured type breast implant. (**z1**) White triangle is thickened capsule with textured type breast implant. (**z2**) White triangle is thickened capsule with textured type breast implant. (**z3**) White triangle is thickened capsule with textured type breast implant. (**z4**) White triangle is thickened capsule with textured type breast implant. (**z5**) White triangle is thickened capsule with smooth type breast implant. (**z6**) White triangle is thickened capsule with textured type breast implant. (**z7**) White triangle is thickened capsule with textured type breast implant. (**z8**) White triangle is thickened capsule with textured type breast implant. (**z9**) White triangle is thickened capsule with textured type breast implant. (**z10**) White triangle is thickened capsule with textured type breast implant. (**z11**) White arrow is thickened capsule with smooth type breast implant. (**z12**) White triangle is thickened capsule with textured type breast implant. (**z13**) White triangle is thickened capsule with textured type breast implant. (**z14**) White triangle is thickened capsule with textured type breast implant. (**z15**) White triangle is thickened capsule with textured type breast implant. (**z16**) White triangle is thickened capsule with textured type breast implant. (**z17**) White triangle is thickened capsule with textured type breast implant. (**z18**) White triangle is thickened capsule with textured type breast implant. (**z19**) White triangle is thickened capsule with textured type breast implant. (**z20**) White triangle is thickened capsule with textured type breast implant. (**z21**) White triangle and arrow is thickened capsule with textured type breast implant. (**z22**) White triangle is thickened capsule with textured type breast implant. (**z23**) White arrow is thickened capsule with textured type breast implant (Polytech anatomical type). (**z24**) White triangle is thickened capsule with smooth type breast implant. (**z25**) White triangle is thickened capsule with smooth type breast implant. (**z26**) White triangle is thickened capsule with textured type breast implant. (**z27**) White triangle is thickened capsule with smooth type breast implant. (**z28**) White triangle is thickened capsule with textured type breast implant. (**z29**) White arrow is thickened capsule with textured type breast implant. (**z30**) White arrow is thickened capsule with textured type breast implant. (**z31**) White triangle is maximal thickened capsule, 3.1 mm with textured type breast implant

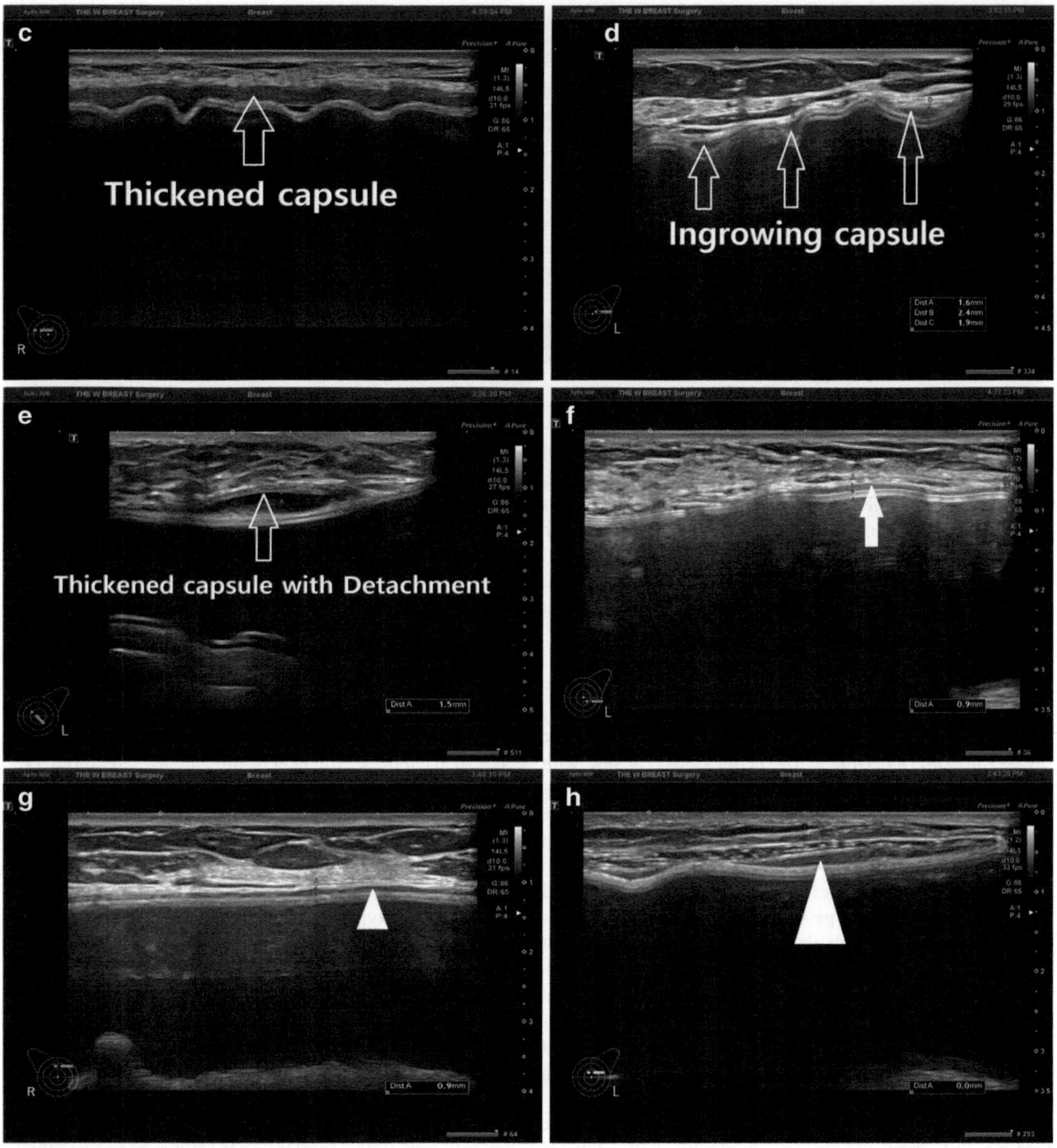

Fig. 5.22 (continued)

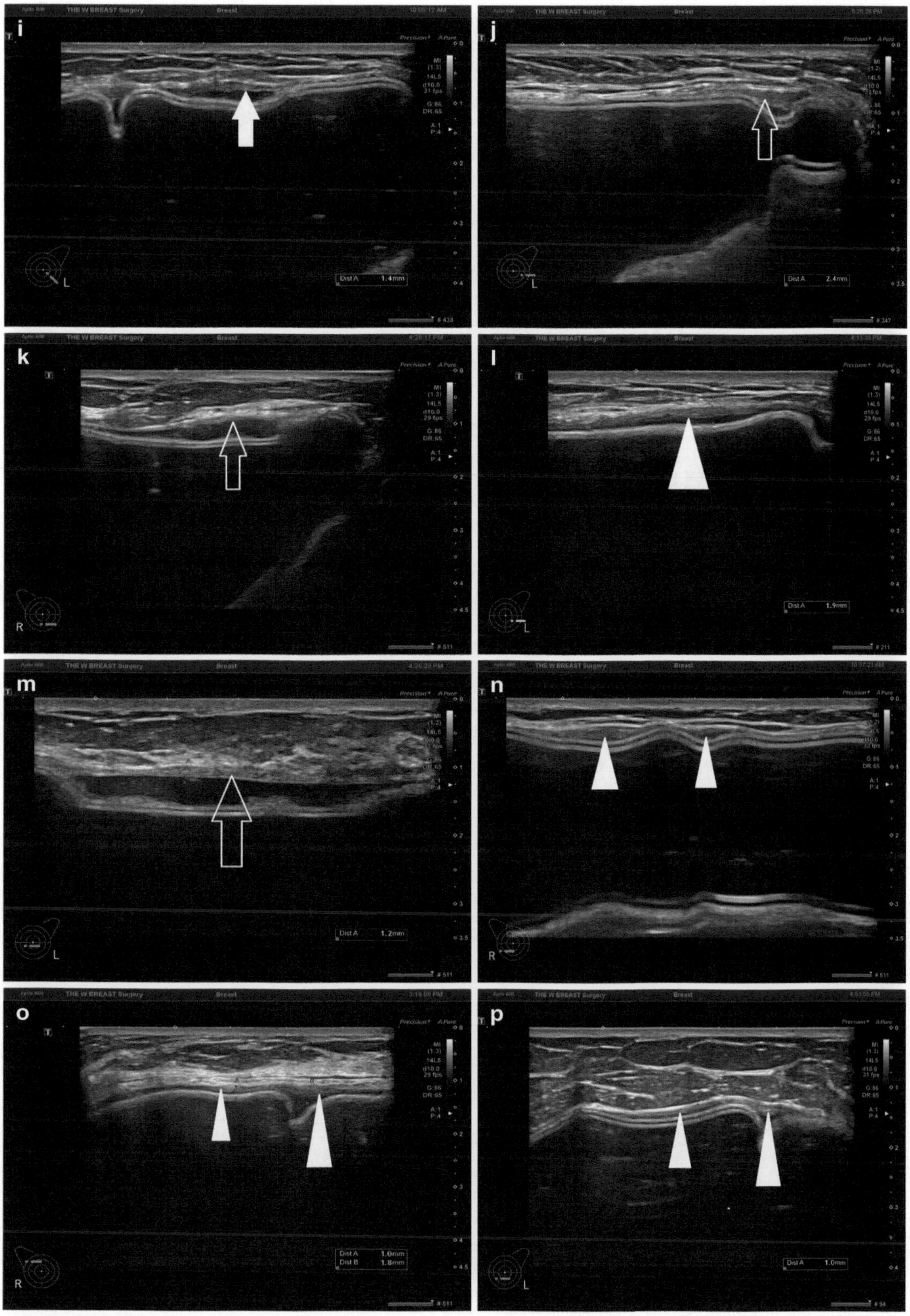

Fig. 5.22 (continued)

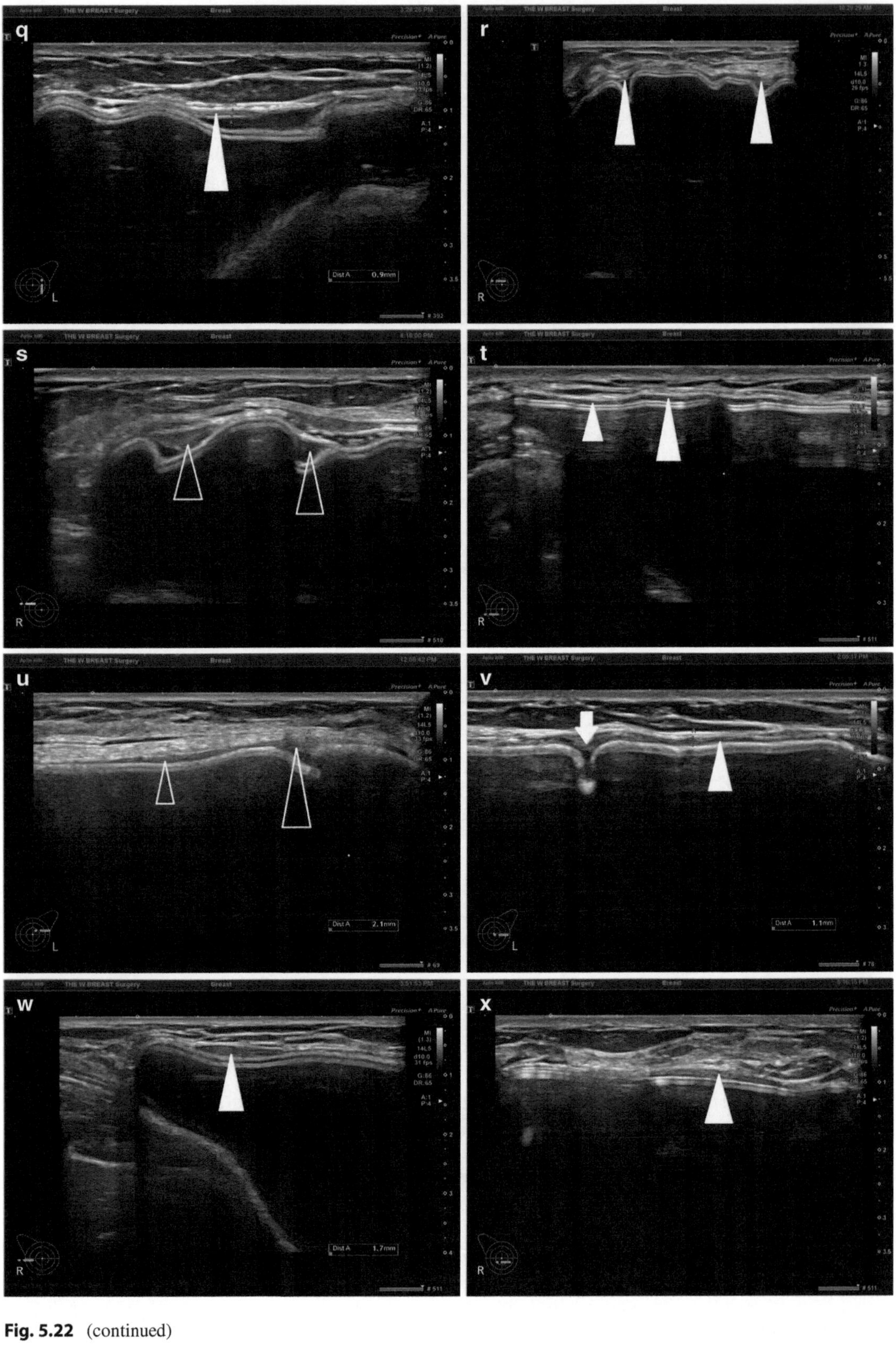

Fig. 5.22 (continued)

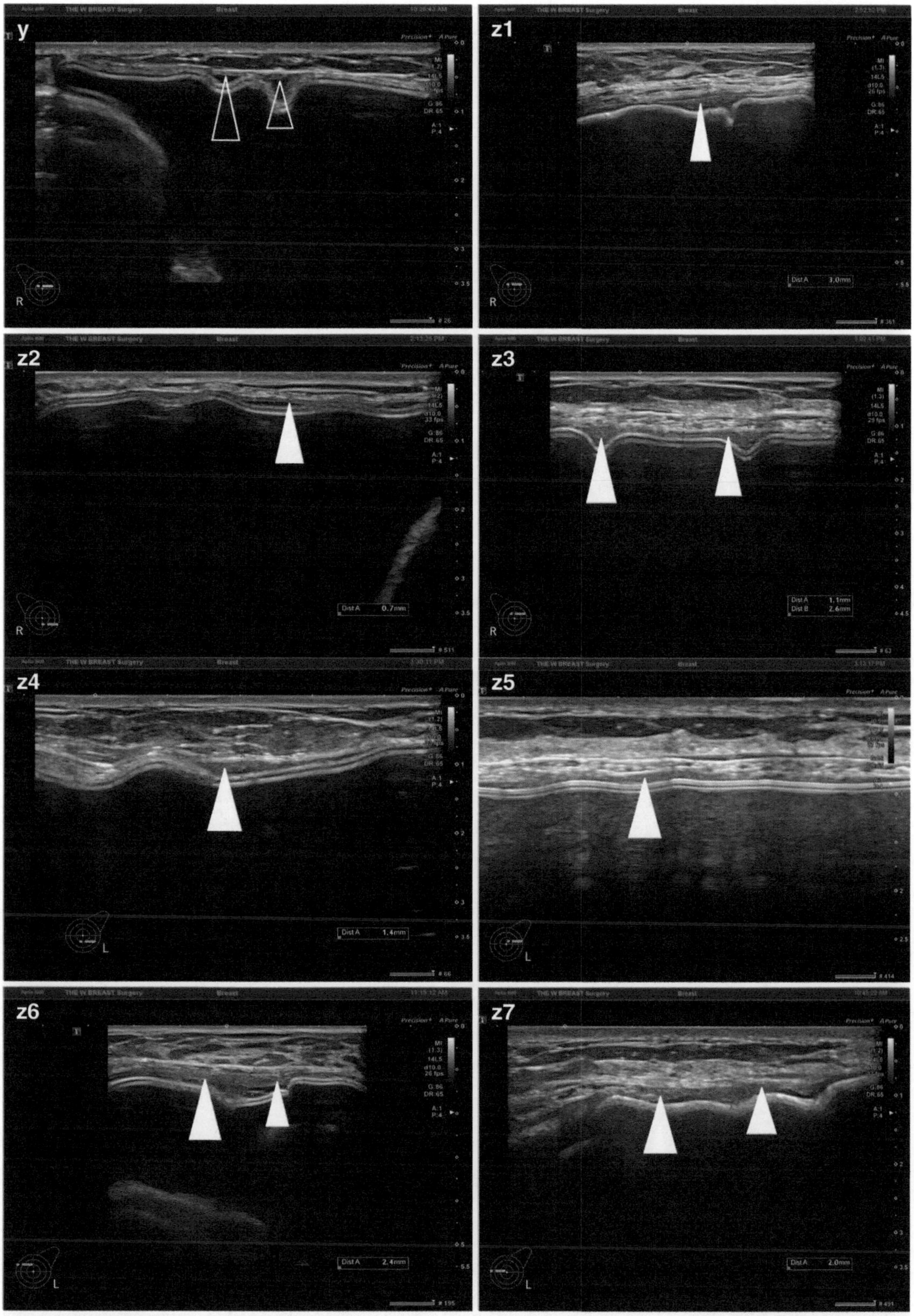

Fig. 5.22 (continued)

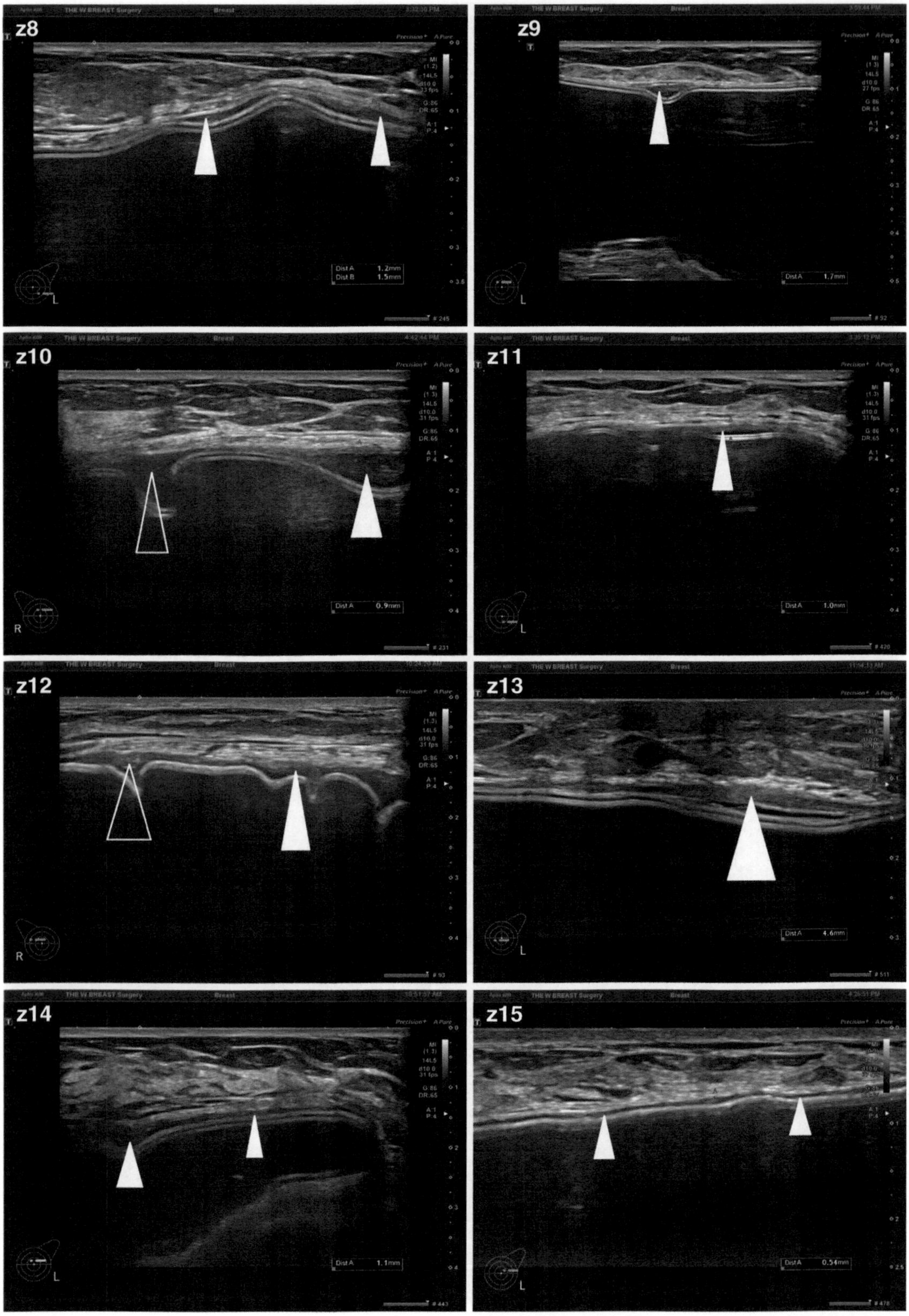

Fig. 5.22 (continued)

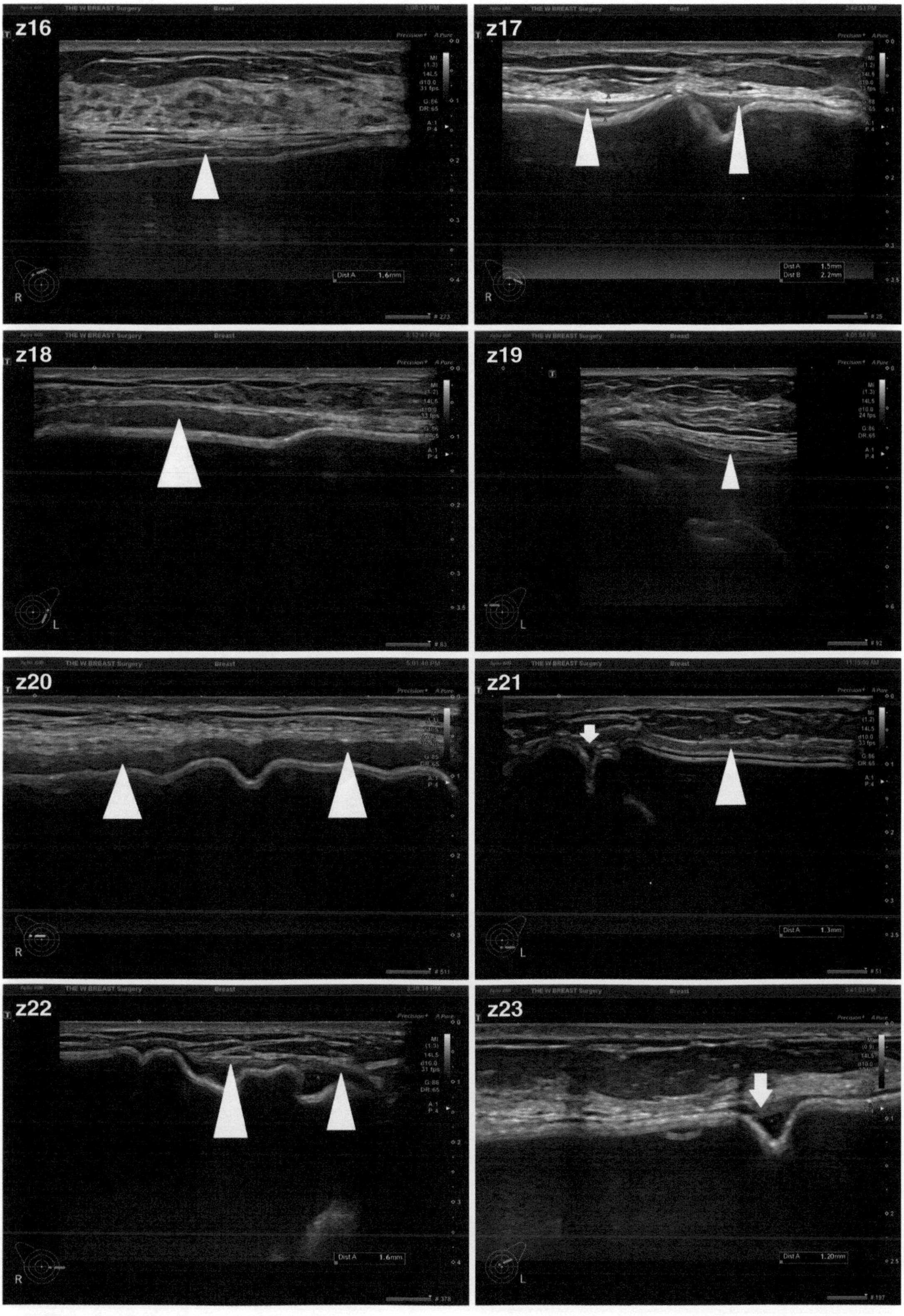

Fig. 5.22 (continued)

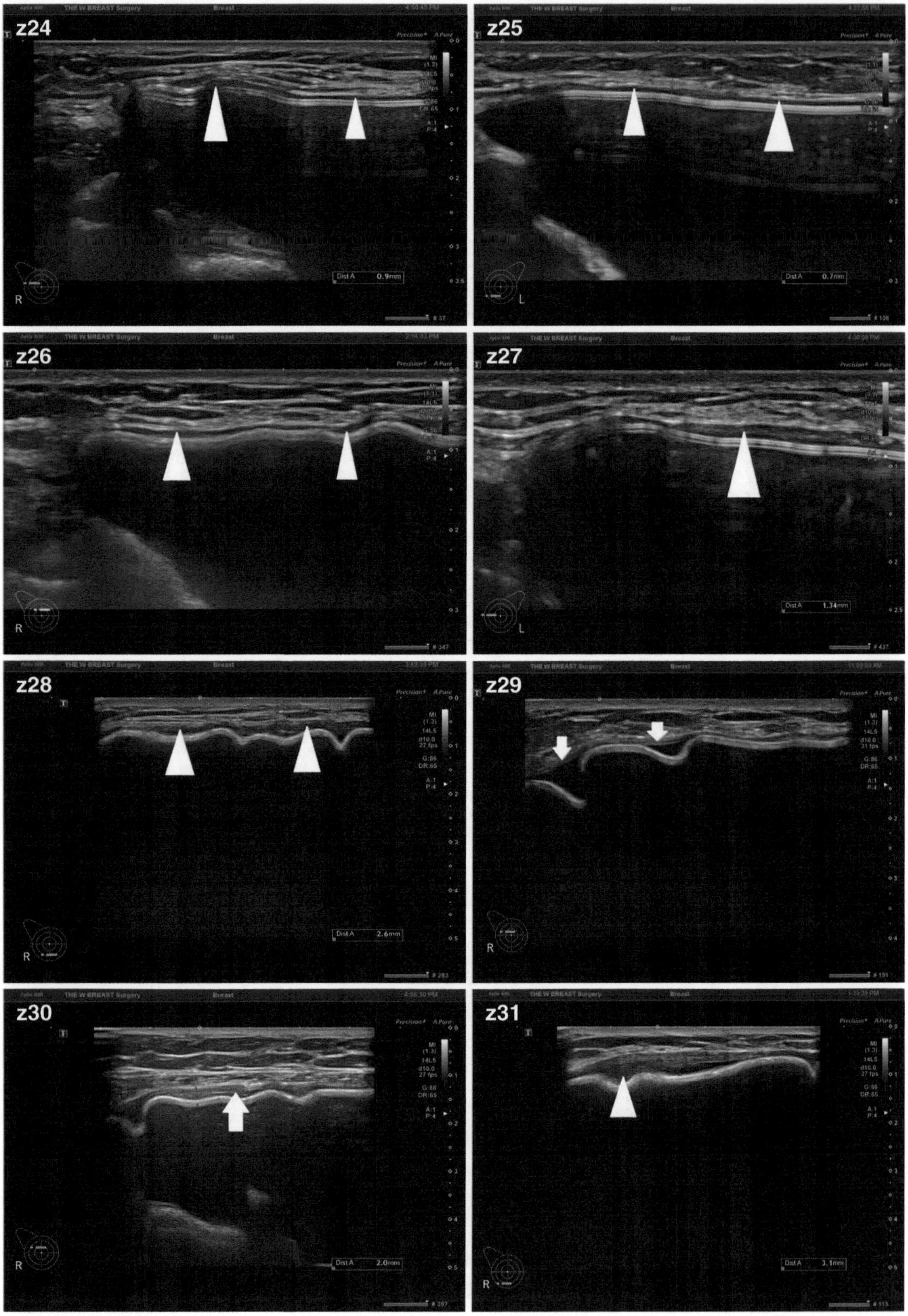

Fig. 5.22 (continued)

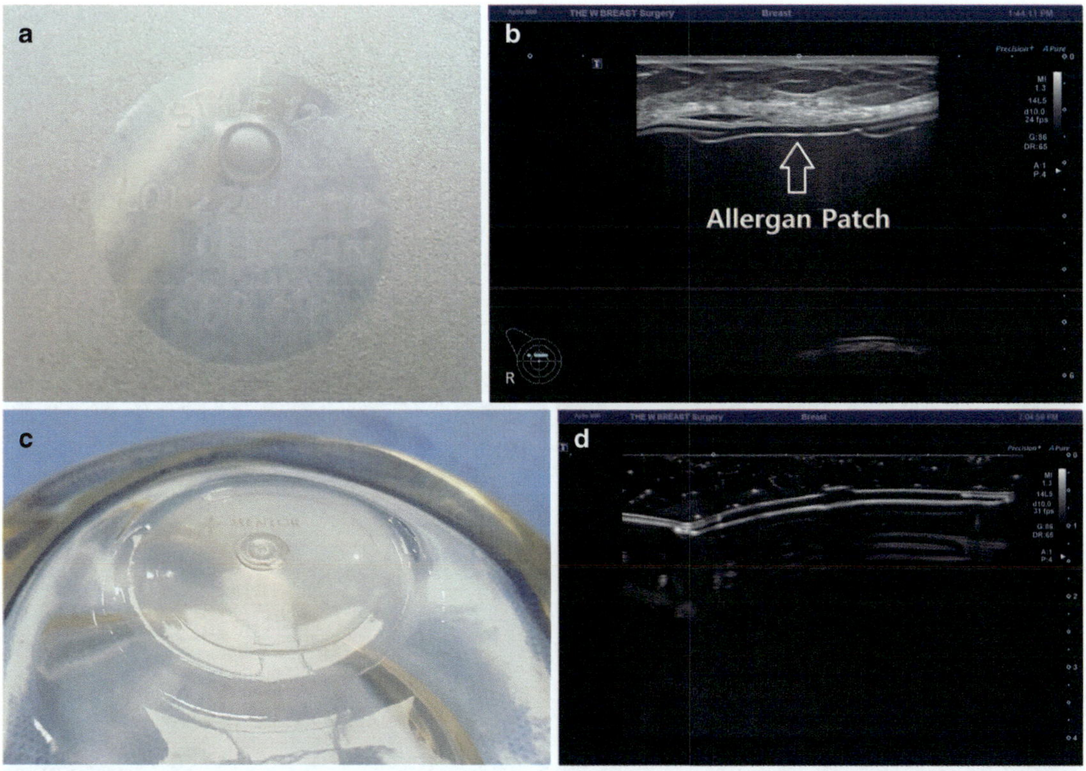

Fig. 5.23 Gross and ultrasonographic finding of various breast implant manufacturers. (**a**, **b**) Gross and ultrasonographic image of Allergan breast implant posterior patch. (**a**) Gross finding of Allergan patch: Dot in patch. (**b**) Ultrasonographic finding of Allergan posterior patch. (**c**–**e**) Gross and ultrasonographic image of Mentor breast implant posterior patch. (**c**) Gross finding of Mentor posterior patch: Dot in center. (**d**) Ultrasonographic image of Mentor posterior patch. (**e**) Ultrasonographic image of Mentor posterior patch. (**f**, **g**, **h**) Gross and ultrasonographic image of Sebbin breast implant. (**f**) Gross finding of Sebbin posterior patch: No dot in patch. (**g**) Ultrasonographic image of Sebbin posterior patch. (**h**) Ultrasonographic image of Sebbin posterior patch. (**i**, **j**, **k**) Gross and ultrasonographic image of Hansbiomed breast implant. (**i**) Gross image of Bellagel patch and US finding: Dot in center. (**j**) Sonographic image of Hansbiomed breast implant posterior patch. (**k**) Sonographic image of Hansbiomed breast implant posterior patch. (**l**, **m**) Gross and ultrasonographic image of Polytech breast implant posterior patch. (**l**) Gross finding of Polytech breast implant posterior patch: No dot in patch. (**m**) Ultrasonographic image of Polytech breast implant posterior patch. (**n**, **o**) Gross and ultrasonographic image of Motiva breast implant posterior patch. (**n**) Gross finding of Motiva breast implant posterior patch. (**o**) Ultrasonographic finding of Motiva breast implant posterior patch. (**p**, **q**) Gross and ultrasonographic image of Eurosilicone breast implant posterior patch. (**p**) Gross finding of Eurosilicone breast implant posterior patch. (**q**) Ultrasonographic image of Eurosilicone breast implant posterior patch

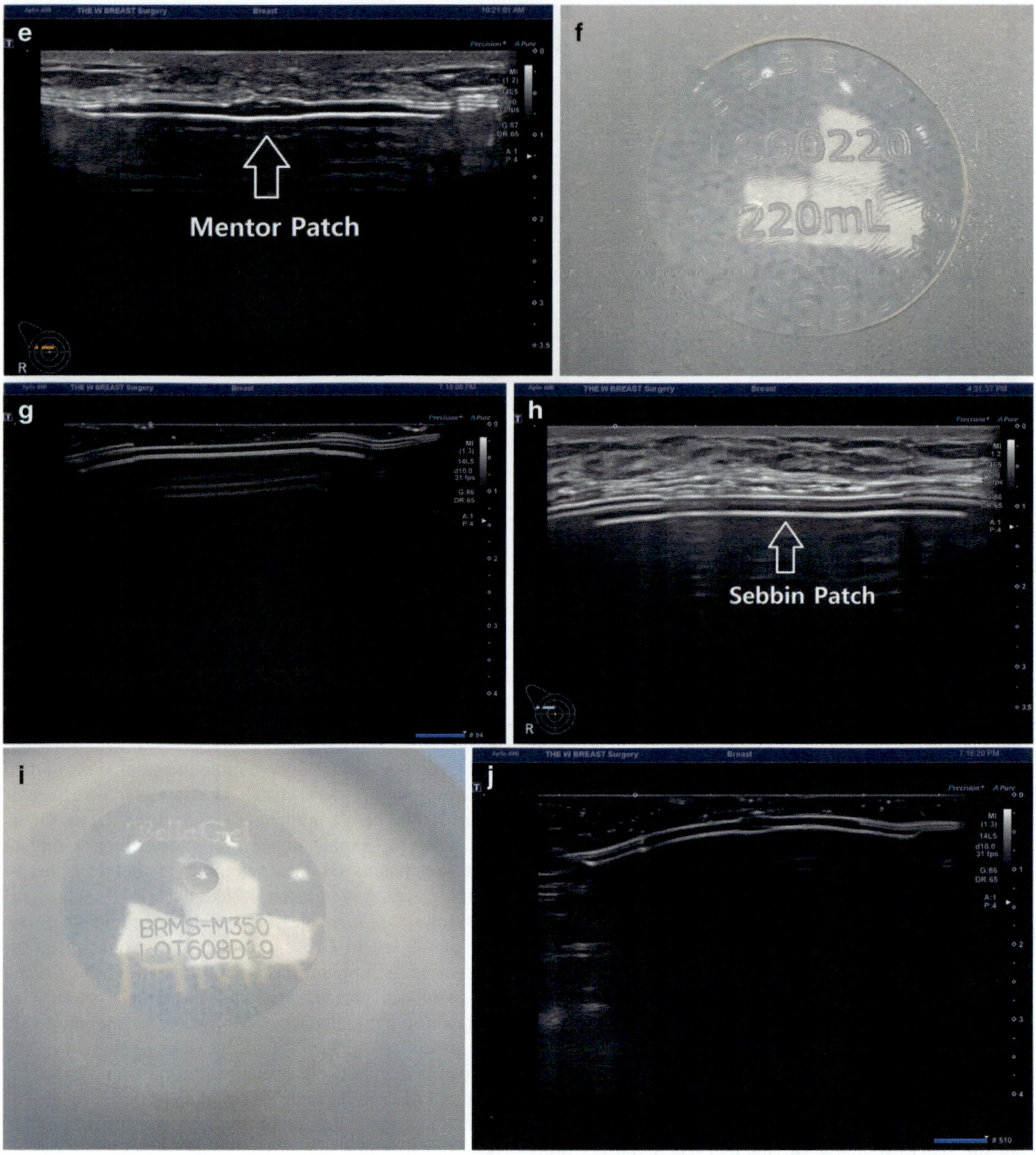

Fig. 5.23 (continued)

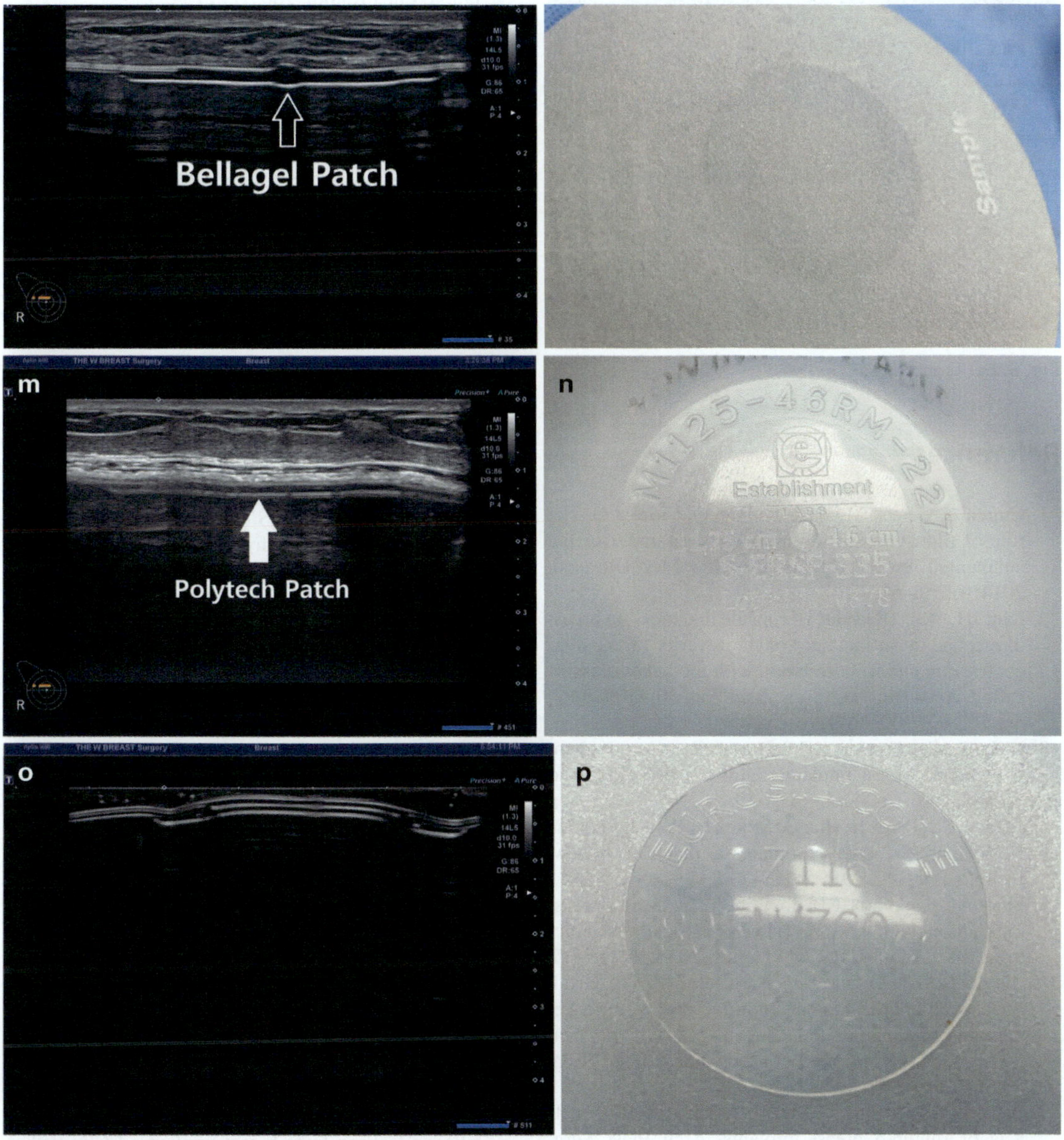

Fig. 5.23 (continued)

Fig. 5.23 (continued)

References

1. Ciurea A, Gersak M, Onoe R, Ivan O, Ciortea C. The role of ultrasound in the imaging assessment of the augmented breast. A pictorial review Med Ultrason. 2014;16:256–61.
2. Kim JH, et al. The value of capsule thickness on breast ultrasound as an indicator of the severity of capsular contracture and its correlation with the baker classification. Aesthetic Plast Surg. 2021 Aug 30; https://doi.org/10.1007/s00266-021-02544-5.
3. Hillard C, Fowler JD, Barta R, Cunningham B. Silicone breast implant rupture: a review. Gland Surg. 2017;6:163–8.
4. Juanpere S, Perez E, Huc O, Motos N, Pont J, Pedraza S. Imaging of breast implants-a pictorial review. Insights Imaging. 2011;2:653–70.
5. Shah AT, Jankharia BB. Imaging of common breast implants and implant- 21 related complications: a pictorial essay. Indian J Radiol Imaging. 2016;26:216–25.
6. Zingaretti N, Fasano D, Baruffaldi PFW, et al. Suspected breast implant rupture: our experience, recommendations on its management and a proposal for a model of informed consent. Eur J Plast Surg. 2020;43:569–76.
7. Baek WY, Lew DH, Lee DW. A retrospective analysis of ruptured breast implants. Arch Plast Surg. 2014;41:734–9.
8. Yang N, Muradali D. The augmented breast: a pictorial review of the abnormal and unusual. AJR Am J Roentgenol. 2011;196:W451–60.
9. Wong T, Lo LW, Fung PY, et al. Magnetic resonance imaging of breast augmentation: a pictorial review. Insights Imaging. 2016;7:399–410.
10. Hölmich LR, Vejborg I, Conrad C, Sletting S, McLaughlin JK. The diagnosis of breast implant rupture: MRI findings compared with findings at explantation. Eur J Radiol. 2005;53:213–25.
11. Berg WA, Caskey CI, Hamper UM, et al. Diagnosing breast implant rupture with MR imaging, US, and mammography. Radiographics. 1993;13:1323–36.
12. Bengtson BP, Eaves FF 3rd. High-resolution ultrasound in the detection of silicone gel breast implant shell failure: background, in vitro studies, and early clinical results. Aesthet Surg J. 2012;32:157–74.
13. Dragoumis DM, Assimaki AS, Vrizas TI, Tsiftsoglou AP. Axillary silicone lymphadenopathy secondary to augmentation mammaplasty. Indian J Plast Surg. 2010;43:206–9.
14. Klang E, Amitai MM, Raskin S, et al. Association between enlarged axillary lymph nodes and silicone breast implant ruptures seen on magnetic resonance imaging. Isr Med Assoc J. 2016;18:719–24.
15. Berg WA, Nguyen TK, Middleton MS, Soo MS, Pennello G, Brown SL. MR imaging of extracapsular silicone from breast implants: diagnostic pitfalls. AJR Am J Roentgenol. 2002;178:465–72.
16. Lee Y, Song SE, Yoon ES, Bae JW, Jung SP. Extensive silicone lymphadenopathy after breast implant insertion mimicking malignant lymphadenopathy. Ann Surg Treat Res. 2017;93:331–5.
17. Zambacos GJ, Molnar C, Mandrekas AD. Silicone lymphadenopathy after breast augmentation: case reports, review of the literature, and current thoughts. Aesthet Plast Surg. 2013;37:278–89.
18. Dragoumis DM, Assimaki AS, Vrizas TI, Tsiftsoglou AP. Axillary silicone lymphadenopathy secondary to augmentation mammaplasty. Indian J Plast Surg. 2010;43:206–9.
19. Omakobia E, Porter G, Armstrong S, Denton K. Silicone lymphadenopathy: an unexpected cause of neck lumps. J Laryngol Otol. 2012;126:970–3.
20. Adams ST, Cox J, Rao GS. Axillary silicone lymphadenopathy presenting with a lump and altered sensation in the breast: a case report. J Med Case Rep. 2009;3:6442.
21. Hausner RJ, Schoen FJ, Mendez-Fernandez MA, Henly WS, Geis RC. Migration of silicone gel to axillary lymph nodes after prosthetic mammoplasty. Arch Pathol Lab Med. 1981;105:371–2.
22. Van Diest PJ, Beekman WH, Hage JJ. Pathology of silicone leakage from breast implants. J Clin Pathol. 1998;51:493–7.
23. Tabatowski K, Elson CE, Johnston WW. Silicone lymphadenopathy in a patient with a mammary prosthesis. Fine needle aspiration cytology, histology and analytical electron microscopy. Acta Cytol. 1990;34:10–4.
24. Kulber DA, Mackenzie D, Steiner JH, Glassman H, Hopp D, et al. Monitoring the axilla in patients with silicone gel implants. Ann Plast Surg. 1995;35:580–4.

6 Breast Implant-Associated Anaplastic Large Cell Lymphoma

6.1 Overview

Both patients' safety and health-related quality of life are essential factors forming the highest priority in an implant-based augmentation mammaplasty [1]. In this context, surgeons, patients, and manufacturers of a breast implant should be aware of detrimental effects of breast implant-associated anaplastic large cell lymphoma (BIA-ALCL); it should be accurately diagnosed at the earliest opportunities possible [2]. Its onset has posed challenges to the safety of a breast implant, that with a textured surface in particular. It should be noted, however, that BIA-ALCL is an extremely rare disease entity with a good prognosis after explantation and capsulectomy [3, 4]. Continuous efforts should therefore be made to update the current treatment strategies for patients with BIA-ALCL.

6.2 A Vicious Circle of Crisis of a Breast Implant

To date, there has been a vicious circle of crisis of breast implant; it has been approved and then removed from the market [5]. This has threatened the safety of patients receiving a breast implant.

The first crisis happened in 1982, when the Dow Corning breast implant was reported to have a causal relationship with autoimmune diseases. In 2010, the second crisis happened in association with the Poly.

Implant Prothèse (PIP) implant that was found to be manufactured using a cheap, non-approved industrial-grade silicone. The number of patients with a past history of receiving the PIP implant was estimated at >600,000 in 65 countries [5].

Recently, the third crisis happened in association with a textured device whose causal relationship with the onset of BIA-ALCL has been well described in the literature [Temp. Ref. 6]. In December 2018, the CE mark for the Biocell and Microcell implants (Allergan, Irvine, CA) was suspended by the French Agency for the Safety of Health Products (ANSM). This has led to the removal of both products from 37 countries [7].

In April 2019, the use of all the macro-textured or polyurethane-coated breast implants was prohibited by the ANSM [7]. In the USA in May 2019, however, the Food and Drug Administration (FDA) issued the letter to the effect that there was no sufficient evidence demonstrating a causal relationship between a textured device and BIA-ALCL; it finally announced that it would not ban it.

As of January 5, 2020, the Food and Drug Administration (FDA) has received a total of 733 US and global medical device reports (MDRs) of breast implant-associated anaplastic large cell lymphoma (BIA-ALCL).

J. H. Kim, *Atlas of Breast Implant Ultrasound*, https://doi.org/10.1007/978-981-16-8282-7_6

6.3 Association Between the Onset of BIA-ALCL and a Textured Implant

It is widely known that the pathogenesis of BIA-ALCL may have a causal relationship with a textured implant, formation of bacterial biofilm, and genetic predispositions of a patient receiving a breast implant [8].

BIA-ALCL is an extremely rare, non-Hodgkin's lymphoma whose characteristics include abnormal growth of T lymphocytes and over-expression of protein cytokine receptor CD30. It annually occurs at an estimated incidence of approximately 3/100 million women in the USA [9]. Possible relationship between vulnerability to BIA-ALCL and placement of a textured breast implant was recently suggested. Ghione et al. prospectively enrolled a cohort of 3546 women receiving 6023 textured implants between 1993 and 2017, all of whom were surgically treated at a median age of 48 (range, 18–89) years old by the same single surgeon and then followed up during a median period of 7 (range, 3 days to 24.7 years). According to these authors, a total of 8 women developed BIA-ALCL after receiving textured implants during a median period of 11.2 (range, 8.3–15.8) years. The reported incidence corresponds to 1/433 women. According to these authors, 96.7% of textured implants were the BioCell (Allergan) [10].

6.4 Approaches to Risk Management for an Early Detection of BIA-ALCL

Currently, manufacturers of a breast implant face a crisis from the emergence of BIA-ALCL; they have been subject to myriads of external forces. To overcome this crisis, possible impacts of BIA-ALCL should be rigorously analyzed and appropriate measures should be taken as promptly as possible. Kim et al. propose the following approaches:

1. Patient data should be prospectively collected. By tracking outcomes and complications of an implant-based augmentation mammaplasty, both high-quality care and patient safety can be ensured.
2. Stakeholders in an implant-based augmentation mammaplasty should collaborate with customers and regulatory authorities.
3. Surgeons should consider applying imaging modalities to an early detection of complications of an implant-based mammaplasty. In this context, a multi-disciplinary, algorithm-based approach deserves special attention. In compliance with the National Comprehensive Cancer Network (NCCN) guidelines, it is recommended that patients with an enlarged breast undergo ultrasound at an initial work-up.

Thus, they should be evaluated for whether they have a fluid collection, a breast mass, or enlarged regional lymph nodes (axillary, supraclavicular, and internal mammary).

Figure 6.1 is 2019 NCCN consensus guidelines on the diagnosis and treatment of breast implant-associated anaplastic large cell lymphoma (BIA-ALCL) [11].

Moreover, it is mandatory to consider the possibility of BIA-ALCL in patients with seroma of non-infectious or non-traumatic origin with a duration of >1 year after an implant-based augmentation mammaplasty. In such patients, an ultrasound-guided fine-needle aspiration biopsy of seroma or surgical biopsy of capsule and seroma should be performed and then evaluated using immunohistochemistry for the purposes of establishing a diagnosis of BIA-ALCL. This should be followed by a positron emission tomography-computed tomography (PET/CT) for the prevention of regional or systemic spread. According to the NCCN, both capsulectomy and implant removal should be considered as first line of treatment for the appropriate management of the affected capsule and a resectable mass. Moreover, chemotherapy should also be performed for patients with an advanced stage of BIA-ALCL involving local lymph or organ metastasis [12].

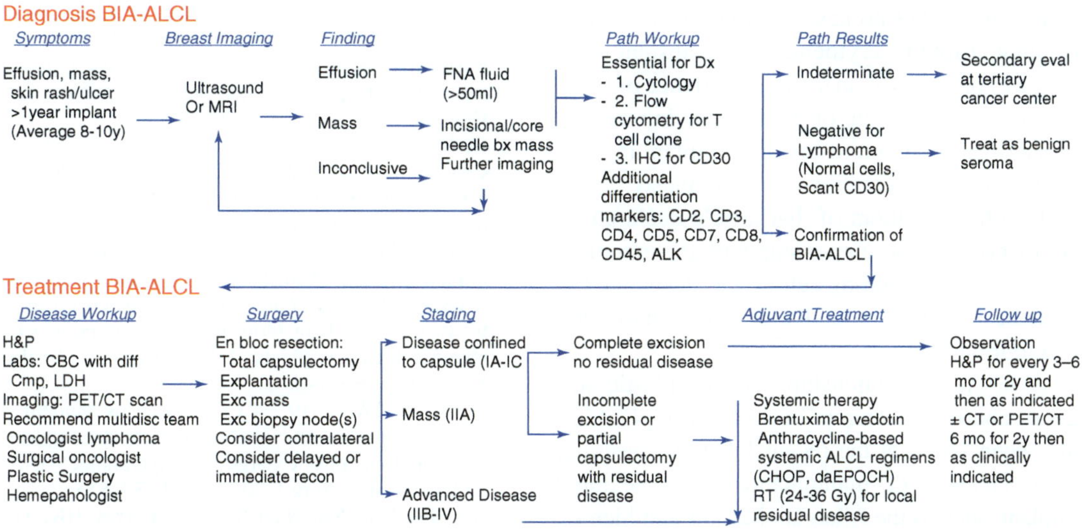

Fig. 6.1 NCCN Guidelines of BIA-ALCL

6.5 Conflict of Interest (COI) in Plastic Surgery and Its Possible Involvement in Crisis of Stakeholders in an Implant-Based Augmentation Mammaplasty

COI is referred to a condition in which professional decision-making in research, involving a primary interest (e.g., patients' safety or welfare or the validity of its design or outcomes) is prone to influence by a secondary one (e.g., financial benefit) [13]. To date, concerns have been raised regarding its potential impacts on patient care, clinical practice and biomedical research; this has been well described in the literature [14, 15].

In the USA in 2007, biomedical and clinical studies were sponsored by industry, and the amount of funding exceeded USD 58 billion. But federal and private foundations paid only USD 36 billion for studies [16]. Moreover, there was a decrease in the amount of federal funding, but that of industrial one rose from 32% to 62% between 1980 and 2000 [17]. As a result, industry-sponsorship has become such a pivotal source of research funding that it has contributed to promoting the delivery of healthcare services and improving treatment outcomes [18]. This is closely associated with the fact that most of the industry-sponsored studies have shown positive findings about their products [19–24].

Disadvantages of shaped breast implants include a high rate of malrotation (42%), palpable margins, the possibility of causing double capsule and seroma, and high cost as compared with their smooth round counterparts [25, 26]. Moreover, a high degree of vulnerability to BIA-ALCL and a lack of aesthetic advantage have also been reported to be problems due to the use of textured breast implants [27–30].

Over decades, however, textured, shaped implants have been reported to be better as compared with their lower-cost counterparts. This is in agreement with a previously published study showing that some plastic surgeons form a favorable relationship with manufacturers of a textured, shaped breast implant and are misled by them [31].

According to Swanson and Brown, the relationship with manufacturers of a breast implant could also be found in an industry-sponsored peer-reviewed article [27]. The authors of that article reported that complications (only one case of hematoma but no cases of malposition, pain, rippling, rupture, erythema, and capsular contracture) occurred at an overall incidence of 0.3% and a reoperation rate of <1% following the use of nano-textured, micro-textured implant in 4103 cases of augmentation mammaplasty [28]. Although the authors of that article declared no conflict of interest relationship with the manufacturer, the corresponding author was designated as a medical advisor immediately after submission to a journal [27].

A favorable relationship between plastic surgeons and manufacturers of a breast implant has also been found at the recent US FDA meeting; representatives of manufactures of a textured implant, such as the Allergan, Mentor and Sientra, maintained that their devices remained commercially available, and plastic surgeons did not recommend that such products be banned from the market [29]. Swanson lamented that plastic surgeons in the USA defended a textured implant, who formerly advocated the use of ultrasound as a first line of screening tool for BIA-ALCL [30, 32].

References

1. Pusic AL, Chen CM, Cano S, et al. Measuring quality of life in cosmetic and reconstructive breast surgery: a systematic review of patient-reported outcomes instruments. Plast Reconstr Surg. 2007;120(4):823–39.
2. Calobrace MB, Schwartz MR, Zeidler KR, et al. Long-term safety of textured and smooth breast implants. Aesthet Surg J. 2017;38:38–48.
3. Mehta-Shah N, Clemens MW, Horwitz SM. How I treat breast implant-associated anaplastic large cell lymphoma. Blood. 2018;132(18):1889–98.
4. Fitzal F, Turner SD, Kenner L. Is breast implant-associated anaplastic large cell lymphoma a hazard of breast implant surgery? Open Biol. 2019;9(4):190006.
5. Deva AK, Cuss A, Magnusson M, Cooter R. The "game of implants": perspective on the crisis-prone history of breast implants. Aesthet Surg J. 2019;39(Suppl_1):S55–65.
6. Collett DJ, Rakhorst H, Lennox P, Magnusson M, Cooter R, Deva AK. Current risk estimate of breast implant-associated anaplastic large cell lymphoma in textured breast implants. Plast Reconstr Surg. 2019;143(3S A Review of Breast Implant-Associated Anaplastic Large Cell Lymphoma):30S–40S.
7. Munhoz AM, Clemens MW, Nahabedian MY. Breast implant surfaces and their impact on current practices: where we are now and where are we going? Plast Reconstr Surg Glob Open. 2019;7(10):e2466.
8. Rastogi P, Deva AK, Prince HM. Breast implant-associated anaplastic large cell lymphoma. Curr Hematol Malig Rep. 2018;13:516–24.
9. Berlin E, Singh K, Mills C, Shapira I, Bakst RL, Chadha M. Breast implant-associated anaplastic large cell lymphoma: case report and review of the literature. Case Rep Hematol. 2018;2018:2414278.
10. Cordeiro PG, Ghione P, Ni A, et al. Risk of breast implant associated anaplastic large cell lymphoma (BIA-ALCL) in a cohort of 3546 women prospectively followed long term after reconstruction with textured breast implants. J Plast Reconstr Aesthet Surg. 2020;73(5):841–6.
11. Clemens MW. 2019 NCCN consensus guidelines on the diagnosis and treatment of breast implant-associated anaplastic large cell lymphoma (BIA-ALCL). Aesthet Surg J. 2019;39(S1):S3–S13.
12. Kim JH, Paik NS, Nam SY, Cho Y, Park HK. The emerging crisis of stakeholders in implant-based augmentation mammaplasty in Korea. J Korean Med Sci. 2020;35(15):e103.
13. Thompson DF. Understanding financial conflicts of interest. N Engl J Med. 1993;329:573–6.
14. Dunn AG, Coiera E, Mandl KD, Bourgeois FT. Conflict of interest disclosure in biomedical research: a review of current practices, biases, and the role of public registries in improving transparency. Res Integr Peer Rev. 2016;1:1.
15. Fabbri A, Parker L, Colombo C, et al. Industry funding of patient and health consumer organisations: systematic review with meta-analysis. BMJ. 2020;368:16925.
16. Dorsey ER, de Roulet J, Thompson JP, et al. Funding of US biomedical research, 2003-2008. JAMA. 2010;303:137–43.
17. Moses H III, Martin JB. Academic relationships with industry: a new model for biomedical research. JAMA. 2001;285:933–5.
18. Santilli J, Vogenberg FR. Key strategic trends that impact healthcare decision-making and stakeholder roles in the new marketplace. Am Health Drug Benefits. 2015;8(1):15–20.
19. Friedman LS, Richter ED. Relationship between conflicts of interest and research results. J Gen Intern Med. 2004;19:51–6.
20. Peppercorn J, Blood E, Winer E, Partridge A. Association between pharmaceutical involvement and outcomes in breast cancer clinical trials. Cancer. 2007;109:1239–46.
21. Bhandari M, Busse JW, Jackowski D, et al. Association between industry funding and statistically significant pro-industry findings in medical and surgical randomized trials. CMAJ. 2004;170:477–80.
22. Kjaergard LL, Als-Nielsen B. Association between competing interests and authors' conclusions: Epidemiological study of randomized clinical trials published in the BMJ. BMJ. 2002;325:249.

23. Leopold SS, Warme WJ, Fritz Braunlich E, Shott S. Association between funding source and study outcome in orthopaedic research. Clin Orthop Relat Res. 2003;415:293–301.
24. Brown A, Kraft D, Schmitz SM, et al. Association of industry sponsorship to published outcomes in gastrointestinal clinical research. Clin Gastroenterol Hepatol. 2006;4:1445–51.
25. Sieber DA, Stark RY, Chase S, Schafer M, Adams WP Jr. Clinical evaluation of shaped gel breast implant rotation using high-resolution ultrasound. Aesthet Surg J. 2017;37(3):290–6.
26. Hall-Findlay EJ. Breast implant complication review: double capsules and late seromas. Plast Reconstr Surg. 2011;127(1):56–66.
27. Swanson E, Brown T. A discussion of conflicts of interest in plastic surgery and possible remedies. Plast Reconstr Surg Glob Open. 2018;6(12):e2043.
28. Sforza M, Zaccheddu R, Alleruzzo A, Seno A, Mileto D, Paganelli A, et al. Preliminary 3-year evaluation of experience with SilkSurface and VelvetSurface Motiva silicone breast implants: a single-center experience with 5813 consecutive breast augmentation cases. Aesthet Surg J. 2018;38(suppl_2):S62–73.
29. Swanson E. Plastic surgeons defend textured breast implants at 2019 U.S. Food and Drug Administration Hearing: why it is time to reconsider. Plast Reconstr Surg Glob Open. 2019;7(8):e2410.
30. Swanson E. The expanding role of diagnostic ultrasound in plastic surgery. Plast Reconstr Surg Glob Open. 2018;6(9):e1911.
31. Hall-Findlay EJ. Discussion: late seromas and breast implants: theory and practice. Plast Reconstr Surg. 2012;130(2):436–8.
32. Swanson E. The textured breast implant crisis: a call for action. Ann Plast Surg. 2019;82:593–4.

7 Usefulness of High-Resolution Ultrasound (HRUS) in Planning Revision or Reoperation for Patients Receiving an Implant-Based Augmentation Mammaplasty

7.1 Overview

Despite the popularity of augmentation mammaplasty, reoperation after primary augmentation remains a serious issue. There is a gradual time-dependent increase in its rate; it rises from 10% by 2 years and reaches approximately 20% by 6–10 years postoperatively [1–4]. Reoperation after primary augmentation mammaplasty is commonly performed due to reasons, such as rupture, capsular contracture (CC), implant malposition, and a patient's wish to change the size or shape of a breast implant [1, 2, 4]. In addition, other reasons for reoperation also include foreign body sensation, dissatisfaction with size, animation deformity, symmastia and neck and shoulder pain, fear of BIA-ALCL, fraud of Hansbiomed breast implant manufacturer [5–7].

7.2 Preoperative Considerations Based on HRUS for Reoperation

For successful reoperation or revisional surgery, surgeons should preoperatively consider the scope of pocket size, position, capsulectomy/capsulotomy (Fig. 7.1).

These important preoperative considerations can be easily achieved by preoperative high-resolution ultrasonography.

The following cases are commonly encountered in a clinical setting, which have incorrectly been planned for reoperation without HRUS.

1. Patients for whom reoperation was planned without an awareness of a breast implant information (shell type, shape type, manufacturer, etc.)
2. Patients for whom reoperation was planned because upside-down (USD) rotation was misdiagnosed as CC. Thick implant patch is misdiagnosed to CC.
3. Patients for whom reoperation was planned for capsulectomy for suspected presence of breast implant-associated anaplastic large cell lymphoma (BIA-ALCL) although they received a smooth device.
4. Patients for whom reoperation was planned at normal breast. The patient had a softened breast feeling d/t ruptured breast implant in contralateral breast. Then normal breast was misdiagnosed as CC.
5. Patients who have suspicious breast cancer symptoms, actually there were extracapsular siliconoma and axillary lymph node silicone invasion d/t silicone implant rupture.

HRUS-assisted reoperation should be performed in an algorithm-based manner, for which surgeons should consider factors associated with it.

Supplementary Information The online version contains supplementary material available at (https://doi.org/10.1007/978-981-16-8282-7_7).

J. H. Kim, *Atlas of Breast Implant Ultrasound*, https://doi.org/10.1007/978-981-16-8282-7_7

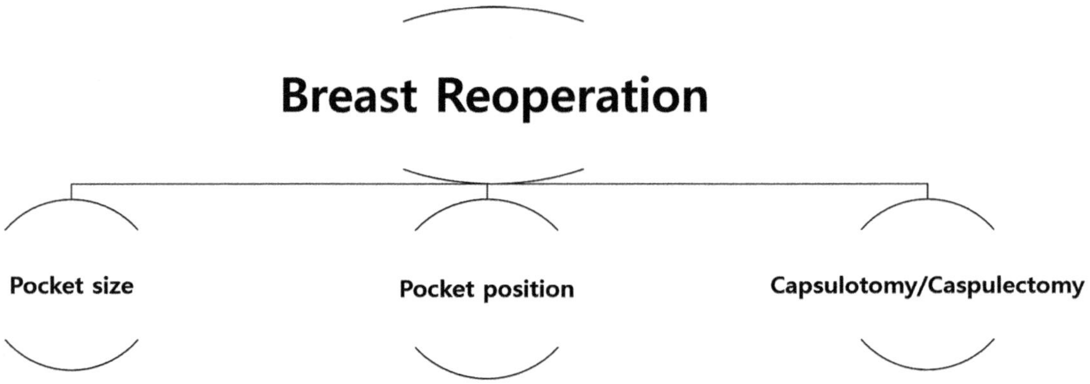

Fig. 7.1 Three point of reoperation plan

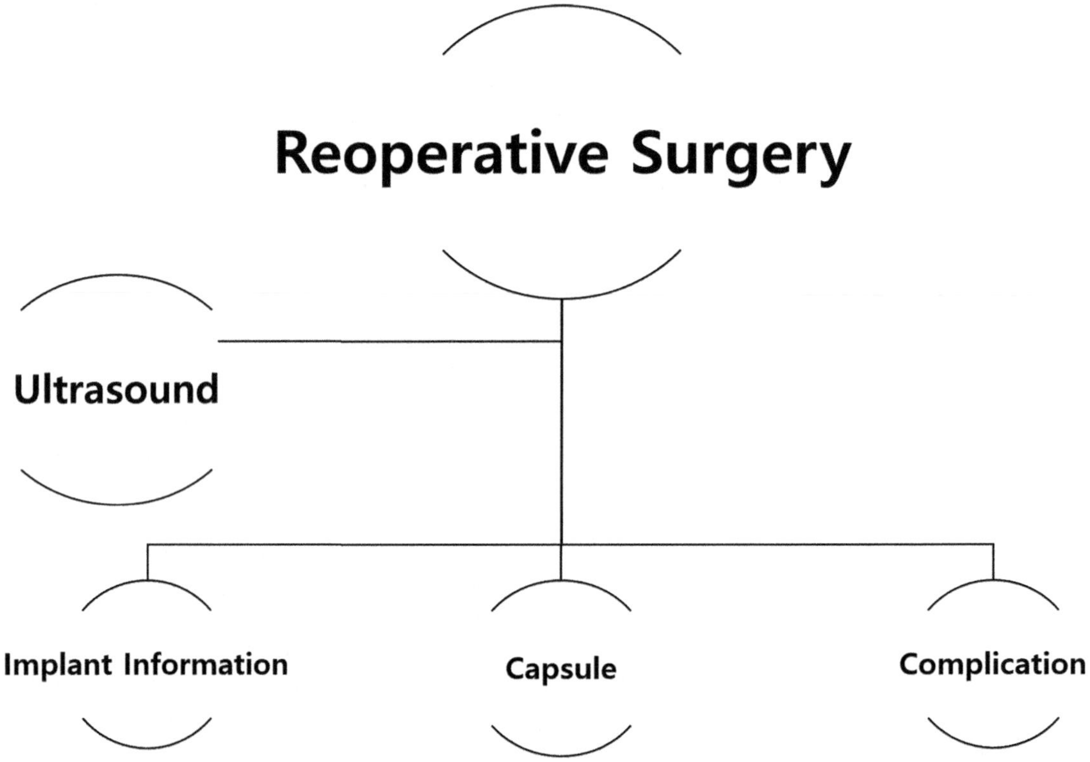

Fig. 7.2 Checkpoint of preoperative HRUS

Such factors include (1) the location of a pocket, (2) surface topography of the shell, (3) the status of a capsule, (4) implant-related complications, and (5) previous surgical approaches (Fig. 7.2). All of these factors are interrelated. That is, the status of a capsule is a determinant of whether a patient should undergo capsulectomy, based on which surgeons can predict implant-related complications and length of operation time. This is essential for making an accurate plan for reoperation or revisional surgery. Therefore, rupture deserves special attention as a serious implant-related complication.

7.3 An Algorithm-Based Approach to HRUS-Assisted Reoperation

7.3.1 Location of a Pocket

Patients complaining of dissatisfaction with shape or CC may require a change in the location of a pocket. In these patients, HRUS is a useful modality in examining whether a breast implant is placed above or below the pectoralis major muscle. Therefore, the location of a pocket cannot be accurately determined using the tactile sense of a surgeon.

The following two cases were treated with pocket position change using preoperative ultrasonography which shows subpectoral pocket (Figs. 7.3 and 7.4).

A 26-year-old woman complained of dissatisfaction with shape arising from a long nipple-to-inframammary fold (N-IMF) distance; the patient had a history of receiving an implant-based augmentation mammaplasty using a round textured device (Silimed Inc., Rio de Janeiro, Brazil; 390 cc) in the subpectoral pocket *via* a trans-axillary incision 2 years ago at other hospital.

But the patient received ultrasound-assisted reoperation using the BellaGel SmoothFine (BRMZ-H 325 cc) in the subglandular pocket *via* a previous axillary scar.

A 25-year-old woman complained of symmastia with a 0.8-cm distance between the two sides of the breast, who had a history of receiving an implant-based augmentation mammaplasty using the BellaGel SmoothFine (BRMZ-H 325 cc) in the subpectoral pocket *via* a trans-axillary incision 8 months ago.

The patient received endoscopy assisted reoperation by pocket position changes to the subglandular pocket *via* a previous axillary scar.

7.3.2 Surface Topography of the Shell of a Breast Implant

There were a total of three Korean cases of BIA-ALCL; it was reported on August 16 and December 24, 2019 and October 5, 2020. All of these three patients had a history of receiving an implant-based augmentation mammaplasty using a textured device (Allergan Inc., Irvine, CA). Therefore, the type of a breast implant should be identified based on its surface topography.

After the onset of the first case of BIA-ALCL in Korea, there were many patients who suffered from a difficulty in identifying characteristics of a breast implant they received; hospitals where they received a surgery did not exist or their medical records were missing. Of patients who were aware of characteristics of a breast implant they received, if ever, those receiving a textured device were in need of explantation or replacement of the device with other brands of a breast implant. There were also some patients who were in need of capsulectomy. But patients who were unaware of characteristics of a breast implant they received could not decide on how they are managed. Use of HRUS is a useful modality in confirming the type of shell and thereby providing information that is essential for planning a reoperation, such as explantation or capsulectomy, for them.

If a smooth breast implant can be identified on ultrasound, the corresponding patients would not be in need of explantation and capsulectomy and would not be concerned about a risk of BIA-ALCL.

HRUS-assisted characterization of a manufacturer of a breast implant is clinically useful due to the following reasons:

An anatomical breast implant can be identified based on its own specific orientation mark, based on which the corresponding manufacturer can be characterized. This may be a key clue to identification or characterization of the manufacturer to researchers in the field of breast implant, thus helping them study complications, including BIA-ALCL, that are specific to each manufacturer.

7.3.3 Status of a Capsule

One of the important points of plan for reoperation is to choose either capsulectomy or capsulotomy.

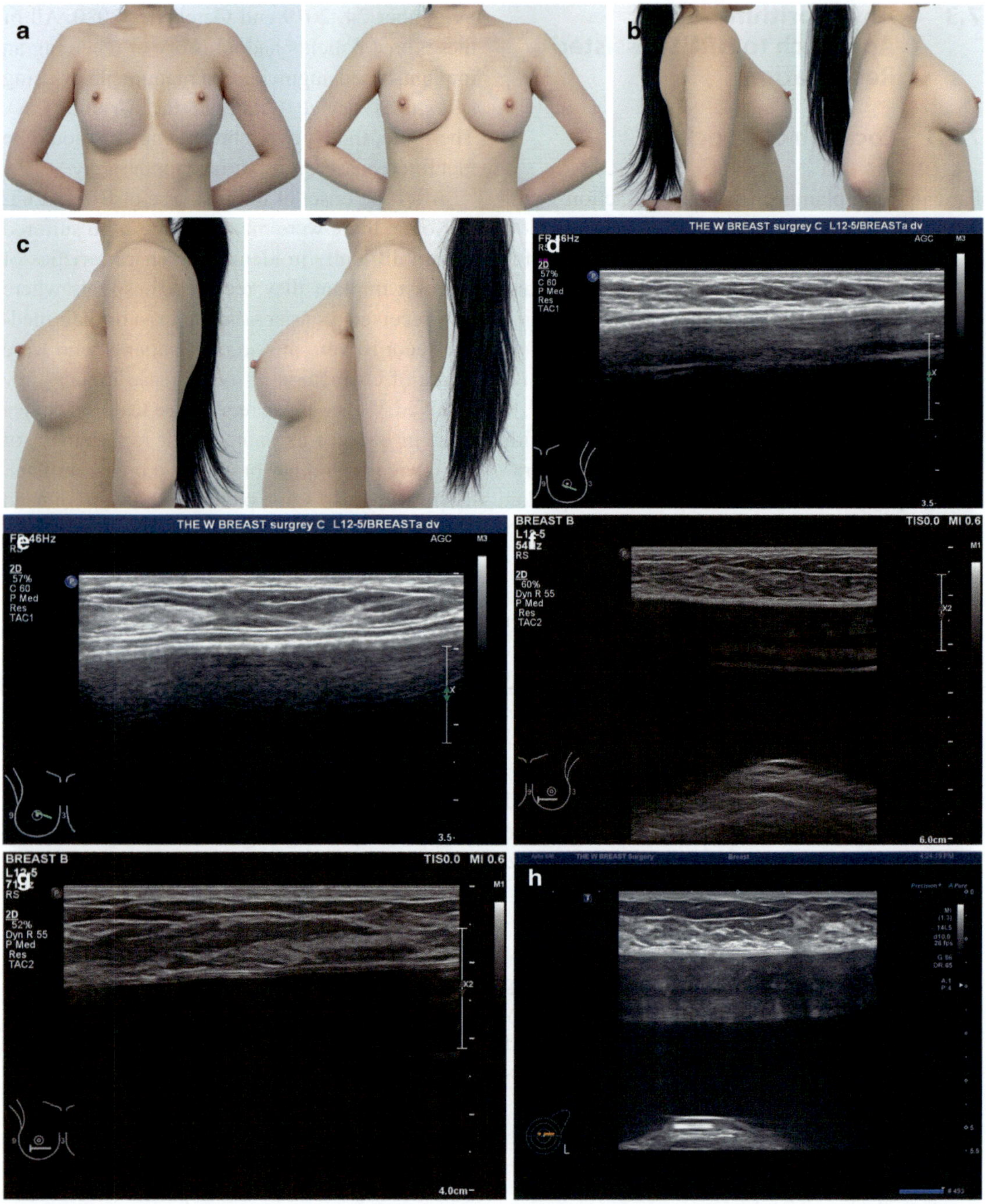

Fig. 7.3 (**A–C**) Preoperative and postoperative view, POD #1 yr. (**D**, **E**) Preoperative US finding. (**F–I**) Postoperative US finding: (a) front view, (b) right side view, (c) left side view, (d) left textured shell type breast implant in subpectoral pocket in preoperative sonography, (e) right textured shell type breast implant in subpectoral pocket in preoperative sonography, (f) left smooth shell type breast implant in subglandular pocket, POD #161, (g) right smooth shell type breast implant in subglandular pocket, POD #161, (h) left smooth shell type breast implant in subglandular pocket, POD #341, (i) right smooth shell type breast implant in subglandular pocket, POD #34

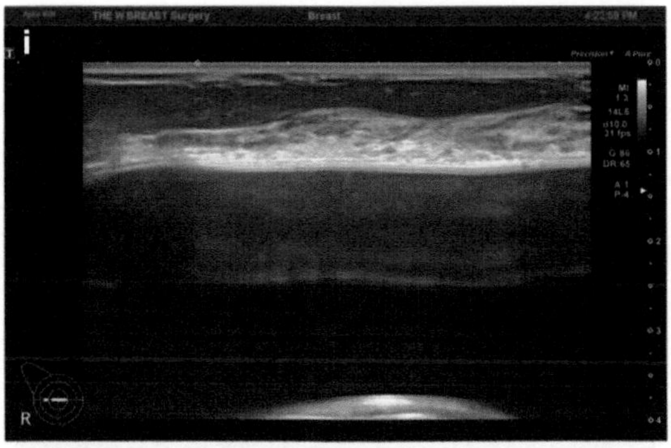

Fig. 7.3 (continued)

If HRUS confirms the presence of thickened capsule following the onset of CC, it becomes possible to inform patients of the importance of capsulectomy. This may also explain the reasons that no capsulectomy can be performed for patients with no thickened capsule or those receiving a smooth breast implant. If a surgeon preoperatively decides whether to perform capsulectomy or capsulotomy or not, this would be of great help for predicting and informing a patient of the possible occurrence of complications, adjusting the operation time and outpatient schedule and monitoring the postoperative course.

The following five cases display patients receiving capsulectomy at reoperation following the confirmation of thickened capsule on preoperative ultrasonography (Fig. 7.5 through 7.9).

A 42-year-old woman received the BellaGel SmoothFine (HansBiomed Co. Ltd, Seoul, Korea; BRMZ-H) (volume: 350 cc for the right breast and 325 cc for the left breast) in the subpectoral pocket *via* a trans-axillary incision 1 year ago. Due to the presence of thickened capsule, the patient underwent subtotal capsulectomy accompanied by replacement of the device with the BellaGel SmoothFine (BRMZ-H) (volume: 350 cc for the right breast and 325 cc for the left breast) in the subpectoral pocket *via* a previous trans-axillary incision.

Preoperatively, the patient had a thickened capsule measuring as 1.1 and 2.3 mm in the left breast on HRUS (Fig. 7.5).

A 53-year-old woman received the Mentor saline-filled breast implant with a round shape and a smooth surface (volume: 225 cc for the right breast and 250 cc for the left breast) in the subpectoral pocket *via* a trans-axillary incision 12 years ago. Due to the presence of thickened capsule, the patient underwent subtotal capsulectomy accompanied by replacement of the device with the Sebbin Sublimity (Groupe Sebbin SAS, Boissy-l' Aillerie, France; LS 71) (volume: 350 cc) in the subpectoral pocket *via* a previous trans-axillary incision.

Preoperatively, the patient had a thickened capsule measuring as 1.5 mm in the left breast on HRUS (Fig. 7.6).

A 50-year-old woman received a textured shell type saline-filled breast implant with a (volume: 120 cc) in the subpectoral pocket *via* a peri-areolar incision 8 years ago at other hospital.

The patient underwent reoperation with both subtotal capsulectomy accompanied by replacement of the device with the BellaGel SmoothFine (BRMZ-H,275 cc) in the subpectoral pocket *via* a previous peri-areolar incision due to capsular contracture (presence of thickened capsule).

Preoperatively, the patient had textured shell type breast implant placed with thickened periprosthetic capsule in the subpectoral pocket in both breasts on HRUS (Fig. 7.7).

A 45-year-old woman received the Silimed anatomical breast implant (volume: 275 cc) in the subglandular pocket *via* a trans-axillary incision in both breasts 5 years ago at other hospital. Due to the presence of thickened capsule, the patient underwent endoscopy assisted subtotal capsulectomy accompanied by replacement of the device with the Motiva Ergonomix ™ Round Silk Surface (volume: 450 cc) in the subpectoral pocket *via* a previous trans-axillary incision.

Preoperatively, the patient had a device placed in the subglandular pocket in both breasts, as identified by the orientation mark. Moreover, the patient also had a thickened capsule in the left breast accompanied by the folded shell despite the presence of the normal capsule in the right breast on HRUS (Fig. 7.8).

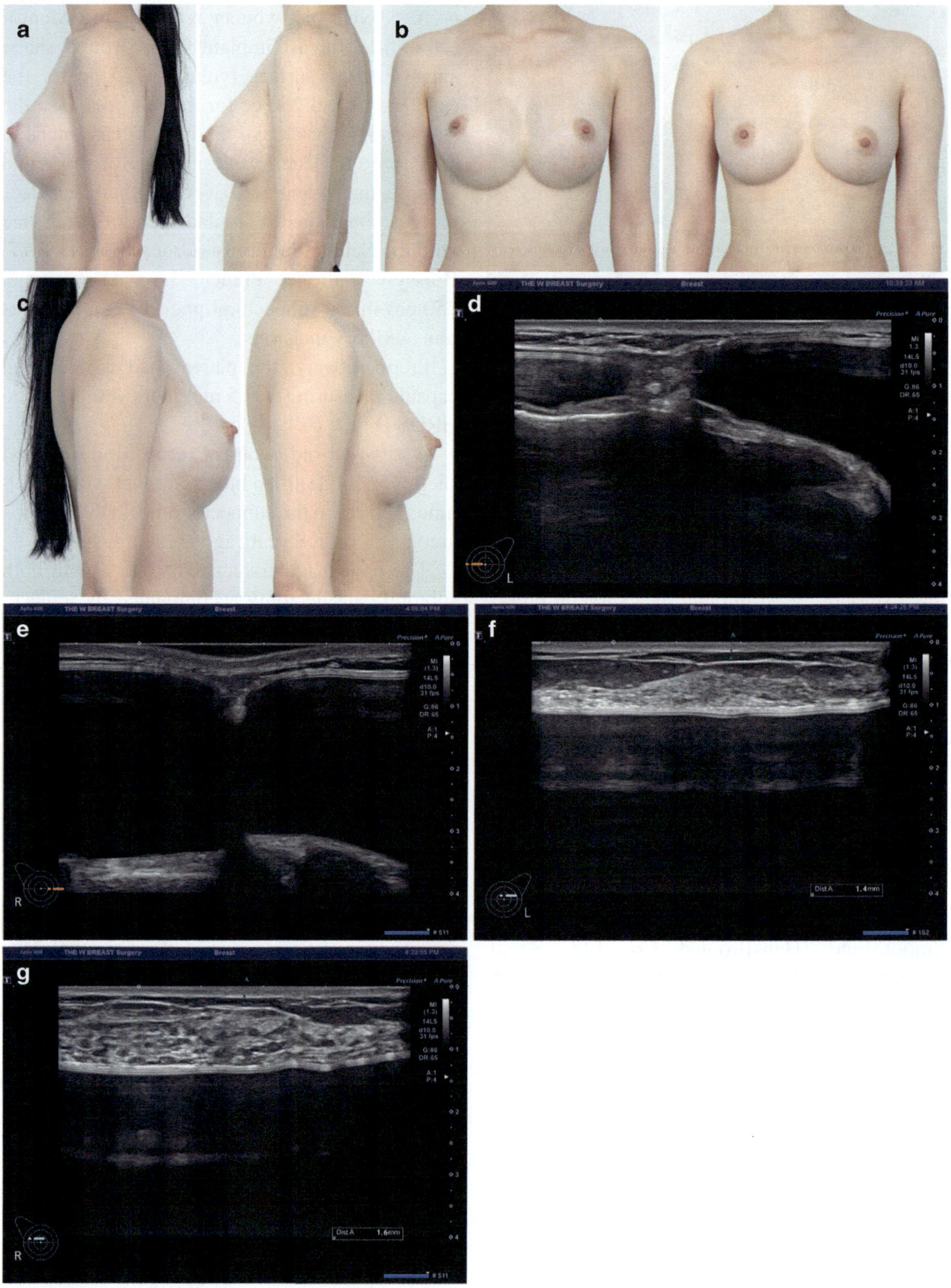

Fig. 7.4 (**A–C**) Preoperative and postoperative view, POD #446. (**D**, **E**) Preoperative ultrasonography. (**F**, **G**) Postoperative ultrasonography: (a) Front view, (b) right side view, (c) left side view, (d) 0.8 cm distance between both breast implant, (e) symmastia sign is checked in pre-operative ultrasonography, (f) left smooth shell type breast implant in subglandular pocket in postoperative US, POD #446, (g) Right smooth shell type breast implant in subglandular pocket in postoperative US, POD #446

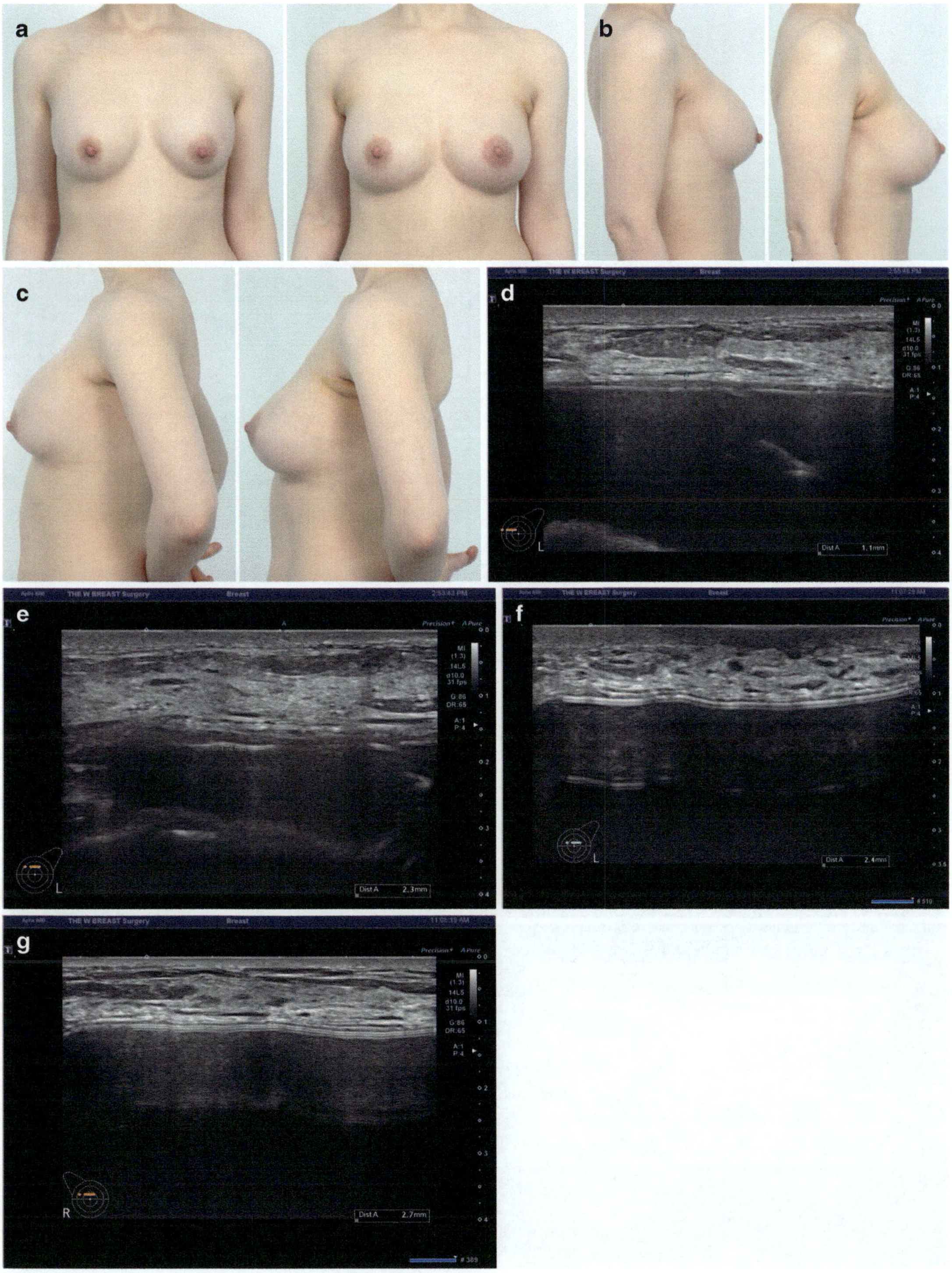

Fig. 7.5 (**A–C**) Preoperative and postoperative view, POD #1 yr. (**D, E**) Preoperative US finding. (**F, G**) Postoperative US finding, POD #72: (a) Front view, (b) right side view, (c) left side view, (d) left thickened capsule, 1.1 mm, is checked in preoperative sonography, (e) left thickened capsule, 2.3 mm, is checked in preoperative sonography, (f) left smooth shell type breast implant with normal periprosthetic capsule, POD #72, (g) right smooth shell type breast implant with normal periprosthetic capsule, POD #72

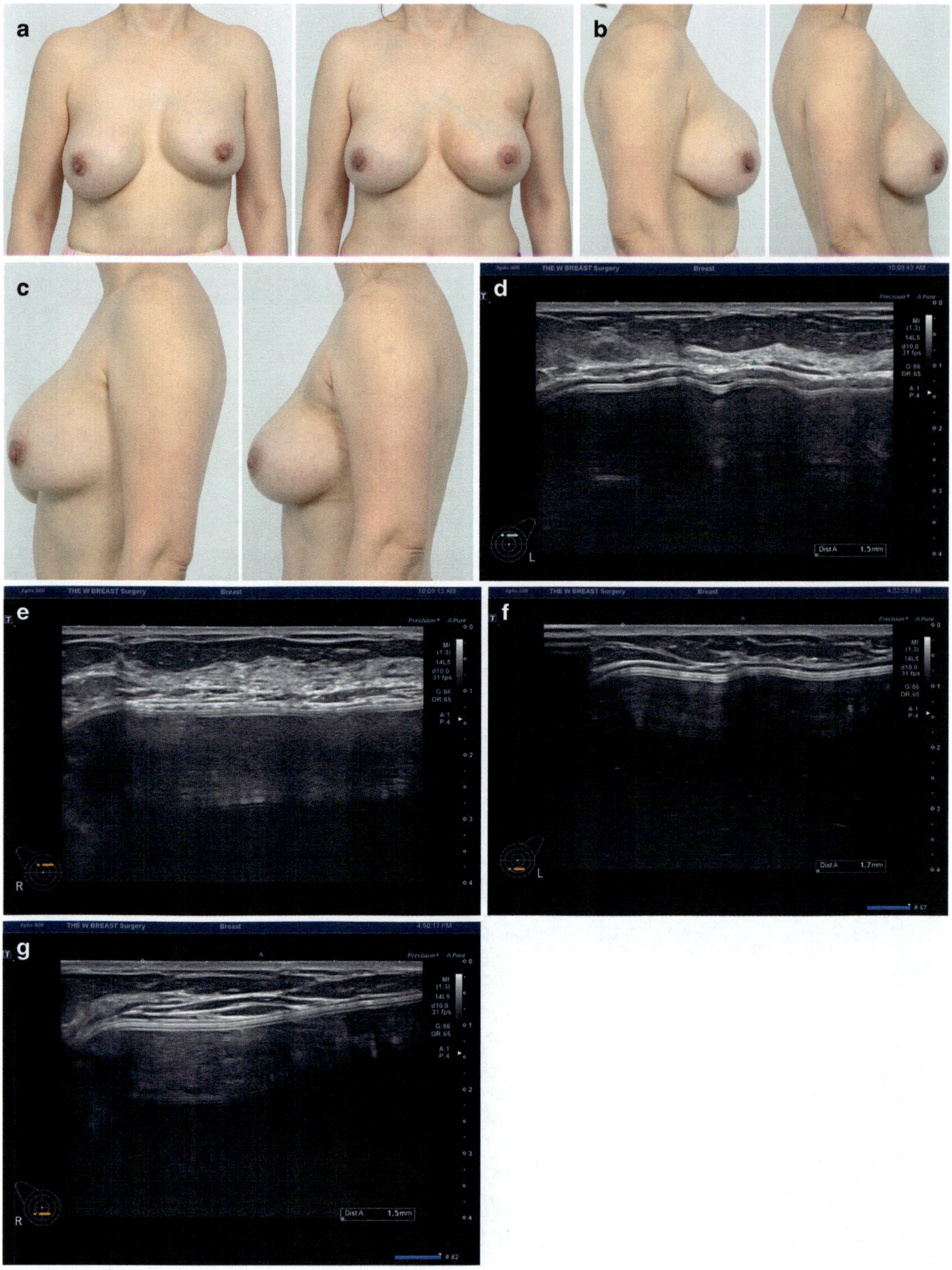

Fig. 7.6 (**A–C**) Preoperative and postoperative view, POD #365. (**D, E**) Preoperative US finding. (**F, G**) Postoperative US finding, POD #365: (a) front view, (b) right side view, (c) left side view, (d) left thickened capsule, 1.5 mm, is checked in preoperative sonography, (e) right smooth shell type breast implant with normal periprosthetic capsule is checked in preoperative sonography, (f) left smooth shell type breast implant with normal periprosthetic capsule, POD #365, (g) right smooth shell type breast implant with normal periprosthetic capsule, POD #365

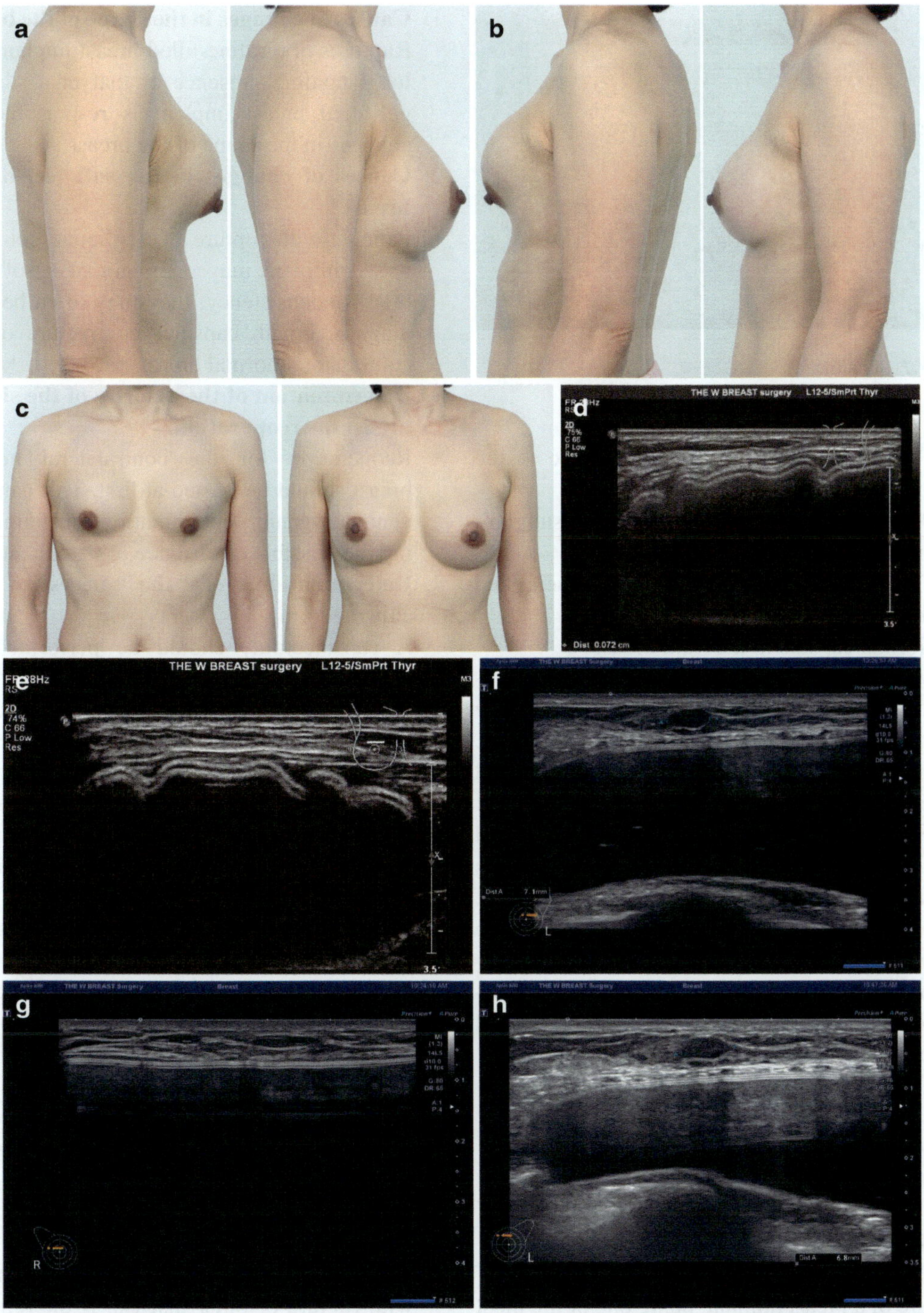

Fig. 7.7 (**A–C**) Preoperative and postoperative view, POD #189. (**D, E**) Preoperative US finding. (**F–I**) Postoperative US finding: (a) front view, (b) right side view, (c) left side view, (d) left thickened capsule, 1.5 mm, is checked in preoperative sonography, (e) right textured shell type breast implant with thickened periprosthetic capsule is checked in preoperative sonography, (f) left smooth shell type breast implant with normal periprosthetic capsule, POD #84, (g) right smooth shell type breast implant with normal periprosthetic capsule, POD #84, (h) left smooth shell type breast implant with normal periprosthetic capsule, POD #189, (i) right smooth shell type breast implant with normal periprosthetic capsule, POD #189

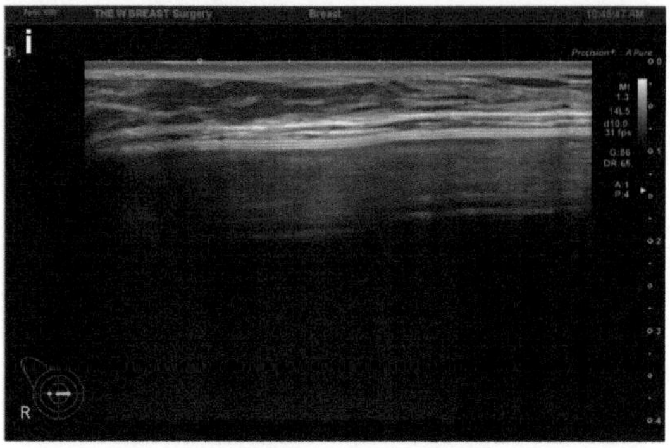

Fig. 7.7 (continued)

1. The orientation mark that is specific to the Silimed breast implant
2. Placement of a breast implant in the subglandular pocket in both breasts
3. Thickened capsule accompanied by the folded shell in the left breast
4. Normal capsule in the right breast

A 58-year-old woman visited shape deformity after explantation 1 year ago at other hospital. There were remnant thickened capsule and fluid collection in the subglandular pocket. The patient underwent subtotal capsulectomy accompanied by adhesiolysis. In this patient, the device was replaced with the Allergan anatomical type implant FX 350 cc in the subglandular pocket *via* a previous peri-areolar incision.

Preoperatively, the patient had both periprosthetic fluid collection and a remnant thickened capsule in both breasts on HRUS (Fig. 7.9).

7.3.4 Implant-Related Complications

7.3.4.1 Rupture

Preoperative ultrasound-assisted diagnosis of rupture of a breast implant, being one of the most common causes of reoperation, is a clinically useful strategy, and it is very important due to the following reasons:

1. **Causes of changes in the shape of the breast**
   Ruptures of a saline-filled breast implant or a long-standing presence of that of a silicone gel-filled breast implant is responsible for changes in the shape of the breast.
2. **Causes of changes in the soft feel of the breast**
   Patients with rupture of a silicone gel-filled breast implant may complain of a softened breast inconsistency; they may often be misdiagnosed with capsular contracture of the contralateral normal breast.
3. **Determination of the priority of the side of breast for reoperation**
   Reoperation for the contralateral normal breast should be started at first. This can prevent iatrogenic contamination and minimizing the possible occurrence of complications.
4. **Determination of the necessity for capsulectomy**
   A capsulectomy should be performed for patients with rupture of a silicone gel-filled breast implant presenting with an intracapsular infiltration of the silicone. In these cases, by predicting a prolonged operation time due to capsulectomy, outpatient schedule can be adjusted. Moreover, patients can be informed of the possibility of bleeding and seroma secondary to capsulectomy.
5. **Preparation of surgical instruments for operation**
   Preoperative information about presence of rupture is checked, it would be helpful to staff nurses who are in charge of operation preparation.
6. **Informed consent about possibility of residual silicone contents after reoperation**
   In extracapsular rupture with or without axillary lymph node silicone invasion, surgeon cannot eliminate all free silicone, then after the breast exam, patient can be misdiagnosed with rupture or other disease. If the remnant free silicone is recorded and informed to a patient, the possibility of misdiagnosis at future breast examinations can be minimized.

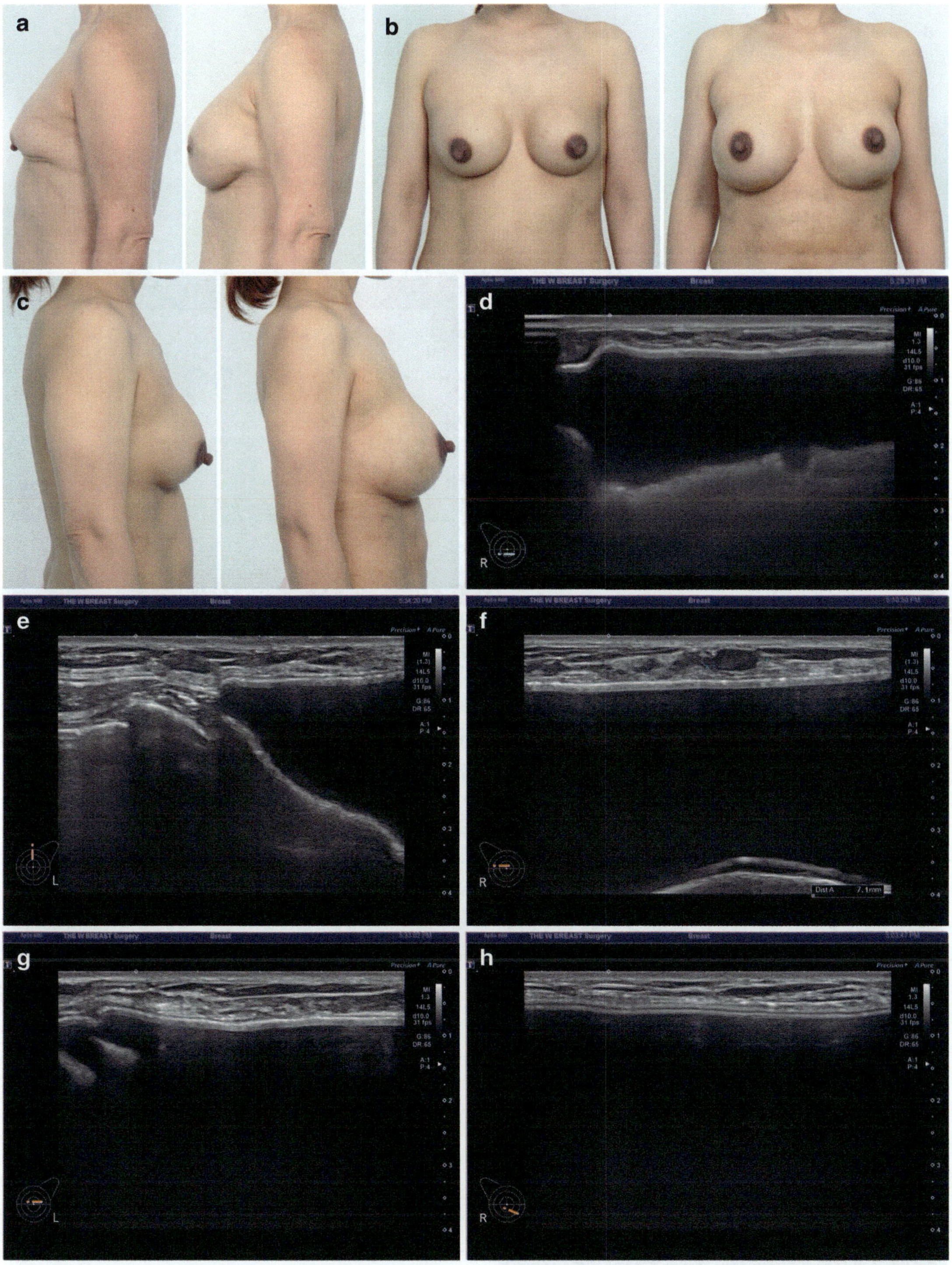

Fig. 7.8 (**A–C**) Preoperative and postoperative view, POD #180. (**D–G**) Preoperative US finding: (a) Front view, (b) right side view, (c) left side view, (d) inferior orientation dot of Silimed anatomical type breast implant is checked in preoperative sonography, (e) left breast implant in subglandular pocket is checked in preoperative sonography, (f) right textured shell type breast implant in subglandular pocket is checked in preoperative sonography, (g) folded shell of left breast implant is checked in preoperative sonography, (h) texture shell type breast implant with normal periprosthetic capsule

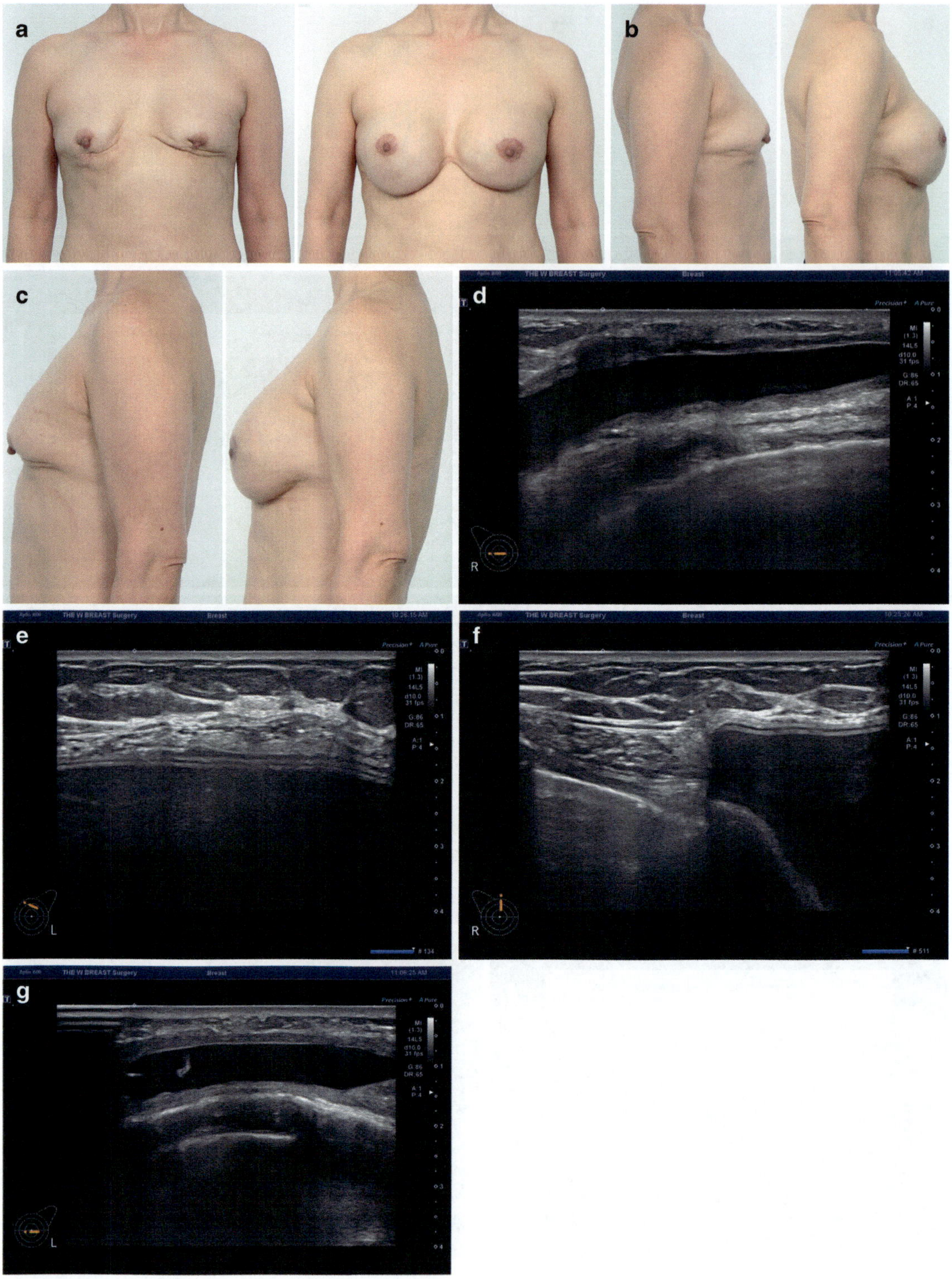

Fig. 7.9 (**A–C**) Preoperative and postoperative view (POD 15 month). (**D–G**) Preoperative US finding: (a) front view, (b) right side view, (c) left side view, (d) fluid collection and remnant thickened capsule in the left subglandular space are checked in preoperative sonography. There was no breast implant, (e) fluid collection and remnant thickened capsule in the right subglandular space are checked in preoperative sonography. There was no breast implant. (f) left breast implant with normal periprosthetic capsule is checked in postoperative sonography, (g) right breast implant with normal periprosthetic capsule in subglandular pocket in postoperative sonography

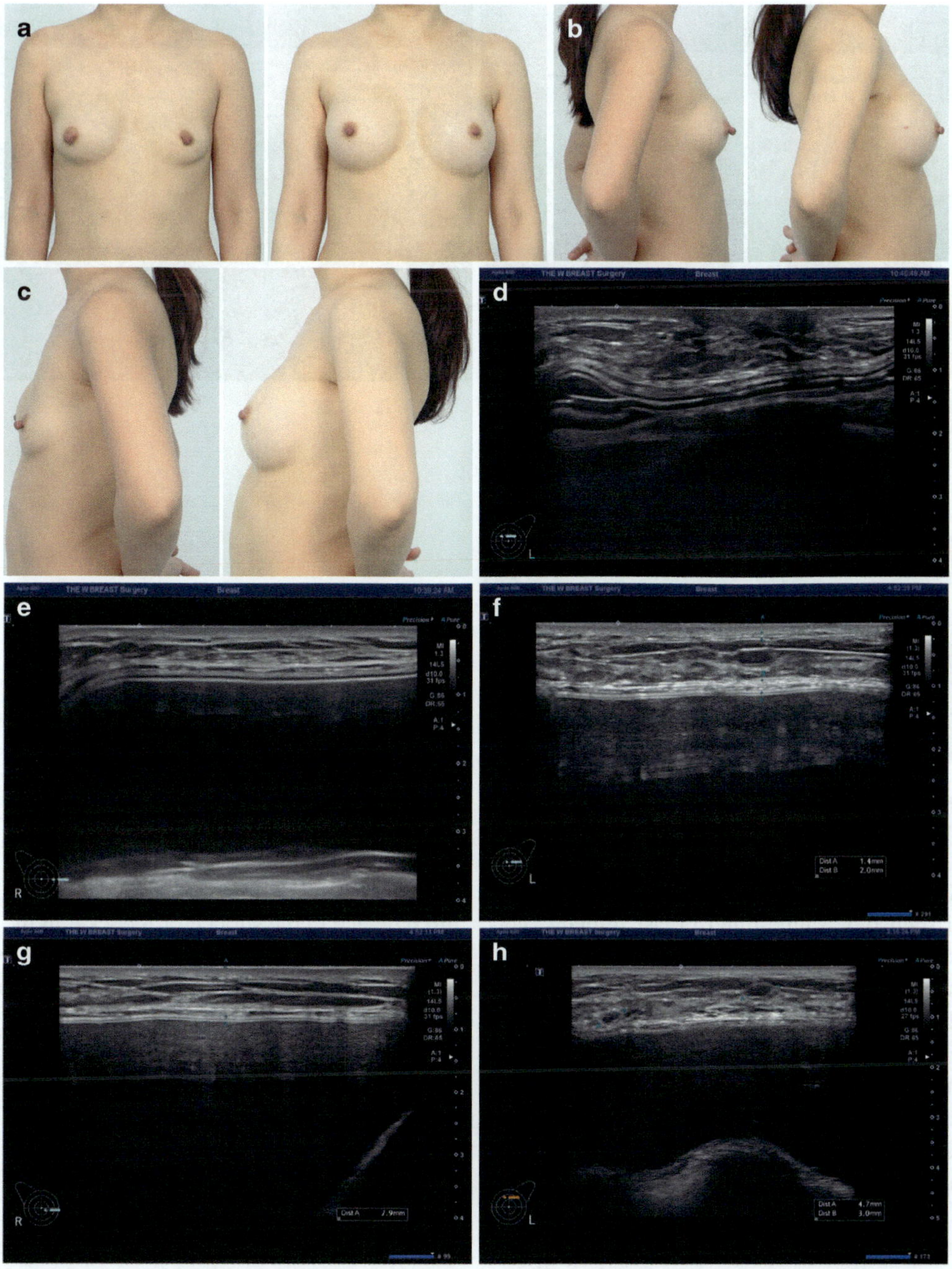

Fig. 7.10 (**A–C**) Preoperative and postoperative view, POD #1 yr. (**D, E**) Preoperative US finding. (**F–K**) Postoperative US finding: (a) front view, (b) right side view, (c) left side view, (d) Left ruptured saline breast implant is seen in preoperative sonography, (e) right normal round textured shell type breast implant in subpectoral pocket is checked in preoperative sonography, (f) left breast implant with normal periprosthetic capsule is checked in postoperative sonography, pod #89, (g) right breast implant with normal periprosthetic capsule in subpectoral pocket in postoperative sonography, pod #89, (h) left breast implant with normal periprosthetic capsule is checked in postoperative sonography, pod #178, (i) right breast implant with normal periprosthetic capsule in subpecotral pocket in postoperative sonography, pod #178, (j) left breast implant with normal periprosthetic capsule is checked in postoperative sonography, pod #367, (k) right breast implant with normal periprosthetic capsule in subpectoral pocket in postoperative sonography, pod #367

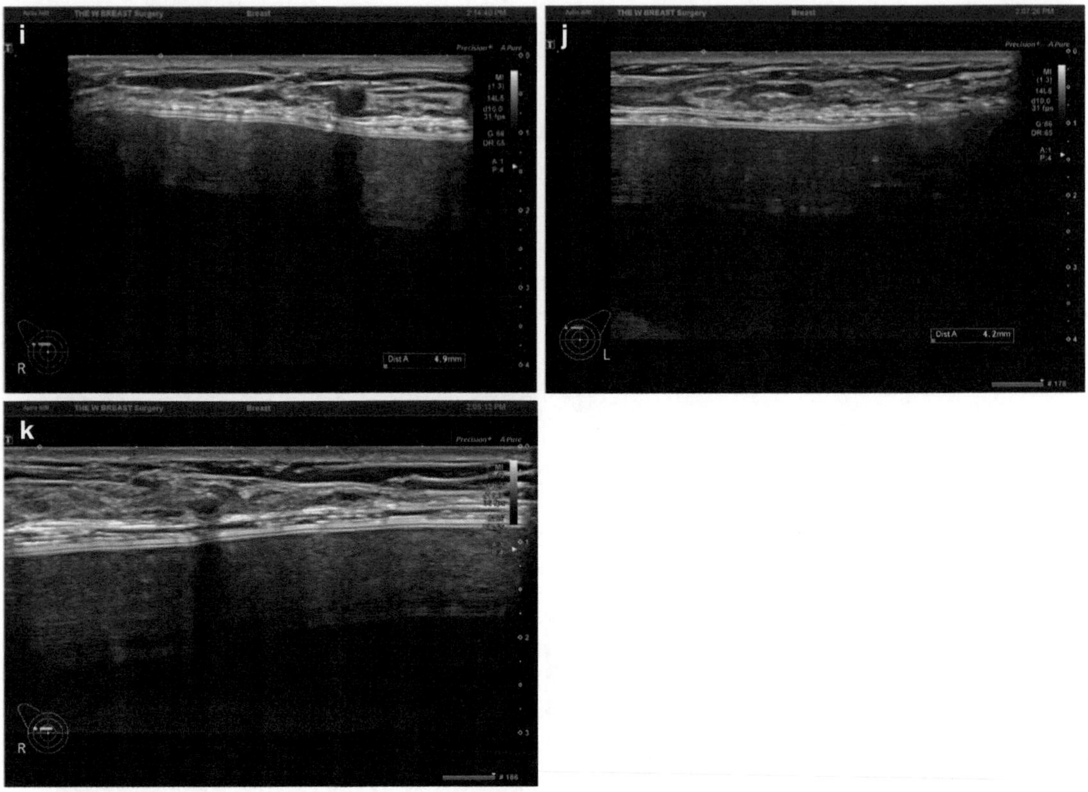

Fig. 7.10 (continued)

A 42-year-old woman had received round textured shell type saline-filled breast implant (volume: 200 cc) in the subpectoral pocket *via* trans-axillary incision 4 years ago at other hospital. Due to a rupture of left breast implant, the patient underwent endoscopy assisted subtotal capsulectomy accompanied by replacement of the device with the Motiva Ergonomix ™ Round Silk Surface (ERSF 315 cc) in the subpectoral pocket *via* a previous trans-axillary incision (Fig. 7.10).

A 44-year-old woman received a round, textured saline-filled breast implant (volume: 250 cc) in the subpectoral pocket *via* a trans-axillary incision 11 years ago at other hospital. Due to a rupture of the left breast implant, the patient underwent endoscopy assisted subtotal capsulectomy accompanied by replacement of the device with the BellaGel SmoothFine (BRMZ-H 375 cc) in the subpectoral pocket *via* a previous trans-axillary incision.

Preoperatively, the patient had a round, textured device in the subpectoral pocket in the right breast and a rupture of a saline-filled breast implant in the subpectoral pocket in the left breast on HRUS (Fig. 7.11).

A 50-year-old woman received a round, smooth shell type silicone gel-filled breast implant (220 cc) in the subpectoral pocket *via* a trans-axillary incision 15 years ago at other hospital. Due to both rupture of silicone gel-filled breast implant, the patient underwent endoscopy assisted subtotal capsulectomy accompanied by replacement of the device with the BellaGel SmoothFine (BRMZ-H 225 cc) in the subpectoral pocket *via* a previous trans-axillary incision.

Grossly, the patient had no notable findings but complained of alterations in the soft feel. Therefore, the patient received HRUS-assisted examination of the breast, rupture sign was checked in ultrasonography (Fig. 7.12).

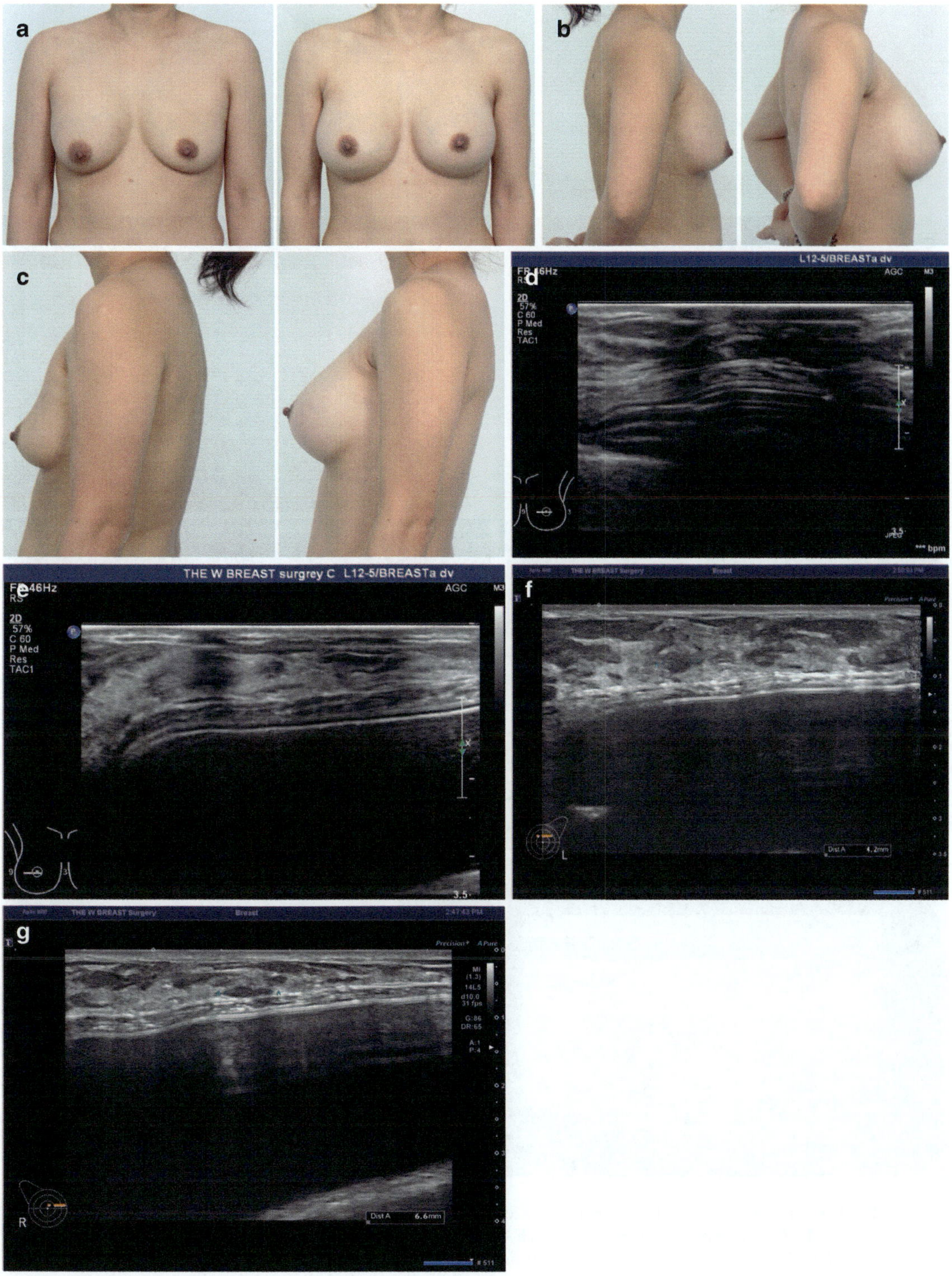

Fig. 7.11 (**A–C**) Preoperative and postoperative view (POD #268). (**D**, **E**) Preoperative US finding. (**F**, **G**) Postoperative US finding: (a) front view, (b) right side view, (c) left side view, (d) left ruptured saline breast implant in subpectoral pocket is checked in preoperative sonography, (e) right normal round textured shell type breast implant in subpectoral pocket is checked in preoperative sonography, (f) left smooth shell type breast implant with normal periprosthetic capsule is checked in postoperative sonography, pod #268, (g) right smooth shell type breast implant with normal periprosthetic capsule in subpectoral pocket in postoperative sonography, pod #268

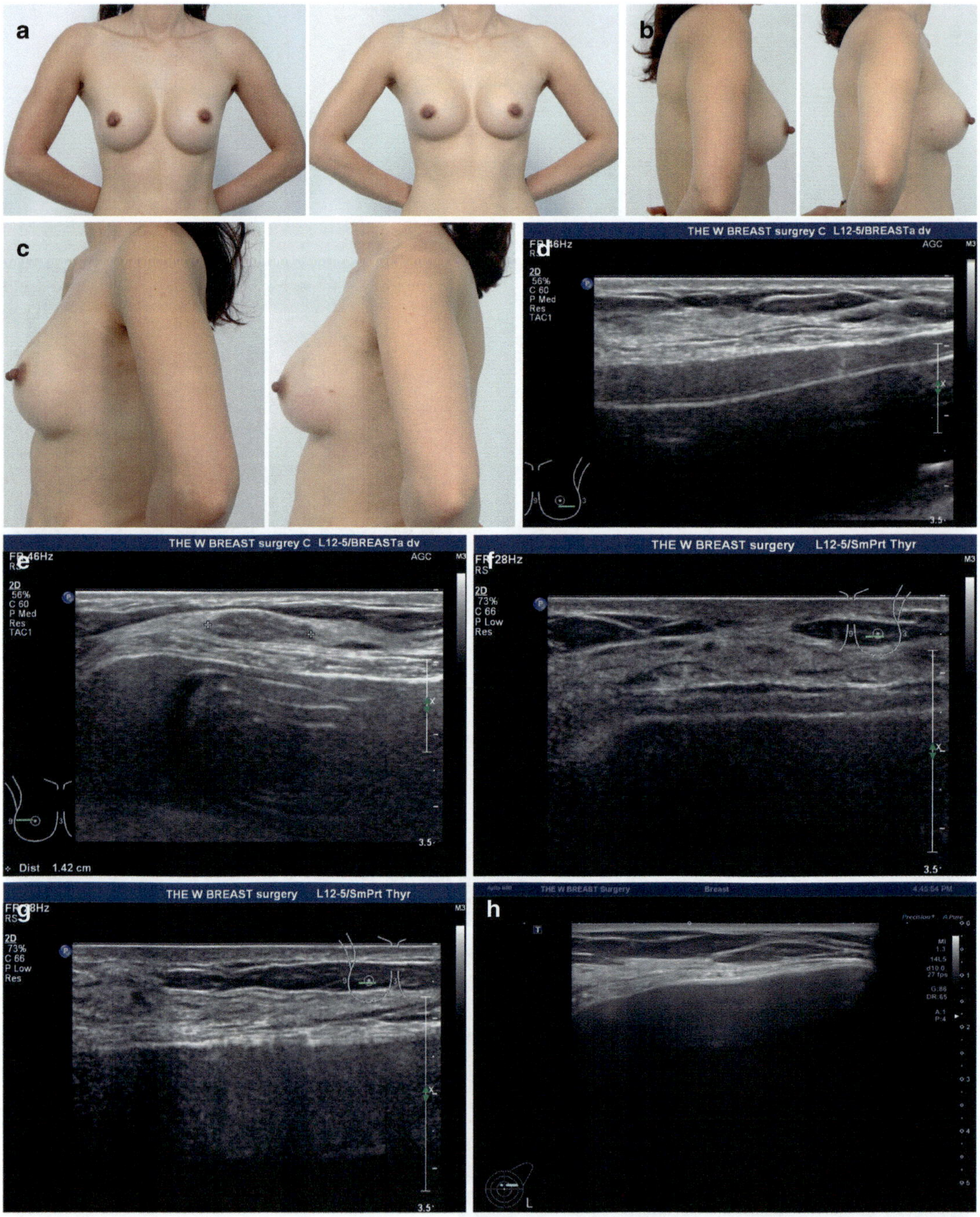

Fig. 7.12 (**A–C**) Preoperative and postoperative view (POD #730). (**D, E**) Preoperative US finding. (**F–I**) Postoperative US finding: (a) front view, (b) right side view, (c) left side view, (d) left ruptured silicone breast implant in subpectoral pocket is checked in preoperative sonography, (e) right ruptured breast implant in subpectoral pocket and breast benign mass were checked in preoperative sonography, (f) left smooth shell type breast implant with normal periprosthetic capsule is checked in postoperative sonography, pod #90, (g) right smooth shell type breast implant with normal periprosthetic capsule in subpectoral pocket in postoperative sonography, pod #90, (h) left smooth shell type breast implant with normal periprosthetic capsule is checked in postoperative sonography, pod #730, (i) right smooth shell type breast implant with normal periprosthetic capsule in subpectoral pocket in postoperative sonography, pod #730

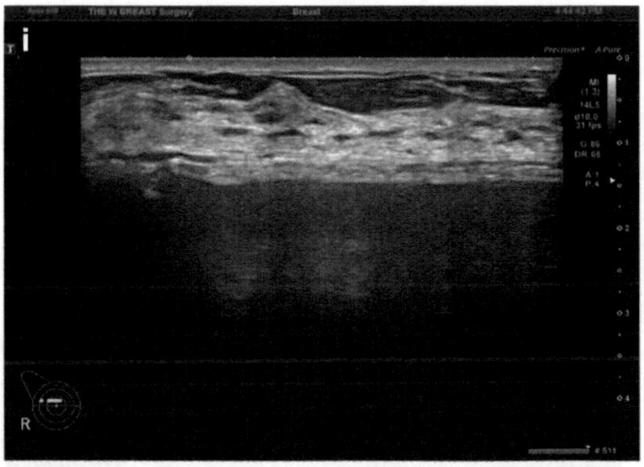

Fig. 7.12 (continued)

As described herein, most cases of the rupture are asymptomatic in nature and are not accompanied by alterations in the gross appearance and volume of the breast. It is therefore mandatory to perform an ultrasound-assisted examination of the breast on a regular basis. Indeed, considering that breast cancer examination is annually recommended, a patient receiving an ultrasound-assisted examination of the breast can be diagnosed with rupture of a breast implant at the earliest opportunities possible.

A 36-year-old woman received a round, textured silicone gel-filled breast implant (Allergan; 310 cc) in the subpectoral pocket *via* an inframammary fold (IMF) incision 5 years ago at other hospital. Due to the presence of a rupture of the left breast implant, the patient underwent subtotal capsulectomy accompanied by replacement of the device with the Natrelle INSPIRA (Allergan; high profile 365 cc) in the subpectoral pocket *via* a previous inframammary fold incision.

Preoperatively, the patient had a normal breast implant in the subpectoral pocket and a breast mass in the right breast and an intracapsular rupture of the device in the left breast on HRUS (Fig. 7.13).

Grossly, the patient had a slight spread of the left breast although she did not perceive it.

A 44-year-old woman received the Allergan anatomical breast implant (MM; volume:280 cc) in the subpectoral pocket *via* a trans-axillary incision in both breasts 6 years ago at other hospital. Due to the presence of thickened capsule in the right breast and a minor rupture of the device with gel bleed in the left breast, the patient underwent endoscopy assisted subtotal capsulectomy accompanied by replacement of the device with the Motiva Ergonomix™ Round SilkSurface (ERSF; volume: 355 cc) in the subpectoral pocket *via* a previous trans-axillary incision in both breasts.

Preoperatively, the patient had a thickened capsule in the right breast and a minor rupture of the device with gel bleed in the left breast on HRUS (Fig. 7.14).

Any rupture or thickened capsule is indication for capsulectomy. Trans-axillary endoscopic total capsulectomy is performed for the patient with rupture or TC, even though breast implant was in subpectoral pocket (Videos 7.1, 7.2, 7.3, and 7.4).

7.3.4.2 USD Rotation

An ultrasound-assisted diagnosis of USD rotation is a clinically useful strategy. A single presence of the USD rotation does not lead to reoperation in a patient complaining of severe symptoms. But severe cases of symptoms in a patient with USD of textured shell type breast implant may be managed with reoperation. An ultrasound-assisted diagnosis of USD rotation can be helpful for the following cases:

1. **Causes of changes in the shape of breast:** Both USD rotation and rupture of a device can cause changes in the shape of breast.
2. **Causes of pain:** Patients who are suspected of having capsular contracture should be differentially diagnosed from USD rotation of a device. The patch is the cause of pain d/t thickened area.
3. **Initial sonographic evidences of USD rotation:** Any lawsuits or litigations for USD rotation occurring over time can be defended based on its initial sonographic evidences.
4. **Characterization of a manufacturer of a breast implant:** Even a round breast implant is equipped with its own patch that is specific to the manufacturer. This is helpful for identification of the manufacturer of a device (Allergan, Mentor, Sebbin, Hansbiomed, Polytech, Motiva).

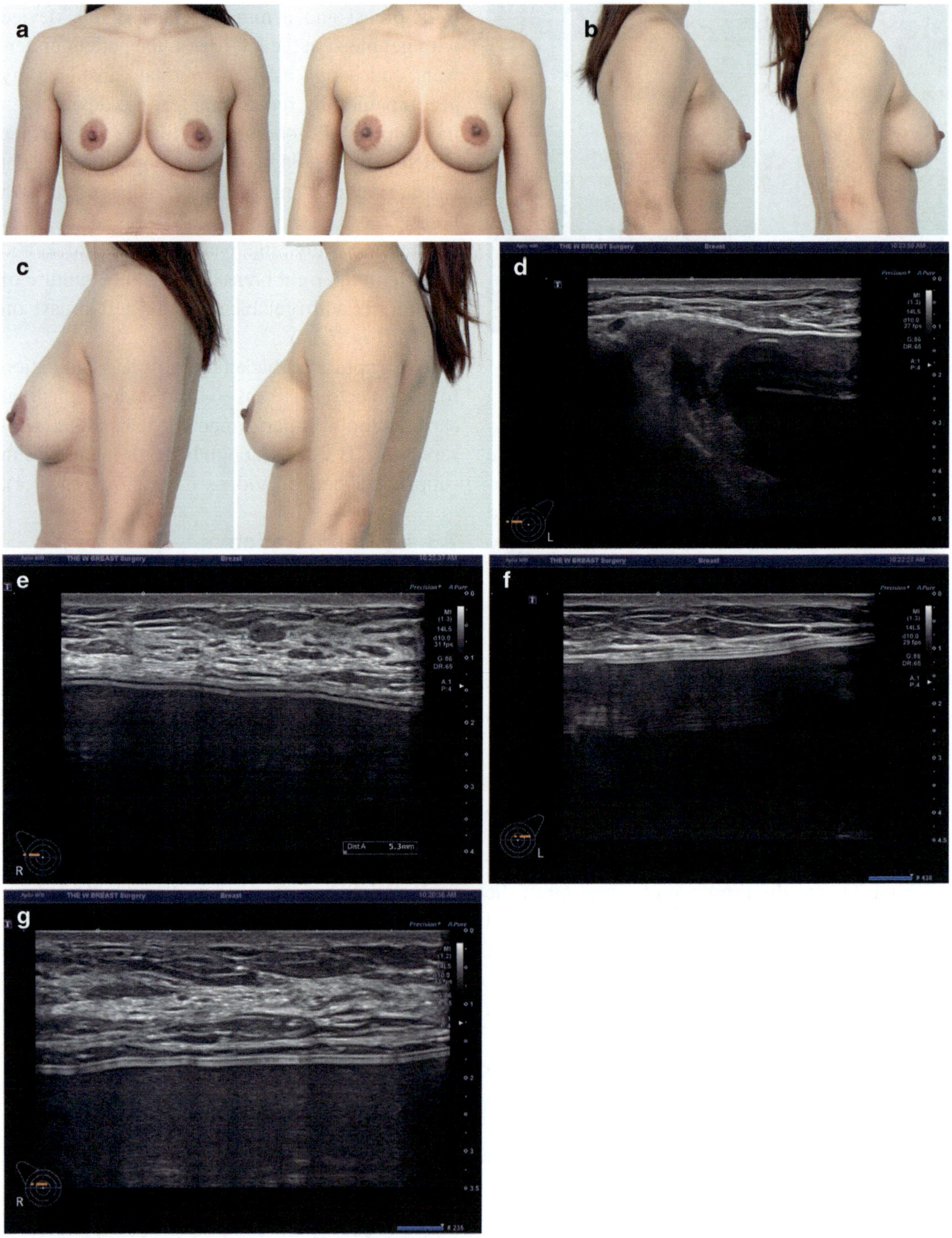

Fig. 7.13 (**A–C**) Preoperative and postoperative view, POD #93. (**D**, **E**) Preoperative US finding. (**F**, **G**) Postoperative US finding: (a) front view, (b) right side view, (c) left side view, (d) left ruptured silicone breast implant in subpectoral pocket is checked in preoperative sonography, (e) right textured shell type breast implant in subpectoral pocket and breast benign mass were checked in preoperative sonography, (f) left smooth shell type breast implant with normal periprosthetic capsule is checked in postoperative sonography, pod #93, (g) right smooth shell type breast implant with normal periprosthetic capsule in subpectoral pocket in postoperative sonography, pod #93

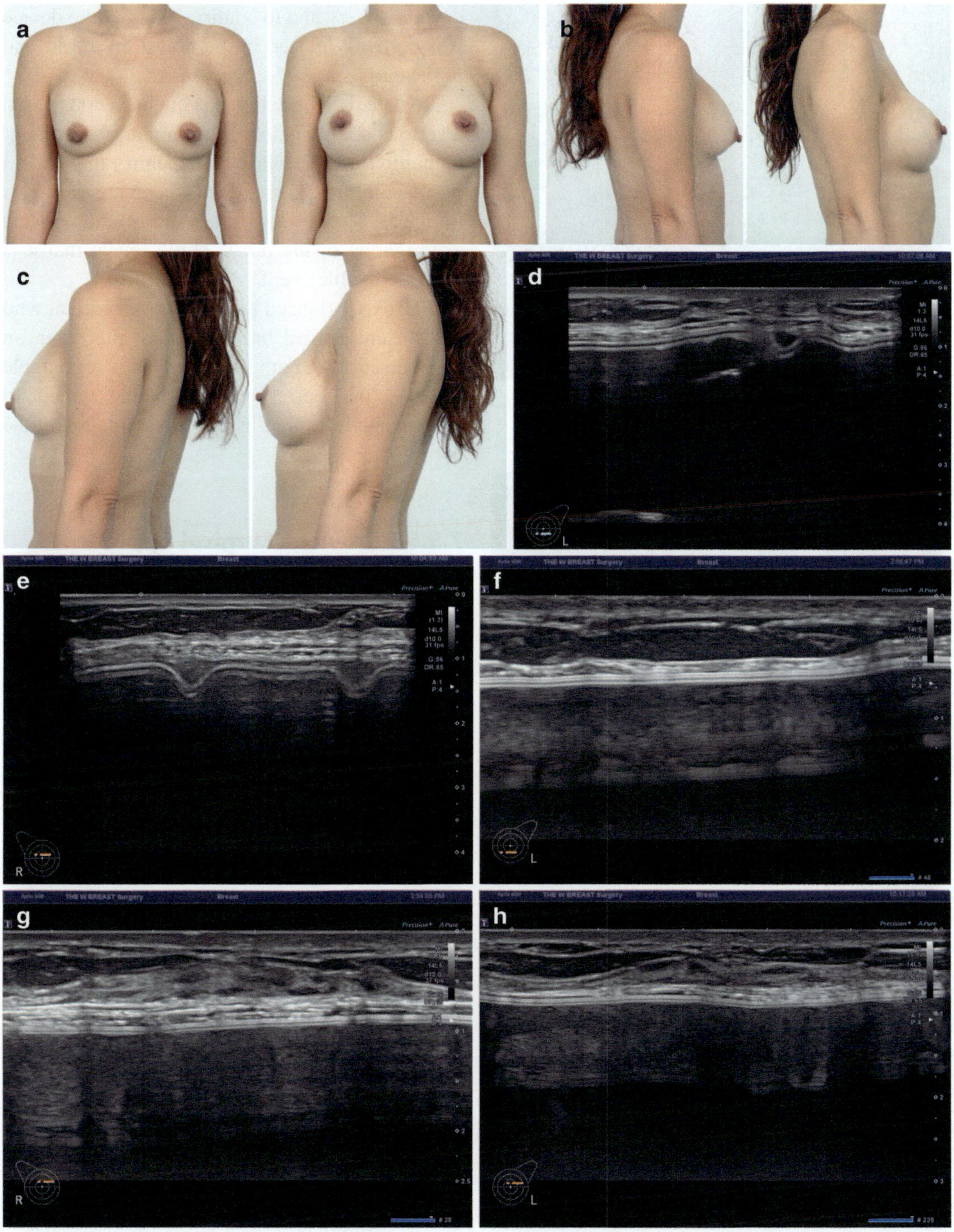

Fig. 7.14 (**A–C**) Preoperative and postoperative view (POD #185). (**D**, **E**) Preoperative US finding. (**F–I**) Postoperative US finding: (a) front view, (b) right side view, (c) left side view, (d) gel bleed of the left textured shell type silicone breast implant in subpectoral pocket is checked in preoperative sonography, (e) right textured shell type breast implant in subpectoral pocket was checked in preoperative sonography, (f) left smooth shell type breast implant with normal periprosthetic capsule is checked in postoperative sonography, pod #84, (g) right smooth shell type breast implant with normal periprosthetic capsule in subpectoral pocket in postoperative sonography, pod #84, (h) left smooth shell type breast implant with normal periprosthetic capsule is checked in postoperative sonography, pod #185, (i) right smooth shell type breast implant with normal periprosthetic capsule in subpectoral pocket in postoperative sonography, pod #185

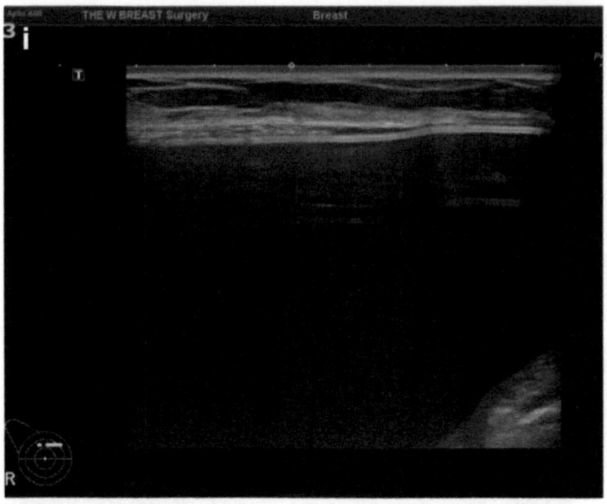

Fig. 7.14 (continued)

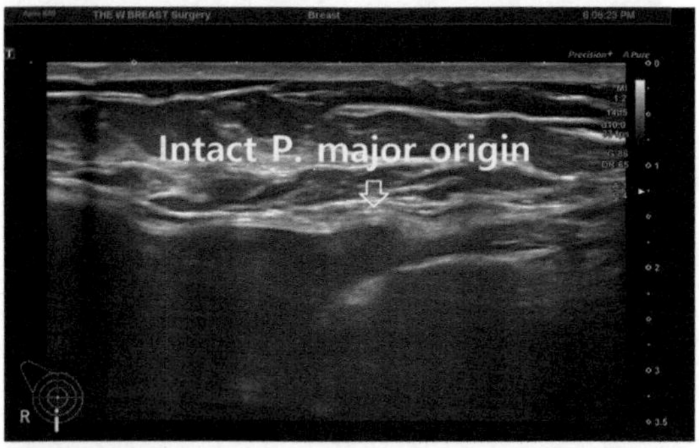

Fig. 7.15 White arrow shows intact inf. origin of P. major muscle. Intact P. major origin is a reason of malpositioning induced upper pole fullness

USD rotation also occurs in a patient receiving a textured breast implant, which is notably seen in a device with a poor texturing or initial wrong setting. It is therefore probable that a smooth breast implant with a high profile is more vulnerable to USD rotation as compared with a device with other types of surface topography.

I have checked a total of 21 cases of USD rotation, comprising 18 patients receiving a textured breast implant and 3 receiving a smooth device in 800 patients who had received breast implant surgery at other hospital for 3 years. This suggests that surgeons should therefore make it a rule to check the upper and lower part of a breast implant during surgery and to confirm whether the device was correctly placed in the breast on ultrasound in the early stage of surgery.

To date, USD rotation has not been considered a serious complication of an implant-based augmentation mammaplasty. To identify any causes of discomfort in a patient receiving a breast implant, however, an ultrasound-assisted examination of the breast could reveal that it is not a negligible event.

I also experienced a rare case of a patient who had an anatomical breast implant placed in an USD position in both breasts. This is regrettable because the corresponding patient failed to receive an ultrasound-assisted examination of the breast.

7.3.5 Previous Surgical Approaches

It is necessary to examine whether there is under-dissection of the pectoralis major muscle origin in patients who has excessive upper pole fullness. If there are upper pole fullness with intact P. major origin in inferior breast, a complete dissection of inferior part of pectoralis major muscle should be achieved. The following sonographic findings show that no dissection of the origin of pectoralis major muscle was achieved at 6 o'clock position of the breast (Fig. 7.15).

References

1. Stevens WG, Harrington J, Alizadeh K, Broadway D, Zeidler K, Godinez TB. Eight-year follow-up data from the U.S. clinical trial for Sientra's FDA-approved round and shaped implants with high-strength cohesive silicone gel. Aesthet Surg J. 2015;35(Suppl 1):S3–10.
2. Maxwell GP, Van Natta BW, Murphy DK, Slicton A, Bengtson BP. Natrelle style 410 form-stable silicone breast implants: core study results at 6 years. Aesthet Surg J. 2012;32(6):709–17.
3. Adams WP Jr, Mallucci P. Breast augmentation. Plast Reconstr Surg. 2012;130(4):597e–611e.
4. Stevens WG, Calobrace MB, Harrington J, Alizadeh K, Zeidler KR, d'Incelli RC. Nine-year core study

data for Sientra's FDA-approved round and shaped implants with high-strength cohesive silicone gel. Aesthet Surg J. 2016;36(4):404–16.
5. Oo M, Myint Z, Sakakibara T, Kasai Y. Relationship between brassiere cup size and shoulder-neck pain in women. Open Orthop J. 2012;6:140–2.
6. Nicoletti G, Mandrini S, Finotti V, Dall'Angelo A, Malovini A, Chierico S, Faga A, Dalla Toffola E. Objective clinical assessment of posture patterns after implant breast augmentation. Plast Reconstr Surg. 2015;136(2):162e–70e.
7. Swanson E. Prospective photographic measurement study of 196 cases of breast augmentation, mastopexy, augmentation/mastopexy, and breast reduction. Plast Reconstr Surg. 2013;131(5):802e–19e.

8 Clinical Presentation

8.1 Overview

Postoperative course was meticulously monitored through our multi-disciplinary, algorithm-based approach to an early detection of complications of an implant-based augmentation mammaplasty, as previously described [1, 2].

Since 2017, more than 1000 patients with a history of receiving surgery at other hospitals have also visited the outpatient clinic. Especially after the Allergan textured implant worldwide recall and Hansbiomed fraud. On history taking and physical examination, the patients were evaluated for whether they were in healthy conditions. Furthermore, the patients were also evaluated for their subjective awareness of the manufacturer, surface and shape of a breast implant [2], and ultrasonographic finding using breast implant checklist (see Chap. 3).

The following 52 cases, comprising both, highlight the importance of ultrasound-assisted diagnosis of complications in patients receiving a breast implant.

Supplementary Information The online version contains supplementary material available at [https://doi.org/10.1007/978-981-16-8282-7_8].

8.2 Illustrative Cases

8.2.1 Case 1

On physical examination and history taking, a 28-year-old woman complained of a change in the shape of the right breast. On preoperative ultrasonography, the patient was found to have subpectoral fat grafted to the pectoralis major, accompanied by the presence of a round smooth silicone gel-filled device in the subpectoral pocket. Breast ultrasound showed rupture of breast implant on the right side, but the patient had no findings that are suggestive of folding, seroma, thickened capsule, upside-down rotation, and capsular mass. The patient underwent explantation via previous axillary incision. And there were right chronic inflammation and fibrosis and left focal chronic inflammation and mild fibrosis in capsule pathology (Fig. 8.1) (Videos 8.1 and 8.2).

8.2.2 Case 2

On physical examination and history taking, a 28-year-old woman complained of breast hardness. On preoperative ultrasonography, the patient was found to have an anatomical textured silicone gel-filled breast implant (Allergen Inc., Irvine, CA) in the subpectoral pocket. The patient had a thickened capsule which was measured as 0.9 mm on the right side and 1.3 mm on the left

J. H. Kim, *Atlas of Breast Implant Ultrasound*, https://doi.org/10.1007/978-981-16-8282-7_8

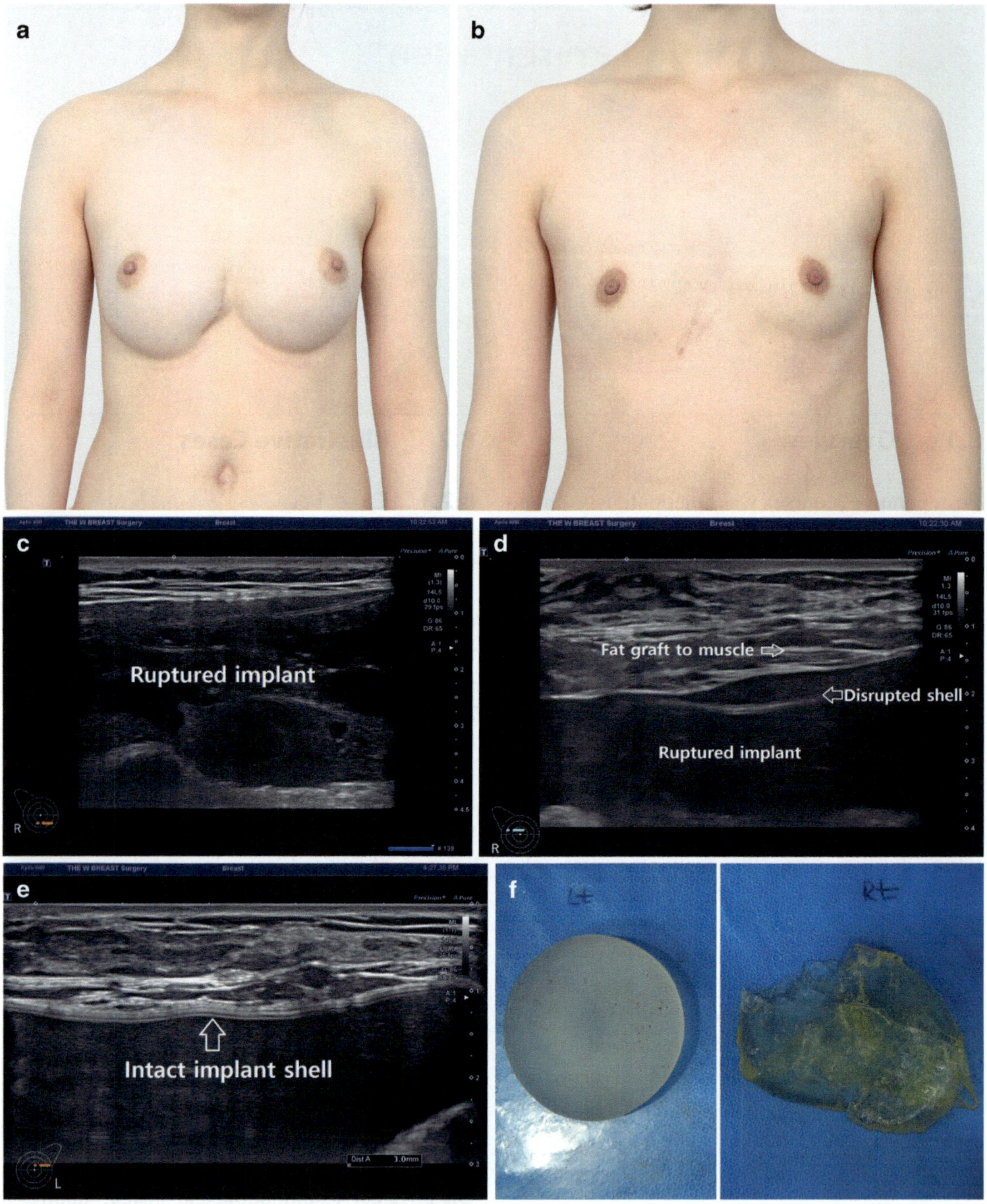

Fig. 8.1 (**a**): A preoperative front view. (**b**) Six-month postoperative view. (**c, d**) Right ruptured breast implant in preoperative ultrasonography. (**e**) Normal left breast implant shell in preoperative ultrasonography. (**f**) Both removed Sebbin (Groupe Sebbin SAS, Boissy-l' Aillerie, France) round micro-textured shell type breast implant, LS 71285 cc. (**g**) Both removed periprosthetic capsule. (**h**) Right intraoperative view of breast pocket before capsulectomy. (**i**) Right intraoperative view of breast pocket after subtotal capsulectomy. (**j**) Left intraoperative view of breast pocket before capsulectomy. (**k**) Left intraoperative view of breast pocket after subtotal capsulectomy. (**l**) Microscopic view of the right capsule. (**m**) Microscopic view of the left capsule

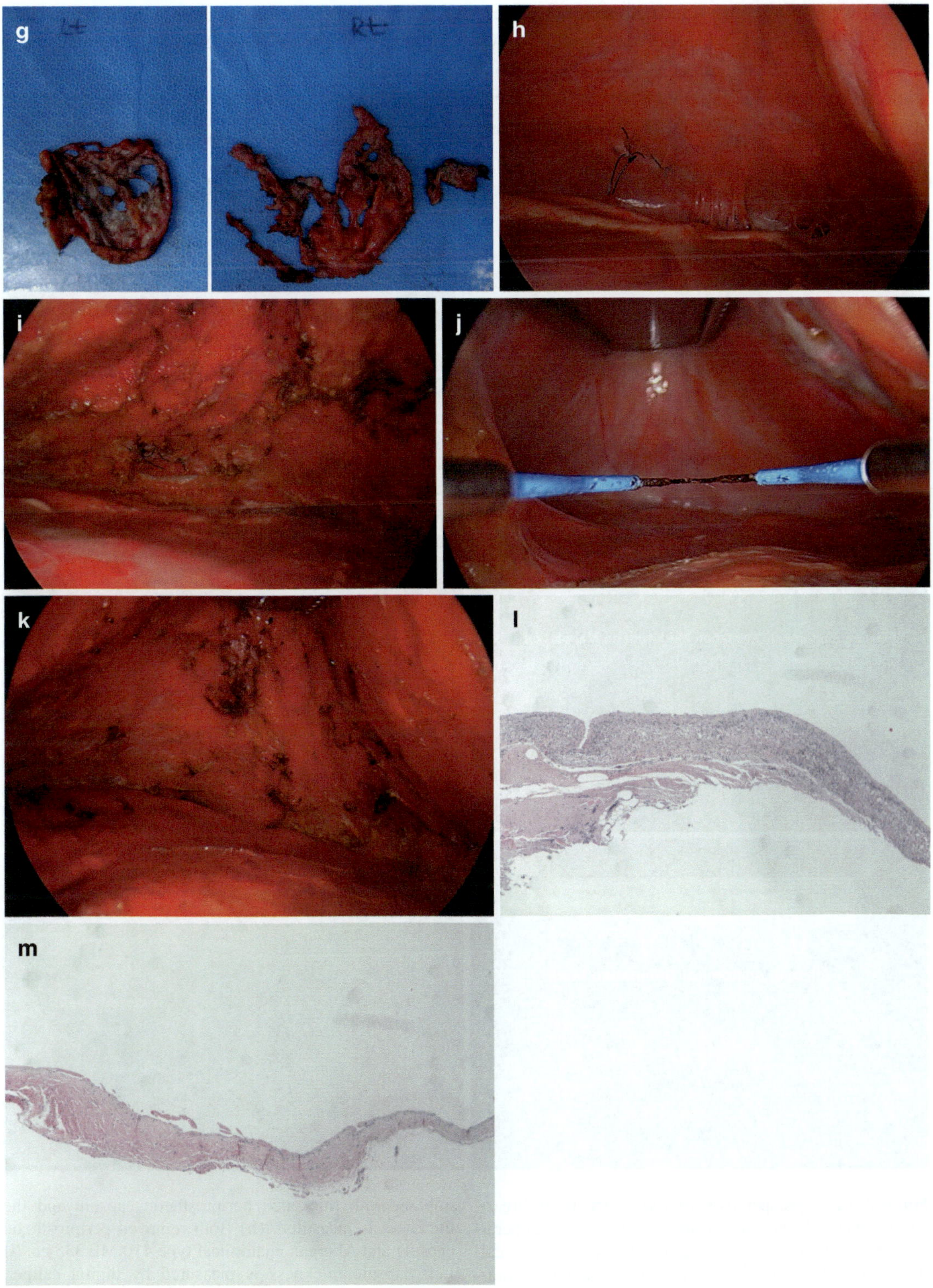

Fig. 8.1 (continued)

side. But there were no findings that are suggestive of malrotation, folding, seroma, upside-down rotation, rupture, and capsular mass. The patient underwent near-total capsulectomy with replacement of the device via a previous inframammary fold scar. Intraoperatively, the patient had a double capsule below the device. There was mild fibrosis in both capsule (Fig. 8.2). And vacuum-assisted breast mass excision was done during the surgery (Video 8.3).

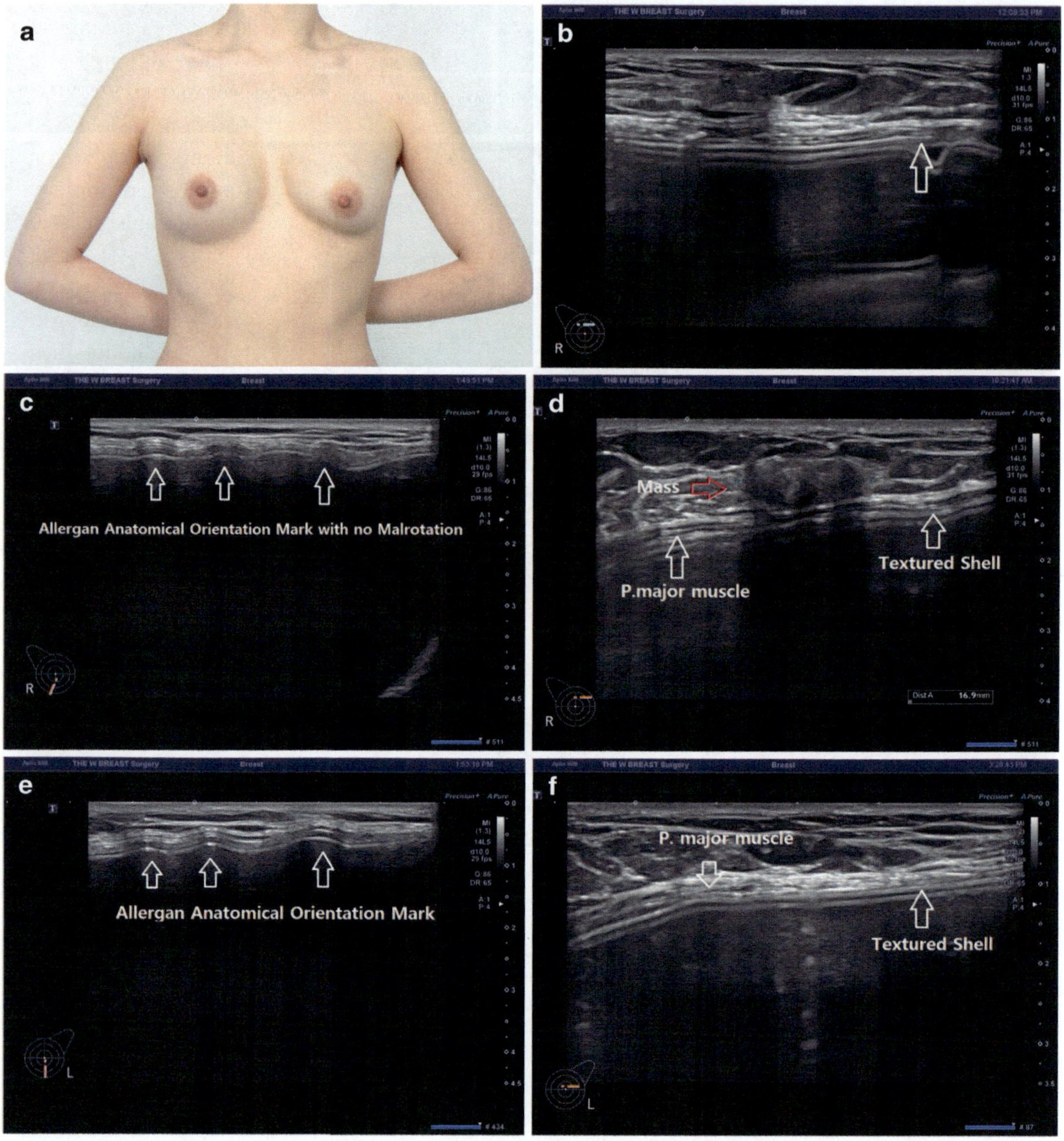

Fig. 8.2 (**a**) A preoperative front view. (**b**) Right breast periprosthetic thickened capsule is checked in preoperative ultrasonography. (**c**) Right Allergan anatomical implant orientation mark is checked in preoperative ultrasonography. (**d**) Right textured shell type breast implant in subpectoral pocket and breast mass. (**e**) Left Allergan anatomical type breast implant orientation mark is checked. (**f**) Left textured shell type breast implant in subpectoral pocket is checked in ultrasonography. (**g**) Left breast implant with thickened periprosthetic capsule and the thickness is measured. (**h**) Both removed periprosthetic capsule and Allergan anatomical type 410 MF 335 cc. (**i**) Left capsule thickness is measured by digital caliper, 1.5 mm. (**j**) Right capsule thickness is measured by digital caliper, 1.3 mm. (**k**) Microscopic view of the left capsule. (**l**) Microscopic view of the right capsule. (**m**) Microscopic view of removed right breast benign mass

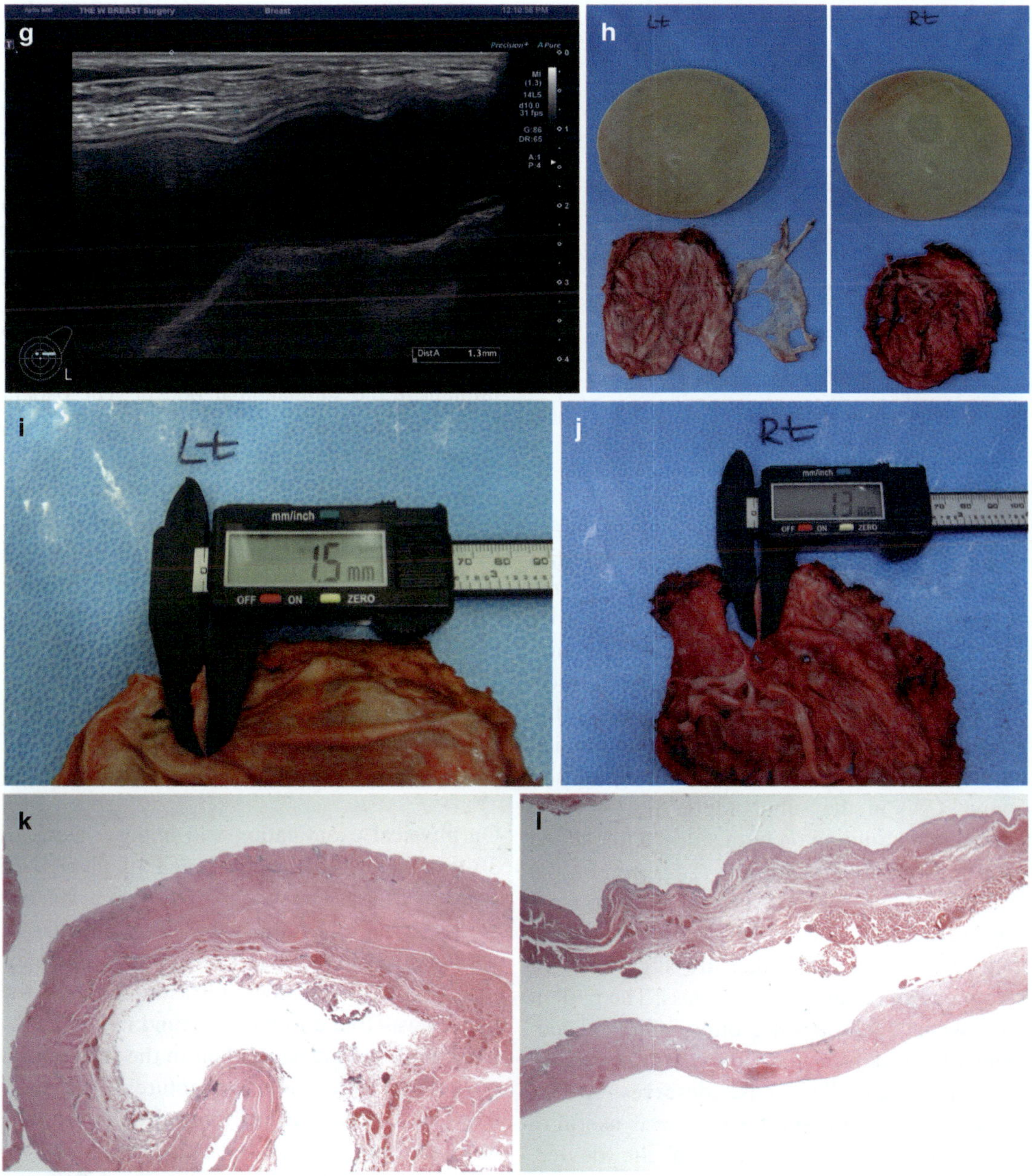

Fig. 8.2 (continued)

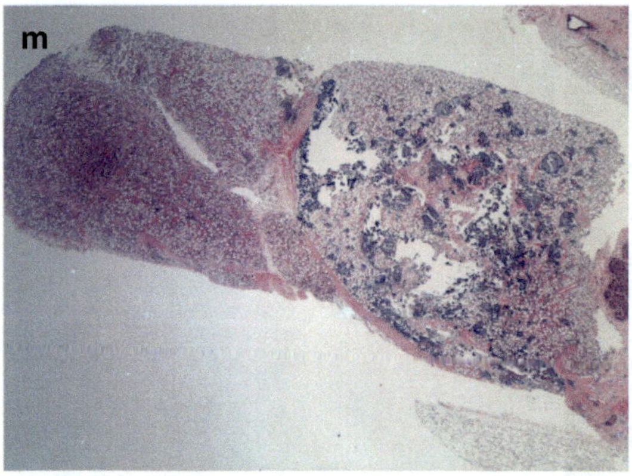

Fig. 8.2 (continued)

8.2.3 Case 3

On physical examination and history taking, a 48-year-old woman complained of breast hardness and pain. The patient had an 8-year history of receiving an implant-based augmentation mammaplasty via an inframammary fold incision. On preoperative ultrasonography, the patient was found to have a round textured silicone gel-filled breast implant (Allergan Inc., Irvine, CA) in the subglandular pocket. The patient had a folding on both sides, a thickened capsule which was measured as 1.3 mm on the left side (Video 8.4) and an upside-down rotation on the right side (Videos 8.5 and 8.6). But there were no findings that are suggestive of seroma, rupture, and capsular mass. The patient underwent total capsulectomy with replacement of the device via a previous inframammary fold scar. This case deserves special attention in that breast ultrasound was useful in identifying the manufacturer of the device. Even though it was round, it was possible to distinguish the manufacturer by using the patch visible when there was USD in the ultrasound. There were right focal degeneration and left focal chronic inflammation with fat necrosis in capsule (Fig. 8.3).

8.2.4 Case 4

On physical examination and history taking, a 49-year-old woman had a 12-year history of receiving an implant-based augmentation mammaplasty in the subpectoral pocket. On preoperative ultrasonography, the patient was found to have a round textured silicone gel-filled breast implant in the subglandular pocket. The patient had a detachment of the device on the left side, accompanied by a minor rupture (gel bleed) on the right side (Videos 8.7 and 8.8). But there were no findings that are suggestive of folding, seroma, thickened capsule, upside-down rotation, and capsular mass. The patient underwent explantation with both total capsulectomy via a previous areolar scar. There was mild fibrosis in both capsule (Fig. 8.4).

8.2.5 Case 5

On physical examination and history taking, a 36-year-old woman complained of change of breast softness. The patient had a 6-year history of receiving an implant-based augmentation mammaplasty via an inframammary fold incision. On preoperative ultrasonography, the patient was found to have a round textured silicone gel-filled breast implant in the subpectoral pocket and there was a left rupture in preoperative US. The patient had multiple oil cysts due to fat grafting on both sides, accompanied by a major rupture of the device on the left breast (Video 8.9). But there were findings that are suggestive of folding, seroma, thickened capsule, upside-down rotation, and capsular mass

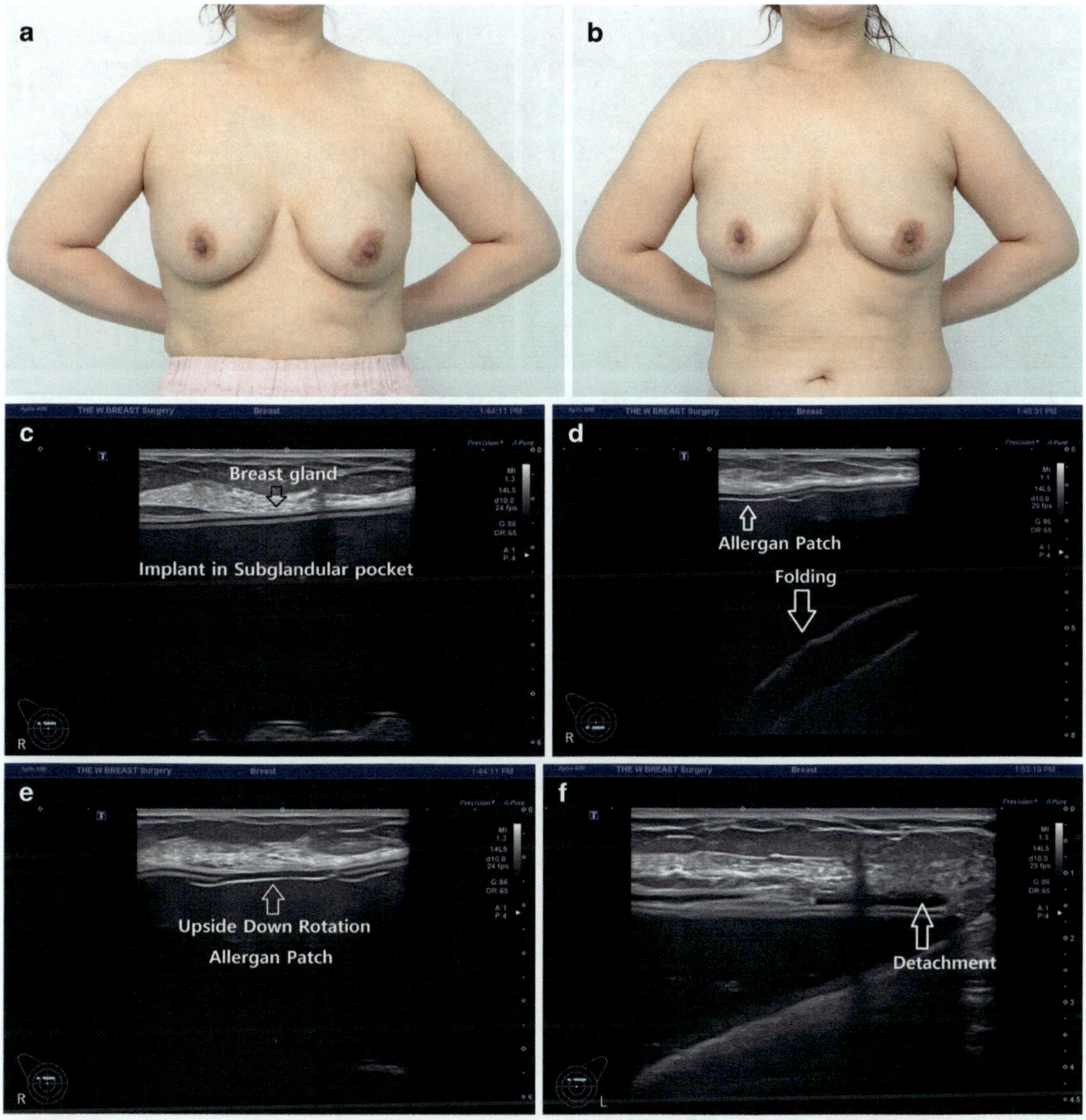

Fig. 8.3 (**a**) A preoperative front view. (**b**) Three-month postoperative view. (**c**) Right textured shell type breast implant in subpectoral pocket is checked in preoperative ultrasonography. (**d, e**) Right breast implant upside-down rotation with folded shell is checked in preoperative ultrasonography. (**f, g, h**) Left breast implant folded shell and detachment, and 1.3 mm thickened periprosthetic capsule is checked in preoperative ultrasonography. (**i**) Both removed periprosthetic capsule by total capsulectomy and Allergan round texture style 120 340 cc. (**j**) Left capsule thickness is measured by digital caliper, 1.5 mm. (**k**) Right capsule thickness is measured by digital caliper, 0.3 mm. (**l**) Microscopic view of the left capsule. (**m**) Microscopic view of the right capsule

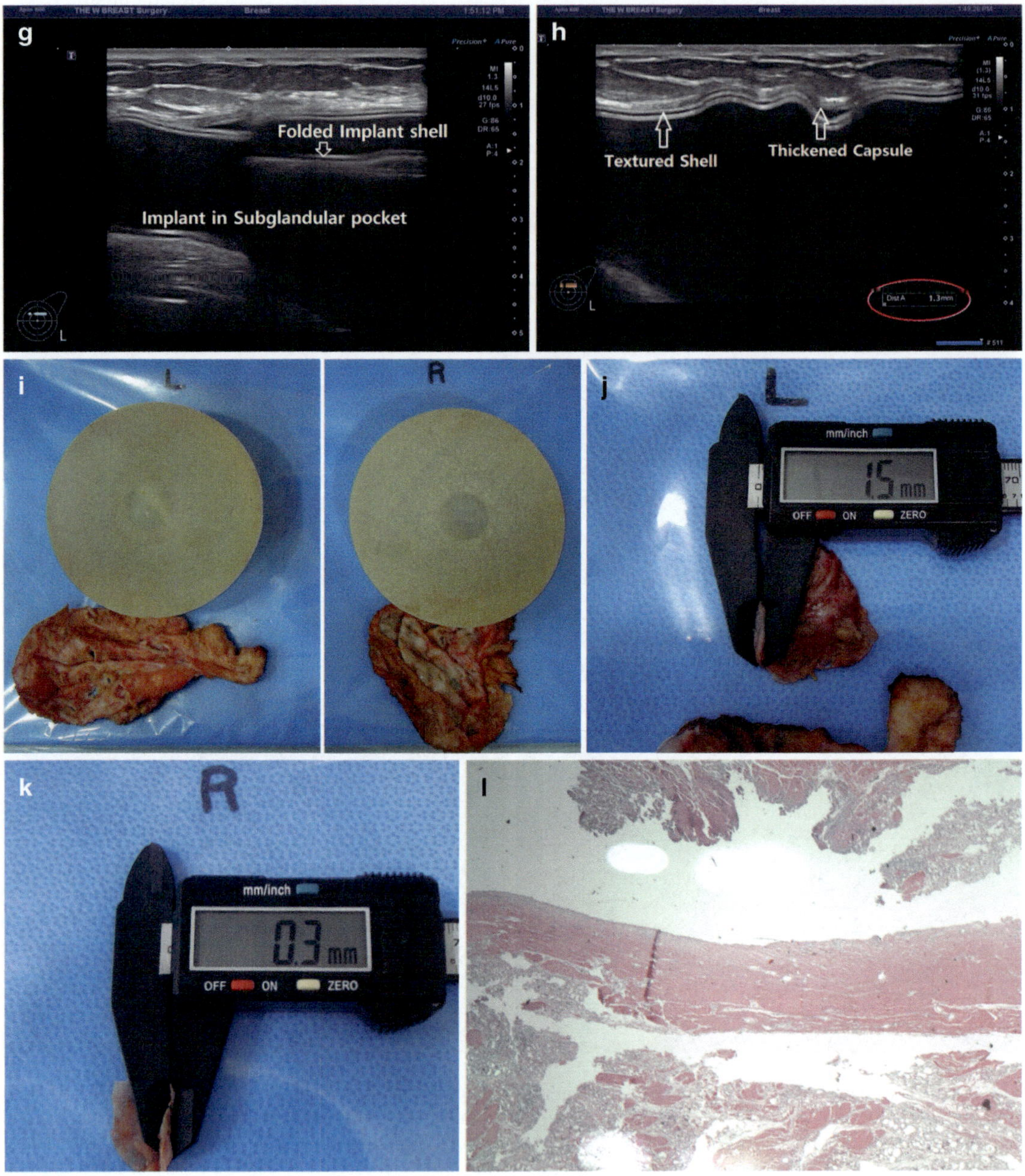

Fig. 8.3 (continued)

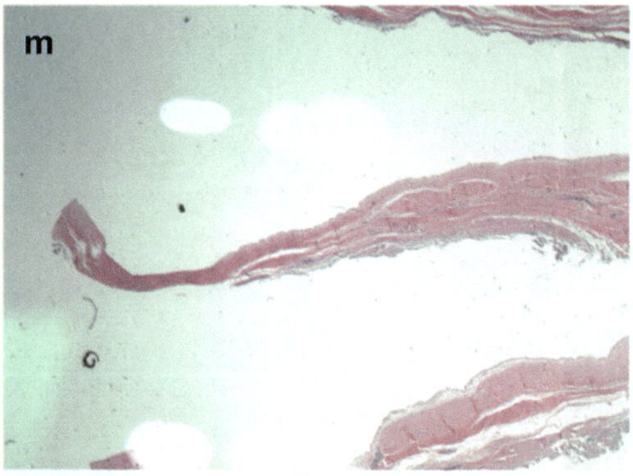

Fig. 8.3 (continued)

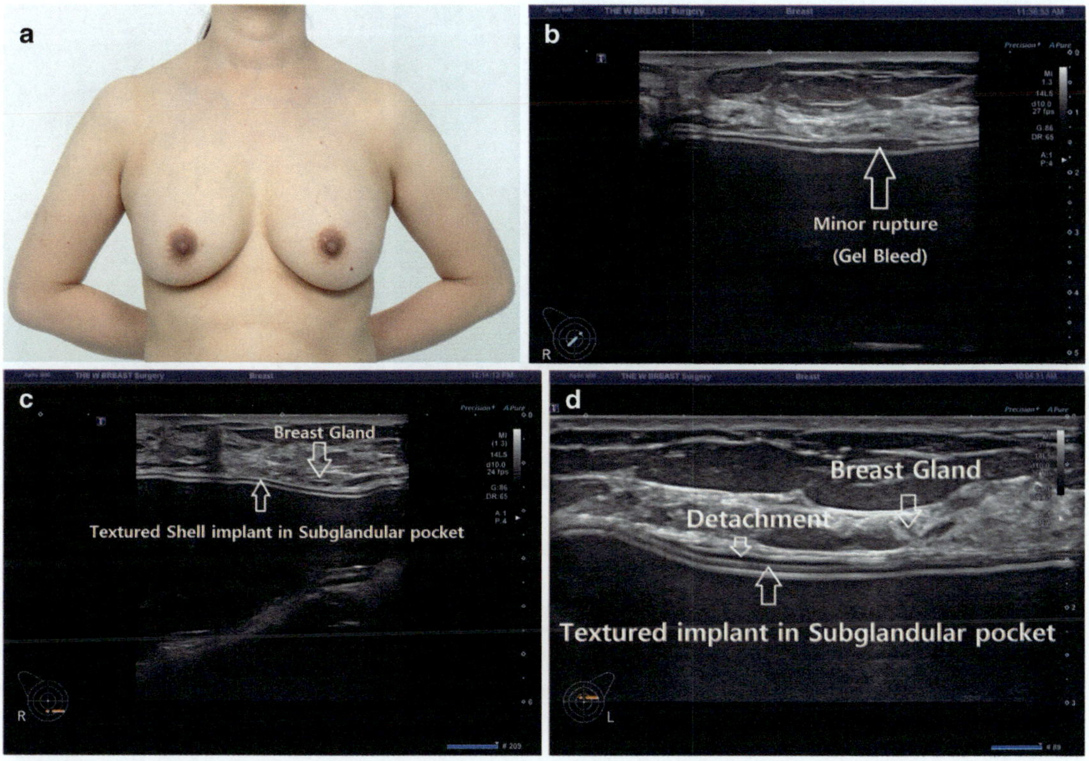

Fig. 8.4 (**a**) A preoperative front view. (**b**) Right textured shell type breast implant in subglandular pocket with gel bleeding is checked in preoperative ultrasonography. (**c**) Right textured shell type breast implant in subglandular pocket is checked in preoperative ultrasonography. (**d, e**) Left breast textured shell type breast implant with detachment in subglandular pocket. (**f, g**) Both removed periprosthetic capsule by total capsulectomy and Mentor round texture type breast implant, 225 cc. (**h**) Right breast implant surface with gel bleed. (**i**) Left capsule thickness is measured by digital caliper, 0.4 mm. (**j**) Right capsule thickness is measured by digital caliper, 0.4 mm. (**k**) Microscopic view of the left capsule. (**l**) Microscopic view of the right capsule

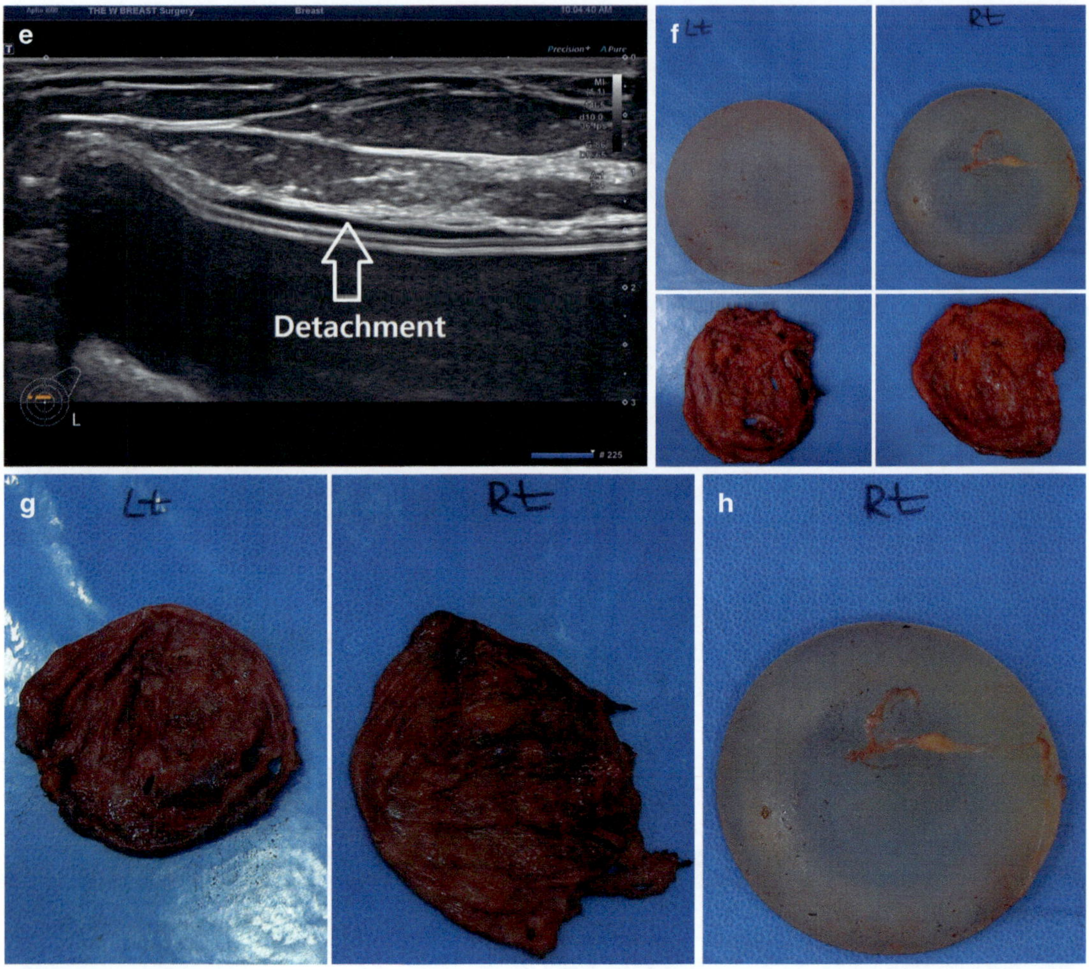

Fig. 8.4 (continued)

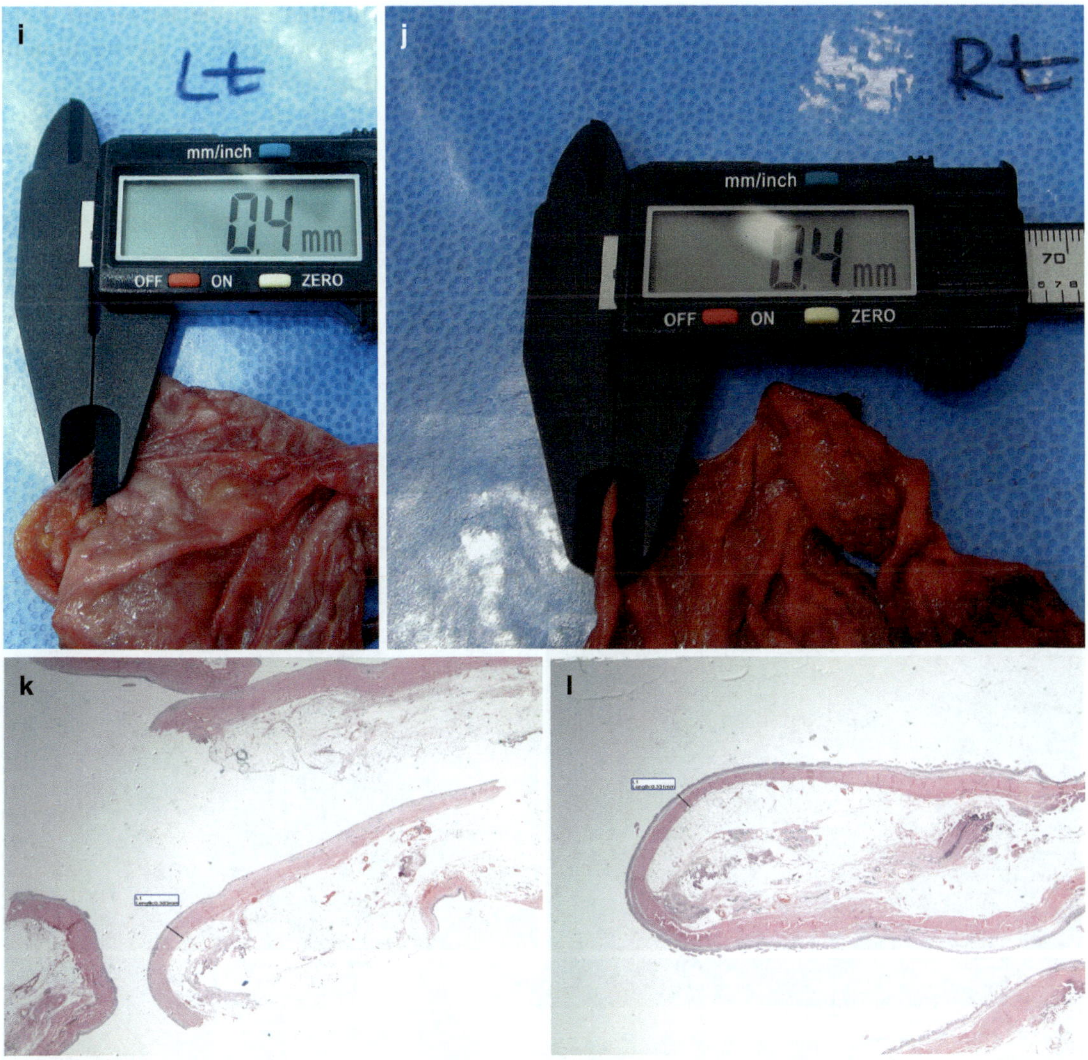

Fig. 8.4 (continued)

on the right breast (Video 8.10). The patient underwent subtotal capsulectomy with replacement of the device via a previous inframammary fold scar on both sides. Intraoperatively, the patient had a double capsule below the right breast implant. There was focal degeneration in both capsule (Fig. 8.5).

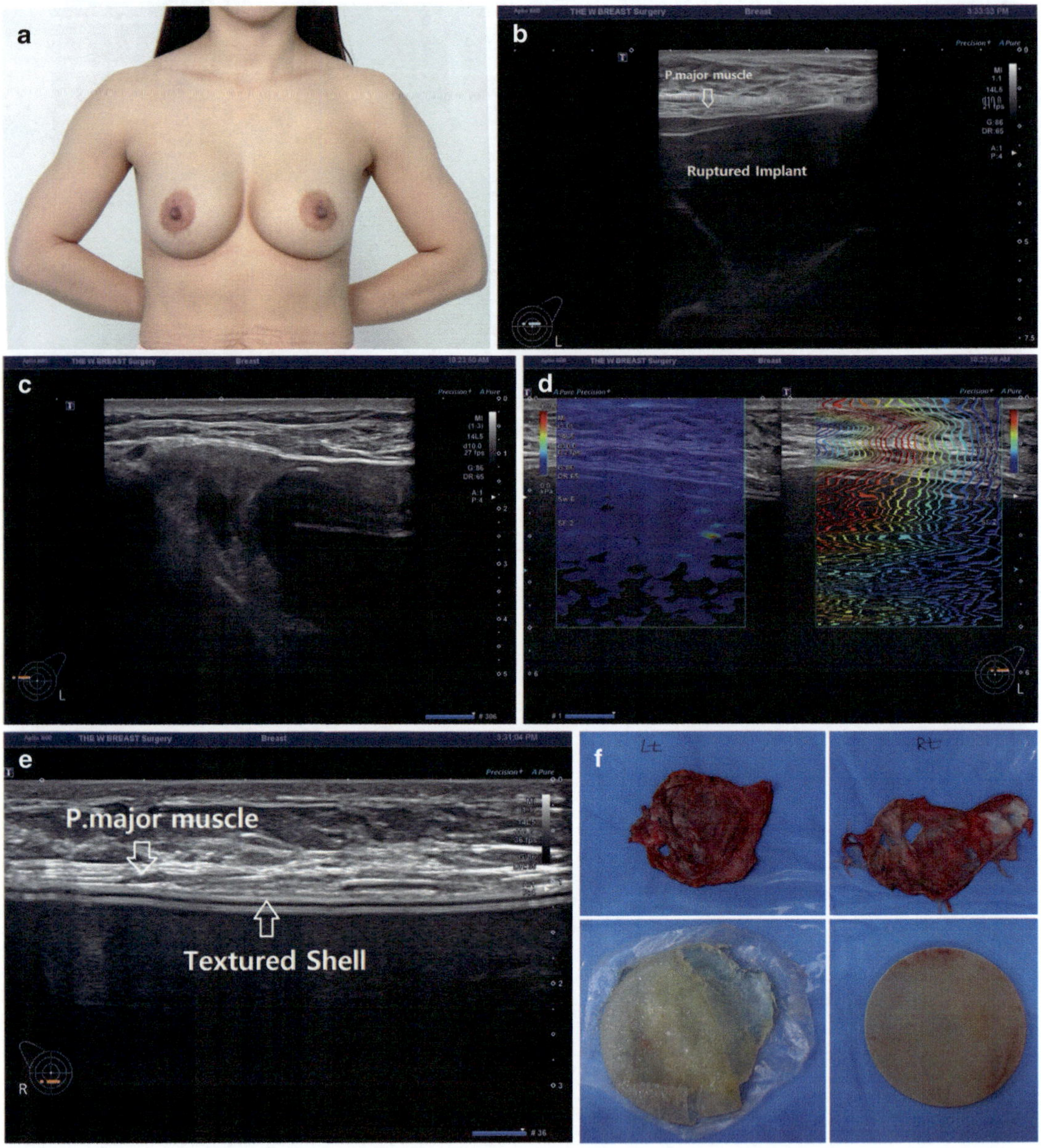

Fig. 8.5 (**a**) A preoperative front view. (**b**, **c**) Left ruptured breast implant in subpectoral pocket is checked in preoperative ultrasonography. (**d**) Shear wave elastography of ruptured left breast implant. (**e**) Right textured shell type breast implant in subpectoral pocket is checked in preoperative ultrasonography. (**f**) Both removed periprosthetic capsule and Allergan round texture type breast implant 310 cc. (**g**) The ruptured left silicone breast implant. (**h**) Both removed periprosthetic capsule by subtotal capsulectomy. (**i**) Left capsule thickness is measured by digital caliper, 0.2 mm. (**j**) Right capsule thickness is measured by digital caliper, 0.3 mm. (**k**) Microscopic view of the left capsule with silicone invasion to capsule. (**l**) Microscopic view of the right capsule

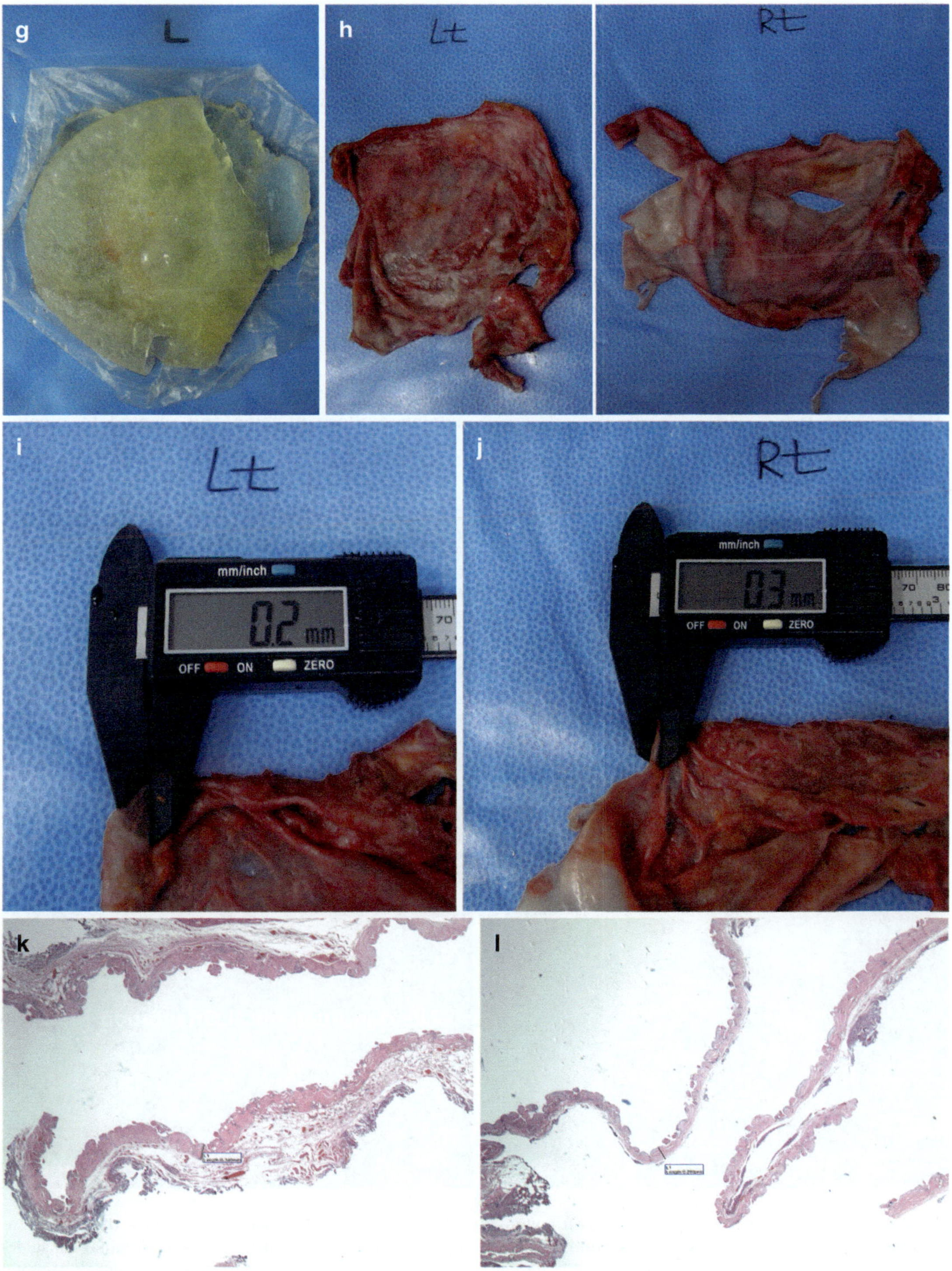

Fig. 8.5 (continued)

8.2.6 Case 6

On physical examination and history taking, a 35-year-old woman complained of foreign body sensation, whose chief complaint was concern for breast implant-associated anaplastic large cell lymphoma (BIA-ALCL). The patient had a 2-year history of receiving an implant-based augmentation mammaplasty *via* an axillary incision. On preoperative ultrasonography, the patient was found to have an anatomical silicone gel-filled breast implant (Allergan Inc., Irvine, CA) in the subpectoral pocket. The patient had a folding on the right side and a minimal seroma in the left axilla. But there were no findings that are suggestive of malrotation, thickened capsule, upside-down rotation, rupture, and capsular mass (Video 8.11).

The patient underwent endoscopic subtotal capsulectomy with replacement of the device *via* a previous axillary scar. There was focal generation of both capsule (Fig. 8.6).

8.2.7 Case 7

On physical examination and history taking, a 33-year-old woman complained of foreign body sensation. The patient had a history of receiving an implant-based augmentation mammaplasty *via* an axillary incision and wanted to receive explantation.

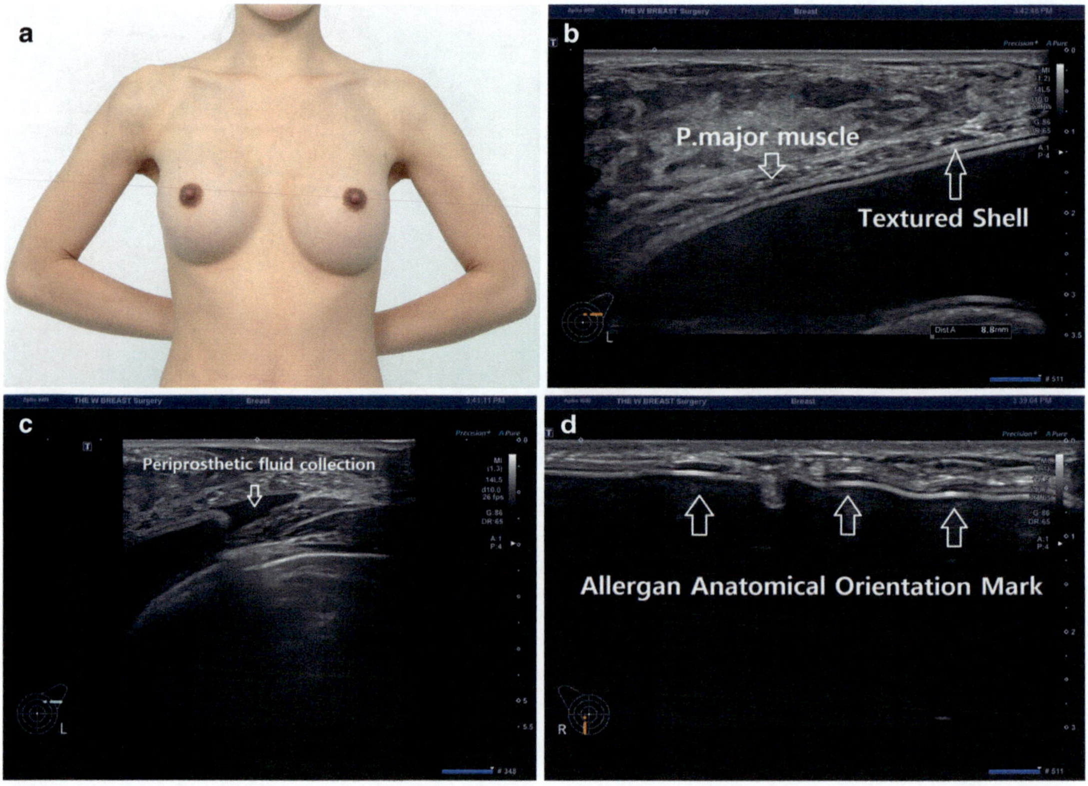

Fig. 8.6 (**a**) A preoperative front view. (**b**) Left textured shell type breast implant in subpectoral pocket is checked in preoperative ultrasonography. (**c**) Sonographic finding of periprosthetic fluid collection in the left axillary area. (**d**) Right Allergan anatomical breast implant is checked in preoperative ultrasonography. (**e**) Left intraoperative view of periprosthetic capsule. (**f**) Right intraoperative view of periprosthetic capsule. (**g**) Left intraoperative view of breast pocket after subtotal capsulectomy. (**h**): Left intraoperative view of breast pocket after subtotal capsulectomy. (**i**) Both removed periprosthetic capsule by subtotal capsulectomy and Allergan anatomical type 410 FX 280 cc. (**j**) Left capsule thickness is measured by digital caliper, 0.3 mm. (**k**) Right capsule thickness is measured by digital caliper, 0.3 mm. (**l**) Microscopic view of left capsule. (**m**) Microscopic view of right capsule

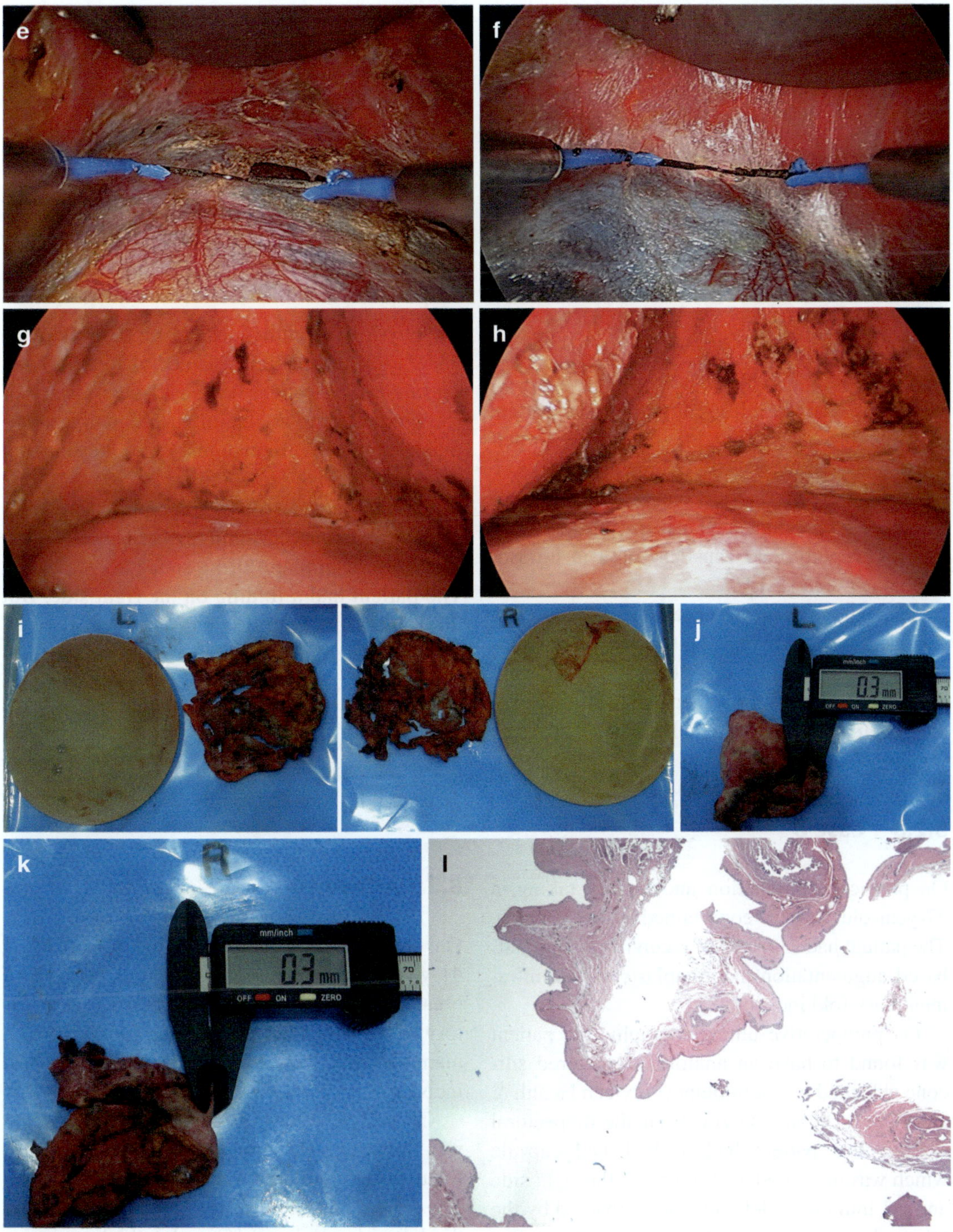

Fig. 8.6 (continued)

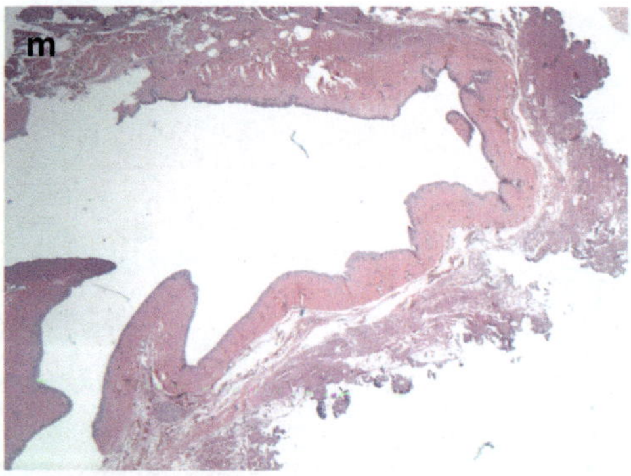

Fig. 8.6 (continued)

On preoperative ultrasonography, the patient was found to have a round textured silicone gel-filled breast implant in the subpectoral pocket. But there were no findings that are suggestive of folding, seroma, thickened capsule, upside-down rotation, rupture, and capsular mass in ultrasonography (Video 8.12).

The patient underwent endoscopic subtotal capsulectomy with explantation *via* a previous axillary scar. There were fibrotic capsule with focal chronic inflammation and some multinucleated giant cells in both capsule (Fig. 8.7).

8.2.8 Case 8

On physical examination and history taking, a 37-year-old woman complained of breast pain. The patient had a history of receiving an implant-based augmentation mammaplasty *via* an inframammary fold incision.

On preoperative ultrasonography, the patient was found to have an anatomical textured silicone gel-filled breast implant (Polytech Health & Aesthetics, Dieburg, Germany) in the subpectoral pocket. The patient had a thickened capsule which was measured as 2.0 mm on the right side and 2.1 mm on the left side, accompanied by the bilateral presence of a folding (Video 8.13). But there were no findings that are suggestive of seroma, upside-down rotation, rupture, and capsular mass.

The patient underwent explantation with both total capsulectomy *via* a previous inframammary fold scar on both sides. There were focal chronic inflammation and fibrosis in both capsule (Fig. 8.8).

8.2.9 Case 9

On physical examination and history taking, a 55-year-old woman complained of foreign body sensation. The patient had an 11-year-history of receiving an implant-based augmentation mammaplasty *via* an inframammary fold incision, but wanted to receive explantation.

On preoperative ultrasonography, the patient was found to have a round textured silicone gel-filled breast implant in the subpectoral pocket. The patient had a folding on the right side. But there were no findings that are suggestive of seroma, thickened capsule, upside-down rotation, rupture, and capsular mass (Video 8.14).

The patient underwent explantation with both subtotal capsulectomy *via* a previous inframammary fold scar on both sides. There was focal degeneration in both capsule (Fig. 8.9).

8.2.10 Case 10

On physical examination and history taking, a 41-year-old woman complained of change of breast tactile sense. The patient had a 7-year history of receiving an implant-based augmentation mammaplasty *via* an inframammary fold incision.

On preoperative ultrasonography, the patient was found to have a round textured silicone gel-filled breast implant in the subpectoral pocket. The patient had an major intracapsular rupture on the left side (Video 8.15) and a thickened capsule, accompanied by capsular ingrowth, on both

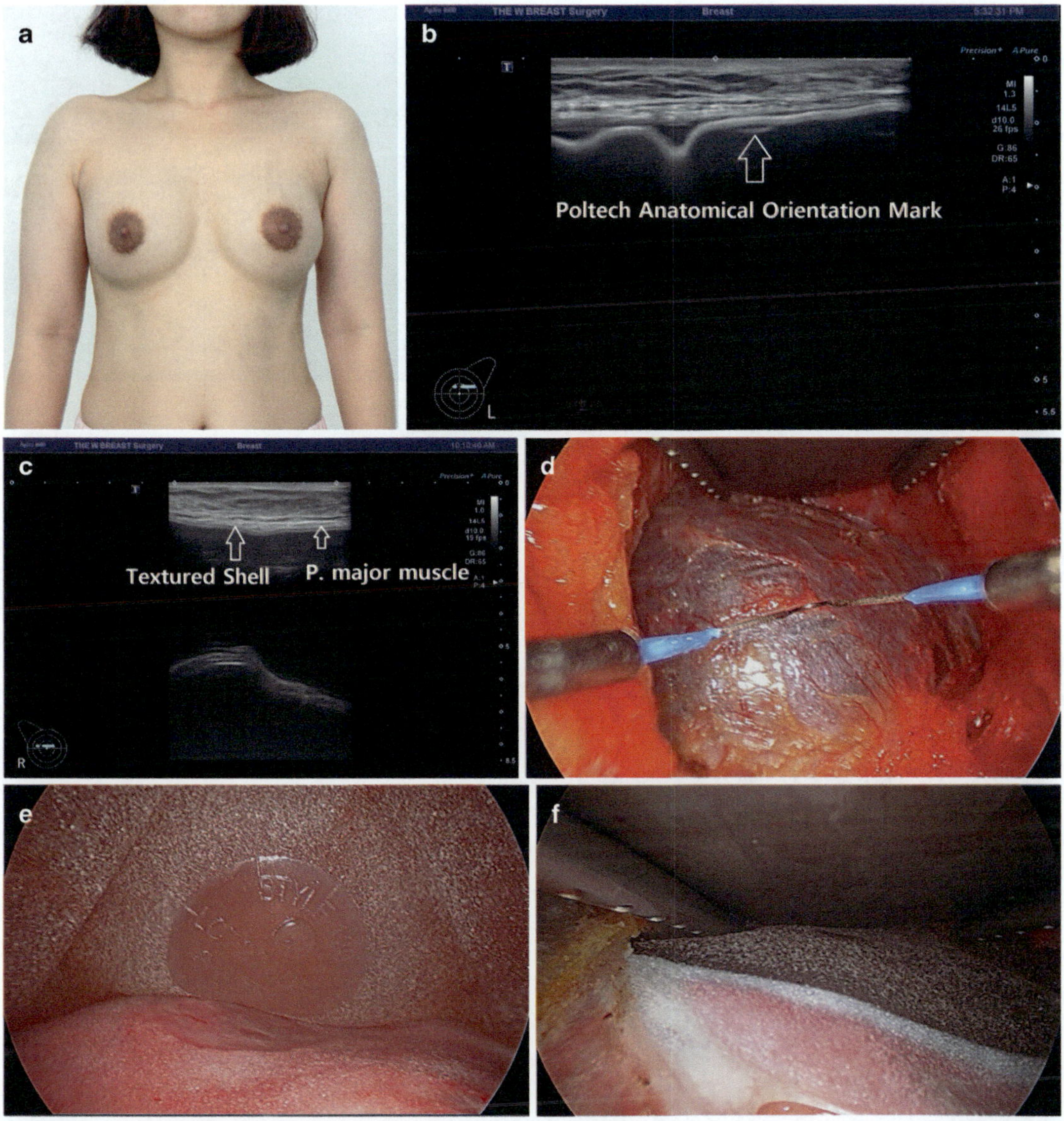

Fig. 8.7 (**a**) A preoperative front view. (**b**) Left textured shell type breast implant in subpectoral pocket is checked in preoperative ultrasonography. (**c**) Preoperative sonographic finding of the right breast textured implant in subpectoral pocket. (**d**) Right intraoperative view of periprosthetic capsule before capsulectomy. (**e**) Right intraoperative view of texture type breast implant, Allergan. (**f**) Right intraoperative view of breast implant texturing between shell and capsule. (**g**) Both removed Allergan round texture type breast implant style 120 300 cc(left), 260 cc(right). (**h**) Left capsule thickness is measured by digital caliper, 0.2 mm. (**i**) Right capsule thickness is measured by digital caliper, 0.3 mm. (**j**) Microscopic view of the left capsule. (**k**) Microscopic view of the right capsule

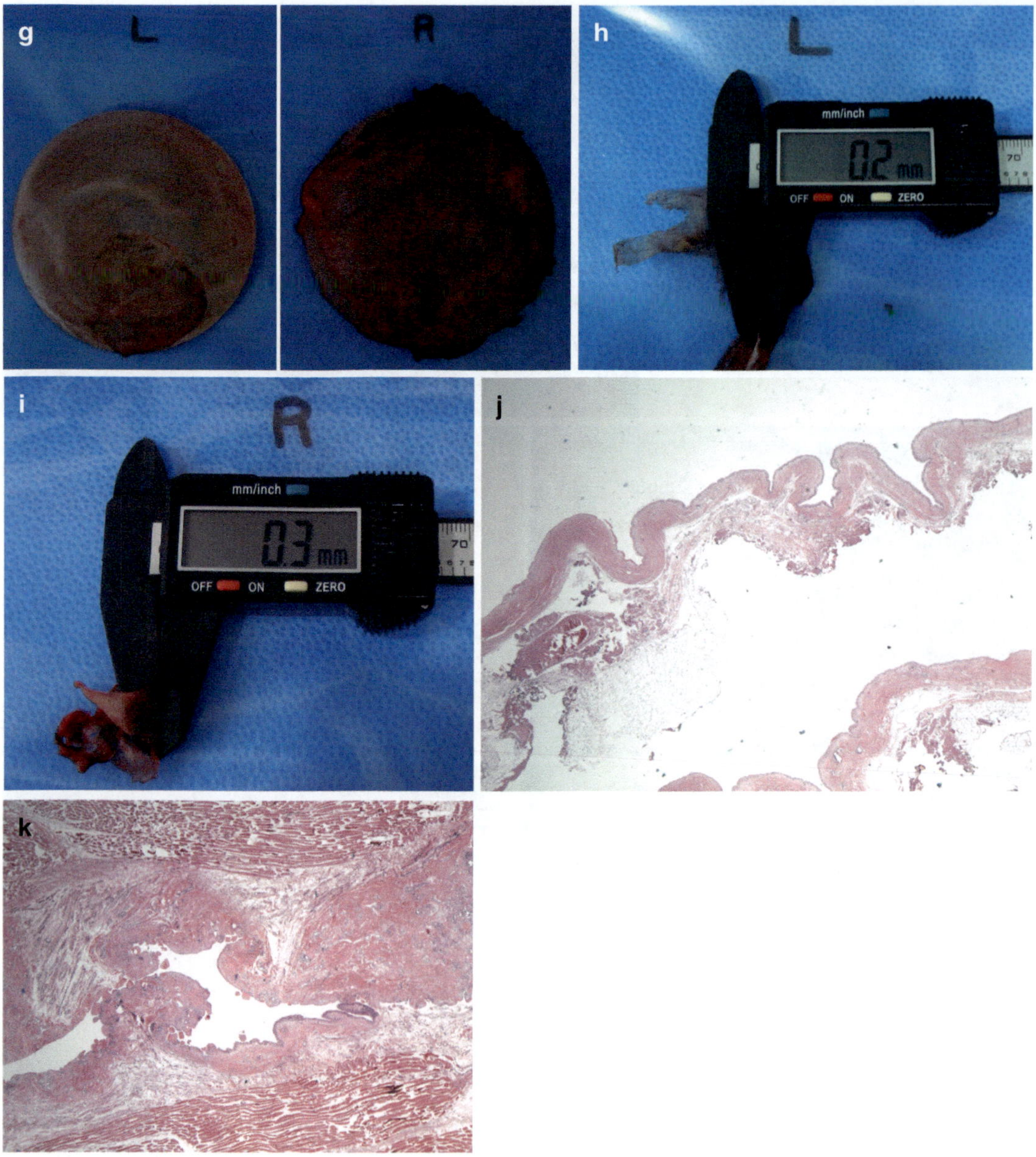

Fig. 8.7 (continued)

sides. But there were no findings that are suggestive of folding, seroma, upside-down rotation, and capsular mass.

The patient underwent explantation with both subtotal capsulectomy *via* a previous inframammary fold scar on both sides. There were focal chronic inflammation in both capsule (Fig. 8.10).

8.2.11 Case 11

On physical examination and history taking, a 59-year-old woman complained of breast hardness. The patient had a 7-year-history of receiving an implant-based augmentation mammaplasty *via* an inframammary fold incision.

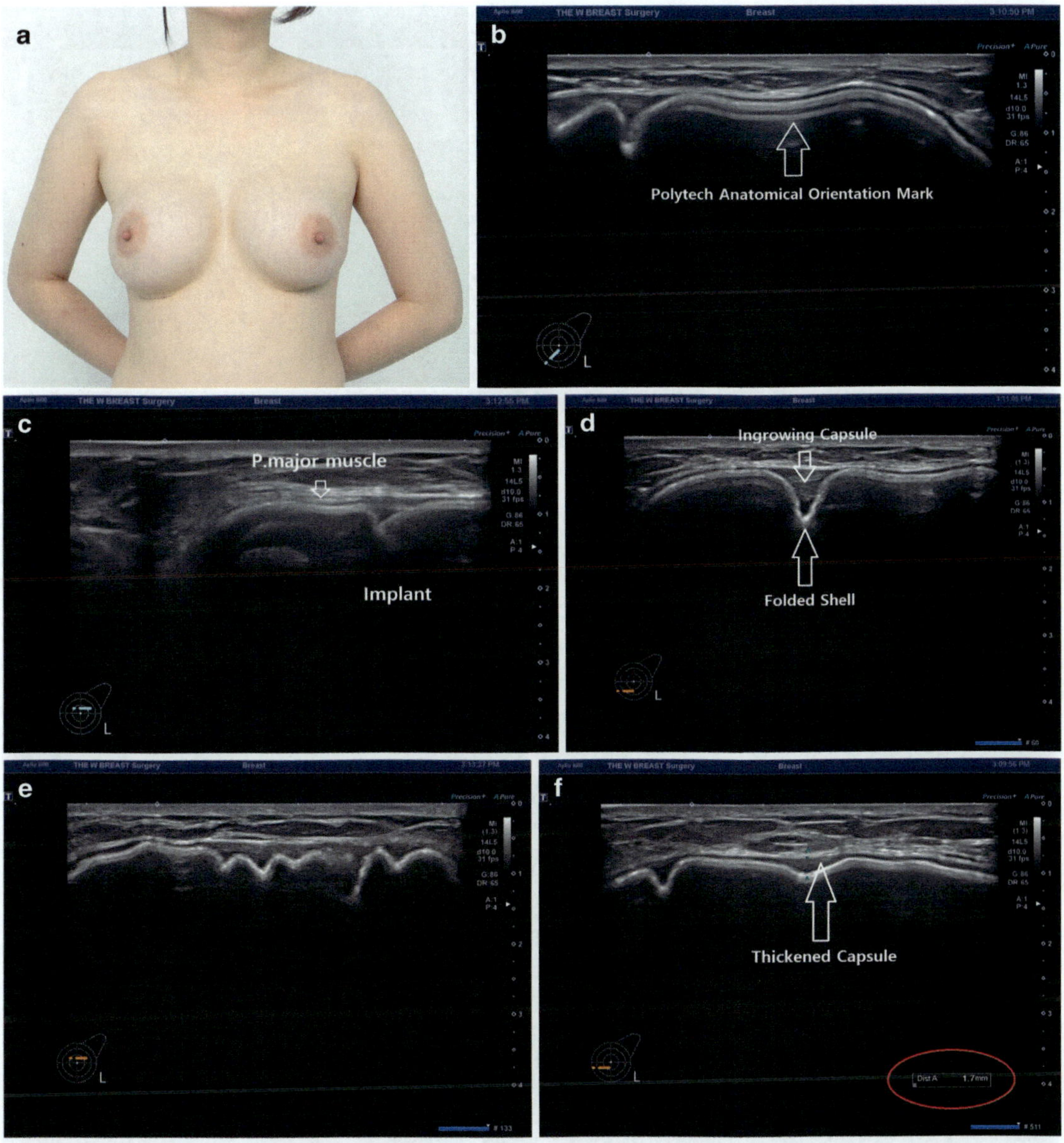

Fig. 8.8 (**a**) A preoperative front view. (**b**) Left Polytech anatomical breast implant in ultrasound is checked in preoperative ultrasonography. (**c**) Left textured shell type breast implant in subpectoral pocket is checked. (**d**) Left breast implant folded shell and ingrowing capsule. (**e, f**) Left periprosthetic thickened capsule, 1.7 mm. (**g, h**) Right textured shell type breast implant in subpectoral pocket with thickened capsule is checked in preoperative ultrasonography. (**i**) Right breast implant folded shell due to thickened capsule is checked. (**j, k**) Right periprosthetic thickened capsule with ingrowing is measured by ultrasound, 2.0 mm. (**l**) Both removed breast implant and periprosthetic capsule by total capsulectomy. (**m**) Left capsule thickness is measured digital caliper, 2.5 mm. (**n–p**) Left capsule with multiple rugae. (**q**) Right capsule thickness is measured by digital caliper, 2.1 mm. (**r**) Right capsule with multiple capsular rugae. (**s**) Microscopic view of the right capsule. (**t**) Microscopic view of the right capsule

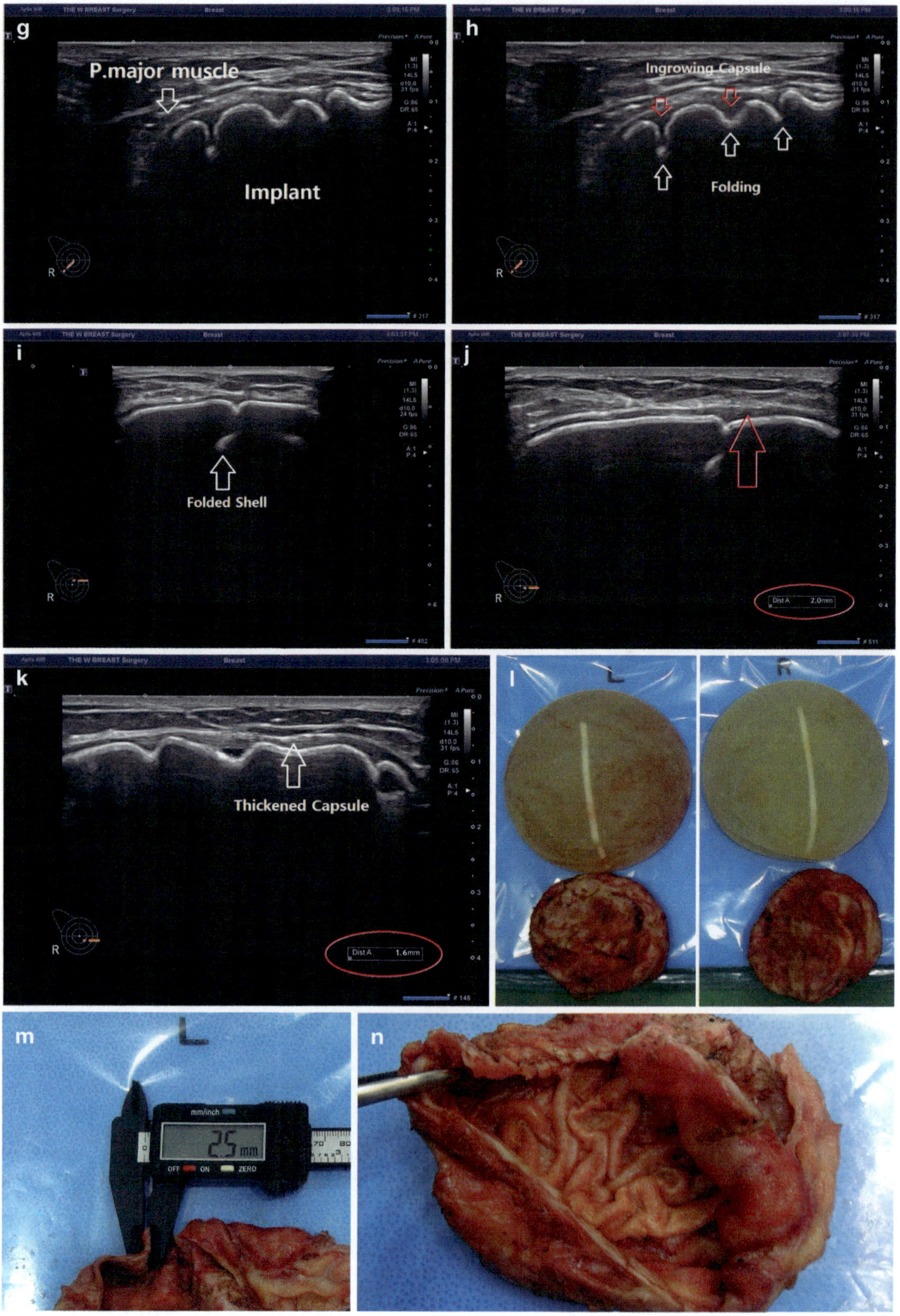

Fig. 8.8 (continued)

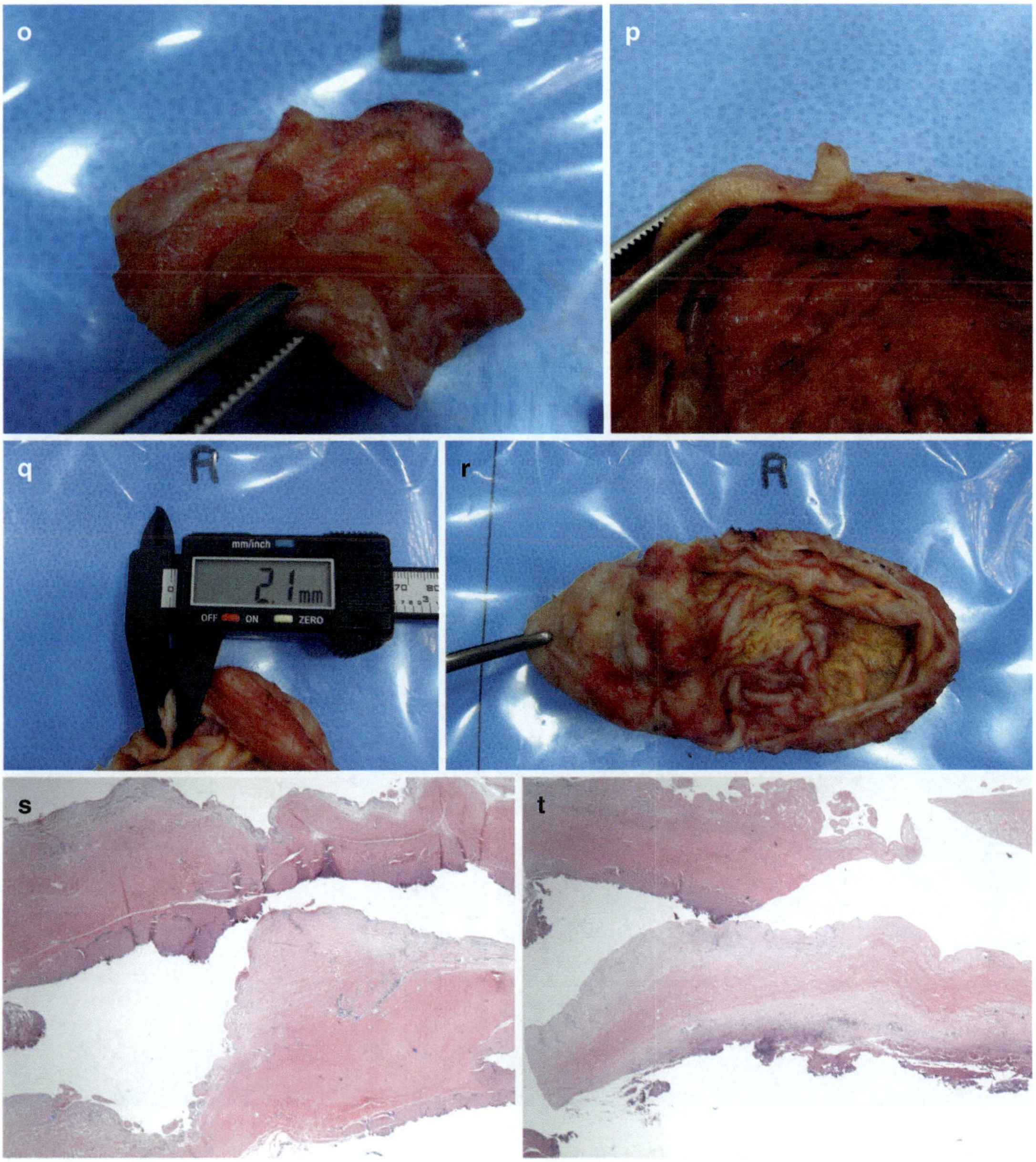

Fig. 8.8 (continued)

On preoperative ultrasonography, the patient was found to have an anatomical silicone gel-filled breast implant (Allergan Inc., Irvine, CA) in the subglandular pocket. The patient had a folding, double capsule, and a thickened capsule which was measured as 1.2 mm on both sides (Video 8.16). But there were no findings that are suggestive of seroma, upside-down rotation, rupture, and capsular mass.

The patient underwent explantation with both total capsulectomy *via* a previous inframammary fold scar on both sides. There were focal chronic inflammation and degeneration in both fibrous capsule (Fig. 8.11).

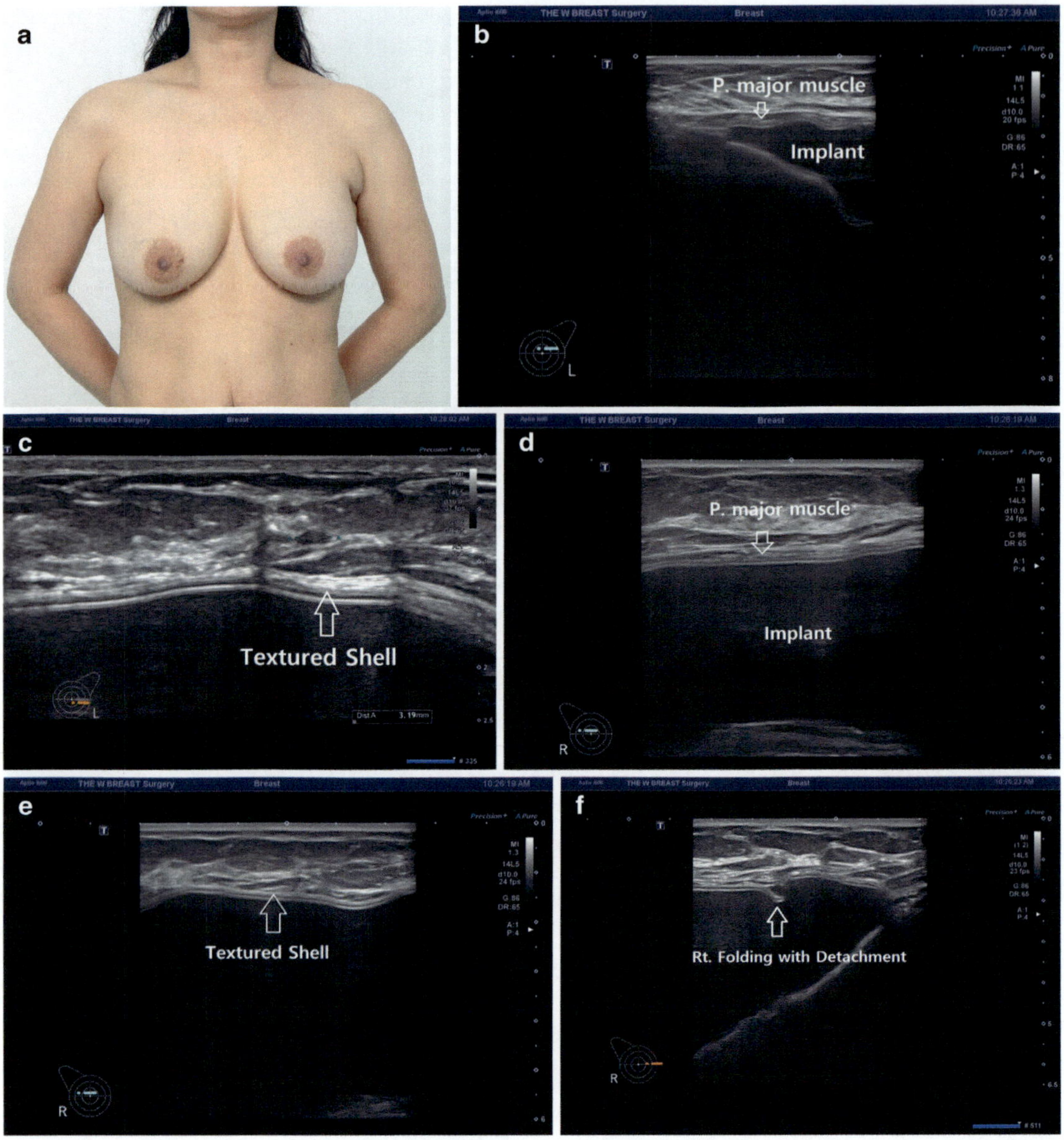

Fig. 8.9 (**a**) A preoperative front view. (**b**) Left breast implant in subpectoral pocket in ultrasound is checked in preoperative ultrasonography. (**c**) Left textured shell type breast implant is checked in preoperative ultrasonography. (**d**) Right breast implant in subpectoral pocket is checked in preoperative ultrasonography. (**e**) Right textured shell type breast implant is checked in preoperative ultrasonography. (**f**): Right breast implant folded shell and detachment is checked in ultrasonography. (**g**) Both removed periprosthetic capsule by subtotal capsulectomy and Mentor round texture type breast implant 225 cc. (**h**) Left capsule thickness is measured by digital caliper, 0.6 mm. (**i**) Right capsule thickness is measured by digital caliper, 0.7 mm. (**j**) Microscopic view of the left capsule. (**k**) Microscopic view of the right capsule

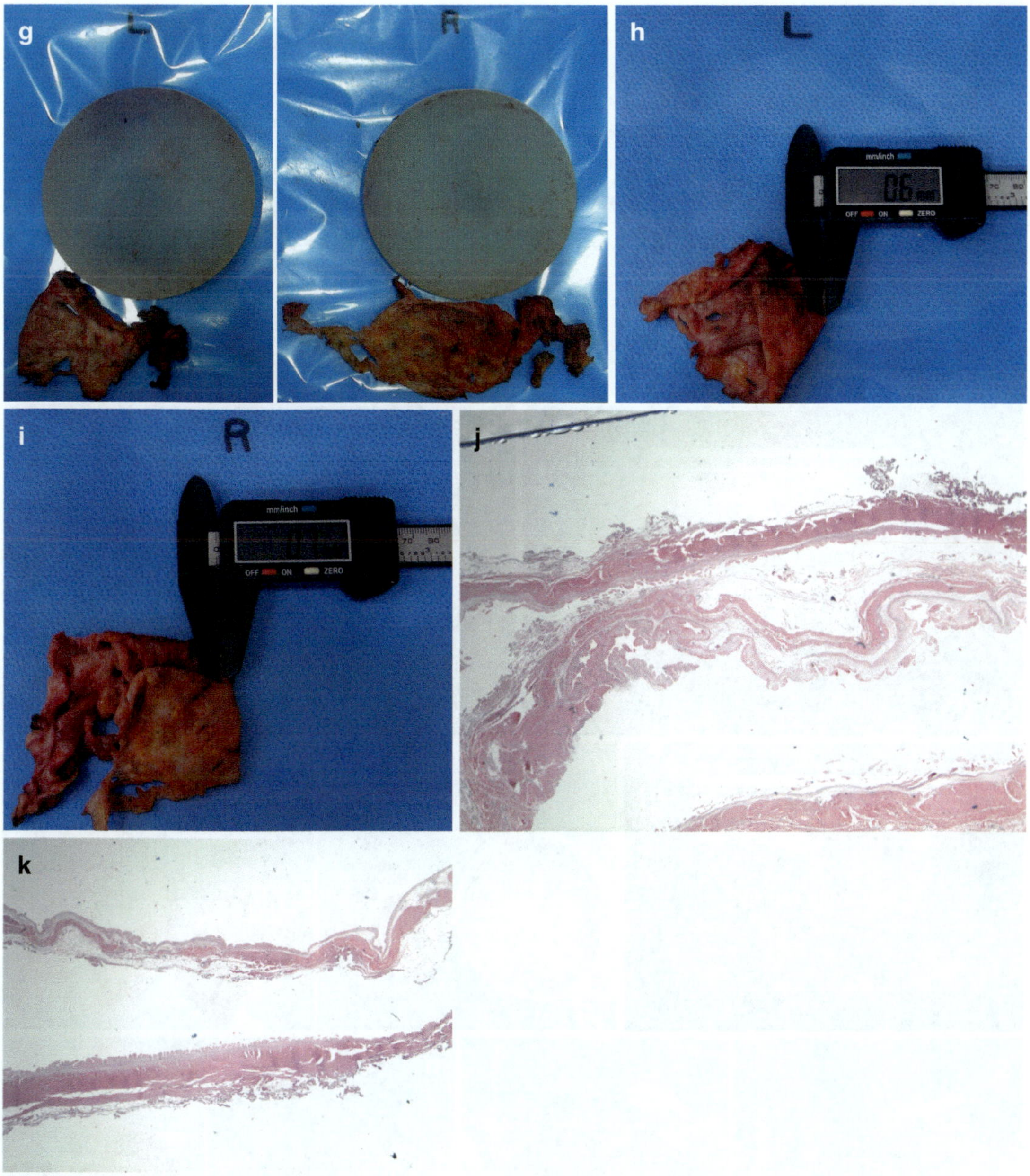

Fig. 8.9 (continued)

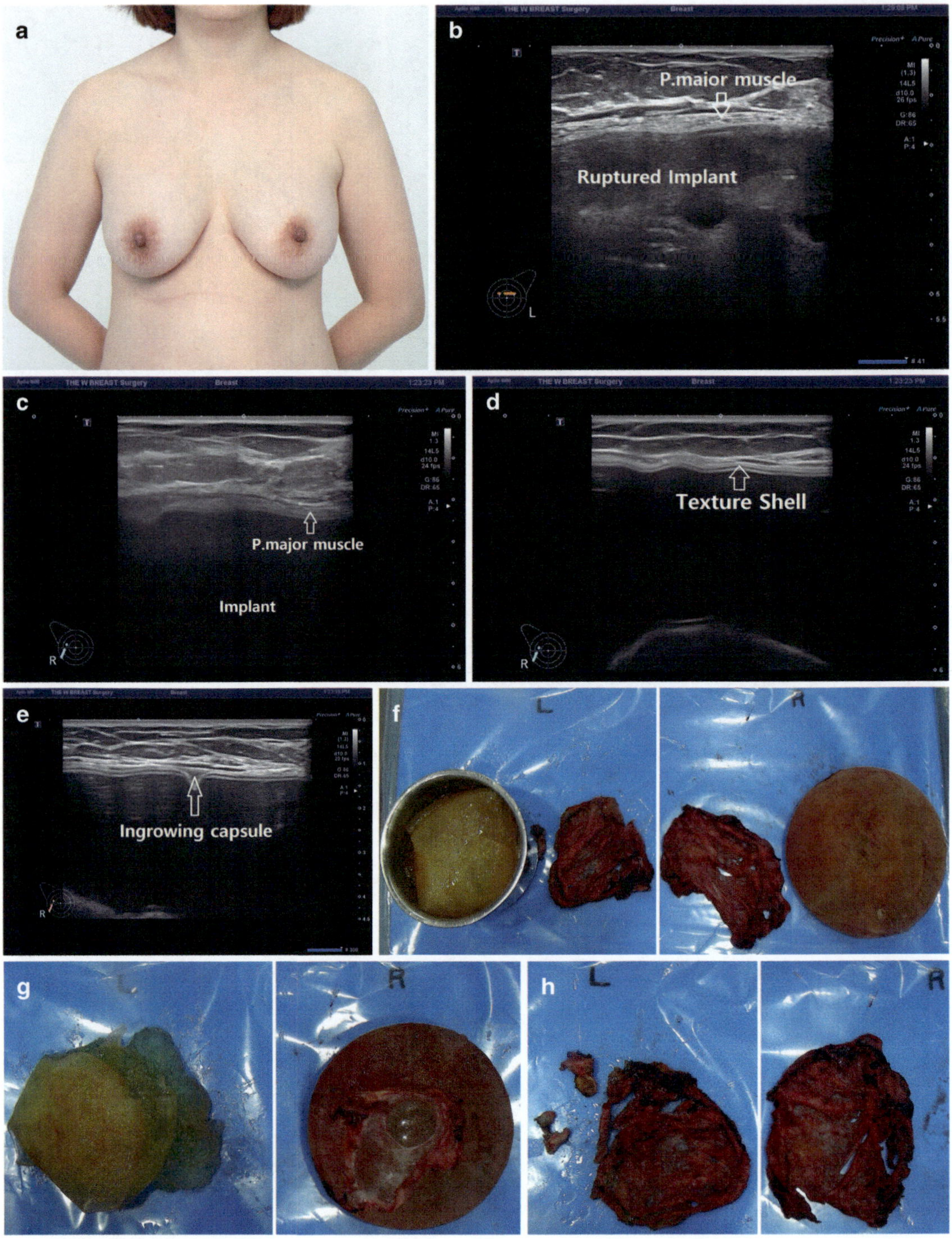

Fig. 8.10 (**a**) A preoperative front view. (**b**) Left ruptured breast implant in subpectoral pocket is checked in preoperative ultrasonography. (**c**) Right breast implant in subpectoral pocket in ultrasonography. (**d**) Right textured shell type breast implant is checked in preoperative ultrasonography. (**e**) Right periprosthetic capsule with ingrowing is checked in ultrasonography. (**f**) Both removed implant and periprosthetic capsule. Gross finding of the right ruptured implant. (**g**) Both removed Allergan round textured shell type breast implant style 115 290 cc (left), 272 cc (right) breast implant. (**h**) Both removed periprosthetic capsule by subtotal capsulectomy. (**i**) Left capsule thickness is measured by digital caliper, 0.6 mm. (**j**) Right capsule thickness is measured by digital caliper, 0.3 mm. (**k**) Right periprosthetic capsule with ingrowing. (**l**) Microscopic view of the left capsule with silicone invasion to capsule. (**m**) Microscopic view of the right capsule

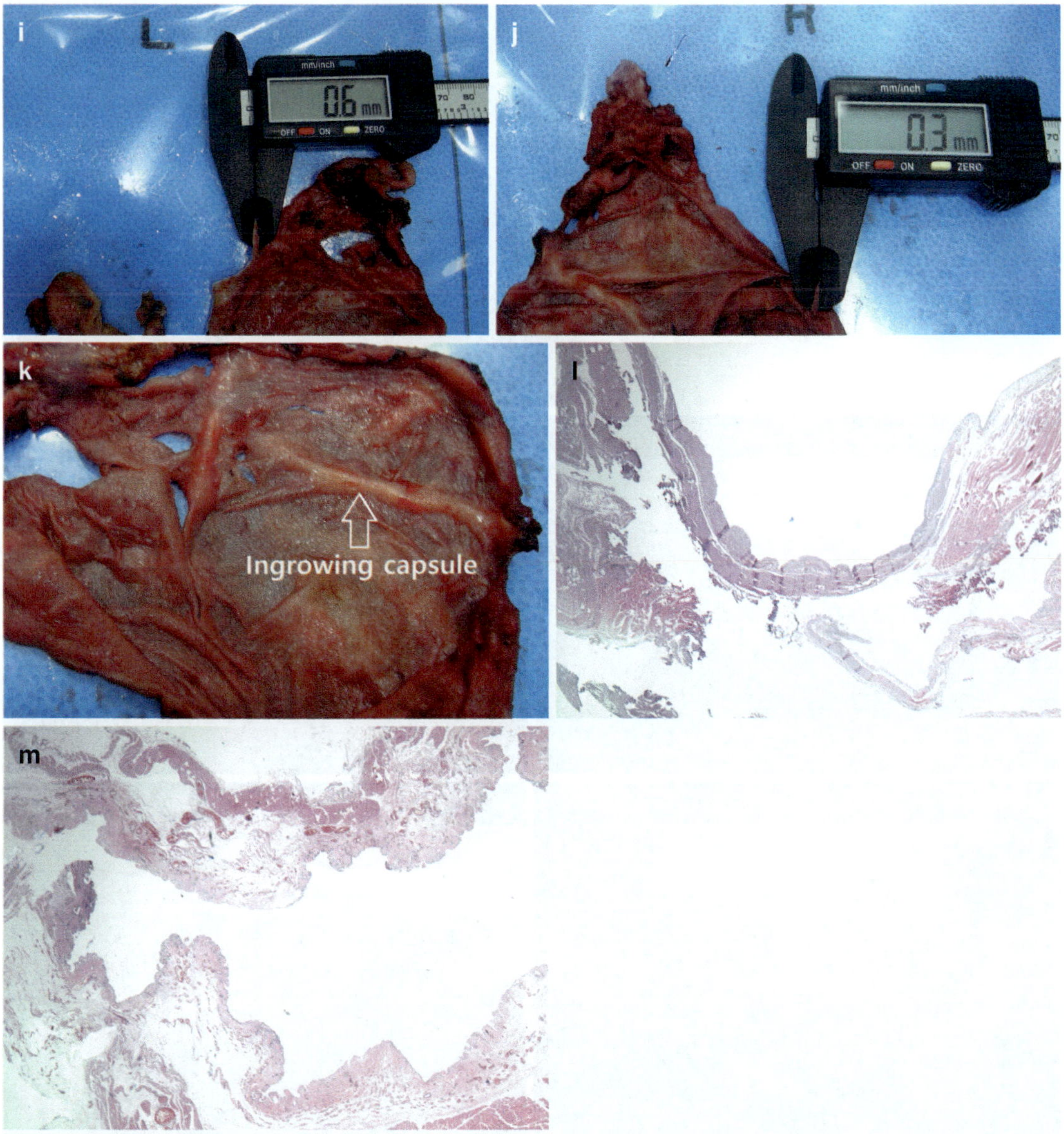

Fig. 8.10 (continued)

8.2.12 Case 12

A 40-year-old woman had an 11-year-history of receiving an implant-based augmentation mammaplasty *via* an axillary incision, but wanted to receive explantation d/t breast discomfort.

On preoperative ultrasound, the patient was found to have a round smooth silicone gel-filled breast implant in the subpectoral pocket. But there were no findings that are suggestive of folding, seroma, thickened capsule, upside-down rotation, rupture, and capsular mass (Video 8.17).

The patient underwent explantation with both subtotal capsulectomy *via* a previous axillary scar on both sides. There were focal chronic inflammation and fibrosis in both capsule (Fig. 8.12).

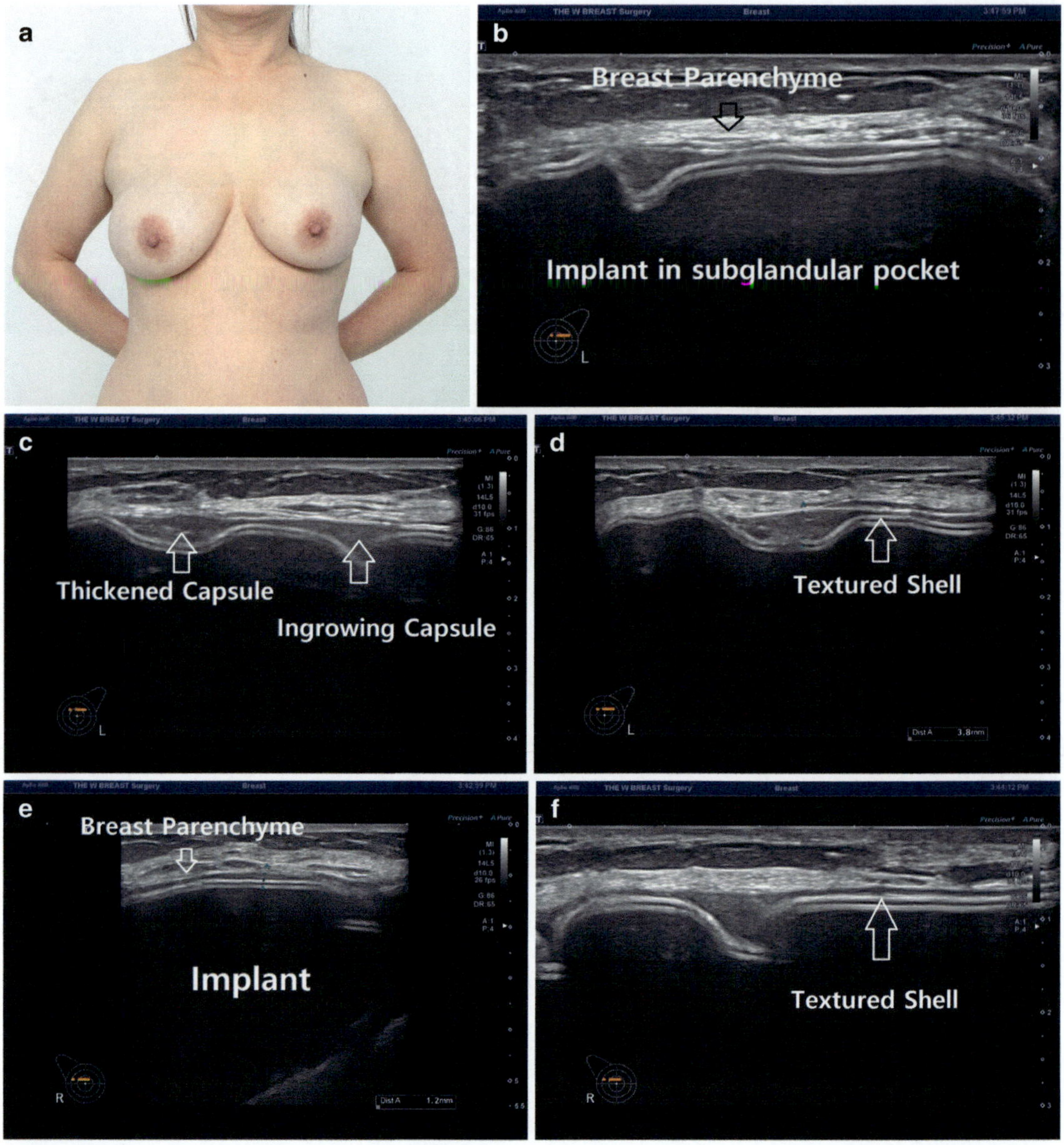

Fig. 8.11 (**a**) A preoperative front view. (**b**) Left breast implant in subglandular pocket in ultrasound is checked in preoperative ultrasonography. (**c**) Left breast implant with thickened capsule is checked. (**d**) Left textured shell type breast implant is checked in preoperative ultrasonography. (**e–i**) Right textured shell type breast implant with thickened capsule and folded shell in subglandular pocket is checked in preoperative ultrasonography. (**j**) Left intraoperative view of breast pocket after total capsulectomy. (**k**) Right intraoperative view of breast pocket after total capsulectomy. (**l**) Both removed periprosthetic capsule and Allergan anatomical type breast implant 410 MM 215 cc. (**m**) Both removed periprosthetic capsule, double capsule by total capsulectomy. (**n, o**) Left removed double capsule. (**p, q**) Left double capsule thickness is measured by digital caliper, 0.9 & 0.3 mm. (**r**) Left periprosthetic capsule thickness with ingrowing is measured, 8 mm. (**s, t**) Right double capsule finding. (**u, v**) Right double capsule thickness is measured by digital caliper, 08 mm & 0.3 mm. (**w**) Right inner capsule thickness is measured, 6 mm. (**x**) Right breast implant with periprosthetic double capsule. (**y**) Microscopic view of the left capsule. (**z**) Microscopic view of the right capsule

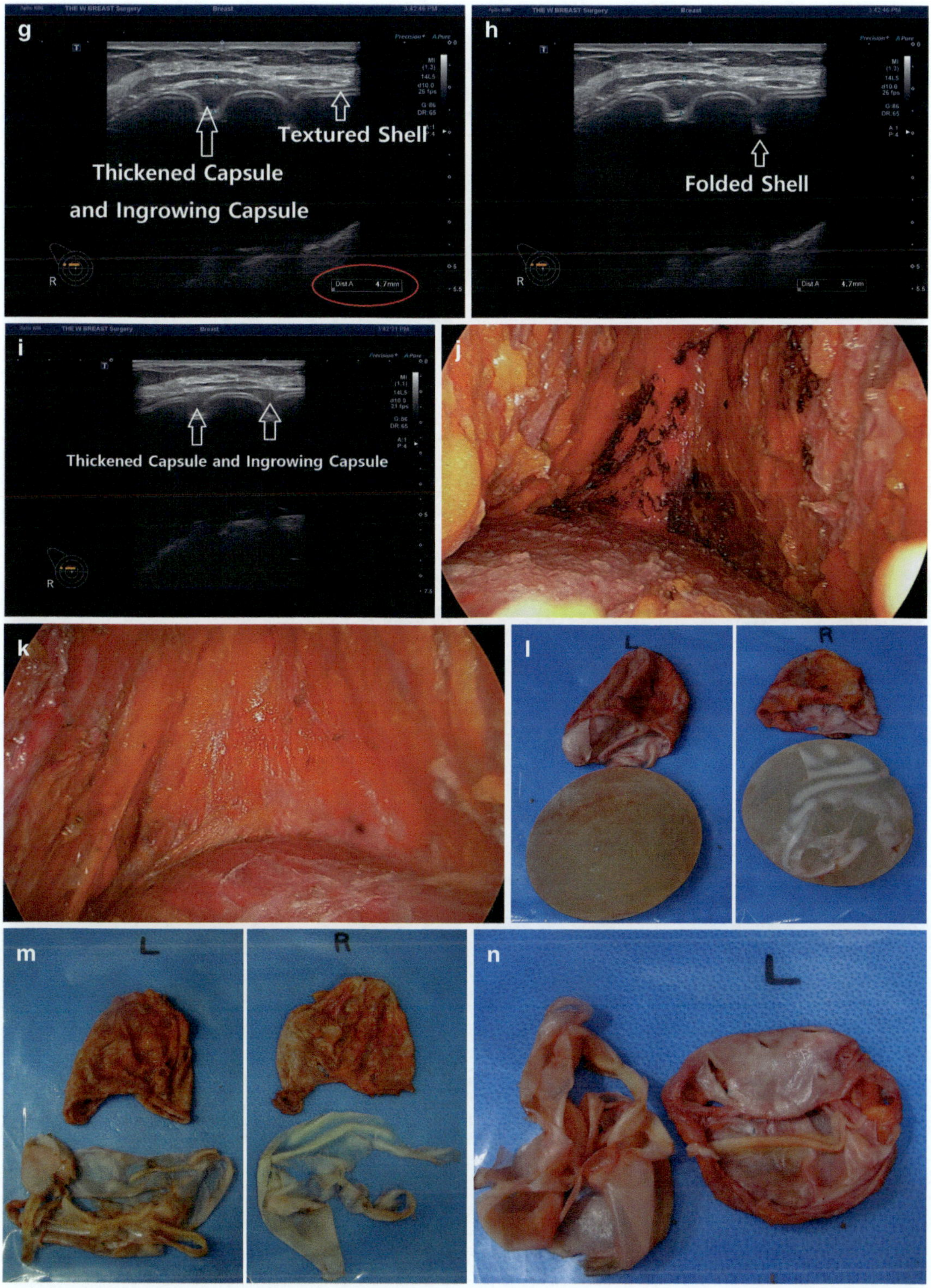

Fig. 8.11 (continued)

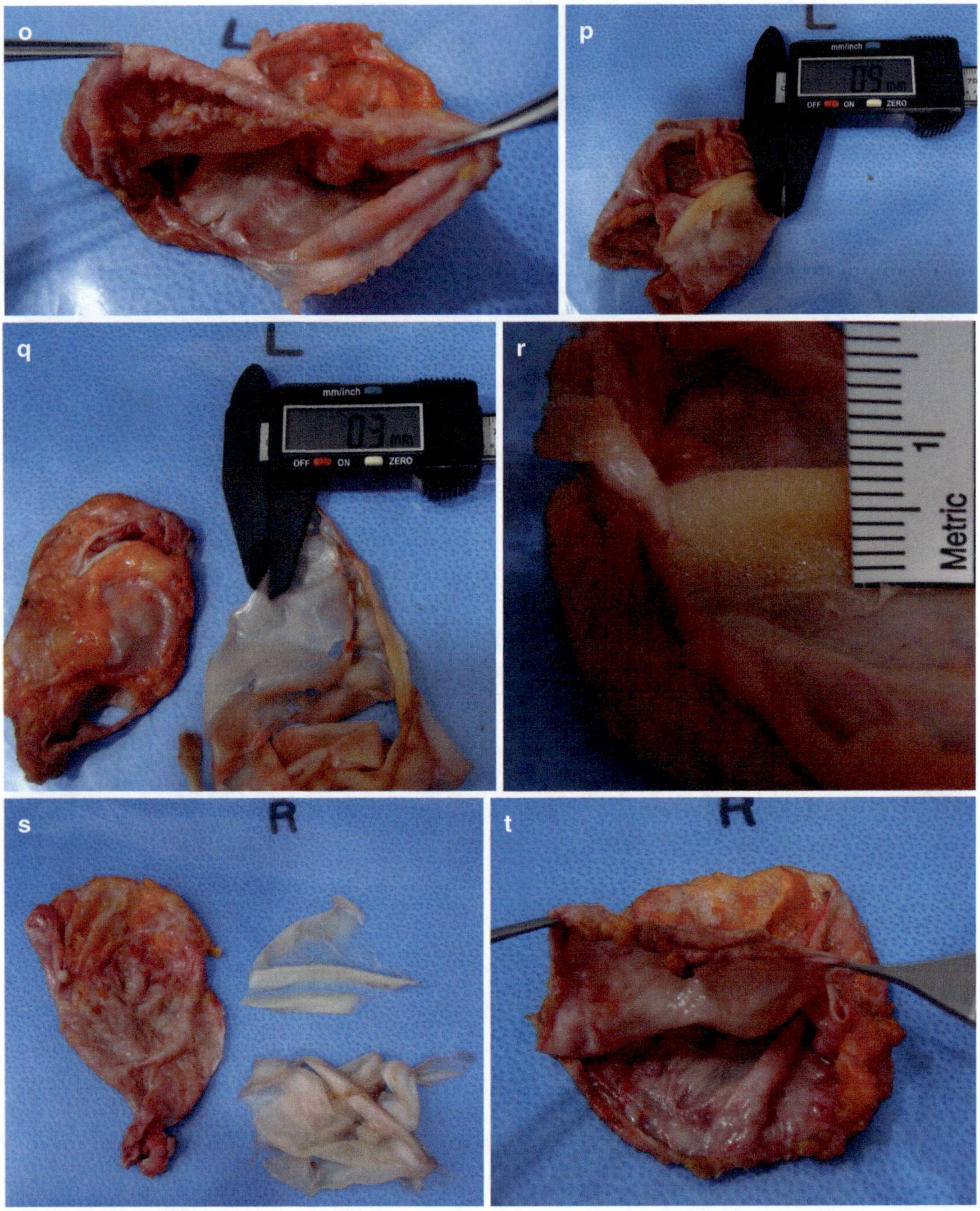

Fig. 8.11 (continued)

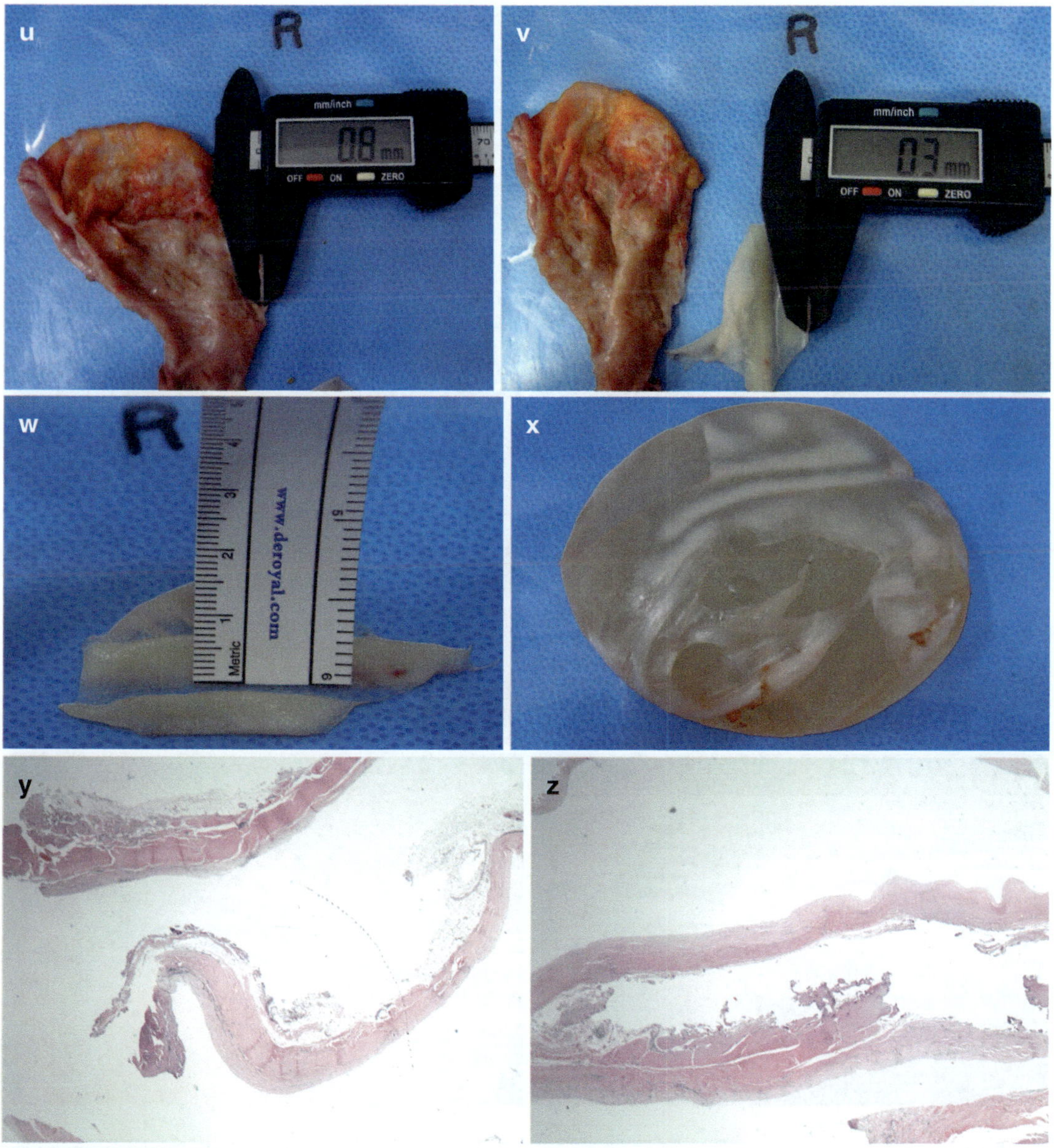

Fig. 8.11 (continued)

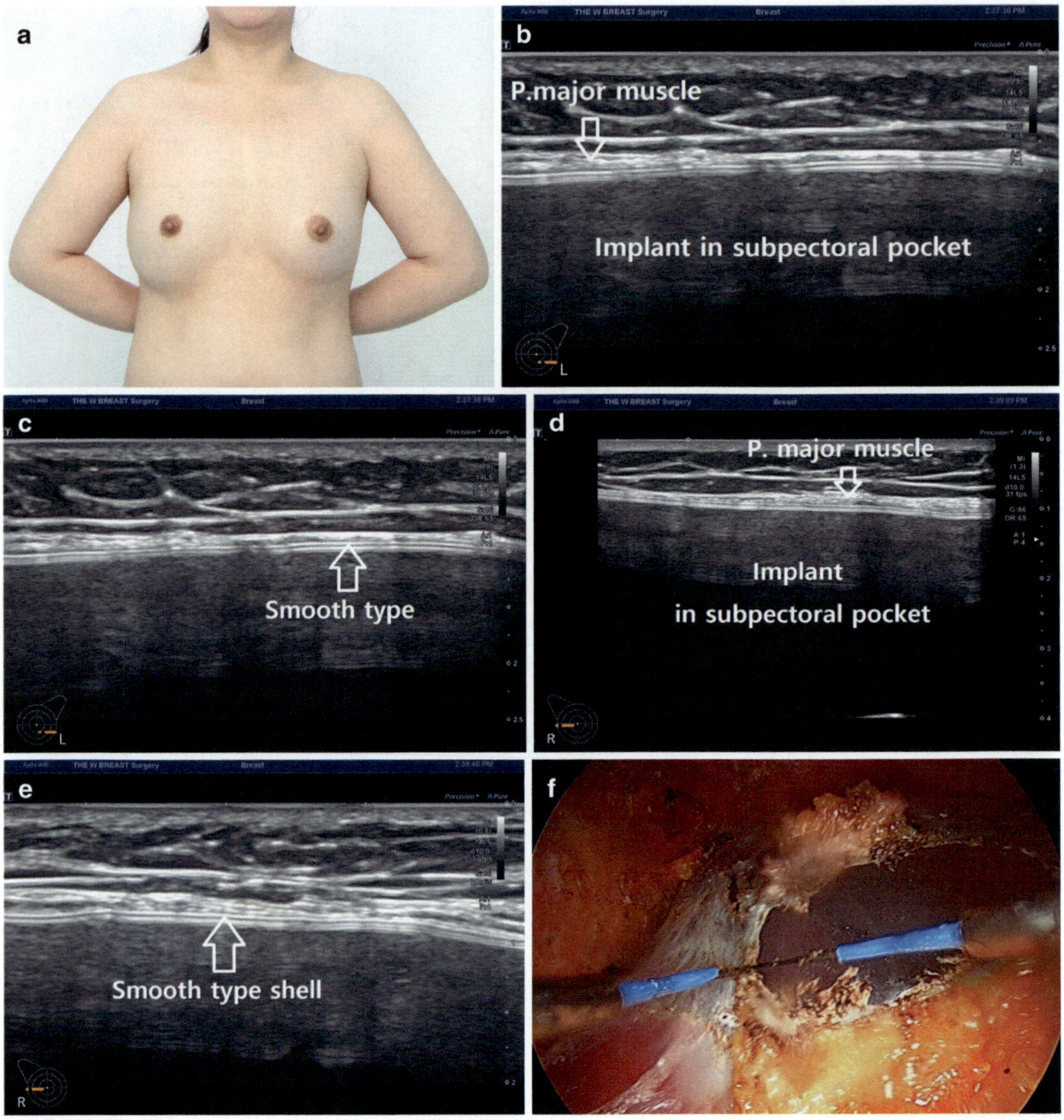

Fig. 8.12 (**a**) A preoperative front view. (**b**) Left breast implant in subpectoral pocket is checked in preoperative ultrasonography. (**c**) Left smooth shell type breast implant is checked in ultrasonography. (**d**) Right breast implant in subpectoral pocket is checked in ultrasonography. (**e**) Right smooth shell type breast implant is checked in ultrasonography. (**f**) Left intraoperative view of smooth type breast implant with periprosthetic capsule. (**g**) Left intraoperative view of breast pocket. (**h**) Left intraoperative view of breast pocket after subtotal capsulectomy. (**i**) Right intraoperative view of periprosthetic capsule. (**j**) Right intraoperative view of breast pocket after subtotal capsulectomy. (**k**) Both removed periprosthetic capsule and Mentor round smooth type breast implant, 250 cc. (**l**) Left removed periprosthetic capsule after subtotal capsulectomy. (**m**) Right removed periprosthetic capsule by subtotal capsulectomy. (**n**) Left capsule thickness is measured by digital caliper, 0.2 mm. (**o**) Right capsule thickness is measured by digital caliper, 0.1 mm. (**p**) Microscopic view of the left capsule. (**q**) Microscopic view of the right capsule

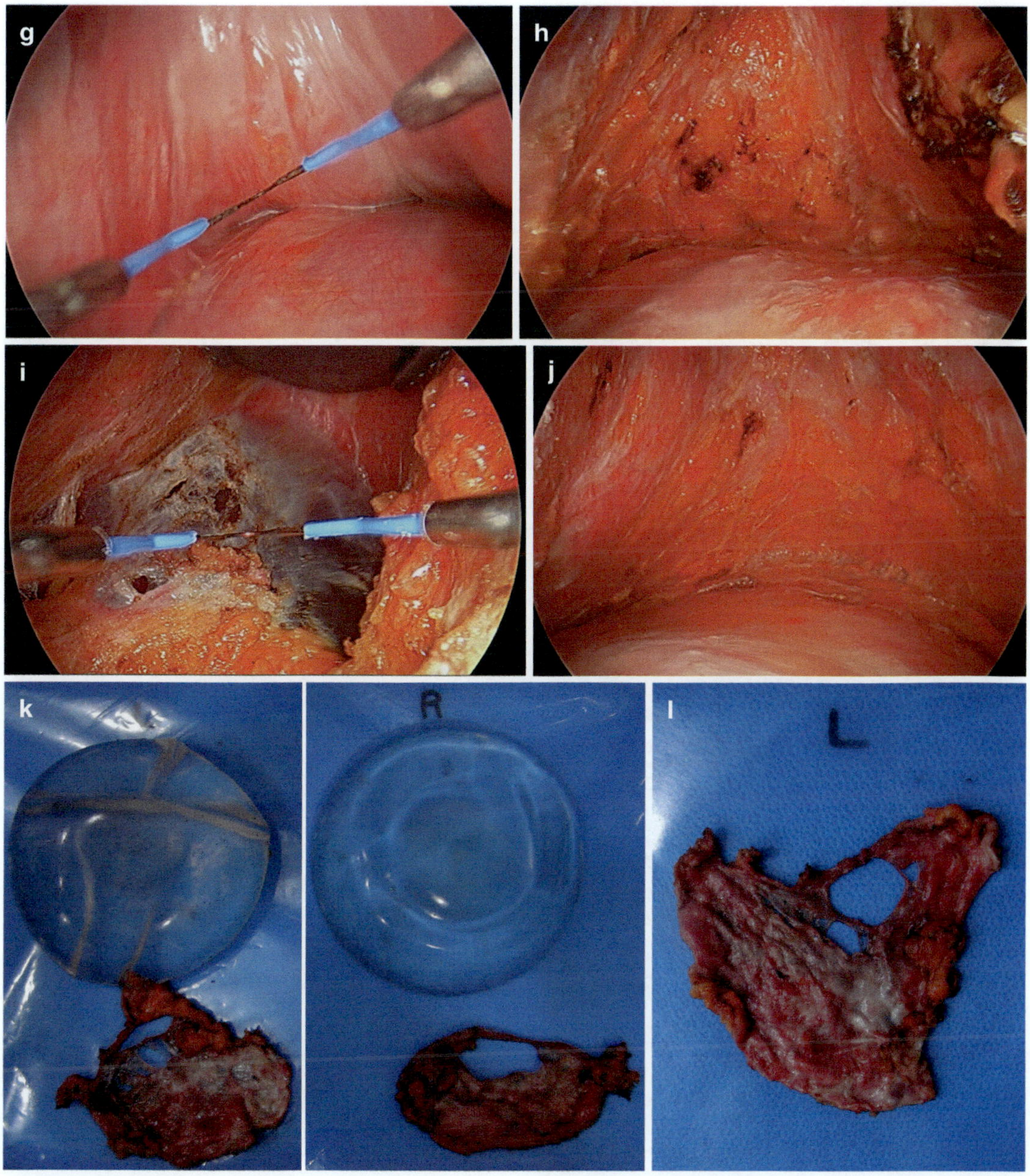

Fig. 8.12 (continued)

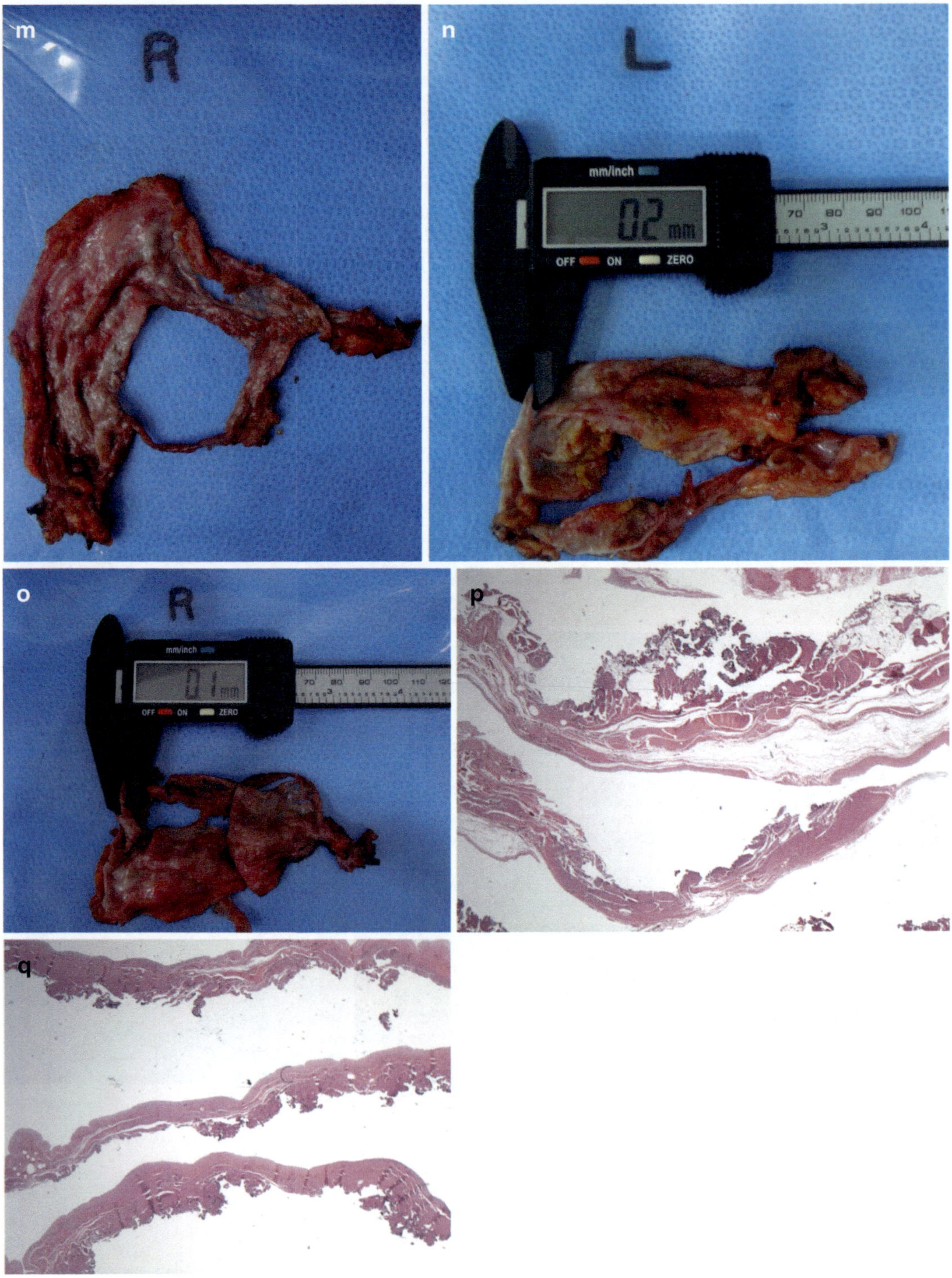

Fig. 8.12 (continued)

8.2.13 Case 13

On physical examination and history taking, a 42-year-old woman complained of breast hardness on both sides. The patient had an 8-year-history of receiving an implant-based augmentation mammaplasty *via* an axillary incision.

On preoperative ultrasonography, the patient was found to have a round textured silicone gel-filled breast implant in the subpectoral pocket. The patient bilaterally had a folding and a thickened capsule which was measured as 1.7 mm on the right side and 1.3 mm on the left side. Moreover, the patient also had a double capsule on the right side. But there were no findings that are suggestive of seroma, upside-down rotation, rupture, and capsular mass (Video 8.18).

The patient underwent explantation with both subtotal capsulectomy *via* a previous axillary scar on both sides. There were focal chronic inflammation in both fibrous capsule (Fig. 8.13).

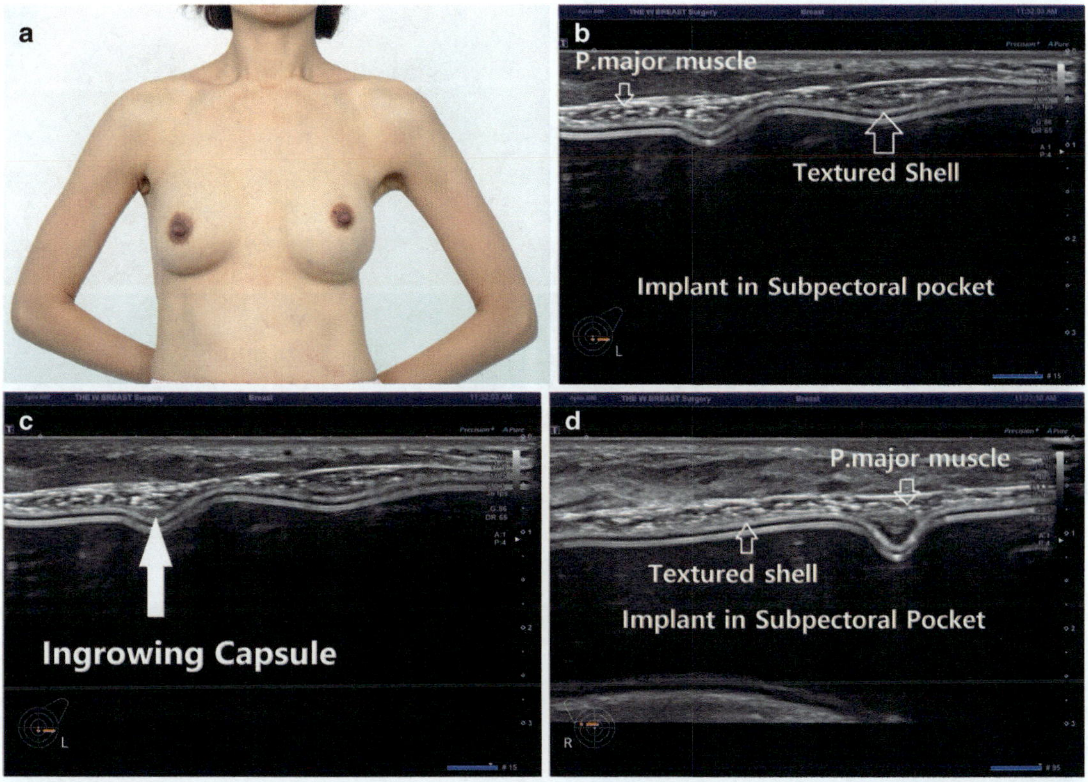

Fig. 8.13 (**a**) A preoperative front view. (**b**) Left textured shell type breast implant in subpectoral pocket is checked in preoperative ultrasonography. (**c**) Left thickened periprosthetic capsule with ingrowing is checked in preoperative ultrasonography. (**d**) Right textured shell type breast implant in subpectoral pocket is checked in preoperative ultrasonography. (**e**) Right thickened periprosthetic capsule with ingrowing is checked in preoperative ultrasonography. (**f**) Left intraoperative view of periprosthetic capsule before capsulectomy. (**g**) Left intraoperative view of breast pocket after subtotal capsulectomy. (**h**) Right intraoperative view of periprosthetic capsule before capsulectomy. (**i**) Right intraoperative view of breast pocket after subtotal capsulectomy. (**j**) Both removed Allergan round texture type breast implant style 115 253 cc. (**k**) Both removed periprosthetic capsule by subtotal capsulectomy. (**l**) Left thickened periprosthetic capsule with ingrowing. (**m**) Right thickened periprosthetic capsule with ingrowing. (**n**) Left capsule thickness is measured by digital caliper, 1.3 mm. (**o**, **p**) Right capsule thickness is measured by digital caliper, 0.5 & 1.7 mm. (**q**) Microscopic view of the left capsule. (**r**) Microscopic view of the right capsule

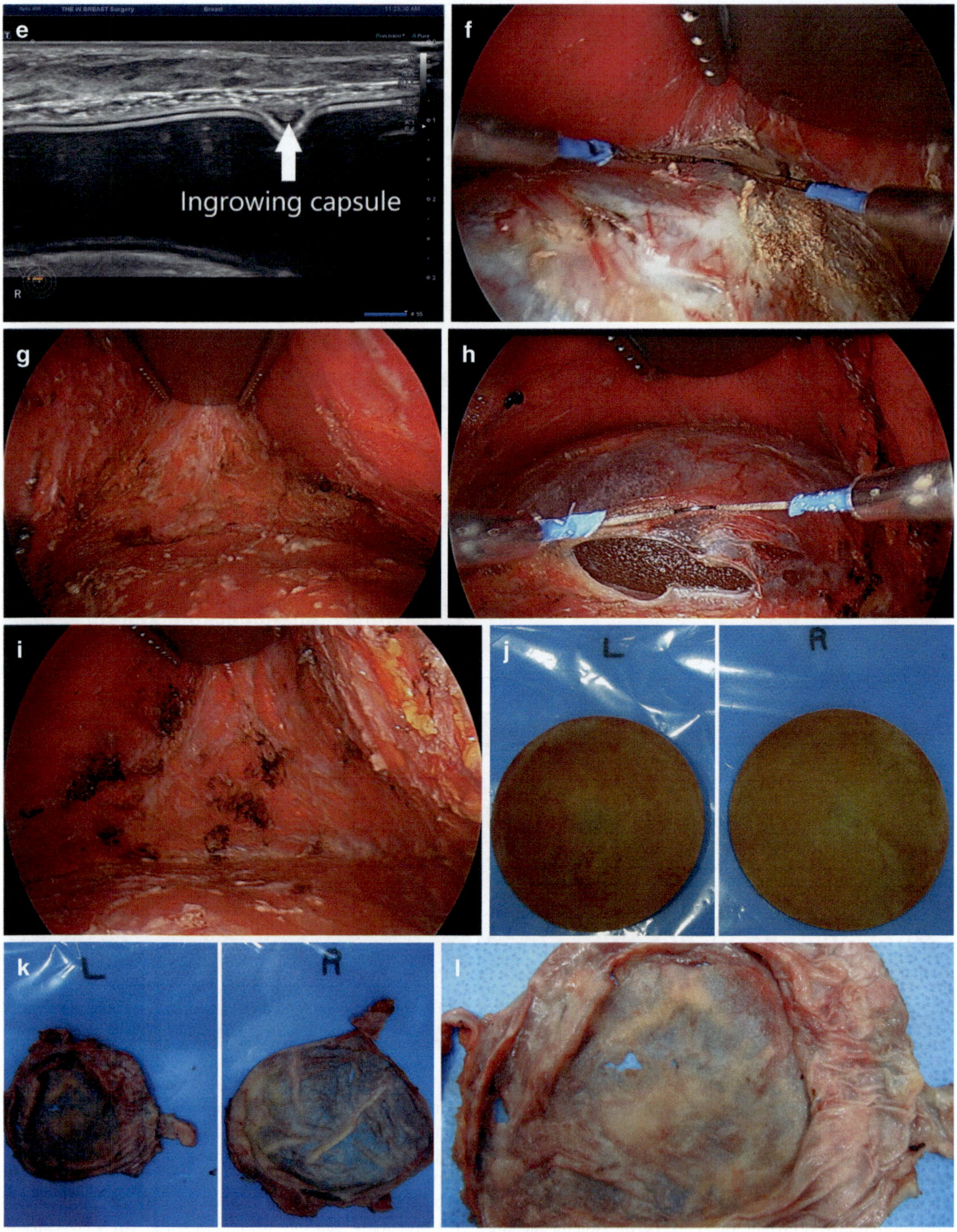

Fig. 8.13 (continued)

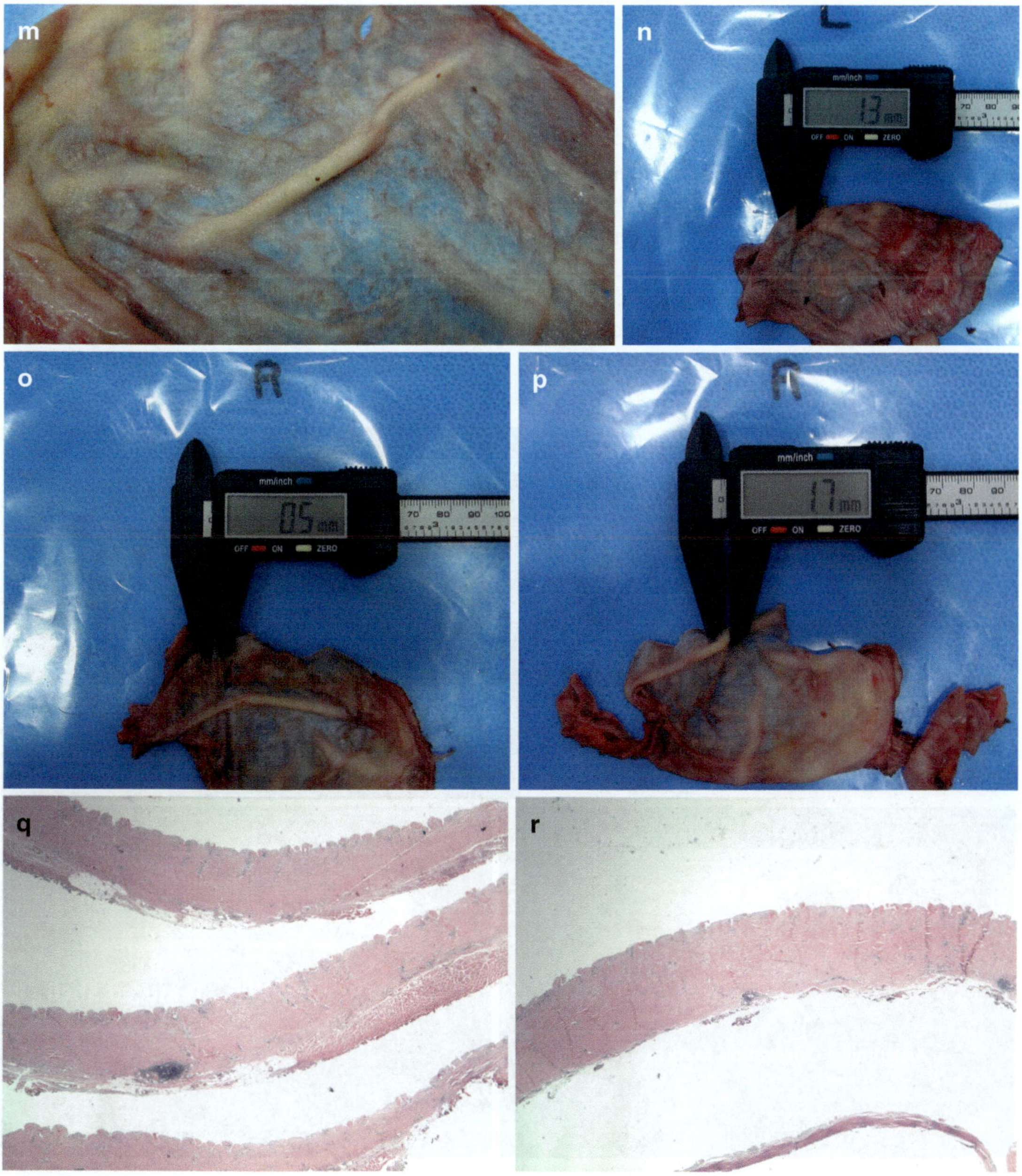

Fig. 8.13 (continued)

8.2.14 Case 14

On physical examination and history taking, a 52-year-old woman complained of breast hardness on both sides. The patient had a 6-year history of receiving an implant-based augmentation mammaplasty *via* an axillary incision.

On preoperative ultrasonography, the patient was found to have an anatomical silicone gel-filled breast implant (Silimed Inc., Rio de Janeiro, Brazil) in the subpectoral pocket. The patient had a folding *as well as* a thickened capsule which was measured as 1.6 mm on both sides, accompanied by the presence of a seroma on the right side (Video 8.19). But there were no findings that are suggestive of upside-down rotation, rupture, and capsular mass.

The patient underwent subtotal capsulectomy with replacement of the device *via* a previous axillary scar on both sides. There were right focal chronic inflammation and hemorrhage and left focal chronic inflammation and subcapsular hemorrhage in capsule (Fig. 8.14).

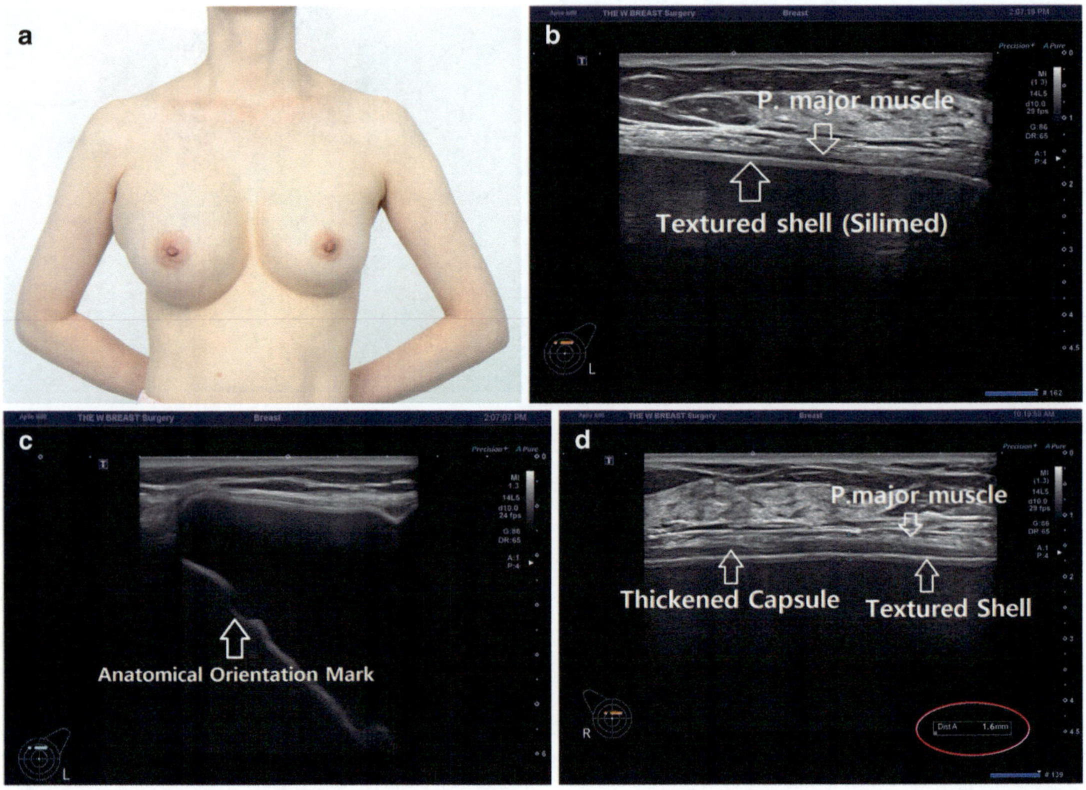

Fig. 8.14 (**a**) A preoperative front view. (**b**) Left textured shell type breast implant in subpectoral pocket is checked in preoperative ultrasonography. (**c**) Left Silimed textured shell type breast implant and inferior orientation mark with thickened capsule is checked in ultrasonography. (**d**) Right textured shell type breast implant in subpectoral pocket with thickened capsule, 1.6 mm is checked in preoperative ultrasonography. (**e**) Right Silimed textured shell type breast implant shell is checked in preoperative ultrasonography. (**f**) Right Silimed anatomical type breast implant with inferior orientation mark is checked preoperative ultrasonography. (**g**) Right breast periprosthetic fluid collection is checked in ultrasonography. (**h**) Both removed breast implant and periprosthetic capsule after subtotal capsulectomy. (**i**) Both removed Silimed anatomical type breast implant, 275 cc. (**j**) Both removed periprosthetic capsule by subtotal capsulectomy. (**k**) Left capsule thickness is measured by digital caliper, 1.6 mm. (**l**) Right capsule thickness is measured by digital caliper, 1.7 mm. (**m**) Microscopic view of the left capsule. (**n**) Microscopic view of the right capsule. (**o**) Right aspirated serous colored periprosthetic fluid

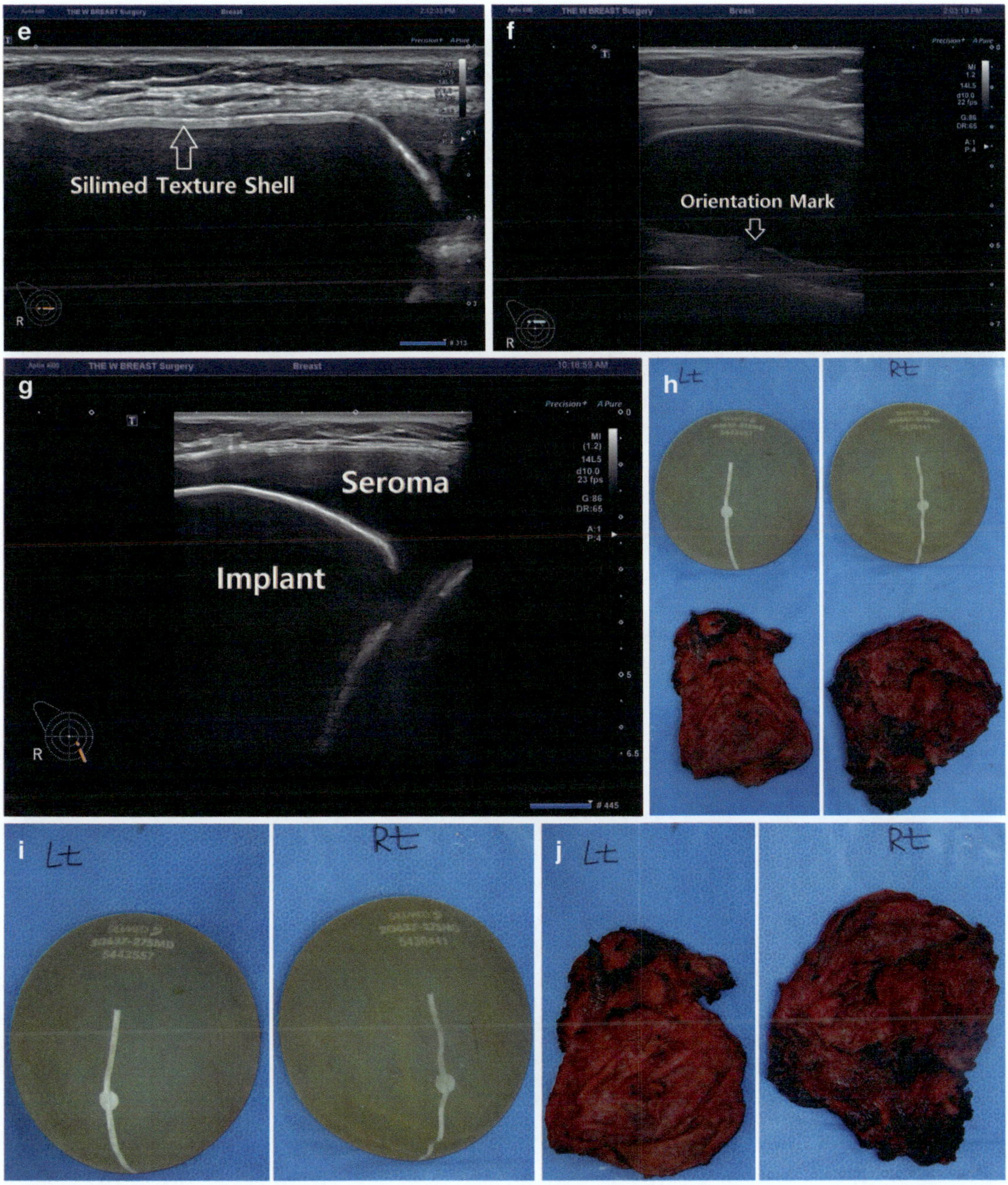

Fig. 8.14 (continued)

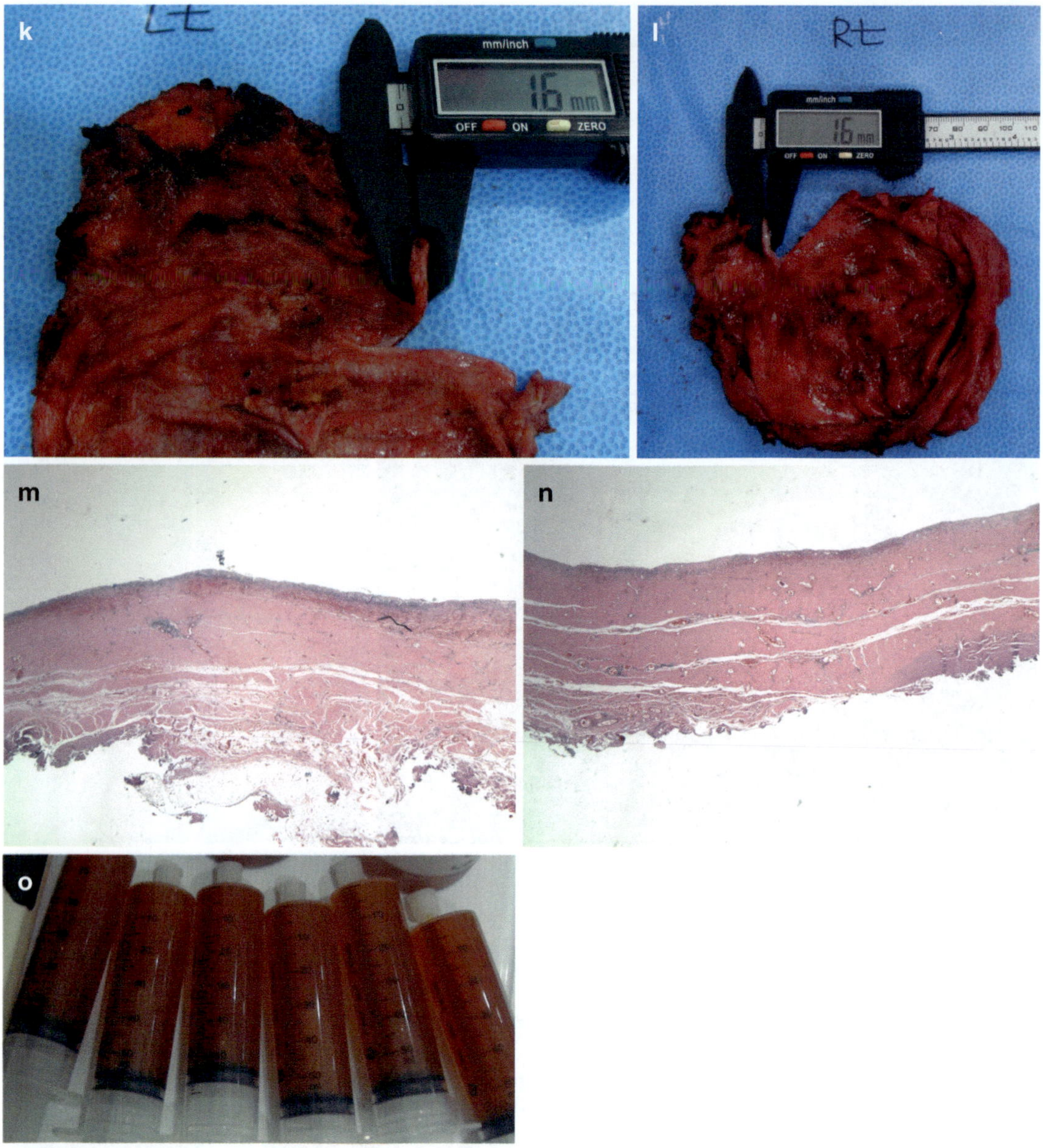

Fig. 8.14 (continued)

8.2.15 Case 15

On physical examination and history taking, a 47-year-old woman complained of breast hardness on the right side. The patient had a 15-year history of receiving an implant-based augmentation mammaplasty.

On preoperative ultrasonography, the patient was found to have a round textured saline-filled breast implant in the subpectoral pocket. The patient had a thickened capsule which was measured as 1.6 mm *as well as* an upside-down rotation on the right side, accompanied by the bilateral presence of a double capsule. But there were no findings that are suggestive of folding, seroma, rupture, and capsular mass.

The patient underwent subtotal capsulectomy with explantation *via* a previous axillary scar on both sides. There was degeneration in both fibrous capsule (Fig. 8.15) (Videos 8.20 and 8.21).

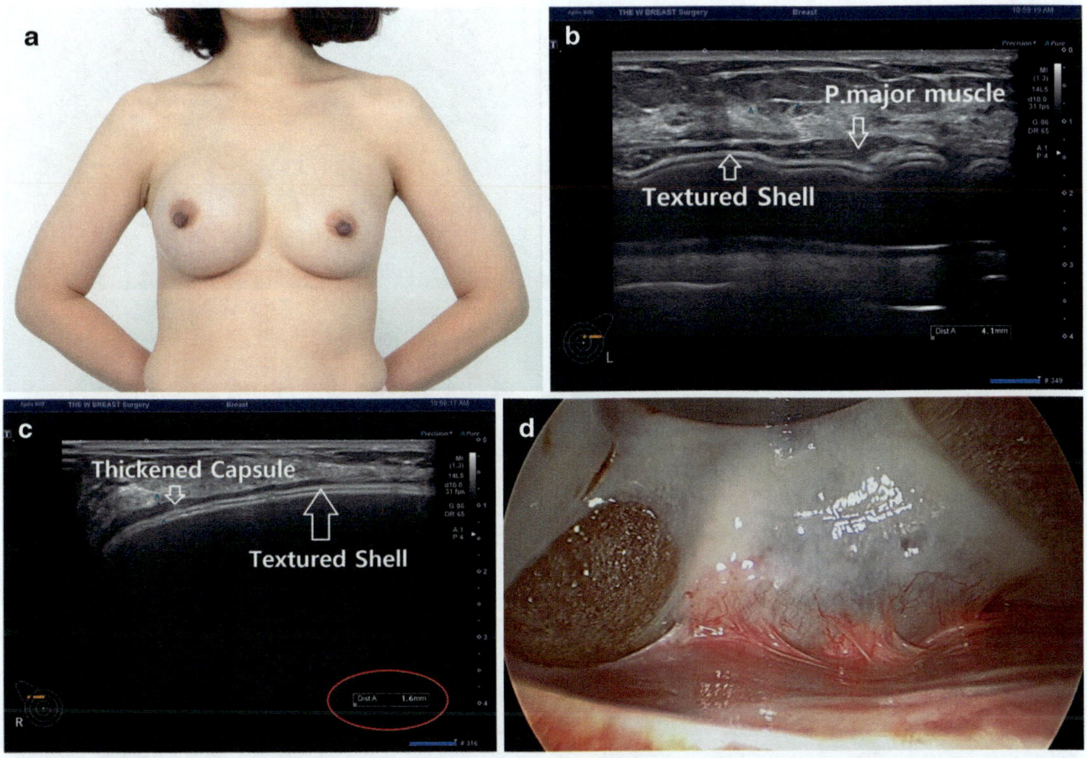

Fig. 8.15 (**a**) A preoperative front view. (**b**) Left textured shell type breast implant in subpectoral pocket is checked in preoperative ultrasonography. (**c**) Right textured shell type breast implant in subpectoral pocket with thickened capsule,1.6 mm is checked in preoperative ultrasonography. (**d**) Left intraoperative view of texture type breast implant with inferior double capsule. (**e**) Right intraoperative view of periprosthetic capsule. (**f**) Right textured shell type breast implant and double capsule. (**g**) Right intraoperative view of intracapsular breast pocket. (**h**) Both removed breast implant and periprosthetic capsule after subtotal capsulectomy. (**i**) Removed round texture type saline implant with port (both unknown manufacturer, 200 cc). (**j**) Right periprosthetic double capsule. (**k**) Left capsule thickness is measured by digital caliper, 0.5 mm. (**l, m**) Right capsule thickness is measured by digital caliper, 0.6 & 1.3 mm. (**n**) Microscopic view of the left capsule. (**o**) Microscopic view of the right inner capsule. (**p**) Microscopic view of the right outer capsule

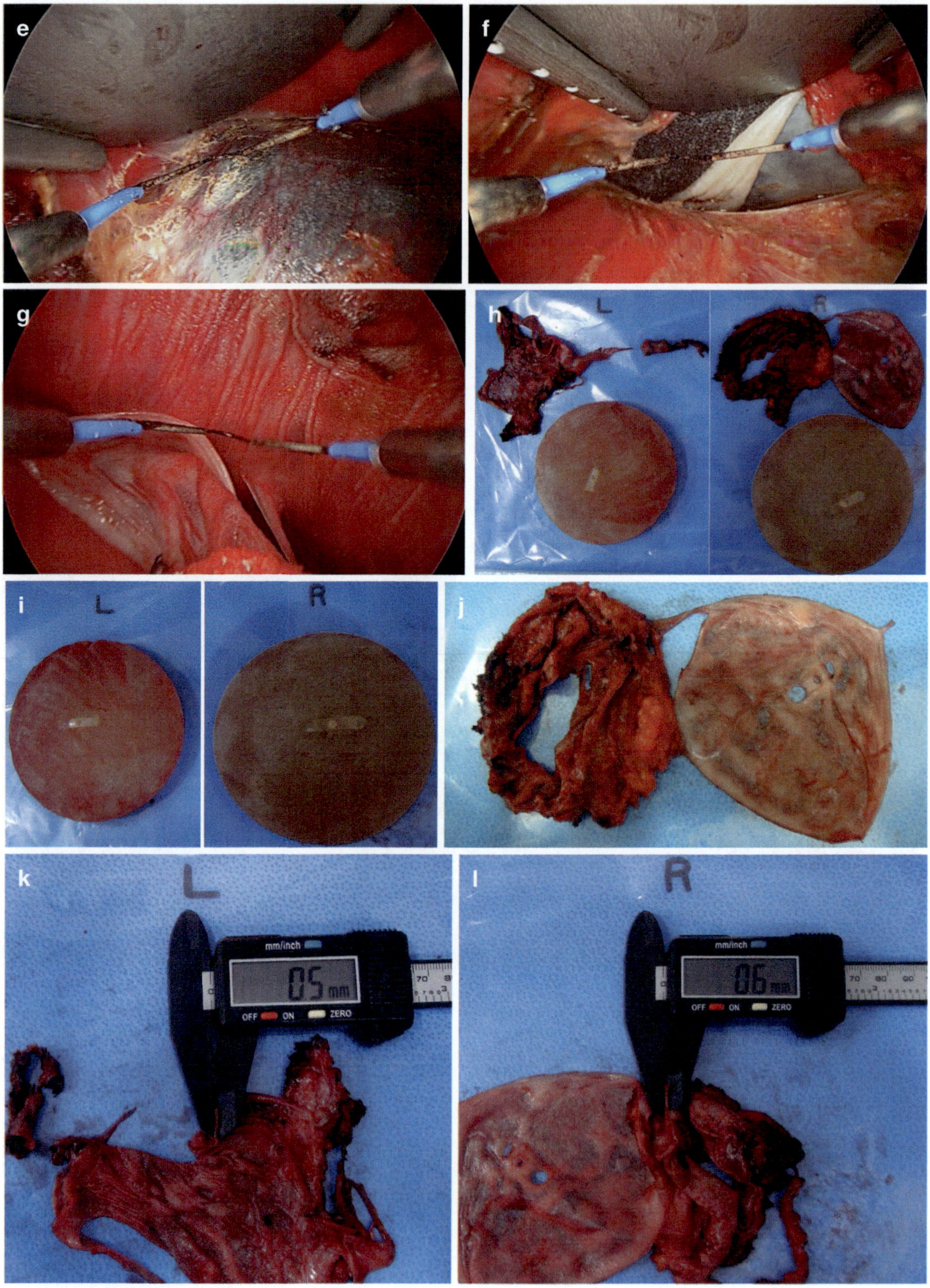

Fig. 8.15 (continued)

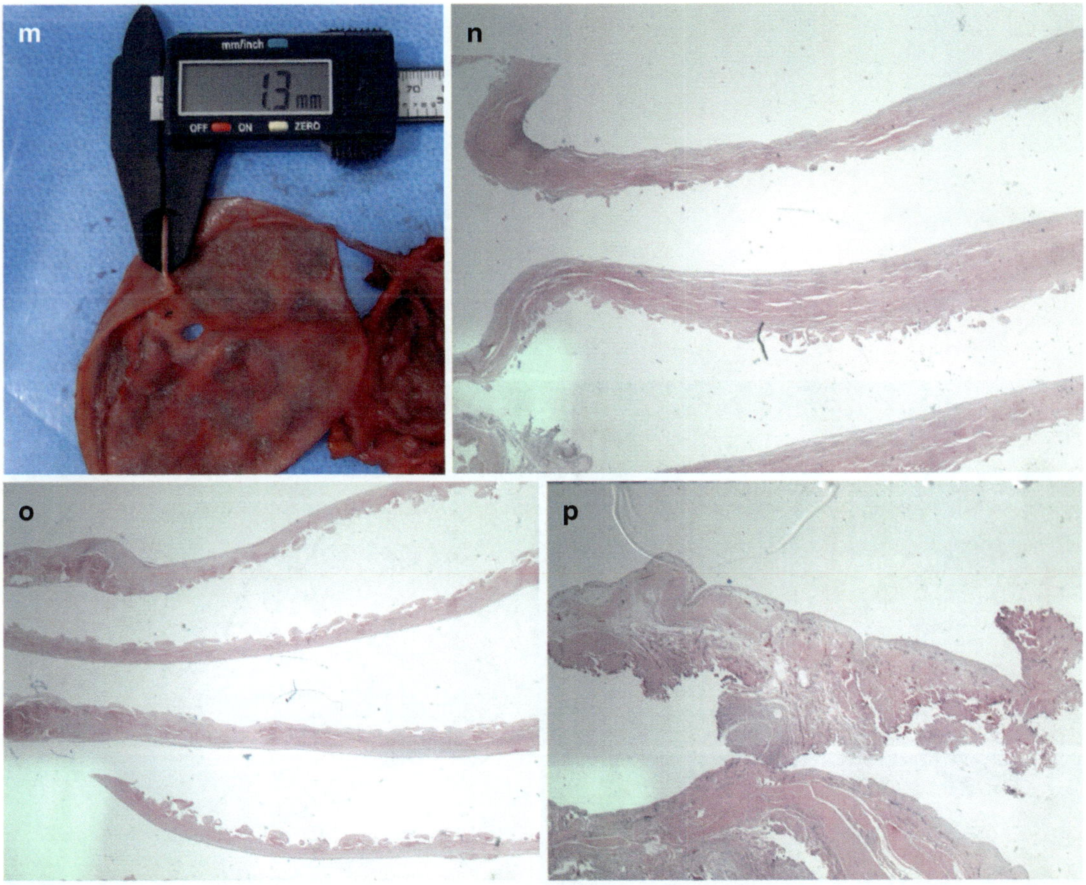

Fig. 8.15 (continued)

8.2.16 Case 16

On physical examination and history taking, a 51-year-old woman complained of shape deformation; the patient was suspected of having a rupture. The patient had an 11-year history of receiving an implant-based augmentation mammaplasty *via* an axillary incision.

On preoperative ultrasonography, the patient was found to have a round textured silicone gel-filled breast implant in the subpectoral pocket. The patient had a rupture on the left side (Videos 8.22 and 8.23). But there were no findings that are suggestive of folding, seroma, thickened capsule, upside-down rotation, and capsular mass.

The patient underwent subtotal capsulectomy with explantation *via* a previous axillary scar on both sides. There was degeneration in both fibrous capsule (Fig. 8.16).

8.2.17 Case 17

On physical examination and history taking, a 41-year-old woman complained of an unpleasant feeling due to a breast implant. The patient had a 5-year-history of receiving an implant-based augmentation mammaplasty *via* an inframammary fold incision.

On preoperative ultrasonography, the patient was found to have an anatomical silicone gel-filled breast implant (Polytech Health & Aesthetics, Dieburg, Germany) in the subpectoral pocket. The patient bilaterally had a folding, a

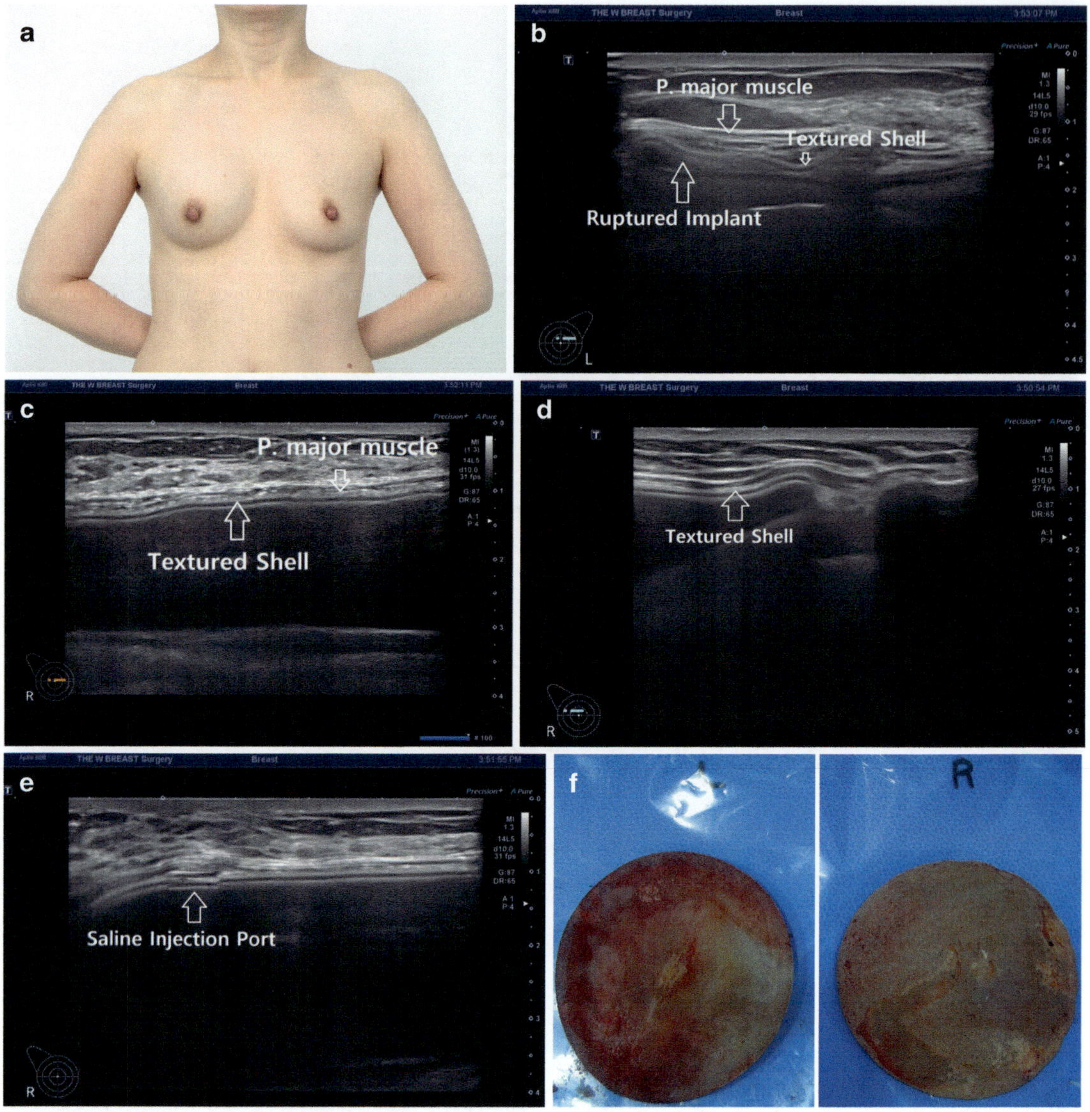

Fig. 8.16 (**a**) A preoperative front view. (**b**) Left textured shell type saline breast implant with rupture in subpectoral pocket is checked in preoperative ultrasonography. (**c**) Right textured shell type breast implant in subpectoral pocket is checked in preoperative ultrasonography. (**d**) Right textured shell type breast implant is checked in ultrasonography. (**e**) Right breast implant saline port is checked in ultrasonography. (**f**) Both removed round texture type breast implant (unknown manufacturer and size). (**g**) Left capsule thickness is measured by digital caliper, 0.3 mm. (**h**) Right capsule thickness is measured by digital caliper, 0.1 mm. (**i**) Microscopic view of the left capsule. (**j**) Microscopic view of the right capsule

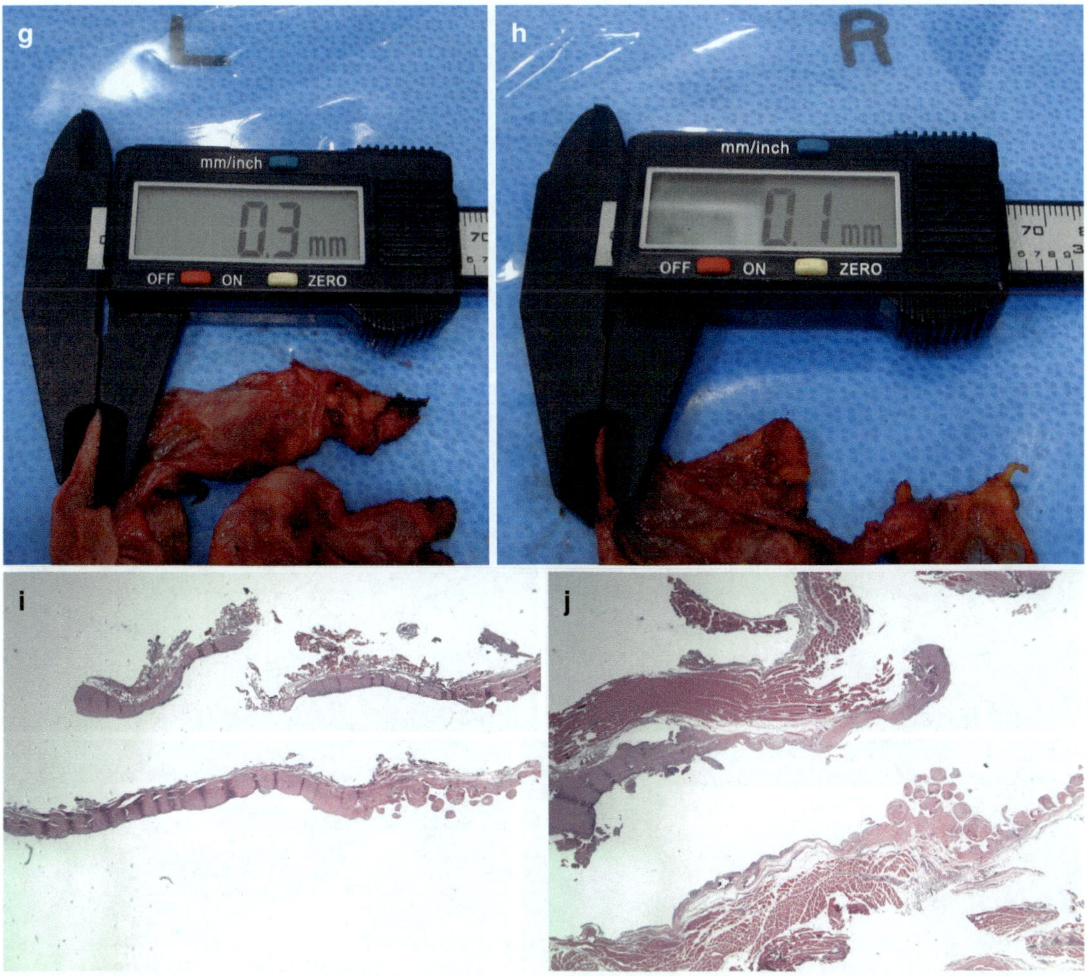

Fig. 8.16 (continued)

seroma, and a thickened capsule which was measured as 1.6 mm on the right side and 1.7 mm on the left side. Moreover, the patient also had a double capsule on the right side (Videos 8.24 and 8.25). But there were no findings that are suggestive of malrotation, upside-down rotation, rupture, and capsular mass.

The patient underwent total capsulectomy on the right side and near-total capsulectomy with explantation *via* a previous axillary scar on the left side. There were right chronic inflammation with lymphoid follicle and focal hemorrhage and left focal chronic inflammation with degeneration (Fig. 8.17).

8.2.18 Case 18

On physical examination and history taking, a 42-year-old woman complained of change of breast softness. The patient had an 11-year, history of receiving an implant-based augmentation mammaplasty.

On preoperative ultrasonography, the patient was found to have a round smooth silicone gel-filled breast implant in the subpectoral pocket. The patient had a intracapsular rupture on the left side (Video 8.26). But there were no findings that are suggestive of folding, seroma, thickened capsule, upside-down rotation, and capsular mass.

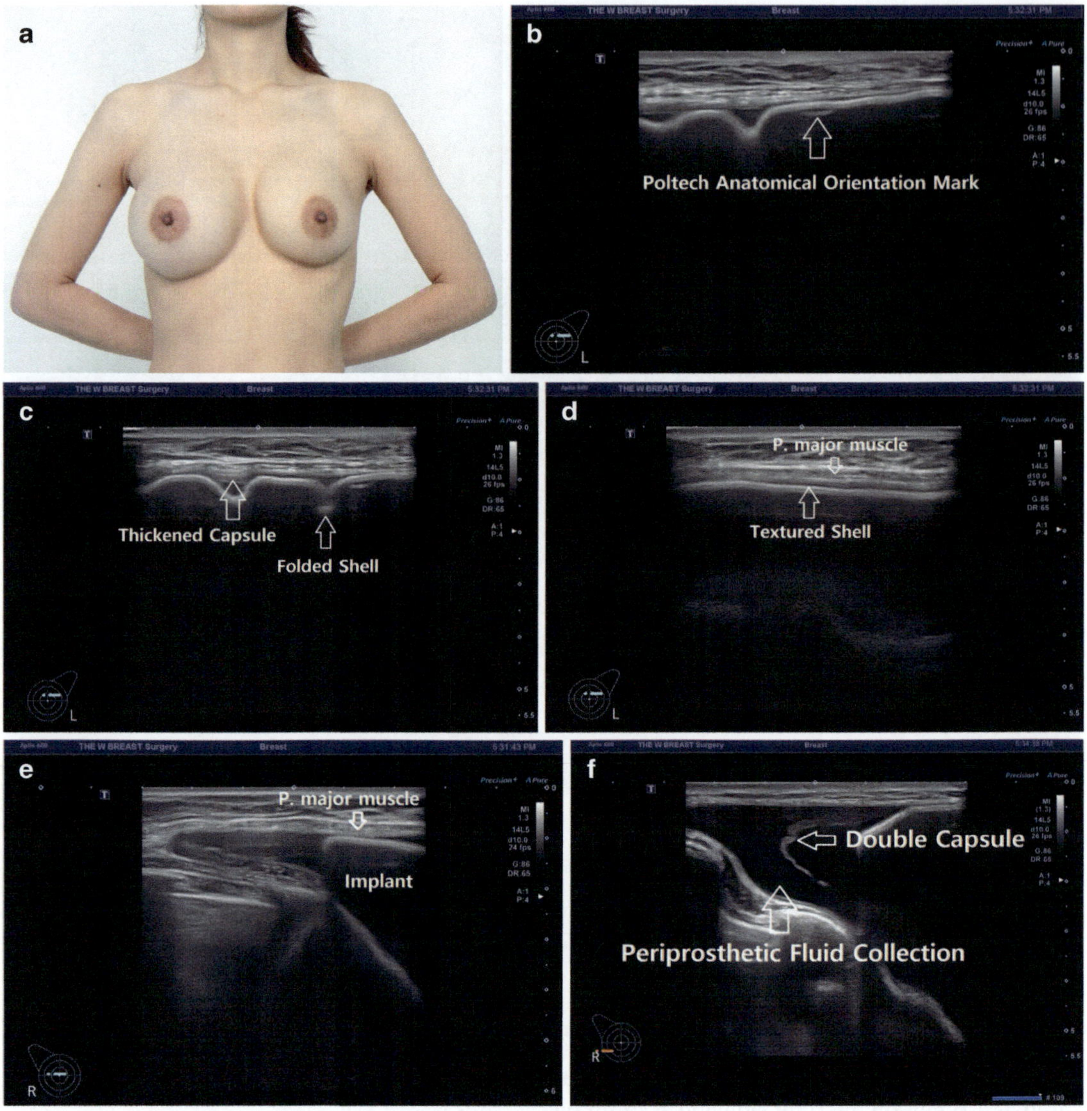

Fig. 8.17 (**a**) A preoperative front view. (**b**) Left Polytech anatomical textured shell type breast implant in subpectoral pocket is checked in preoperative ultrasonography. (**c**) Left periprosthetic thickened capsule and folded shell is checked in ultrasonography. (**d**) Left breast implant in subpectoral pocket is checked in ultrasonography. (**e**) Right textured shell type breast implant in subpectoral pocket is checked in preoperative ultrasonography. (**f**) Right periprosthetic fluid collection and double capsule is checked in ultrasonography. (**g**) Right capsule thickness is measured by ultrasound, 0.8 mm. (**h**) Left intraoperative view of periprosthetic capsule before capsulectomy. (**i, j**) Left intraoperative view of breast pocket after total capsulectomy. (**k**) Both removed breast Polytech anatomical breast implant 305 cc (left), 280 cc (right). (**l**) Left removed breast implant and periprosthetic capsule. (**m**) Right removed breast implant and inner, outer capsule (double capsule) after near-total capsulectomy. (**n**) Right inner capsule. (**o**) Left capsule thickness is measured by digital caliper, 1.9 mm. (**p, q**) Right capsule thickness is measured by digital caliper, 1.8 mm & 0.8 mm. (**r**) Microscopic view of the left capsule. (**s**) Microscopic view of the right capsule

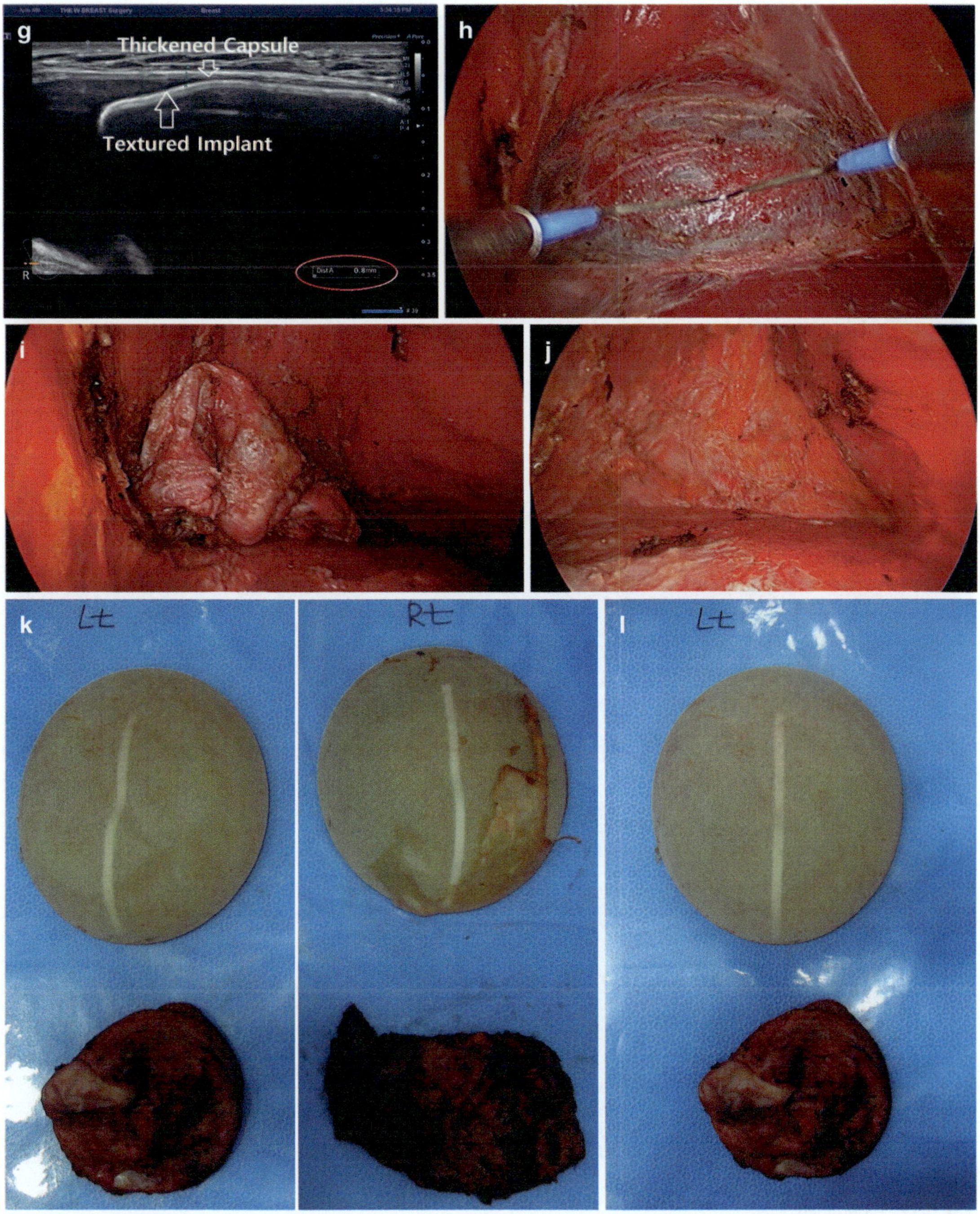

Fig. 8.17 (continued)

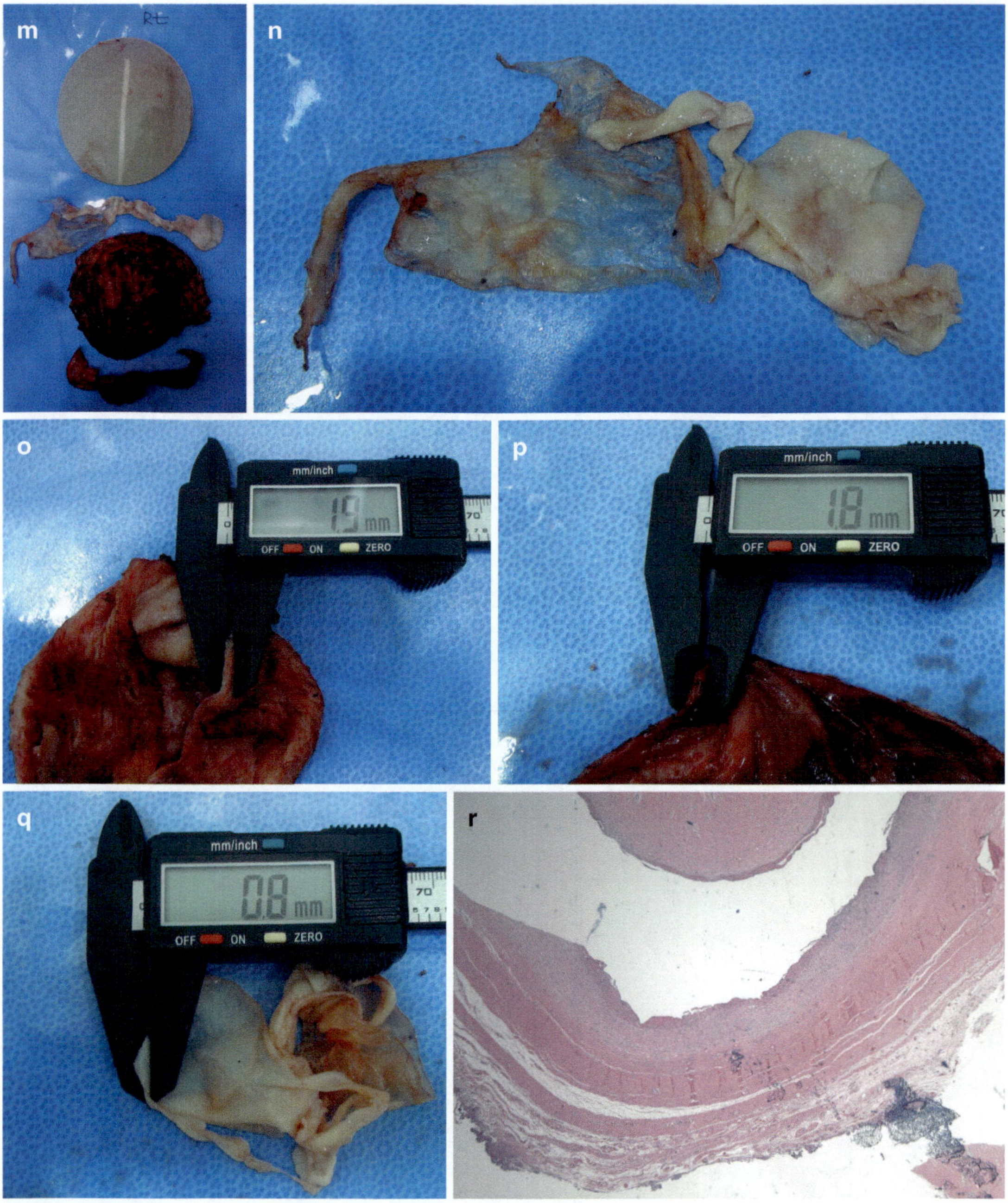

Fig. 8.17 (continued)

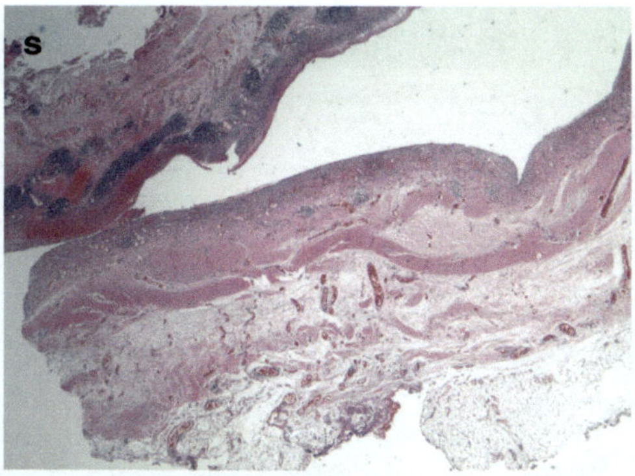

Fig. 8.17 (continued)

The patient underwent subtotal capsulectomy with replacement of the device via a previous axillary scar on both sides. There were focal chronic inflammation and fibrosis in both capsule (Fig. 8.18).

8.2.19 Case 19

On physical examination and history taking, a 32-year-old woman complained of postoperative stiffness of the neck and shoulder. The patient had a 7-year history of receiving an implant-based augmentation mammaplasty *via* an axillary incision.

On preoperative ultrasonography, the patient was found to have a round textured silicone gel-filled breast implant in the subpectoral pocket. The patient had a folding with detachment on the left side. But there were no findings that are suggestive of seroma, thickened capsule, upside-down rotation, and capsular mass.

The patient underwent explantation with both subtotal capsulectomy *via* a previous axillary scar on both sides (Video 8.27). There was focal chronic inflammation in both capsule (Fig. 8.19).

8.2.20 Case 20

On physical examination and history taking, a 54-year-old woman had a 12-year history of receiving an implant-based augmentation mammaplasty *via* an axillary incision.

On preoperative ultrasonography, the patient was found to have a round smooth silicone gel-filled breast implant in the subpectoral pocket. The patient had a major intracapsular rupture on the right side (Video 8.28). But there were no findings that are suggestive of seroma, thickened capsule, upside-down rotation, and capsular mass.

The patient underwent near-total capsulectomy with replacement of the device *via* a previous inframammary fold scar. There were focal chronic inflammation and microcalcification in both capsule (Fig. 8.20).

8.2.21 Case 21

On physical examination and history taking, a 51-year-old woman complained of dissatisfaction with shape. The patient had a 10-year history of receiving an implant-based augmentation mammaplasty *via* an axillary incision.

On preoperative ultrasonography, the patient was found to have a round textured silicone gel-filled breast implant in the subpectoral pocket. But there were no findings that are suggestive of folding, seroma, thickened capsule, upside-down rotation, rupture, and capsular mass (Video 8.29).

The patient underwent subtotal capsulectomy with replacement of the device *via* a previous inframammary fold scar on both sides. There were focal chronic inflammation and fibrosis in both capsule (Fig. 8.21).

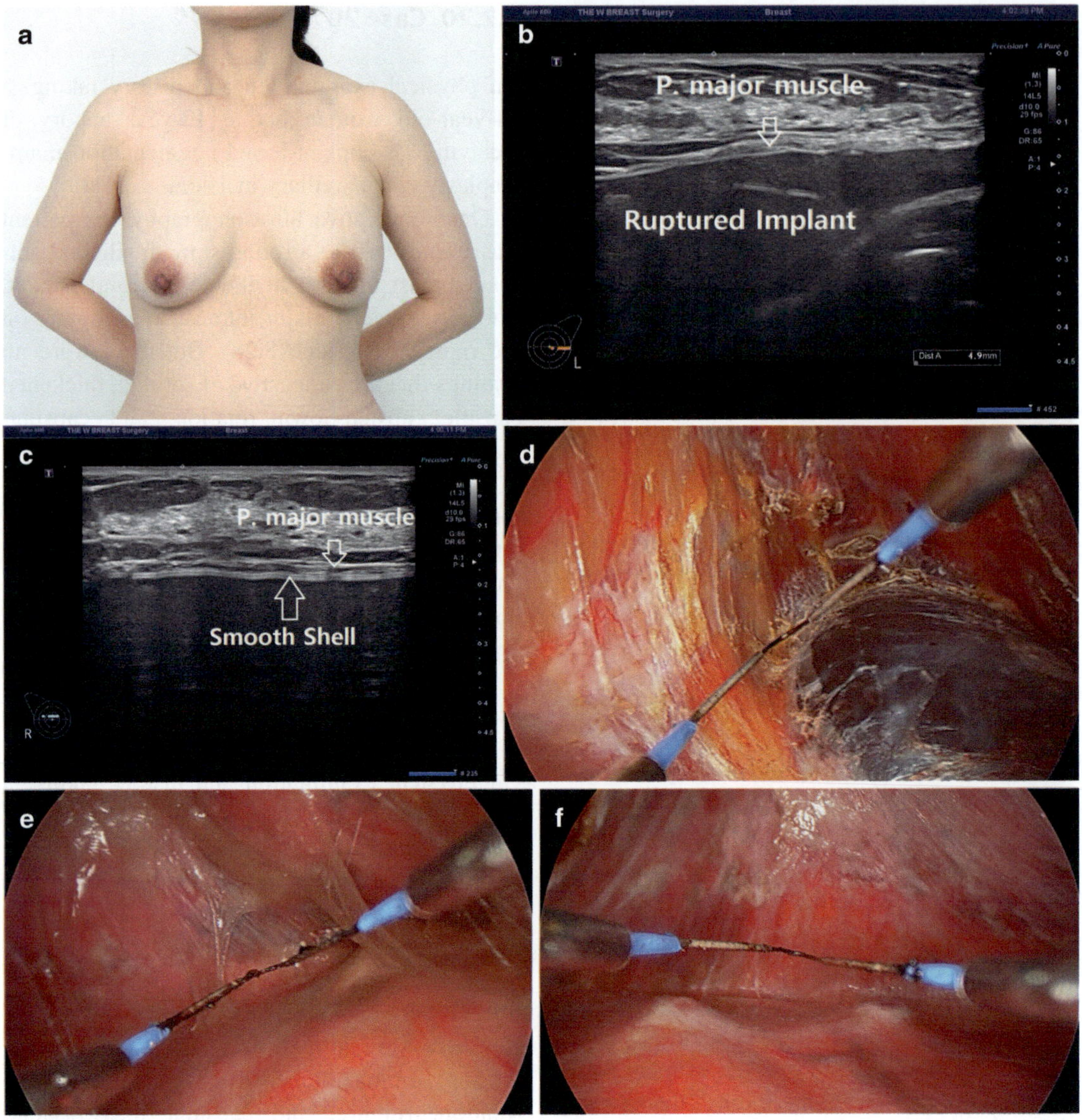

Fig. 8.18 (**a**) A preoperative front view. (**b**) Left ruptured breast implant in subpectoral pocket is checked in preoperative ultrasonography. (**c**) Right breast implant in subpectoral pocket is checked in preoperative ultrasonography. (**d**) Left intraoperative view of breast implant with periprosthetic capsule. (**e**) Left intraoperative view of inner capsule with free silicone. (**f**) Left intraoperative view of inner capsule after gauze irrigation for removal of free silicone. (**g**) Left intraoperative view of breast pocket after subtotal capsulectomy. (**h**) Right intraoperative view of capsulectomy. (**i**) Right intraoperative view of breast pocket after subtotal capsulectomy. (**j**) Both removed Mentor smooth type breast implant, 250 cc. (**k**) Both removed breast implant. (**l**) Both removed periprosthetic capsule by subtotal capsulectomy. (**m**) Left capsule thickness is measured by digital caliper, 0.6 mm. (**n**) Right capsule thickness is measured by digital caliper, 0.3 mm. (**o**) Microscopic view of the left capsule with silicone invasion to capsule. (**p**) Microscopic view of the right capsule

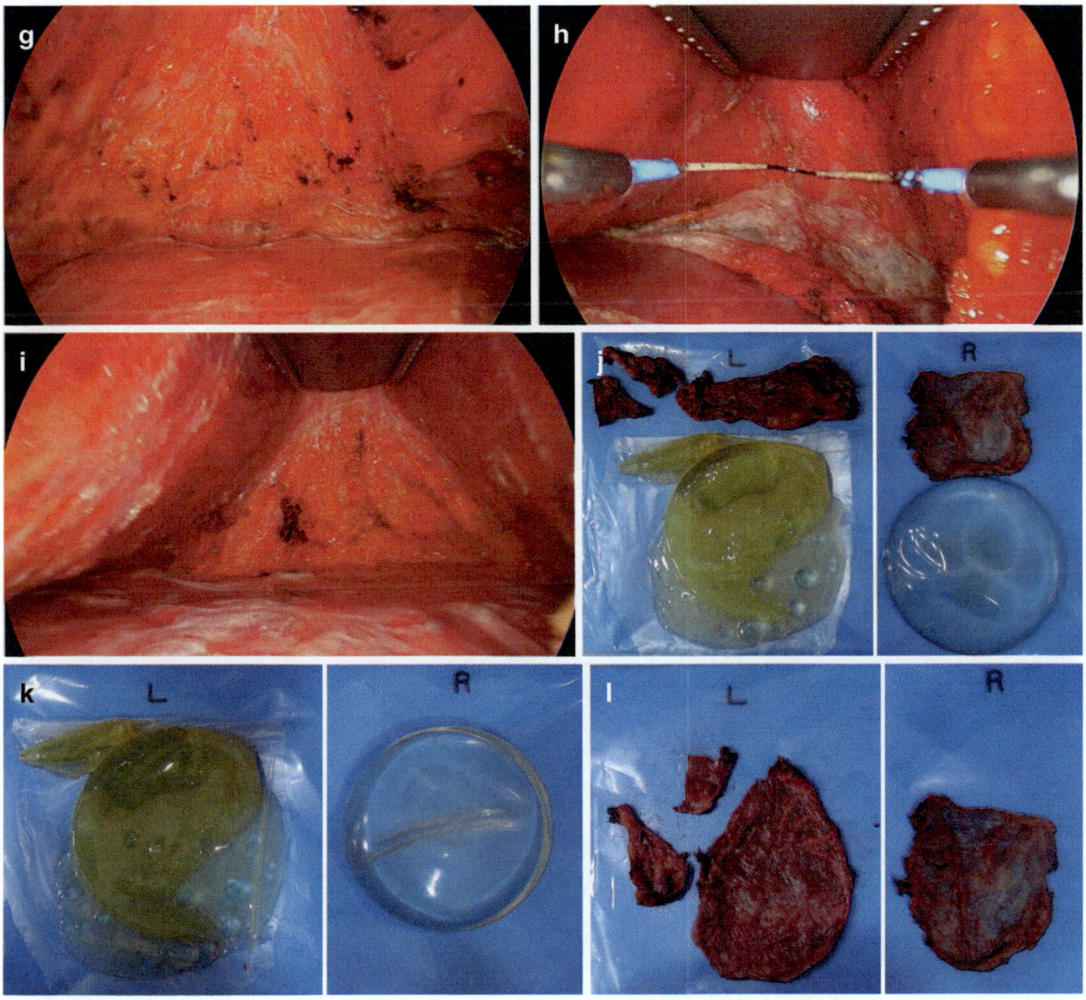

Fig. 8.18 (continued)

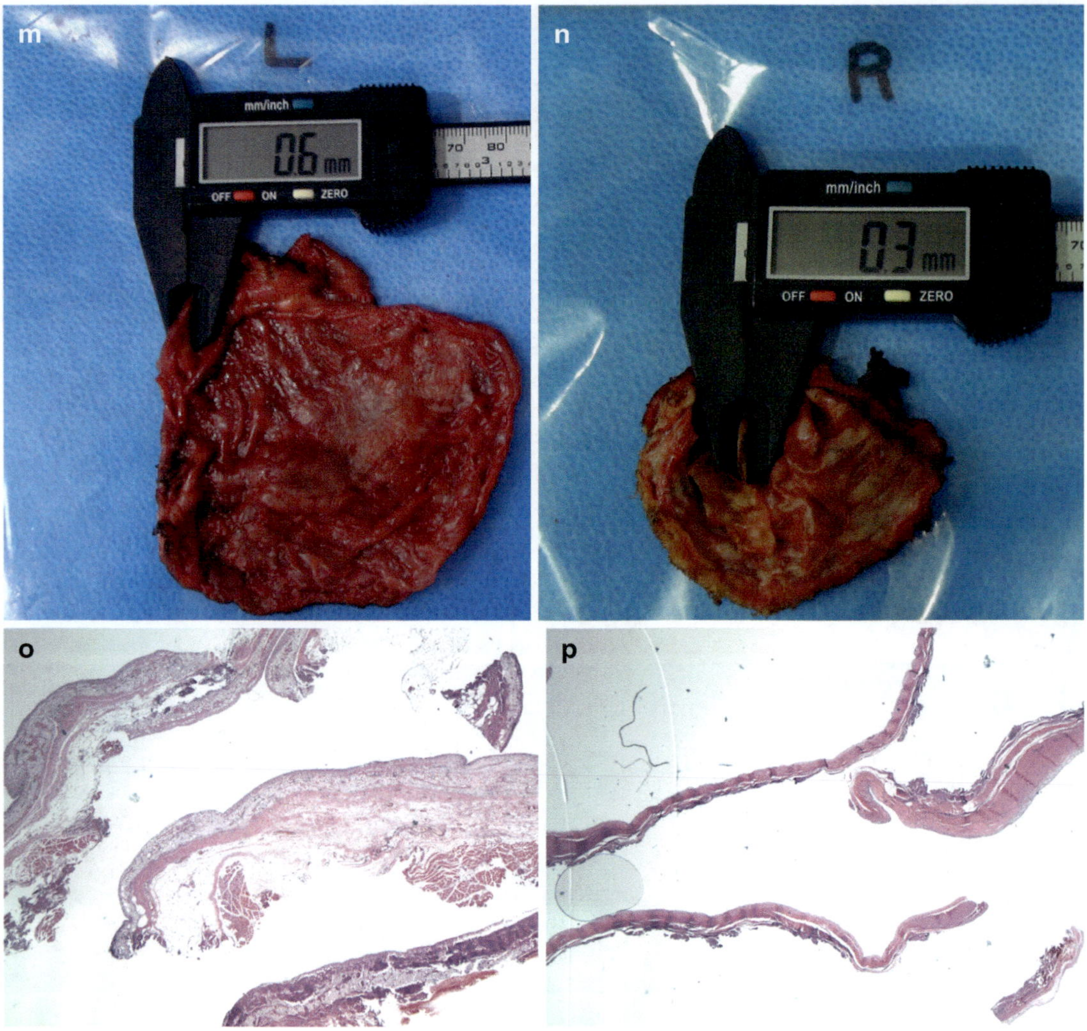

Fig. 8.18 (continued)

8.2.22 Case 22

A 54-year-old woman had a 4-year history of receiving an implant-based augmentation mammaplasty *via* an axillary incision, whose chief complaint was concern for breast implant-associated anaplastic large cell lymphoma (BIA-ALCL).

On preoperative ultrasound, the patient was found to have an anatomical silicone gel-filled breast implant (Allergan Inc., Irvine, CA) in the subpectoral pocket. But there were no findings that are suggestive of malrotation, folding, seroma, thickened capsule, upside-down rotation, rupture, and capsular mass (Video 8.30).

The patient underwent subtotal capsulectomy with explantation *via* a previous axillary scar on both sides. There were focal chronic inflammation and fibrosis in both capsule (Fig. 8.22).

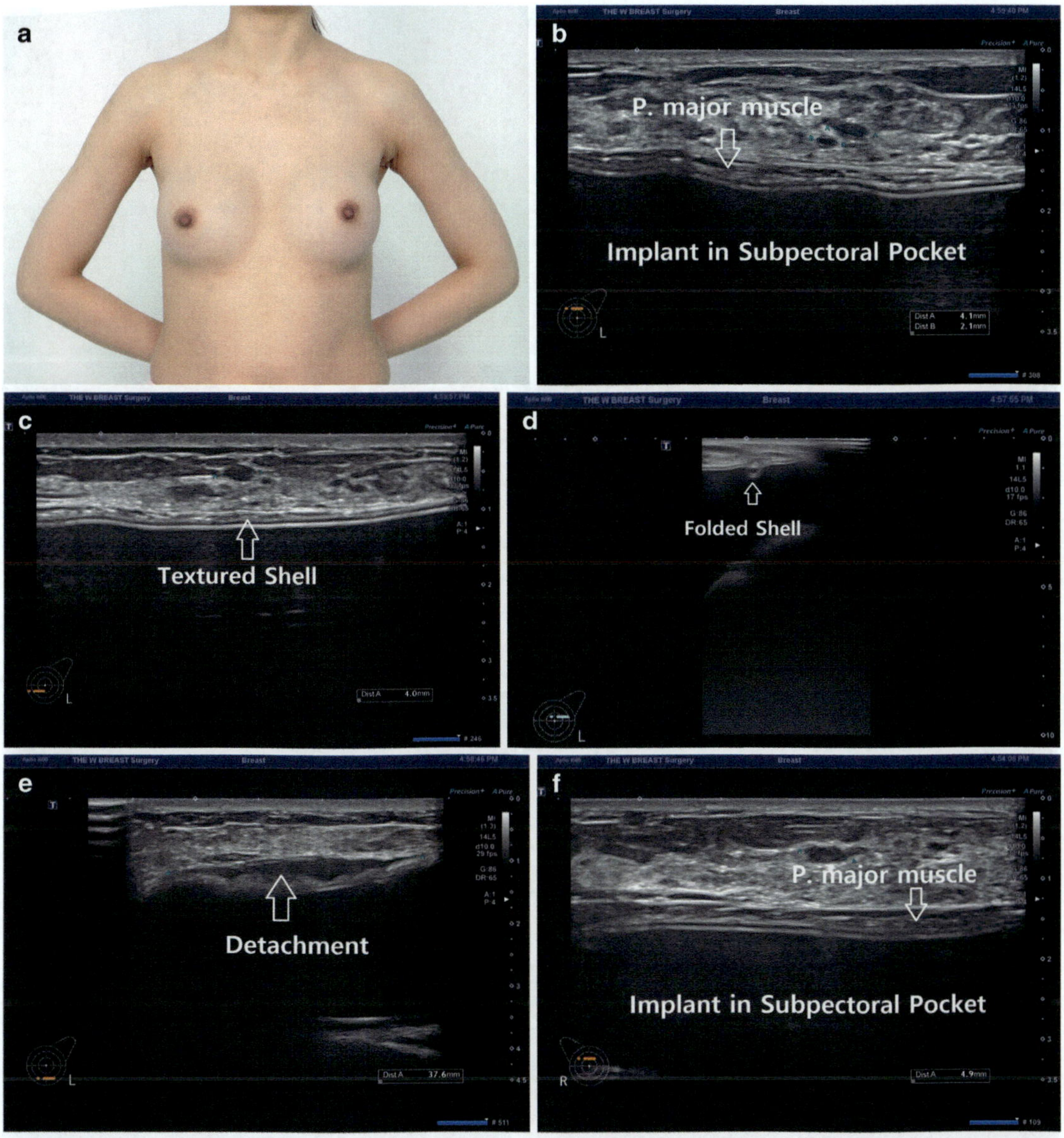

Fig. 8.19 (**a**) A preoperative front view. (**b**) Left breast implant in subpectoral pocket is checked in preoperative ultrasonography. (**c**) Left textured shell type breast implant is checked in preoperative ultrasonography. (**d**) Left breast implant shell folding is checked in ultrasonography. (**e**) Left textured shell type breast implant with detachment is checked in preoperative ultrasonography. (**f**) Right breast implant in subpectoral pocket is checked in ultrasonography. (**g**) Right textured shell type breast implant is checked in ultrasonography. (**h**) Left intraoperative view of breast implant and periprosthetic capsule. (**i**) Left intraoperative view of intracapsular breast pocket. (**j**) Left intraoperative view of breast pocket after subtotal capsulectomy. (**k**) Right intraoperative endoscopic view of breast implant and periprosthetic capsule. (**l**) Right intraoperative view of intracapsular breast pocket. (**m**) Right intraoperative view of breast pocket after subtotal capsulectomy. (**n**) Both removed Mentor round texture type breast implant, 325 cc. (**o**) Both removed periprosthetic capsule after subtotal capsulectomy. (**p**) Left capsule thickness is measured by digital caliper, 0.2 mm. (**q**) Right capsule thickness is measured by digital caliper, 0.3 mm. (**r**) Microscopic view of the left capsule. (**s**) Microscopic view of the right capsule

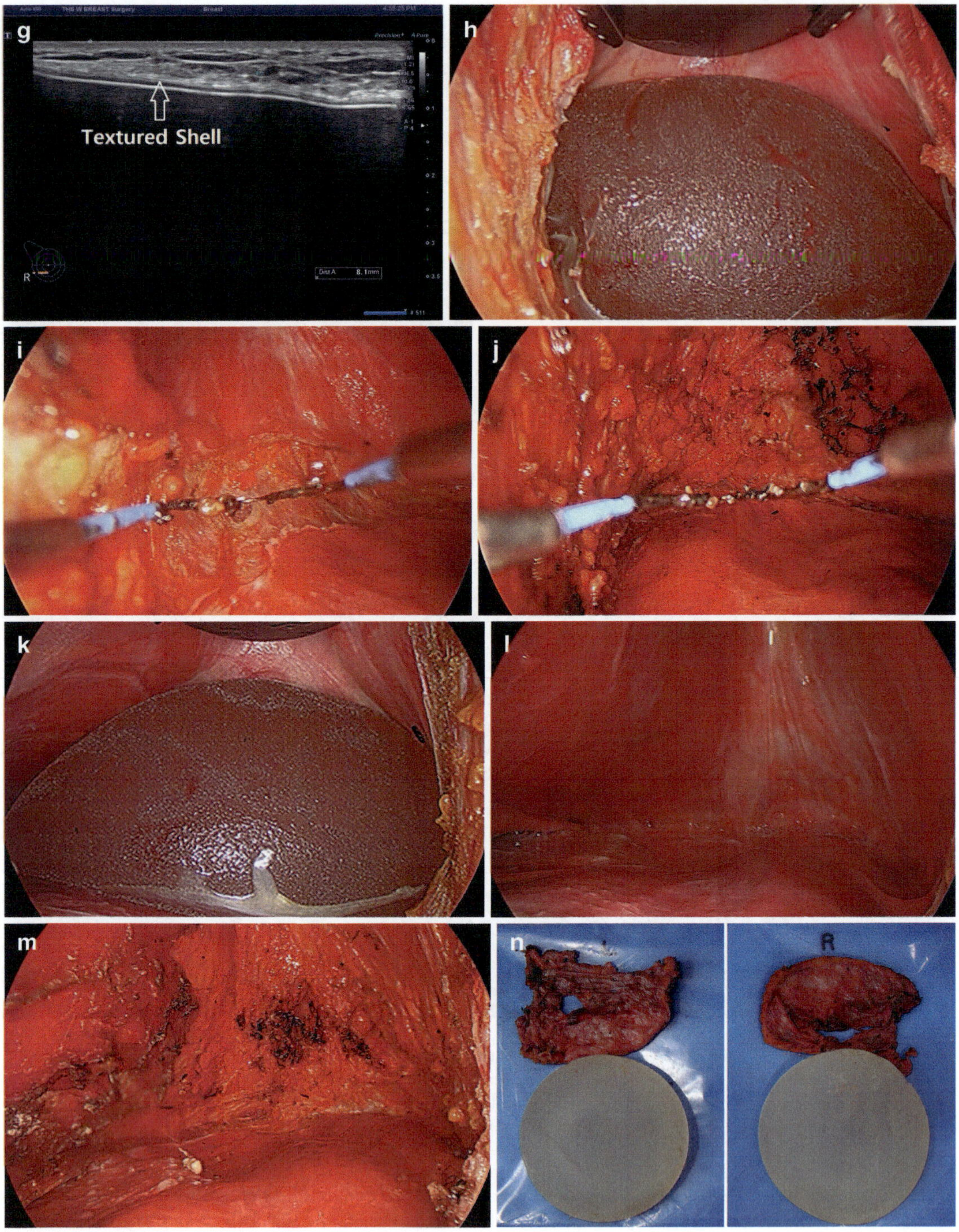

Fig. 8.19 (continued)

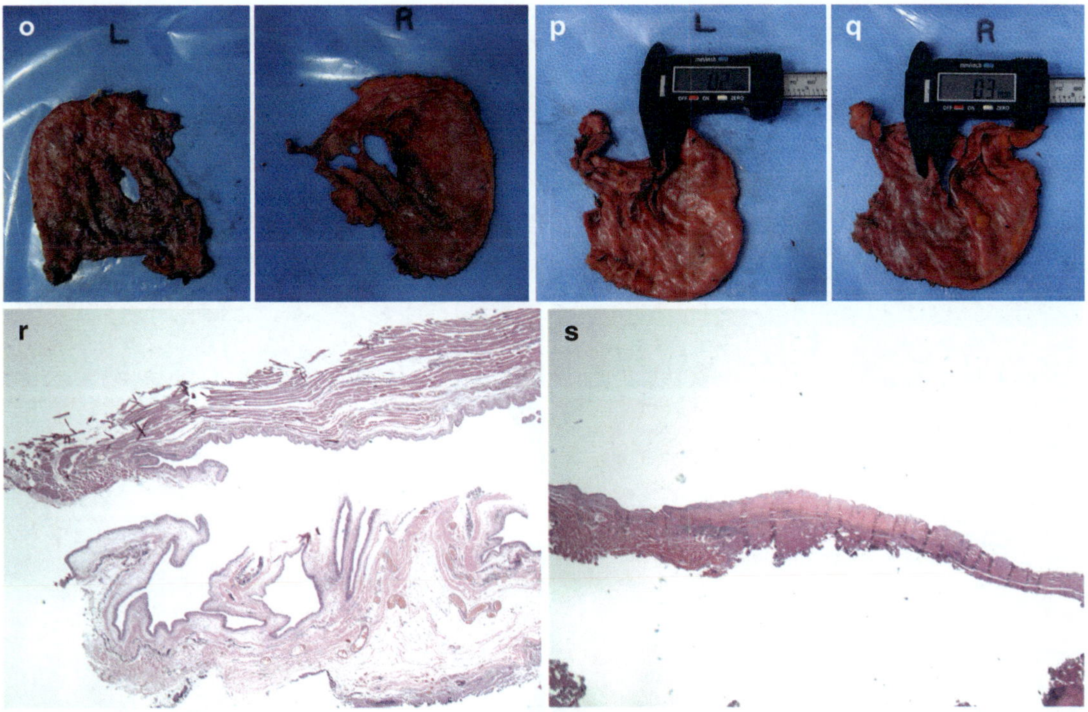

Fig. 8.19 (continued)

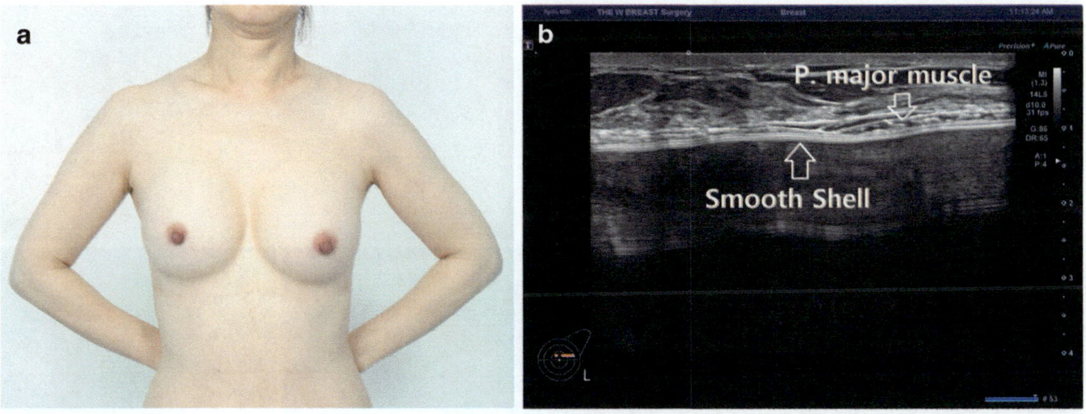

Fig. 8.20 (**a**) A preoperative front view. (**b**) Left smooth shell type breast implant in subpectoral pocket is checked in preoperative ultrasound. (**c, d**) Right ruptured smooth shell type shell type breast implant in subpectoral pocket is checked in preoperative ultrasonography. (**e**) Left intraoperative view of periprosthetic capsule. (**f**) Left intraoperative view of intracapsular breast pocket. (**g**) Left intraoperative view of breast pocket after near-total capsulectomy. (**h**) Right intraoperative view of periprosthetic capsule. (**i**) Right intraoperative view of breast pocket after near-total capsulectomy. (**j**) Both removed Mentor smooth type breast implant, 400 cc. (**k**) Right ruptured breast implant. (**l**) Both removed periprosthetic capsule by near-total capsulectomy. (**m**) Left capsule thickness is measured by digital caliper, 0.5 mm. (**n**) Right capsule thickness is measured by digital caliper, 0.5 mm. (**o**) Microscopic view of the left capsule. (**p**) Microscopic view of the right capsule

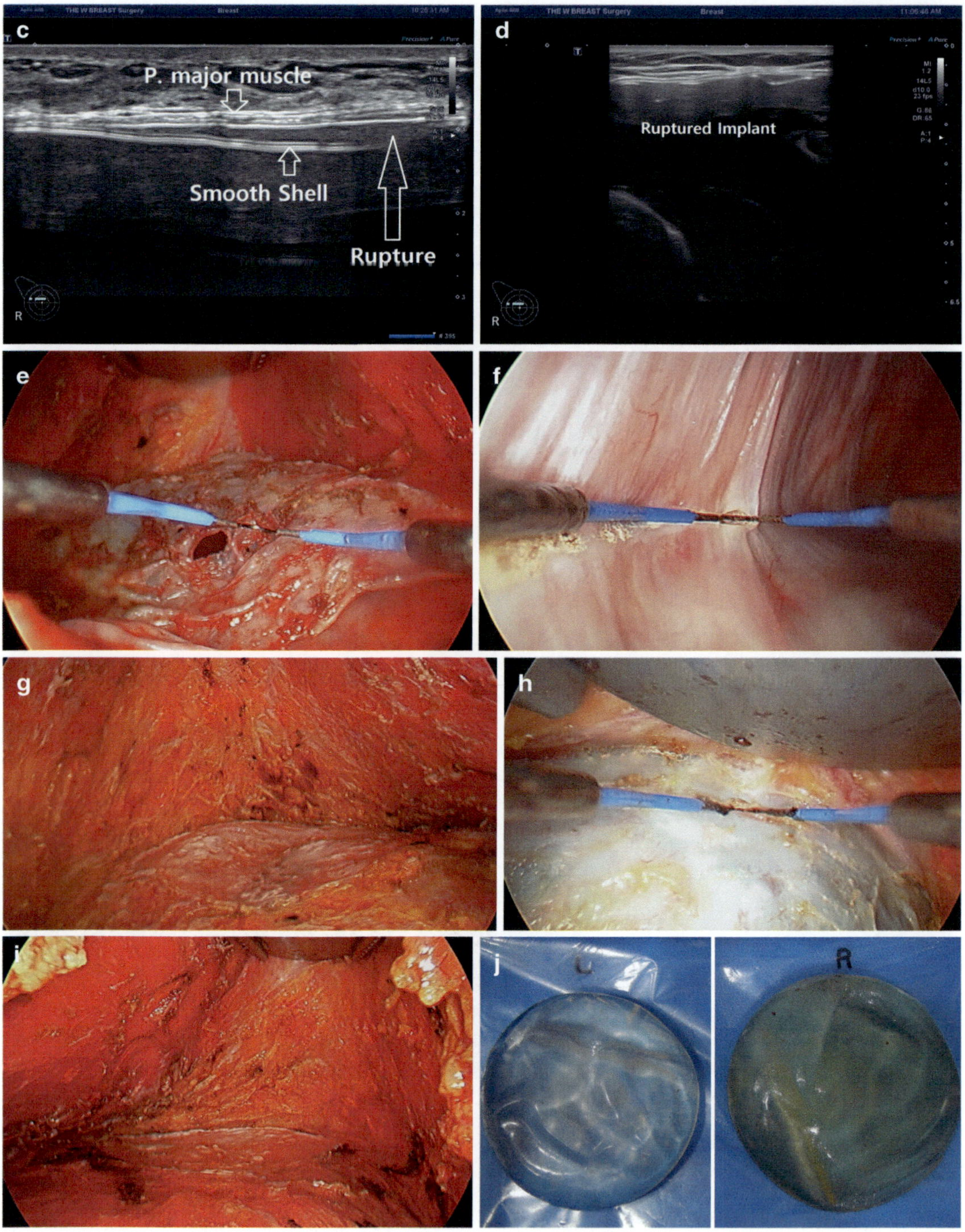

Fig. 8.20 (continued)

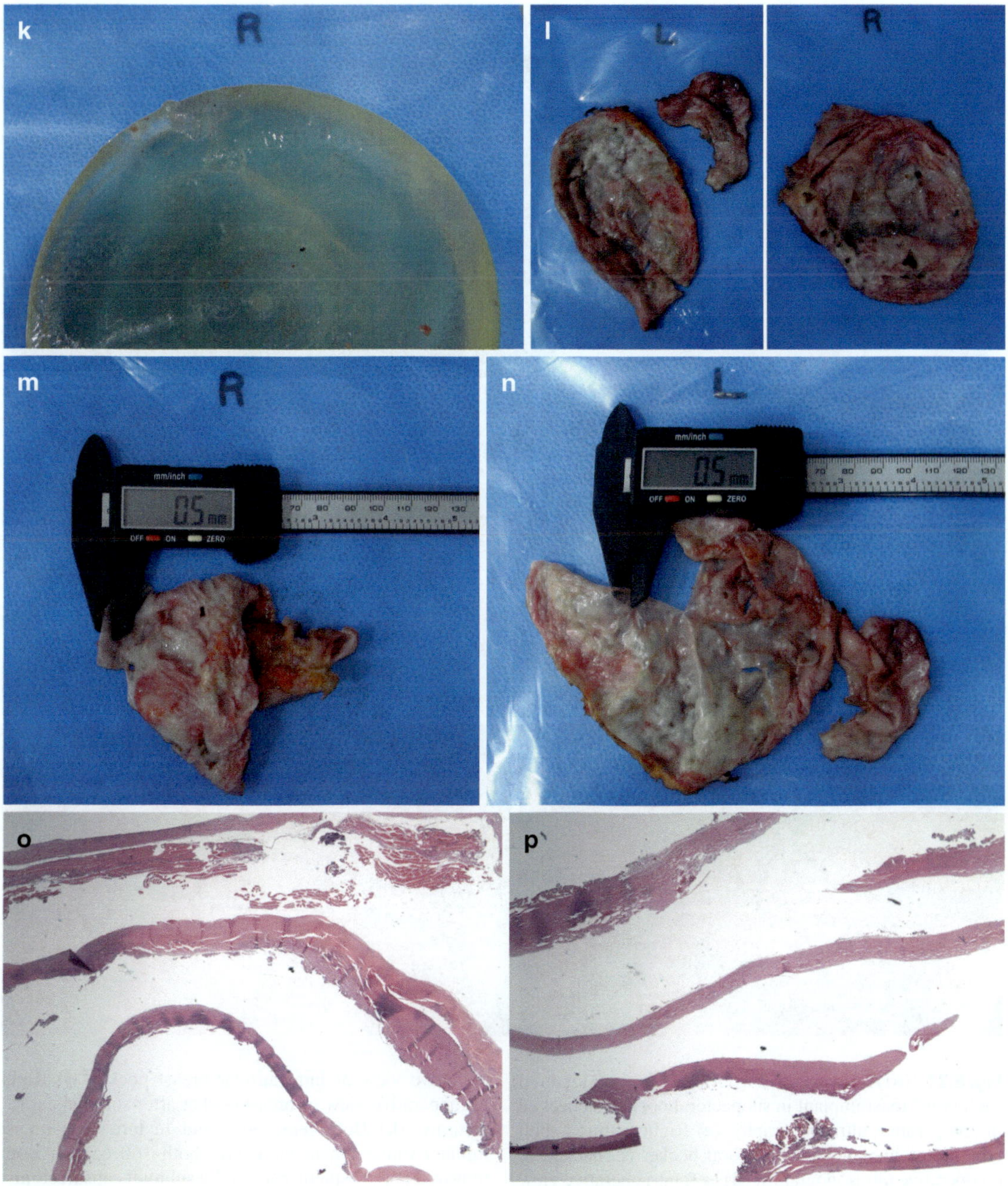

Fig. 8.20 (continued)

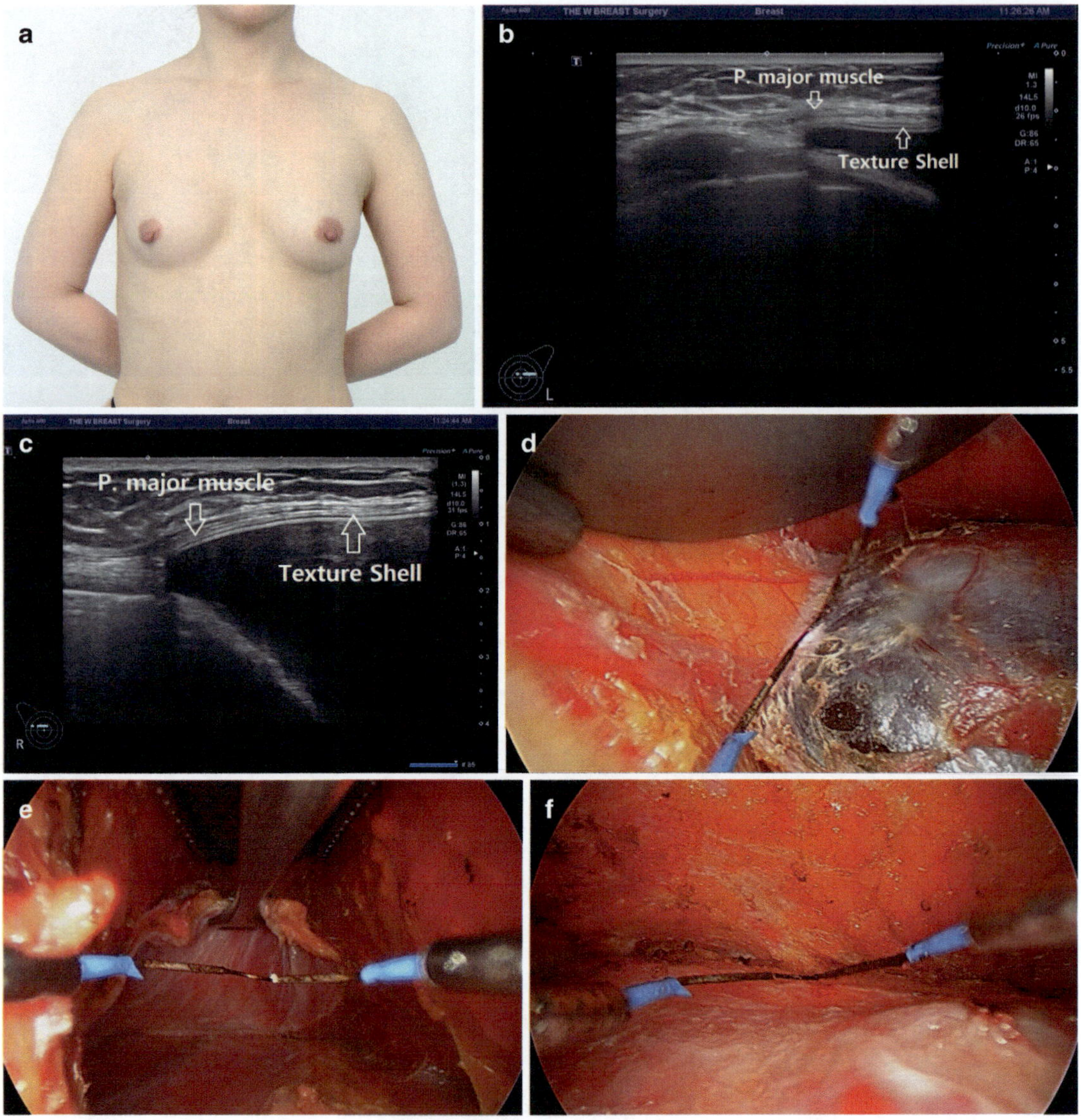

Fig. 8.21 (**a**) A preoperative front view. (**b**) Left textured shell type breast implant in subpectoral pocket is checked in preoperative ultrasonography. (**c**) Right textured shell type breast implant in subpectoral pocket is checked in preoperative ultrasonography. (**d**) Left intraoperative view of breast implant with periprosthetic capsule. (**e**) Left intraoperative view of periprosthetic capsule. (**f**) Left intraoperative view of breast pocket after subtotal capsulectomy. (**g**, **h**) Right intraoperative view of texture type breast implant with periprosthetic capsule. (**i**) Right intraoperative view of intracapsular breast pocket. (**j**) Right intraoperative view of breast pocket after subtotal capsulectomy. (**k**) Both removed round texture type breast implant (unknown manufacturer both 160 cc). (**l**) Both removed periprosthetic capsule by subtotal capsulectomy. (**m**) Left capsule thickness is measured by digital caliper, 0. 3 mm. (**n**) Right capsule thickness is measured by digital caliper, 0.2 mm. (**o**) Microscopic view of the left capsule. (**p**) Microscopic view of the right capsule

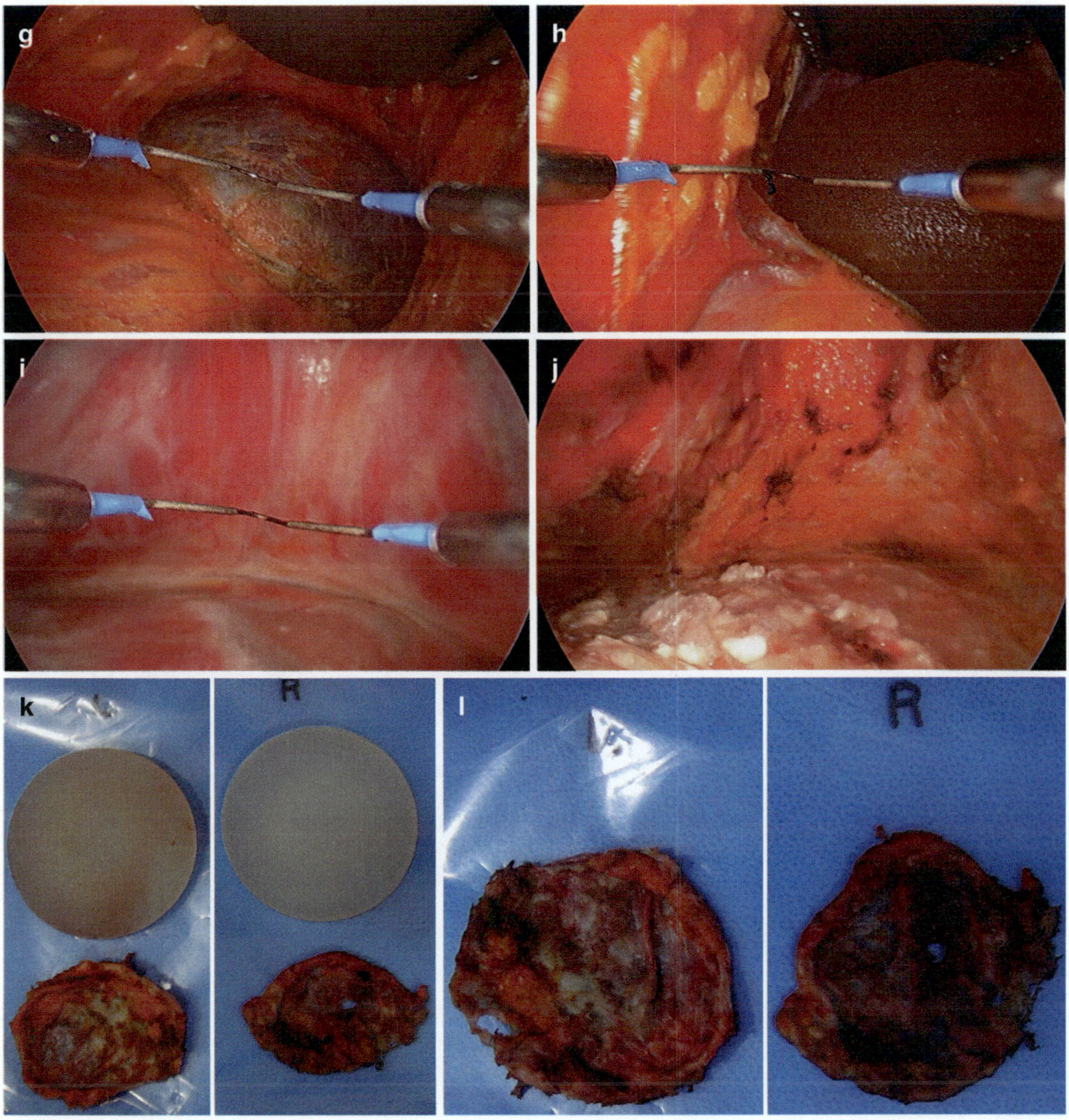

Fig. 8.21 (continued)

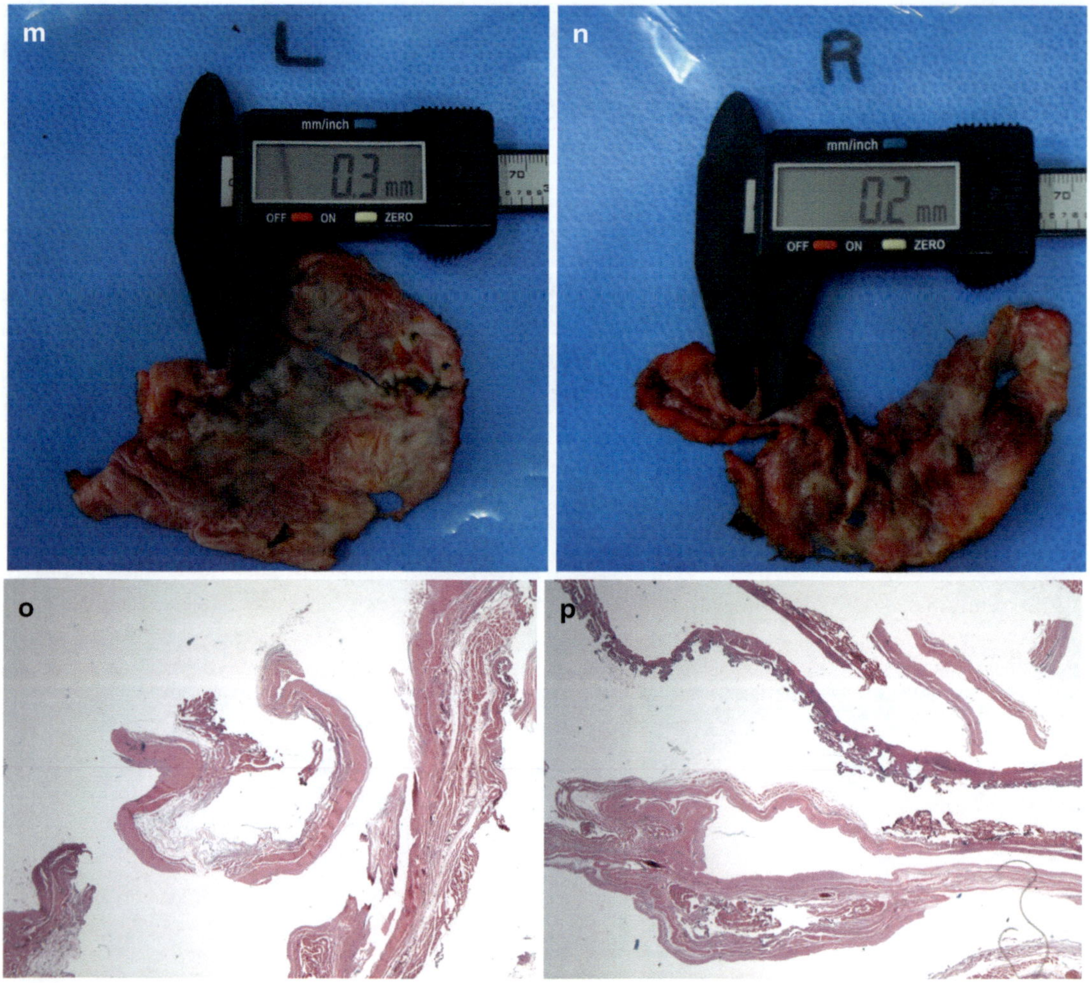

Fig. 8.21 (continued)

8.2.23 Case 23

On physical examination and history taking, a 62-year-old woman complained of dissatisfaction of breast softness; the patient had a suspicion of having a rupture. The patient had a 12-year history of receiving an implant-based augmentation mammaplasty *via* an axillary incision.

On preoperative ultrasonography, the patient was found to have a round smooth saline-filled breast implant in the subpectoral pocket (Video 8.31). The patient had a thickened capsule which was measured as 4.1 mm on the left side (Video 8.32). But there were no findings that are suggestive of folding, seroma, upside-down rotation, rupture, and capsular mass.

The patient underwent explantation with subtotal capsulectomy *via* a previous axillary scar on both sides. There were right focal degeneration and left focal chronic inflammation and fibrosis (Fig. 8.23).

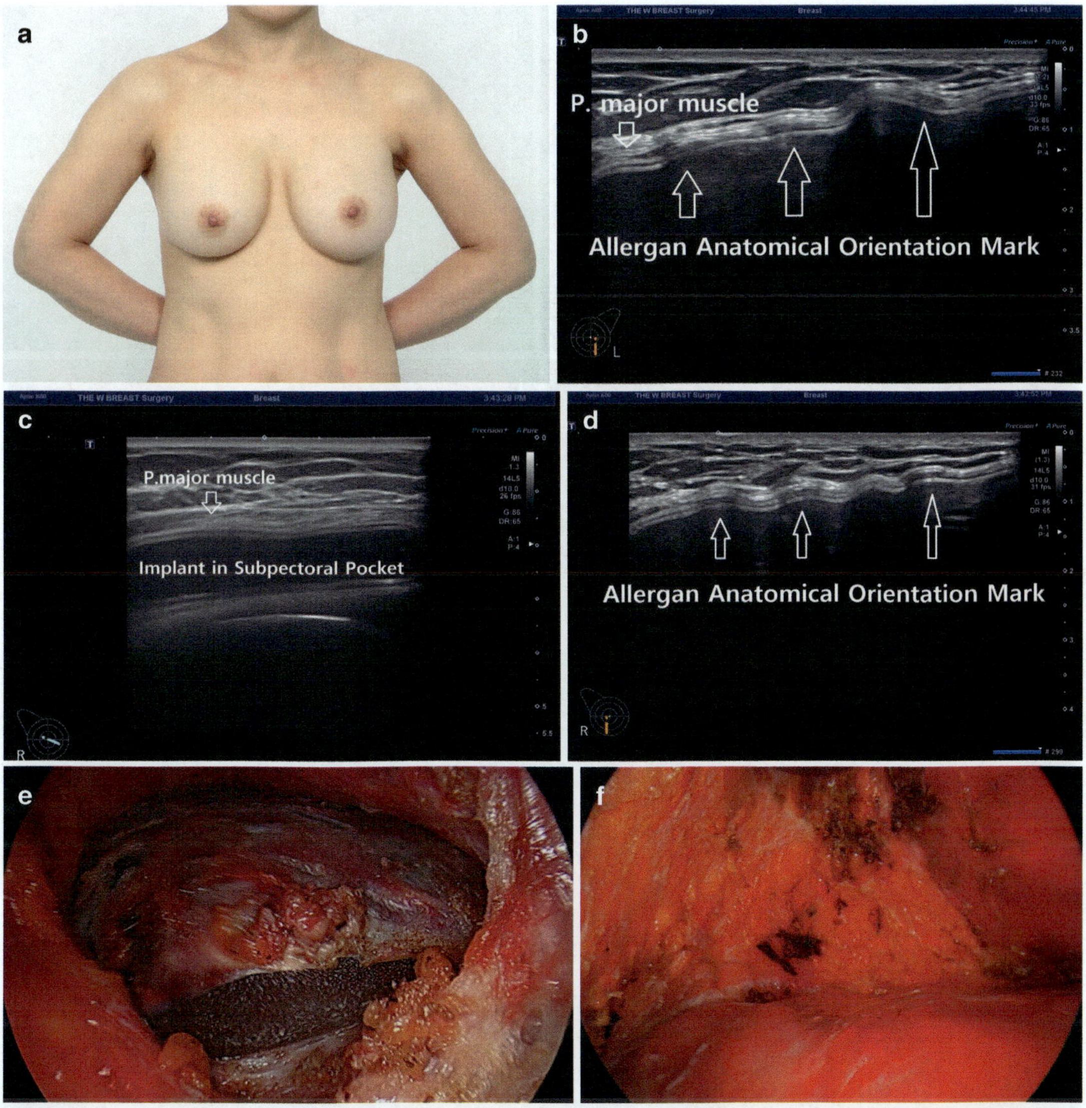

Fig. 8.22 (**a**) A preoperative front view. (**b**) Left Allegan anatomical type breast implant in subpectoral pocket is checked in preoperative ultrasonography. (**c**) Right texture type breast implant in subpectoral pocket is checked in preoperative ultrasonography. (**d**) Right preoperative sonographic findings; Allergan orientation mark; three dots is checked. (**e**) Left intraoperative view of breast implant with periprosthetic capsule. (**f**) Left intraoperative view of breast pocket after subtotal capsulectomy. (**g**) Right intraoperative view of texture type breast implant with periprosthetic capsule. (**h**) Right intraoperative finding of Allergan breast anatomical type implant. (**i**) Right intraoperative view of periprosthetic capsule. (**j**) Right intraoperative view of breast pocket after subtotal capsulectomy. (**k**) Both removed implant and periprosthetic capsule after subtotal capsulectomy. (**l**) Both removed Allergan anatomical type breast implant 410 FM 270 cc. (**m**) Both removed periprosthetic capsule by subtotal capsulectomy. (**n**) Left capsule thickness is measured by digital caliper, 0.4 mm. (**o**) Right capsule thickness is measured by digital caliper, 0.4 mm. (**p**) Microscopic view of the left capsule. (**q**) Microscopic view of the right capsule

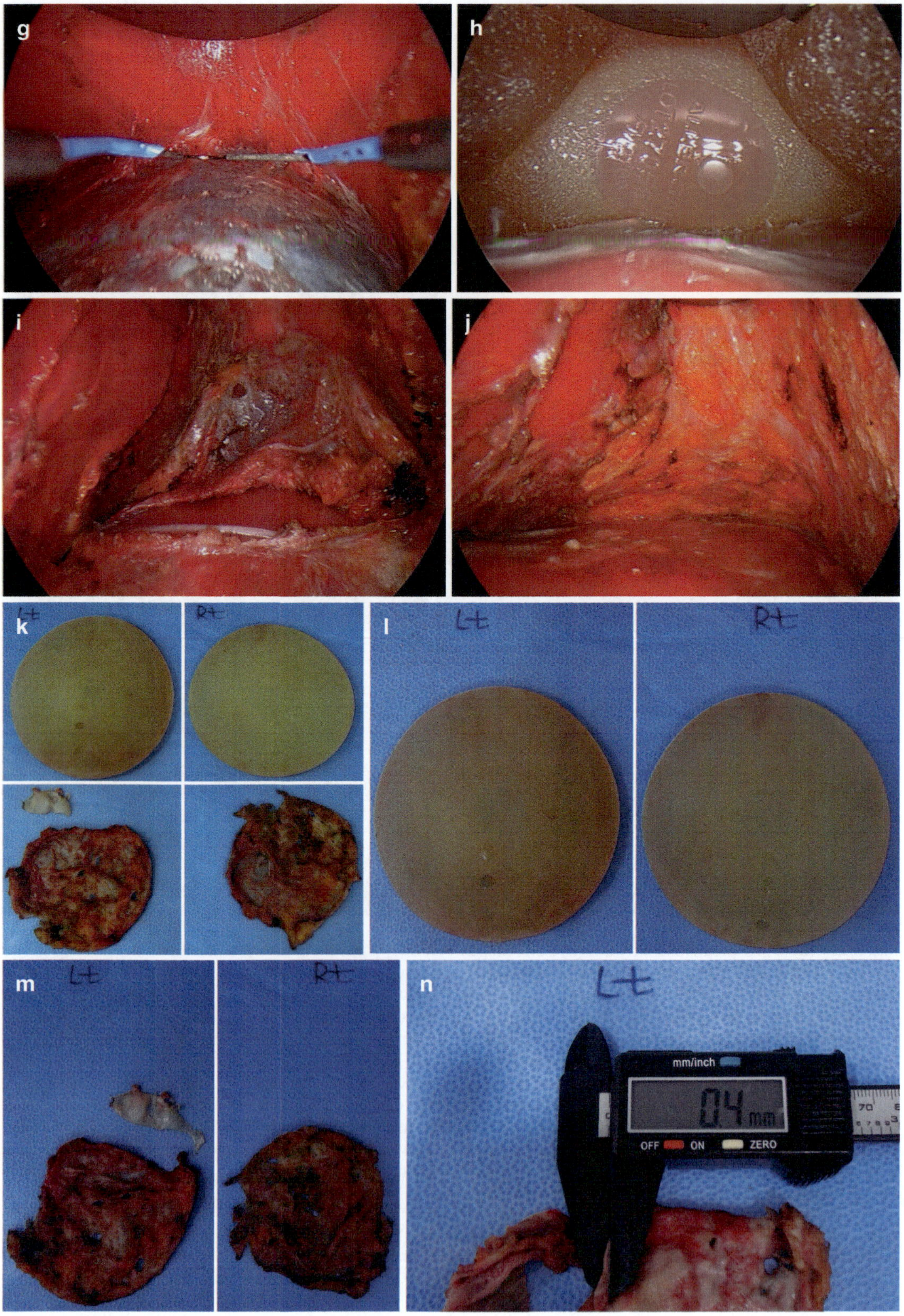

Fig. 8.22 (continued)

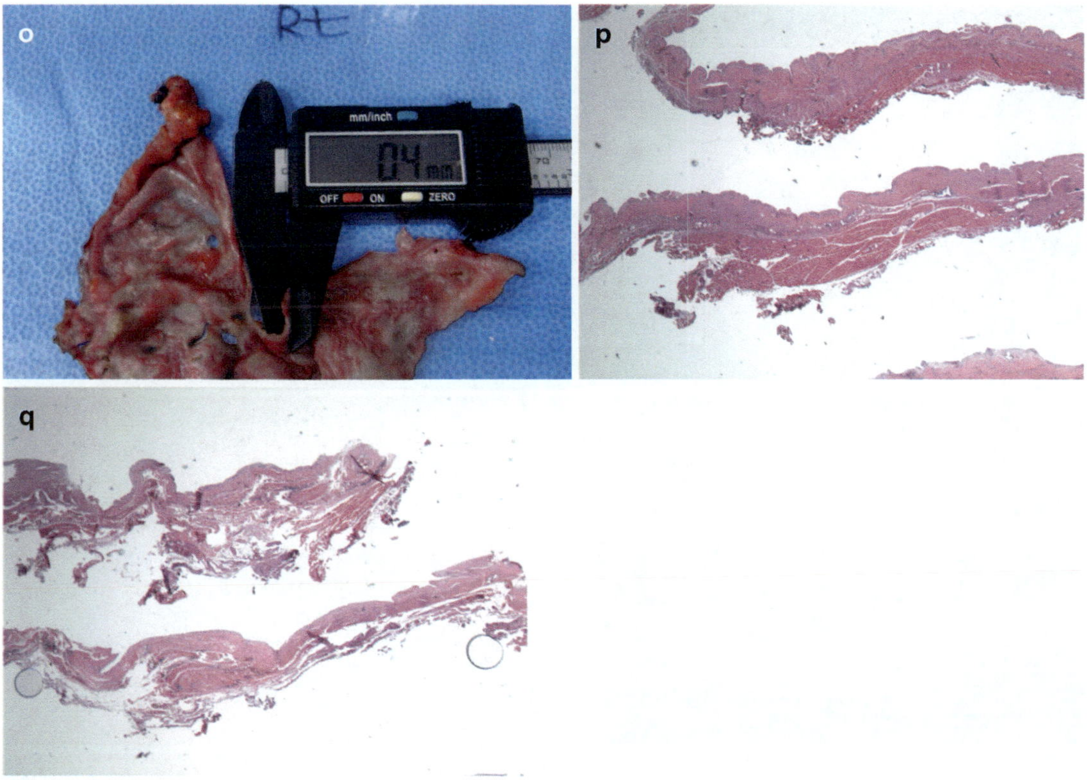

Fig. 8.22 (continued)

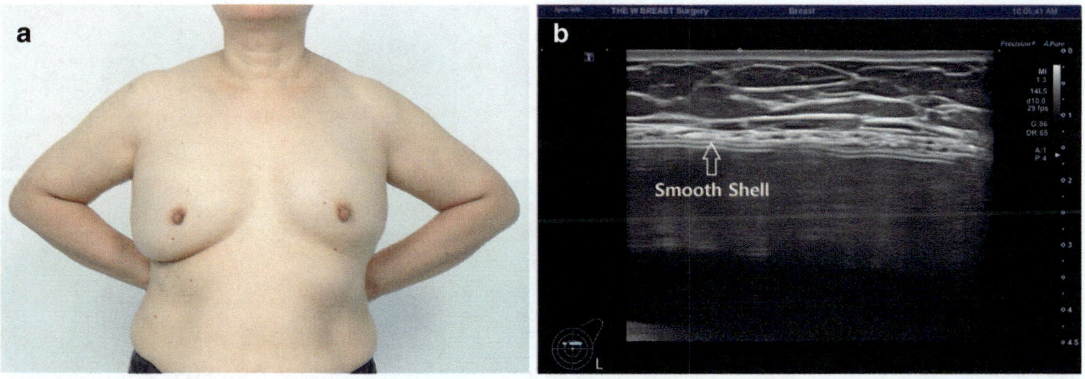

Fig. 8.23 (**a**) A preoperative front view. (**b**) Left smooth shell type breast implant in subpectoral pocket is checked in preoperative ultrasonography. (**c**) Left thickened periprosthetic capsule is measured 4.1 mm in preoperative ultrasonography. (**d**) Shear wave elastography of left breast implant and thickened capsule. It shows hardness (red color means hardness). (**e**) Right smooth type breast implant in subpectoral pocket is checked in preoperative ultrasonography. (**f**) Left intraoperative view of smooth type breast implant with periprosthetic capsule. (**g**) Left intraoperative view of intracapsular breast pocket. (**h**) Left intraoperative view of breast pocket after subtotal capsulectomy. (**i**) Right intraoperative view of intracapsular breast pocket. (**j**) Right intraoperative view after subtotal capsulectomy. (**k**) Both removed Mentor smooth type saline breast implant, 225 cc. (**l**) Both removed breast implant. (**m**) Both removed periprosthetic capsule by subtotal capsulectomy. (**n**) Left capsule thickness is measured by digital caliper, 4.0 mm. (**o**) Right capsule thickness is measured by digital caliper, 0.1 mm. (**p**) Microscopic view of the left capsule. (**q**) Microscopic view of the right capsule

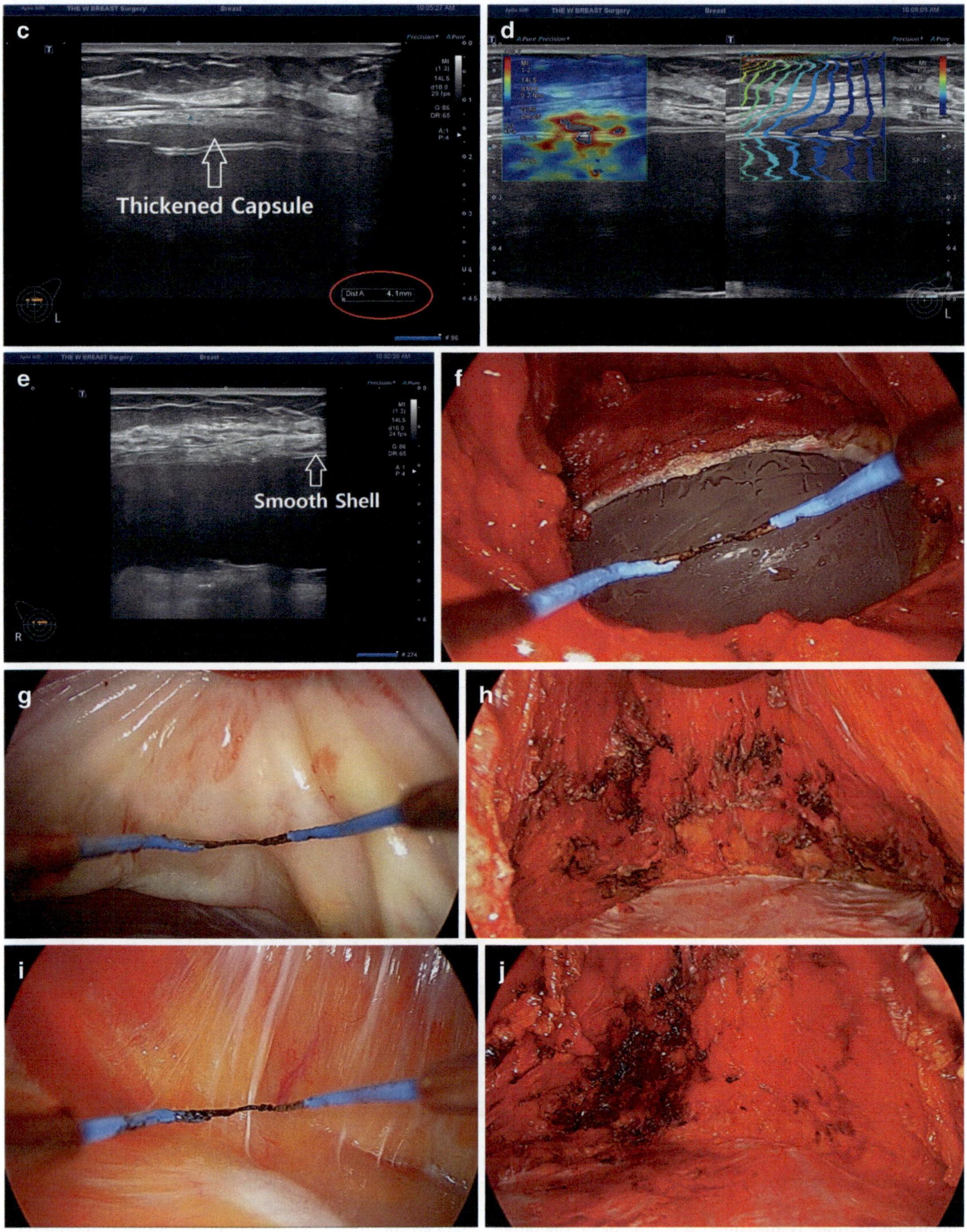

Fig. 8.23 (continued)

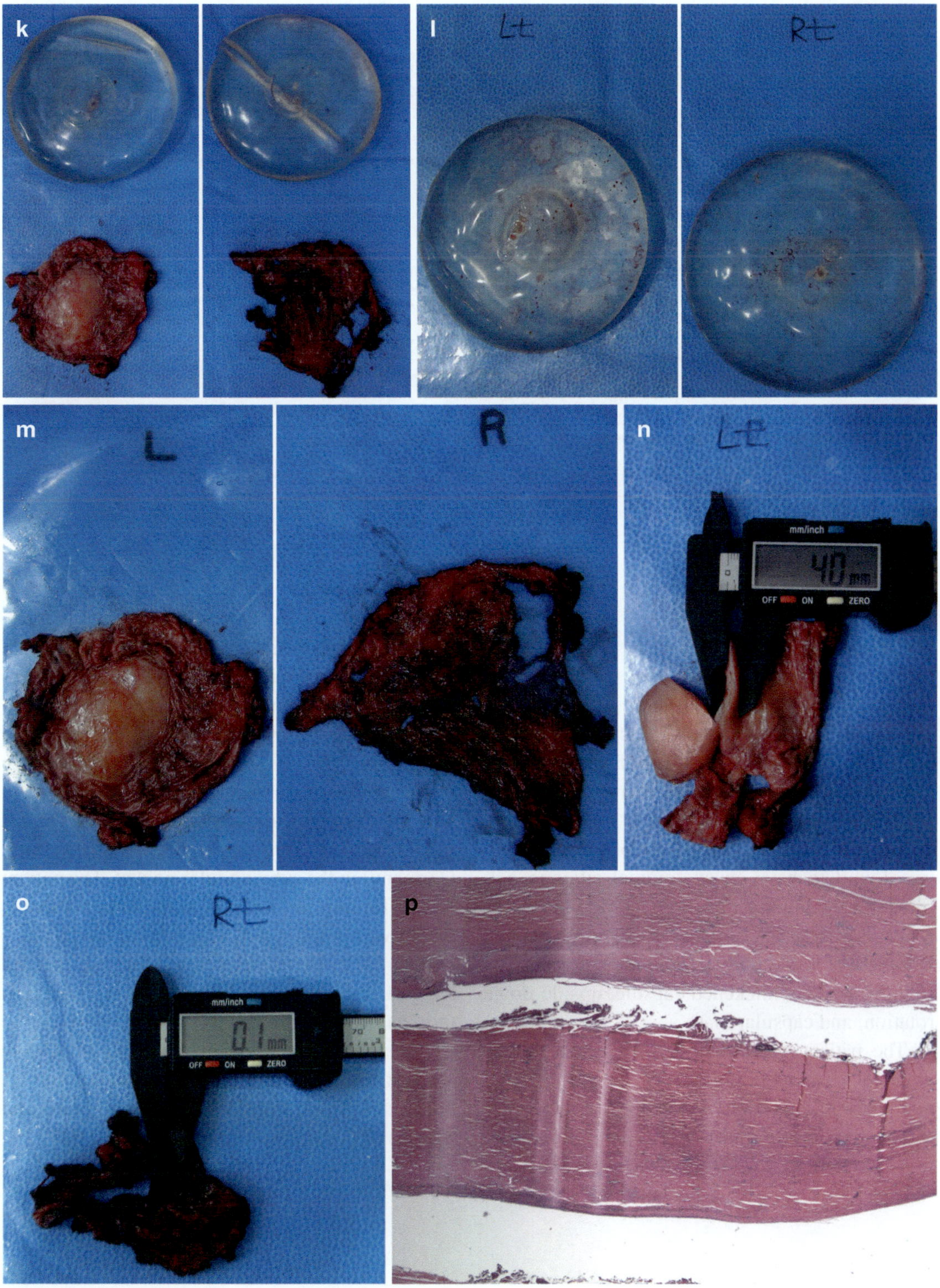

Fig. 8.23 (continued)

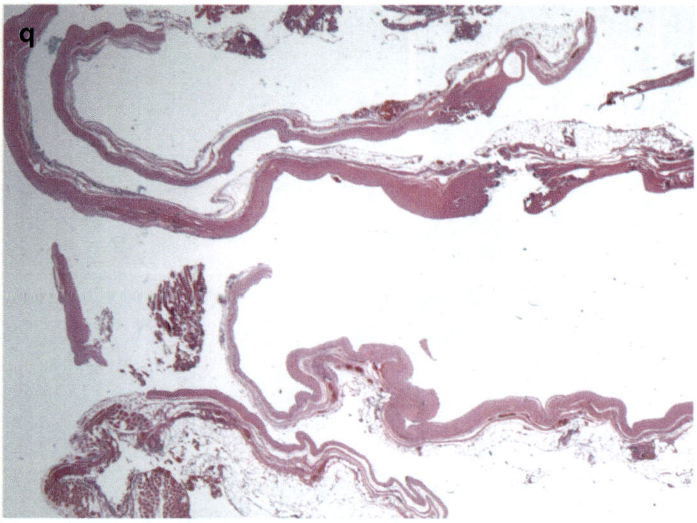

Fig. 8.23 (continued)

8.2.24 Case 24

On physical examination and history taking, a 26-year-old woman complained of dissatisfaction with shape due to rippling *as well as* an unpleasant feeling due to a breast implant. The patient had a 4-year history of receiving an implant-based augmentation mammaplasty *via* an inframammary fold incision.

On preoperative ultrasonography, the patient was found to have an anatomical silicone gel-filled breast implant (Mentor Worldwide LLC, Santa Barbara, CA) in the subpectoral pocket. But there were no findings that are suggestive of folding, seroma, thickened capsule, upside-down rotation, and capsular mass.

The patient underwent subtotal capsulectomy with replacement of the device *via* a previous inframammary fold incision, concurrently with the use of allograft dermal matrix, on both sides. There was mild fibrosis in both capsule (Fig. 8.24).

8.2.25 Case 25

On physical examination and history taking, a 30-year-old woman wanted to receive explantation. The patient had a 6-year history of receiving an implant-based augmentation mammaplasty.

On preoperative ultrasonography, the patient had an anatomical silicone gel-filled breast implant (Polytech Health & Aesthetics, Dieburg, Germany) in the subglandular pocket. The patient had a folding *as well as* a thickened capsule which was measured as 0.6 mm on the left side (Video 8.33). But there were no findings that are suggestive of seroma, upside-down rotation, rupture, and capsular mass.

The patient underwent total capsulectomy with explantation *via* a previous areolar scar on both sides. There were chronic inflammation and fibrosis in both capsule (Fig. 8.25).

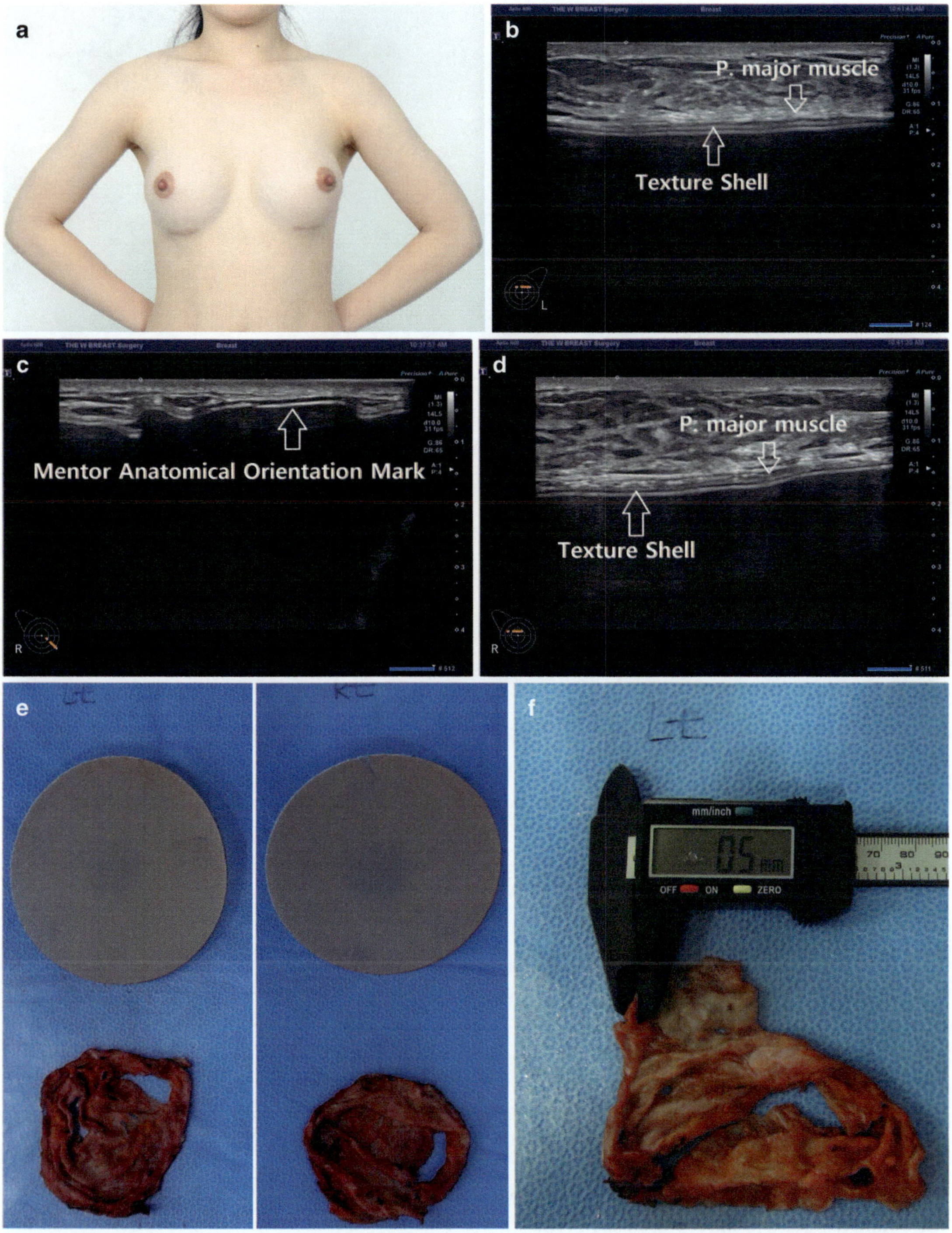

Fig. 8.24 (**a**) A preoperative front view. (**b**) Left textured shell type breast implant in subpectoral pocket is checked in preoperative ultrasonography. (**c**) Right Mentor anatomical type breast implant is checked in preoperative ultrasonography. (**d**) Right textured shell type breast implant in subpectoral pocket. (**e**) Both removed Mentor anatomical breast implant, 295 cc and periprosthetic capsule after subtotal capsulectomy. (**f**) Left capsule thickness is measured by digital caliper, 0.5 mm. (**g**) Right capsule thickness is measured by digital caliper, 0.5 mm. (**h**) Microscopic view of the left capsule. (**i**) Microscopic view of the right capsule

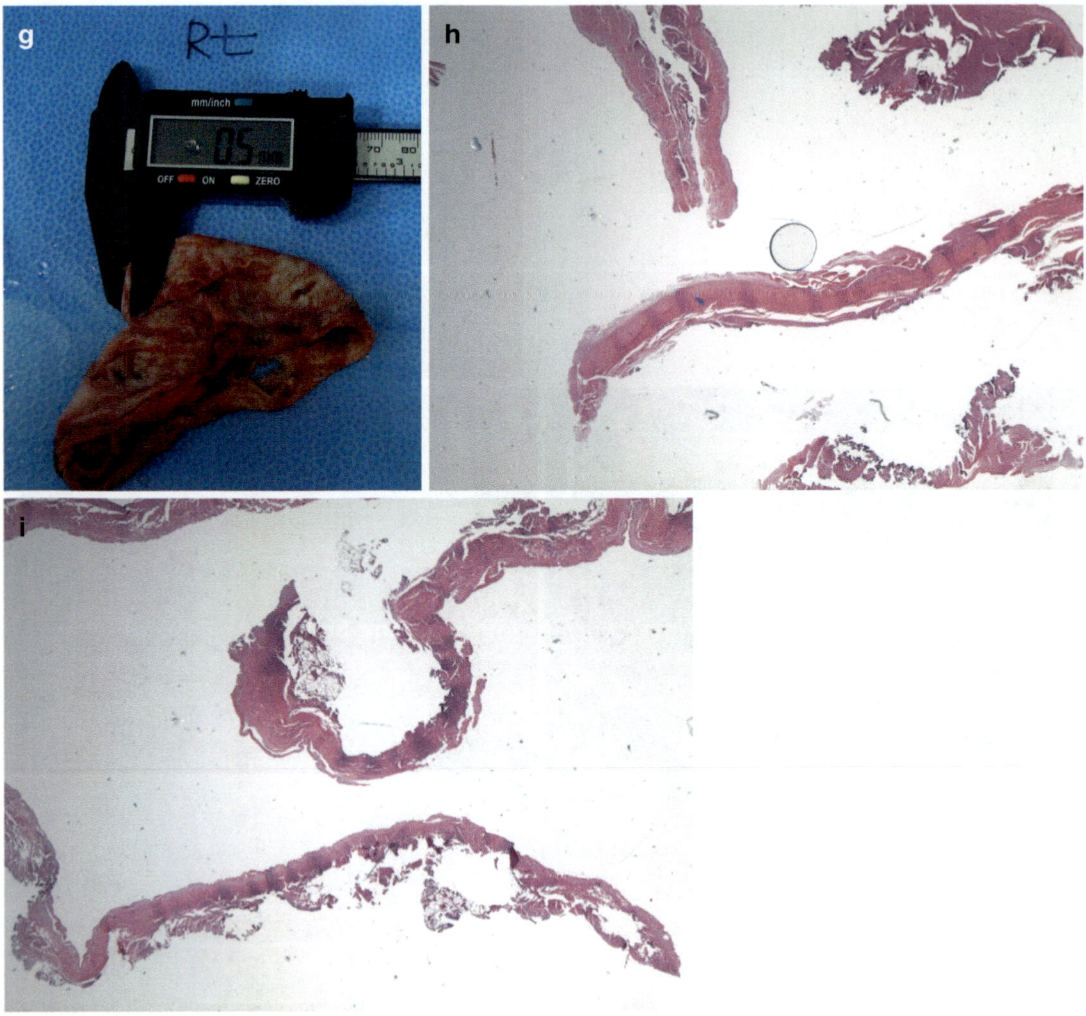

Fig. 8.24 (continued)

8.2.26 Case 26

On physical examination and history taking, a 58-year-old woman complained of breast hardness on the left side. The patient had an 8-year history of receiving an implant-based augmentation mammaplasty.

On preoperative ultrasonography, the patient was found to have a round textured shell type silicone gel-filled breast implant in the subpectoral pocket. The patient had a thickened capsule which was measured as 1.0–2.1 mm on the left side (Video 8.34), accompanied by the bilateral presence of a folding. But there were no findings that are suggestive of seroma, upside-down rotation, rupture, and capsular mass.

The patient underwent near-total capsulectomy on the right side and total capsulectomy with explantation *via* a previous axillary scar on the left side. There were chronic inflammation and fibrosis in both capsule (Fig. 8.26) (Video 8.35).

8.2.27 Case 27

On physical examination and history taking, a 46-year-old woman complained of breast pain. The patient had an 8-year history of receiving an implant-based augmentation mammaplasty.

On preoperative ultrasonography, the patient was found to have a round textured saline-filled breast implant in the subpectoral pocket (Video

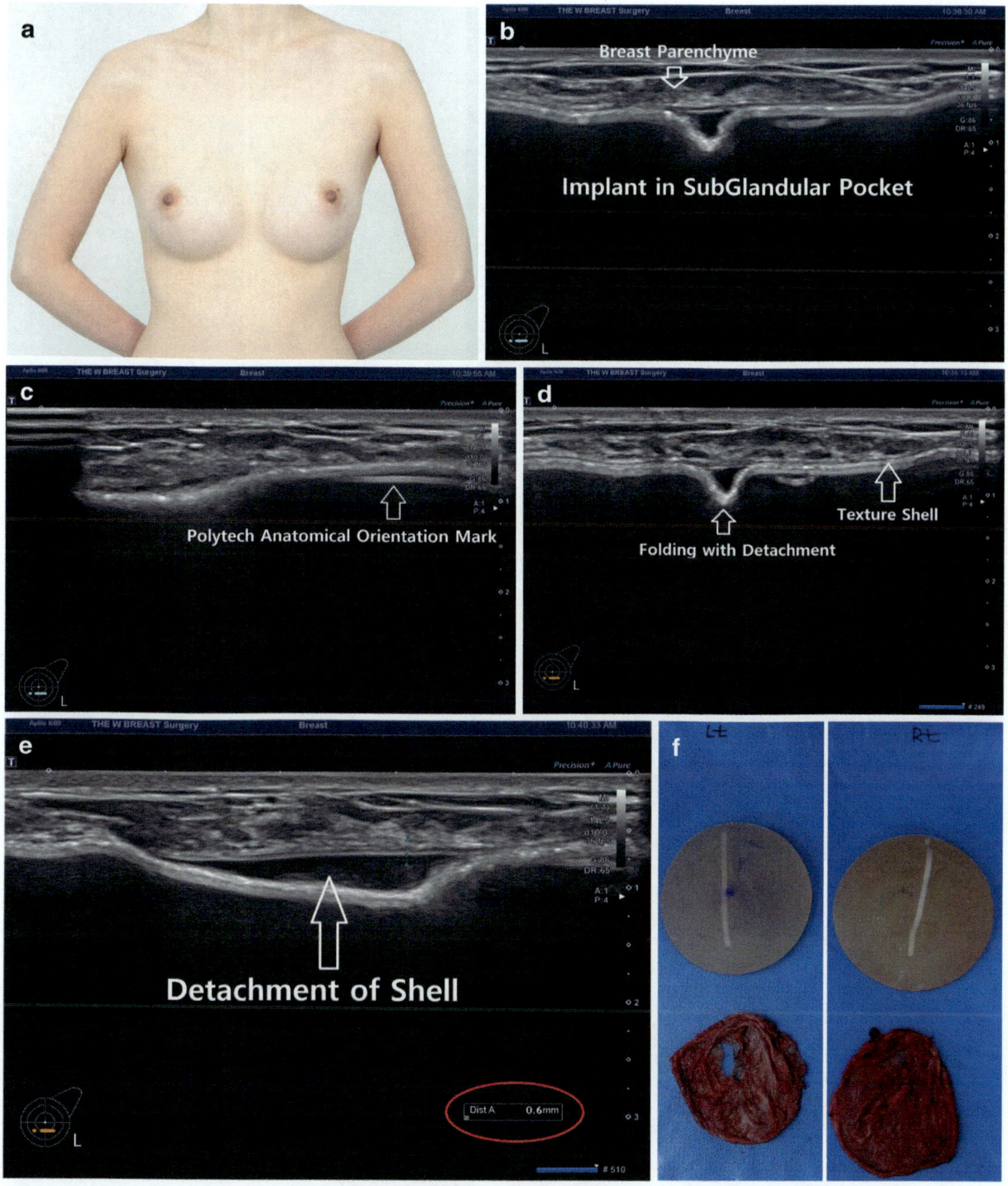

Fig. 8.25 (**a**) A preoperative front view. (**b**) Left textured shell type breast implant in subglandular pocket is checked in preoperative ultrasonography. (**c**): Left Polytech anatomical type breast implant with orientation mark is checked in preoperative ultrasonography. (**d**, **e**) Left breast implant folded shell and detachment is checked in ultrasonography. (**f**) Both removed Polytech anatomical breast implant and periprosthetic capsule. (**g**) Both removed Polytech anatomical breast implant 275 cc. (**h**) Both removed periprosthetic capsule after total capsulectomy. (**i**) Left capsule thickness is measured by digital caliper, 0.7 mm. (**j**) Right capsule thickness is measured by digital caliper, 0.2 mm. (**k**) Microscopic view of the left capsule. (**l**) Microscopic view of the right capsule

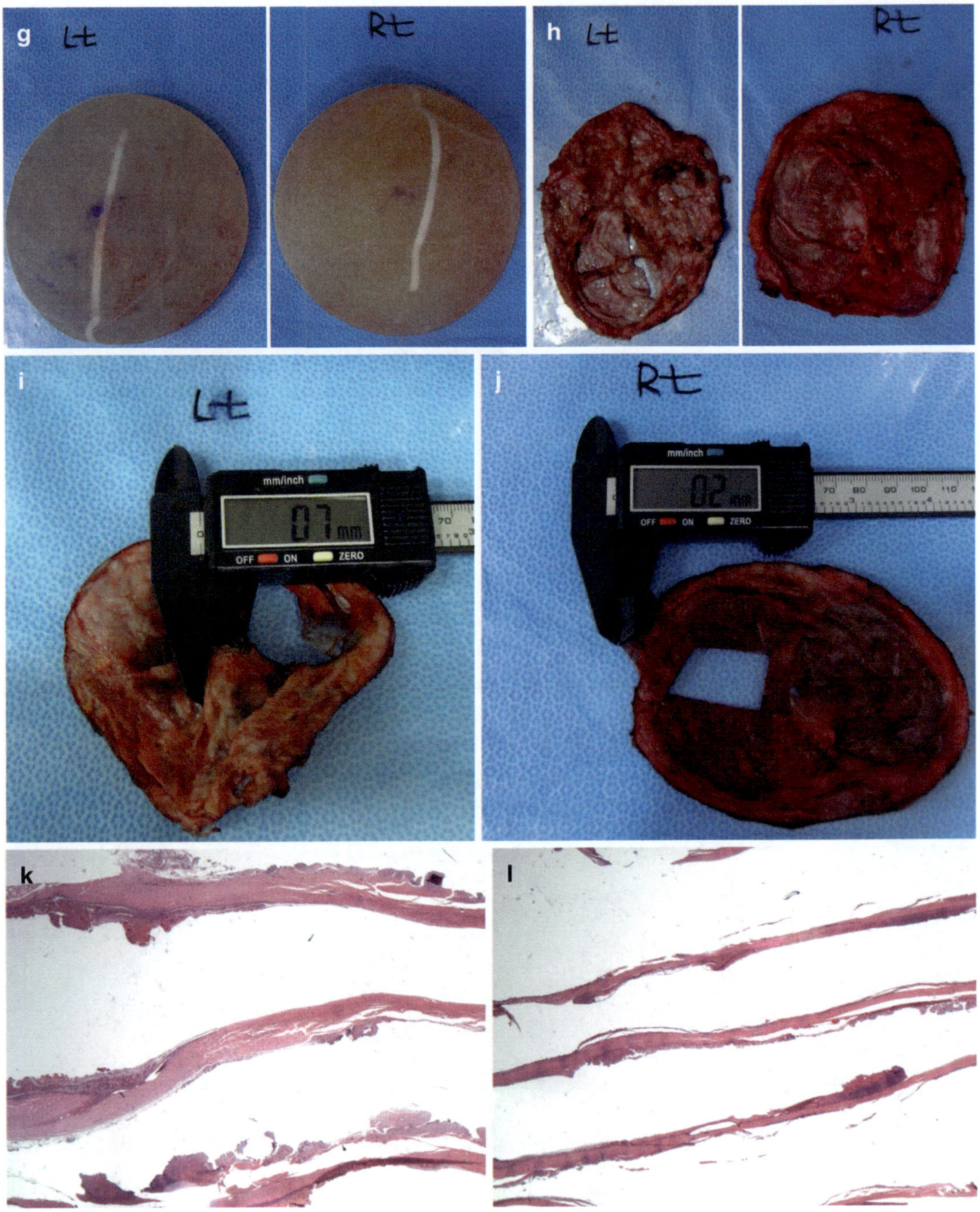

Fig. 8.25 (continued)

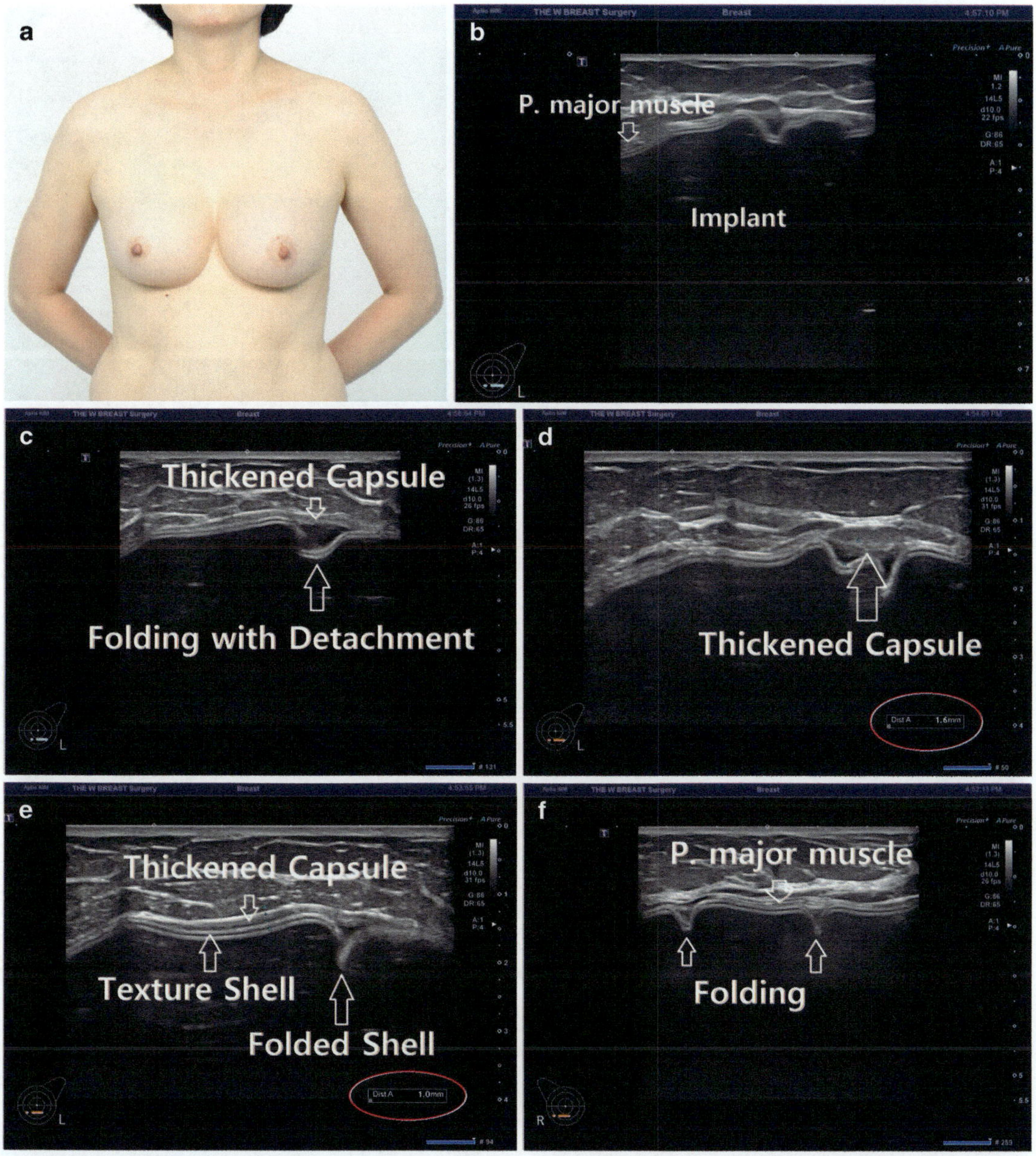

Fig. 8.26 (**a**) A preoperative front view. (**b–e**) Left textured shell type breast implant in subpectoral pocket with folded shell and thickened capsule is checked in preoperative ultrasonography. (**f, g**) Right textured shell type breast implant in subpectoral pocket with folding is checked in preoperative ultrasonography. (**h**) Left intraoperative view of breast implant with periprosthetic capsule. (**i**) Left intraoperative view of periprosthetic capsule. (**j**) Left intraoperative view of breast pocket after total capsulectomy. (**k, l**) Right intraoperative view of breast implant with periprosthetic capsule. (**m**) Right intraoperative view of breast pocket after near-total capsulectomy. (**n**) Both removed Allergan round texture type breast implant style 115 272 cc. (**o–q**) Left capsule thickness is measured by digital caliper, 2.0 mm, 8.9 mm, and 8.4 mm. (**r**) Right capsule thickness is measured by digital caliper, 0.1 mm. (**s**) Microscopic view of the left capsule. (**t**) Microscopic view of the right capsule

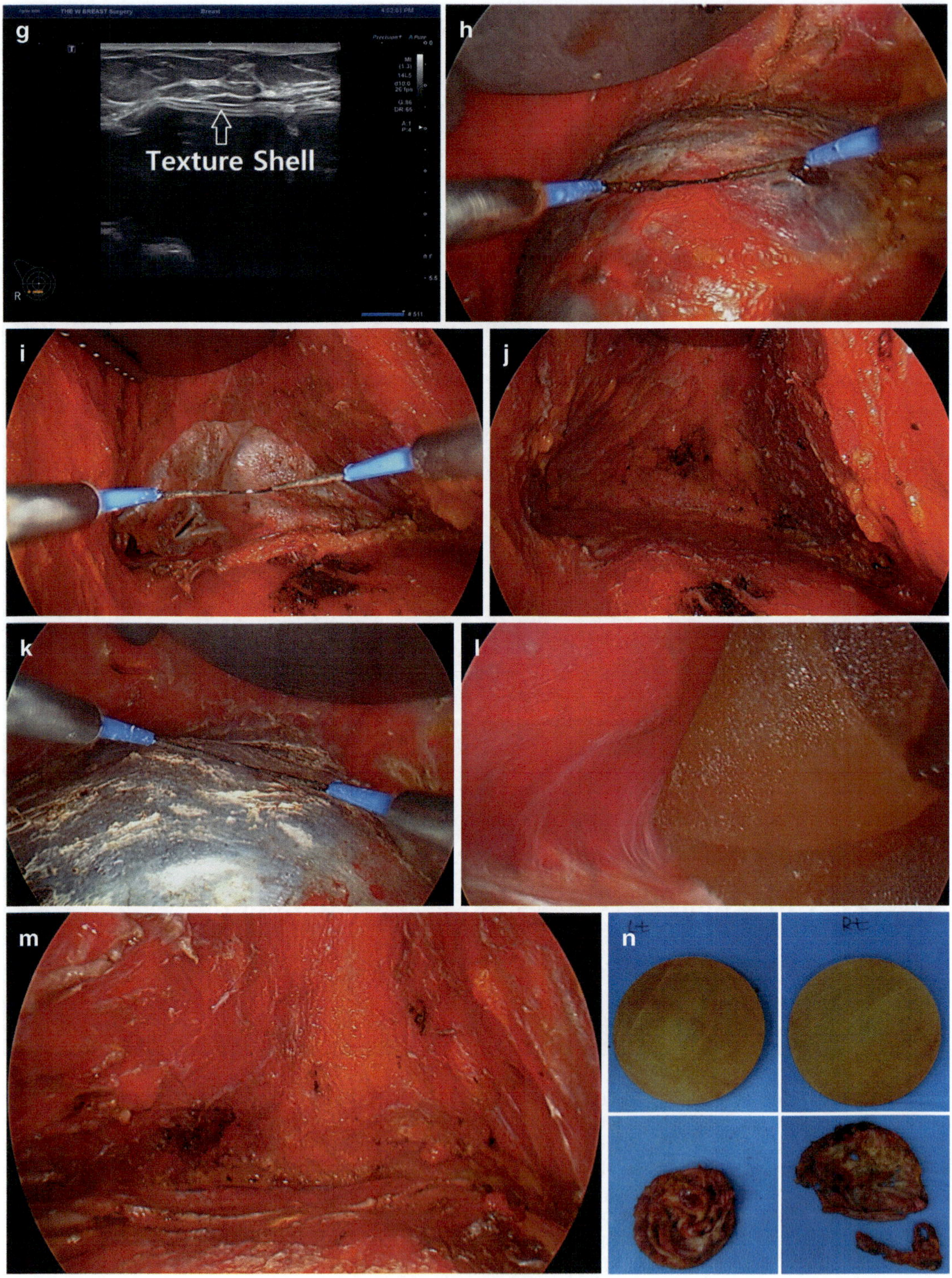

Fig. 8.26 (continued)

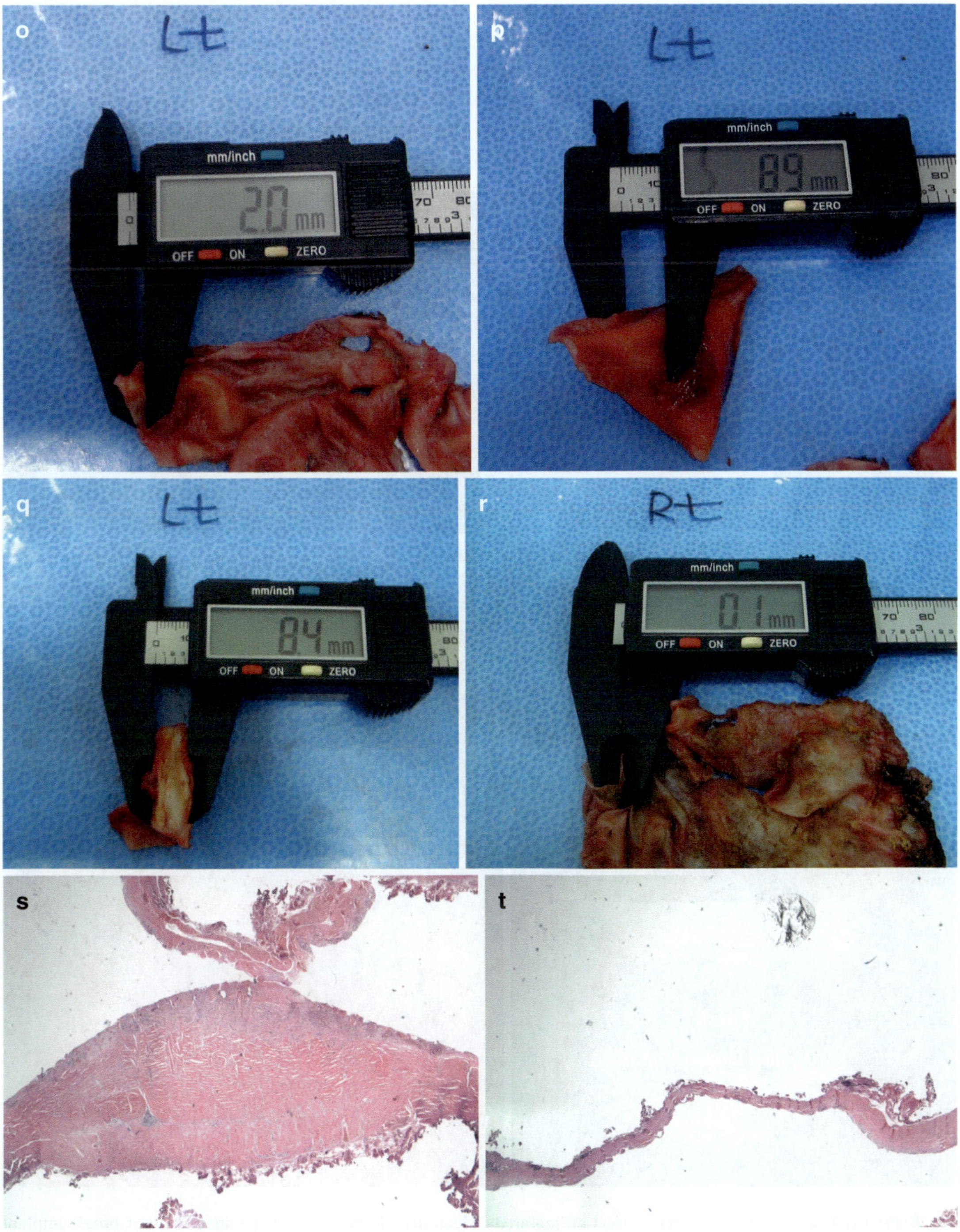

Fig. 8.26 (continued)

8.37). The patient had an upside-down rotation on the right side (Video 8.38). But there were no findings that are suggestive of folding, seroma, thickened capsule, rupture, and capsular mass (Fig. 8.27) (Video 8.36).

The patient underwent near-total capsulectomy on the right side and subtotal capsulectomy on the left side with replacement of the new breast implant *via* a previous axillary scar. There were focal chronic inflammation and fibrosis in both capsule.

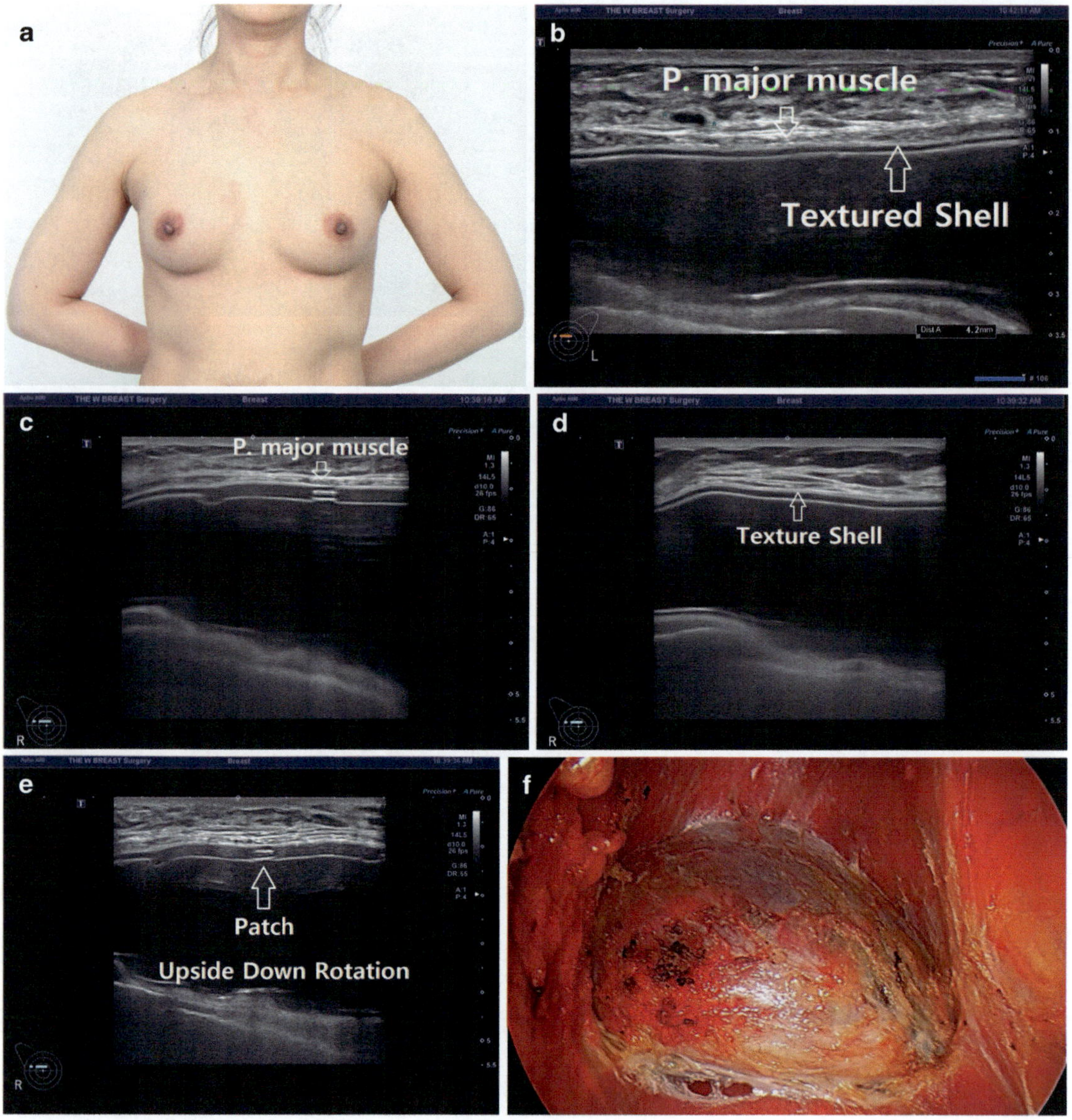

Fig. 8.27 (**a**) A preoperative front view. (**b**) Left textured shell type breast implant in subpectoral pocket is checked in preoperative ultrasonography. (**c**) Right breast implant in subpectoral pocket is checked in preoperative ultrasonography. (**d**) Right textured shell type breast implant is checked in preoperative ultrasonography. (**e**) Right breast implant upside-down rotation is checked by patch in preoperative ultrasonography. (**f**) Left intraoperative view of breast implant with periprosthetic capsule. (**g**) Left Intraoperative view of breast pocket after subtotal capsulectomy. (**h**) Right intraoperative view of breast implant with periprosthetic capsule. (**i**) Right intraoperative view of breast pocket after near-total capsulectomy. (**j**) Both removed breast implant, unknown manufacturer, round texture saline breast implant 200 cc. (**k**) Both removed periprosthetic capsule. (**l**) Left capsule thickness is measured by digital caliper, 0.3 mm. (**m**) Right capsule thickness is measured by digital caliper, 0.3 mm. (**n**) Microscopic view of the left capsule. (**o**) Microscopic view of the right capsule

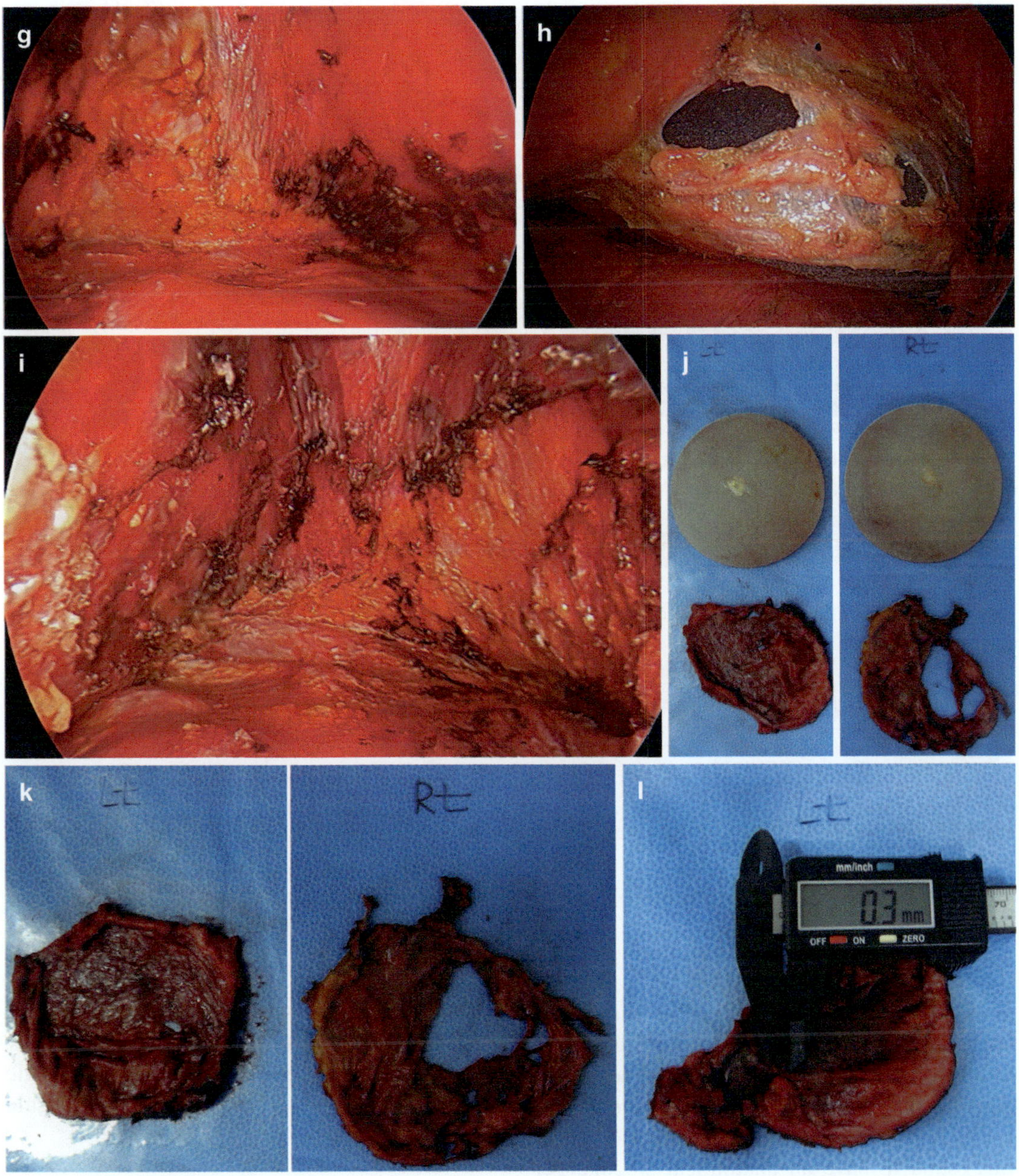

Fig. 8.27 (continued)

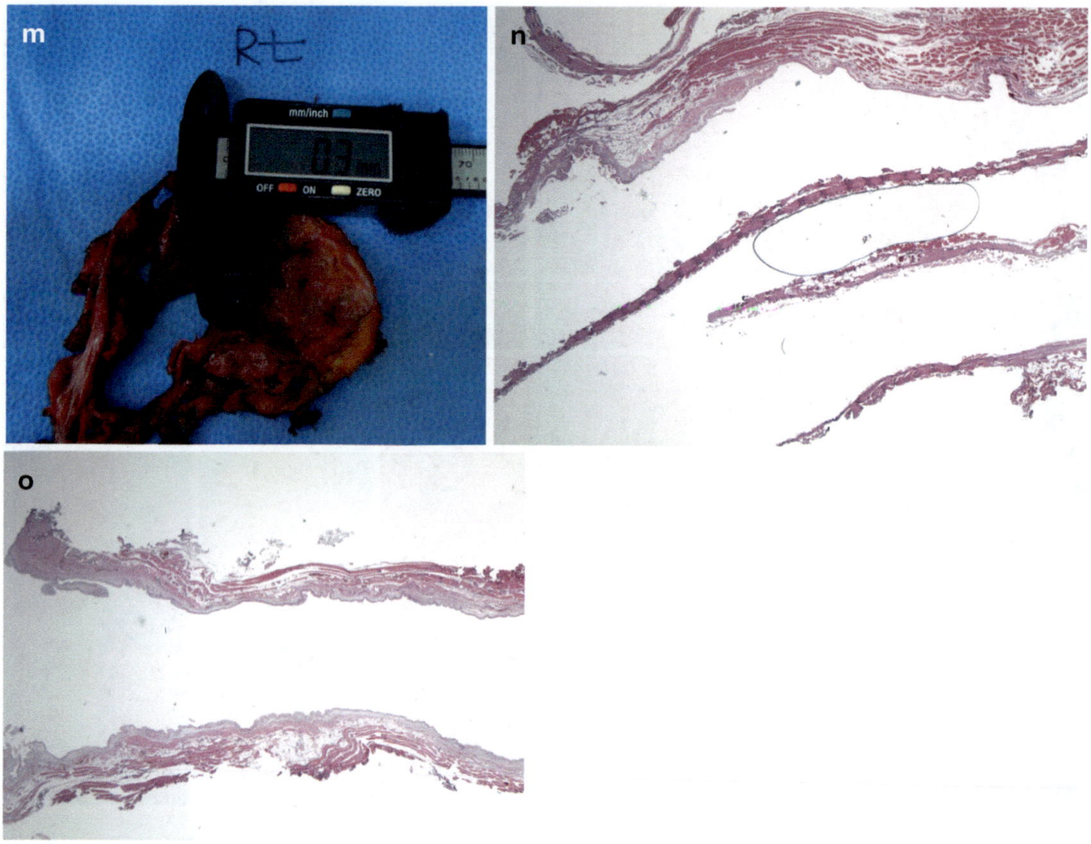

Fig. 8.27 (continued)

8.2.28 Case 28

On physical examination and history taking, a 44-year-old woman complained of dissatisfaction with shape and size. The patient had a 5-year history of receiving an implant-based augmentation mammaplasty *via* an axillary incision.

On preoperative ultrasonography, the patient was found to have an anatomical silicone gel-filled breast implant (Polytech Health & Aesthetics, Dieburg, Germany) in the subpectoral pocket. The patient bilaterally had a folding *as well as* a thickened capsule which was measured as 1.7 mm on the right side and 1.0 mm on the left side (Video 8.39). But there were no findings that are suggestive of malrotation, folding, seroma, thickened capsule, upside-down rotation, rupture, and capsular mass.

The patient underwent near-total capsulectomy on the right side and subtotal capsulectomy with explantation *via* a previous axillary scar on the left side. There were focal chronic inflammation and fibrosis in both capsule (Fig. 8.28).

8.2.29 Case 29

On physical examination and history taking, a 61-year-old woman complained of breast pain. The patient had a 9-year history of receiving an implant-based augmentation mammaplasty.

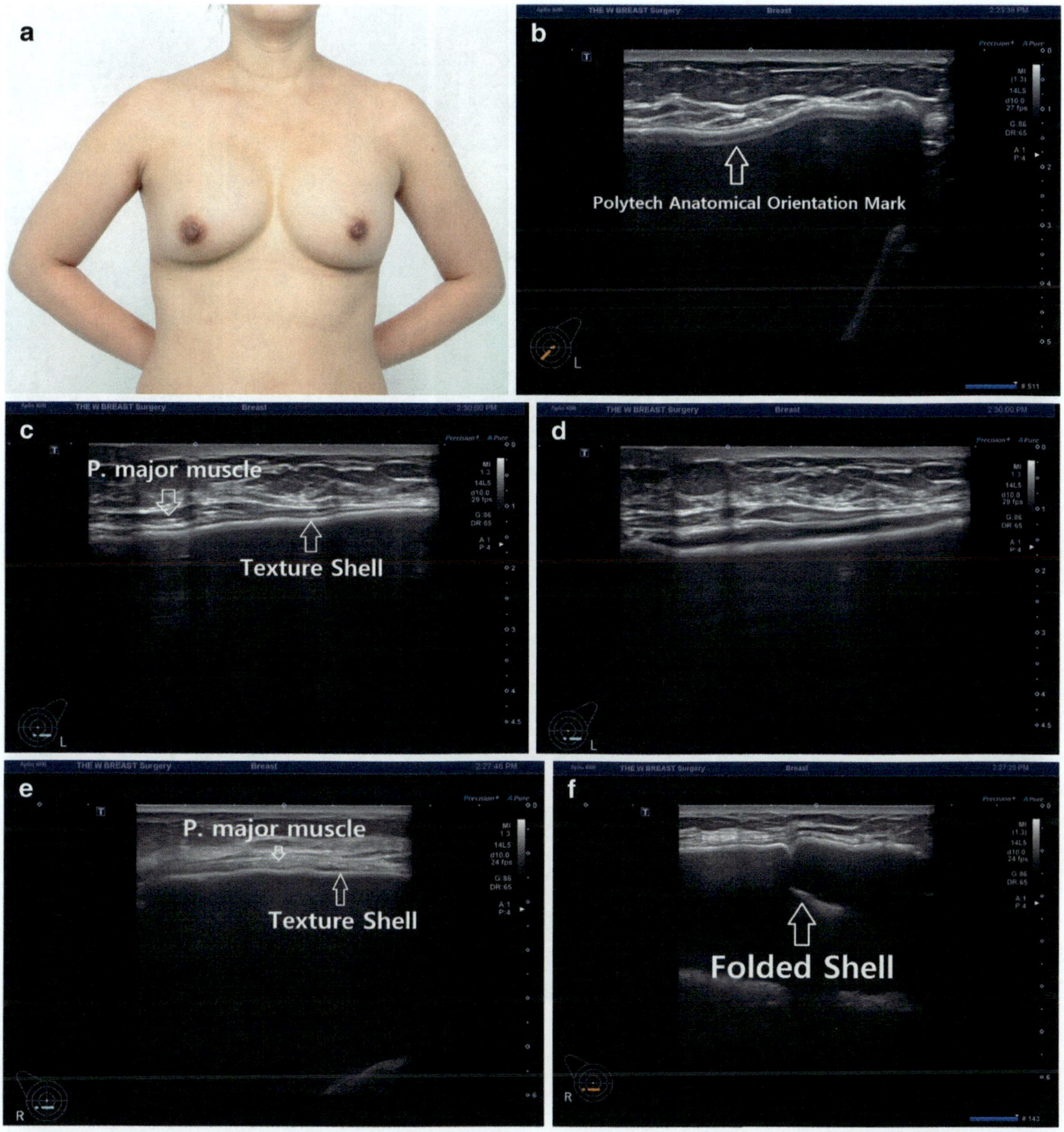

Fig. 8.28 (**a**) A preoperative front view. (**b**) Left Polytech anatomical breast implant is checked in preoperative ultrasonography. (**c**) Left textured shell type breast implant in subpectoral pocket is checked in preoperative ultrasonography. (**d**) Left breast implant shell detachment is checked in preoperative ultrasonography. (**e**) Right textured shell type breast implant in subpectoral pocket is checked in preoperative ultrasonography. (**f**) Right breast implant shell folding is checked in preoperative ultrasonography. (**g**) Right periprosthetic thickened capsule (1.0 mm) is checked in preoperative ultrasonography. (**h**) Both removed breast implant, Polytech anatomical type 300 cc breast implant. (**i**) Both removed periprosthetic capsule. (**j**) Left capsule thickness is measured by digital caliper, 1.1 mm. (**k**) Right capsule thickness is measured by digital caliper, 1.0 mm. (**l**) Microscopic view of the left capsule. (**m**) Microscopic view of the right capsule

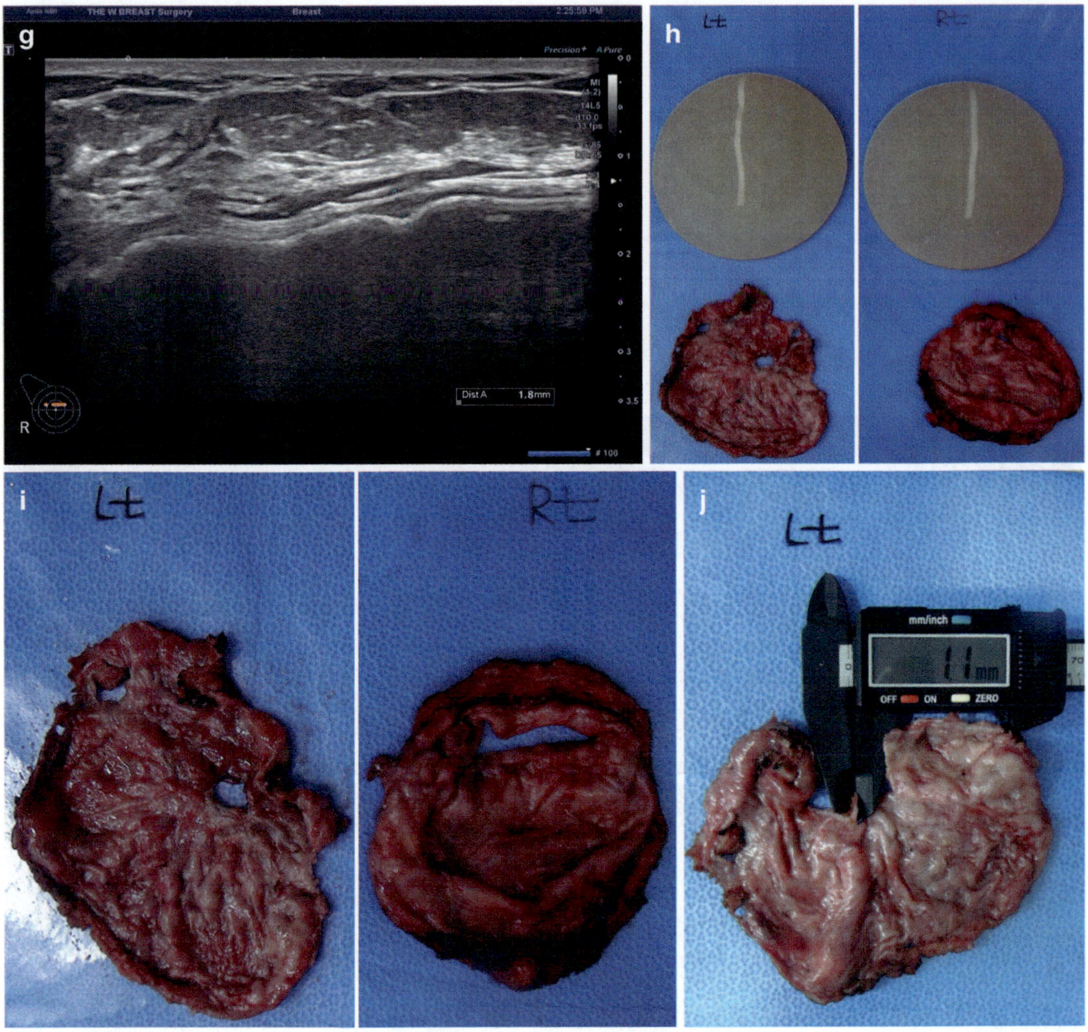

Fig. 8.28 (continued)

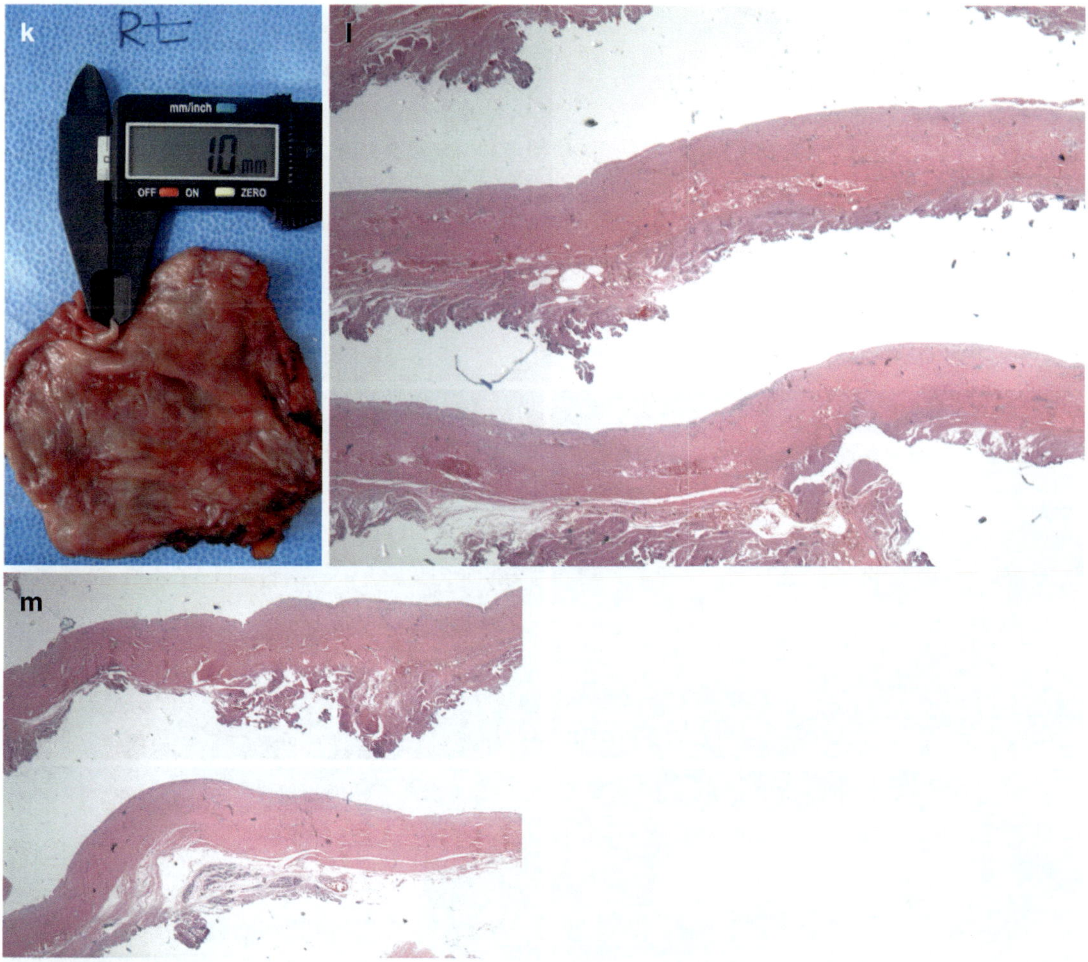

Fig. 8.28 (continued)

On preoperative ultrasonography, the patient was found to have a round smooth shell type saline-filled breast implant in the subpectoral pocket. The patient had an upside-down rotation on both sides (Video 8.40). But there were no findings that are suggestive of folding, seroma, thickened capsule, rupture, and capsular mass.

The patient underwent subtotal capsulectomy with explantation *via* a previous inframammary fold scar on both sides. There were focal chronic inflammation and fibrosis in both capsule (Fig. 8.29).

8.2.30 Case 30

On physical examination and history taking, a 33-year-old woman complained of breast pain. The patient had a 7-year history of receiving an implant-based augmentation mammaplasty.

On preoperative ultrasonography, the patient was found to have an anatomical silicone gel-filled breast implant (Allergan Inc., Irvine, CA) in the subpectoral pocket. But there was no malrotation. The patient had an upside-down rotation

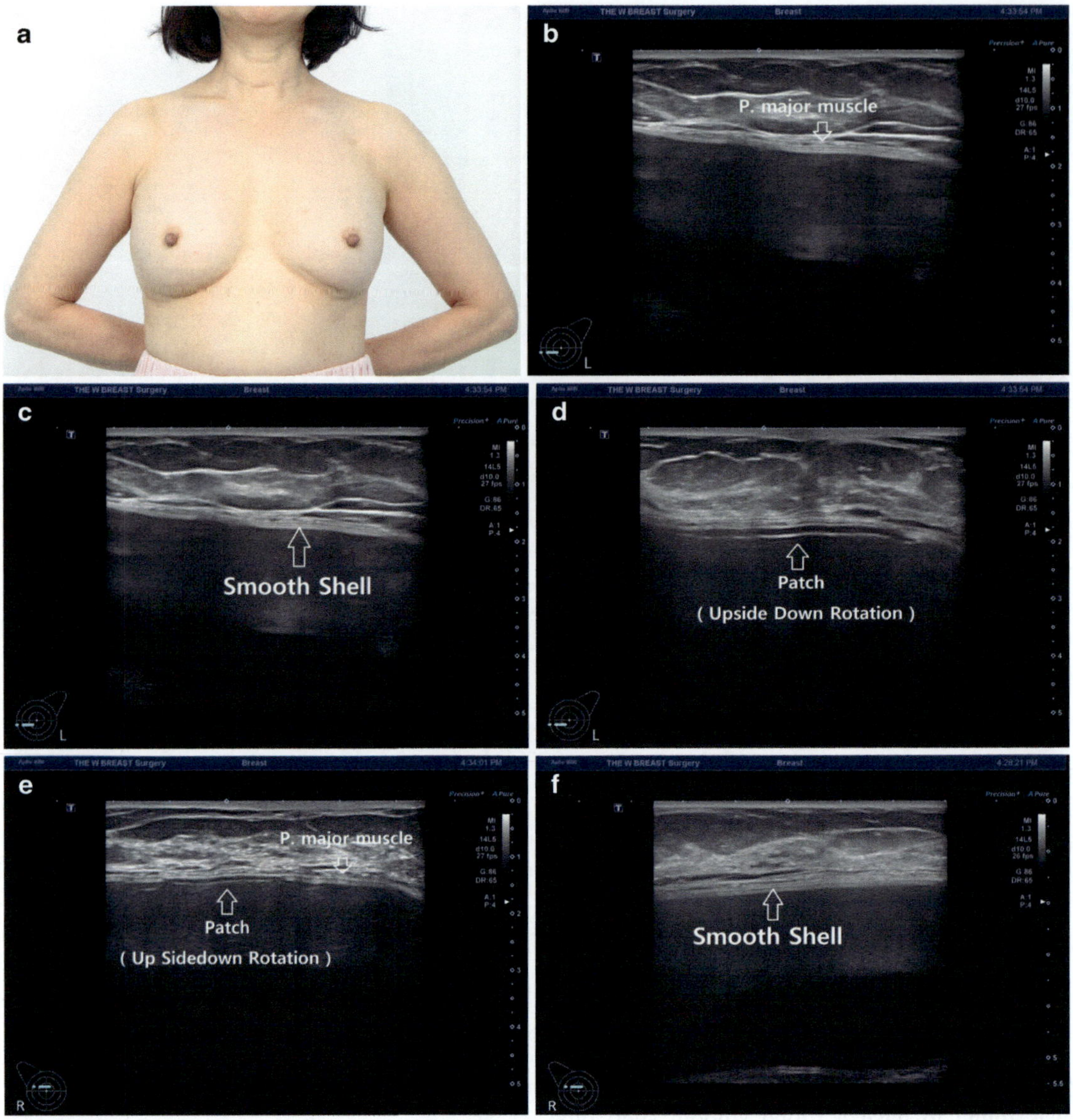

Fig. 8.29 (**a**) A preoperative front view. (**b**): Left breast implant in subpectoral pocket is checked in preoperative ultrasonography. (**c**) Left smooth shell type breast implant is checked in preoperative ultrasonography. (**d**) Left breast implant upside-down rotation is checked in preoperative ultrasonography. (**e**) Right breast implant upside-down rotation is checked in preoperative ultrasonography. (**f**) Right smooth shell type breast implant is checked in preoperative ultrasonography. (**g**) Both removed Mentor smooth shell type breast implant, 200 cc. (**h**) Both removed breast implant and periprosthetic capsule after subtotal capsulectomy. (**i**) Left capsule thickness is measured by digital caliper, 0.2 mm. (**j**) Right capsule thickness is measured by digital caliper, 0.1 mm. (**k**) Microscopic view of the left capsule. (**l**) Microscopic view of the right capsule

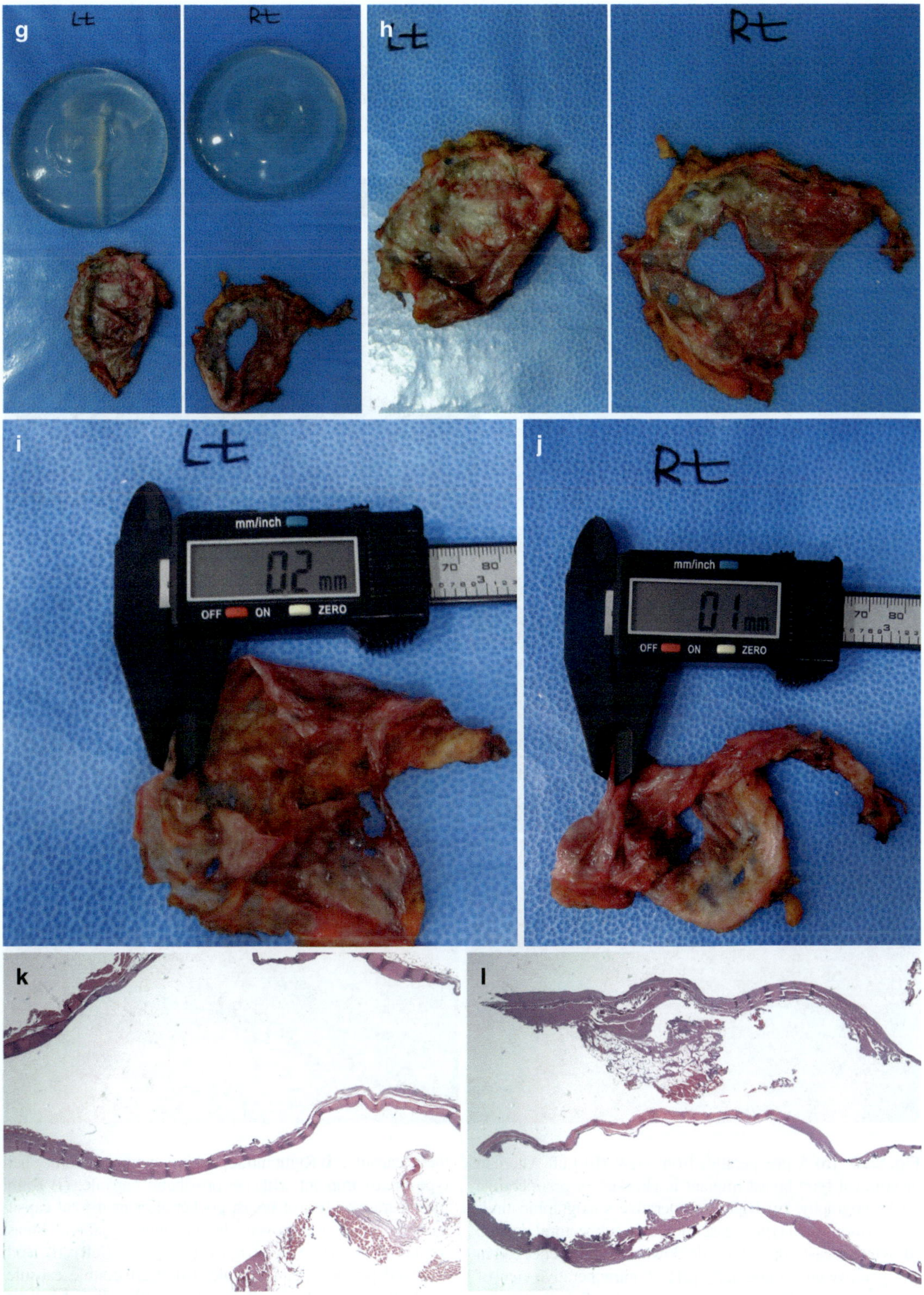

Fig. 8.29 (continued)

on the right side, accompanied by the bilateral presence of a double capsule (Video 8.41). But there were no findings that are suggestive of folding, seroma, thickened capsule, rupture, and capsular mass.

The patient underwent near-total capsulectomy with replacement of the device *via* a previous axillary scar on both sides. There were focal chronic inflammation and fibrosis in both capsule (Fig. 8.30).

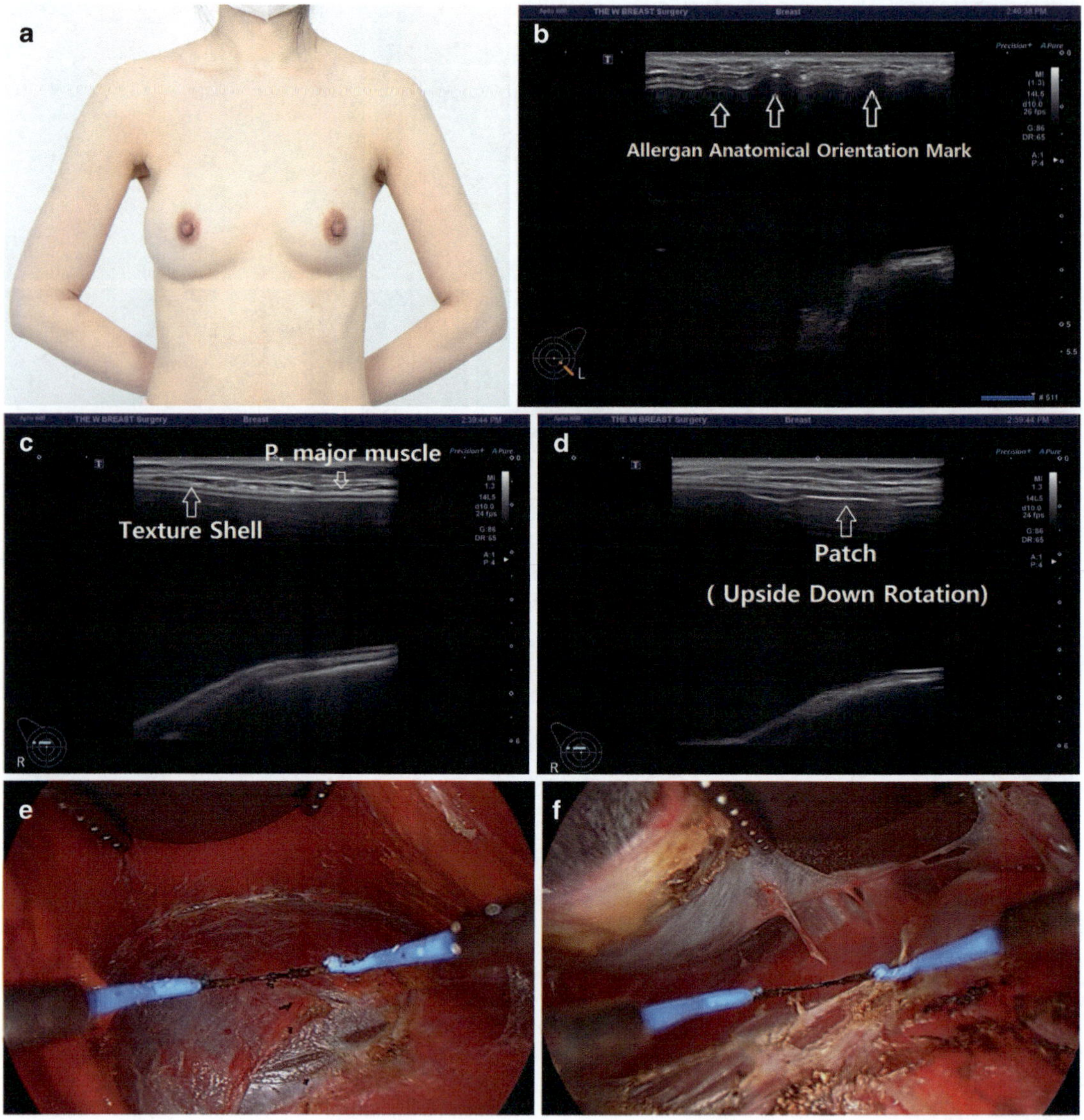

Fig. 8.30 (**a**) A preoperative front view. (**b**) Left Allergan anatomical type breast implant is checked in preoperative ultrasonography. (**c**) Right preoperative sonographic finding; textured shell type breast implant in subpectoral pocket. (**d**) Right breast implant upside-down rotation is checked in preoperative ultrasonography. (**e**) Left intraoperative view of breast implant with periprosthetic capsule. (**f**) Left intraoperative view of inferior double capsule. (**g**) Left intraoperative view of breast pocket after subtotal capsulectomy. (**h**) Right intraoperative view of breast implant with periprosthetic capsule. (**i**) Right intraoperative view of textured shell type breast implant with periprosthetic capsule. (**j**) Right intraoperative view of breast pocket after near-total capsulectomy. (**k**) Both removed Allergan anatomical type breast implant 410 FM 252 cc (right), FF 272 cc (left). (**l**) Both removed periprosthetic capsule. (**m**) Left double capsule. (**n**) Left capsule thickness is measured by digital caliper, 0.3 mm. (**o**) Right capsule thickness is measured by digital caliper, 0.4 mm. (**p**) Microscopic view of the left capsule. (**q**) Microscopic view of the right capsule

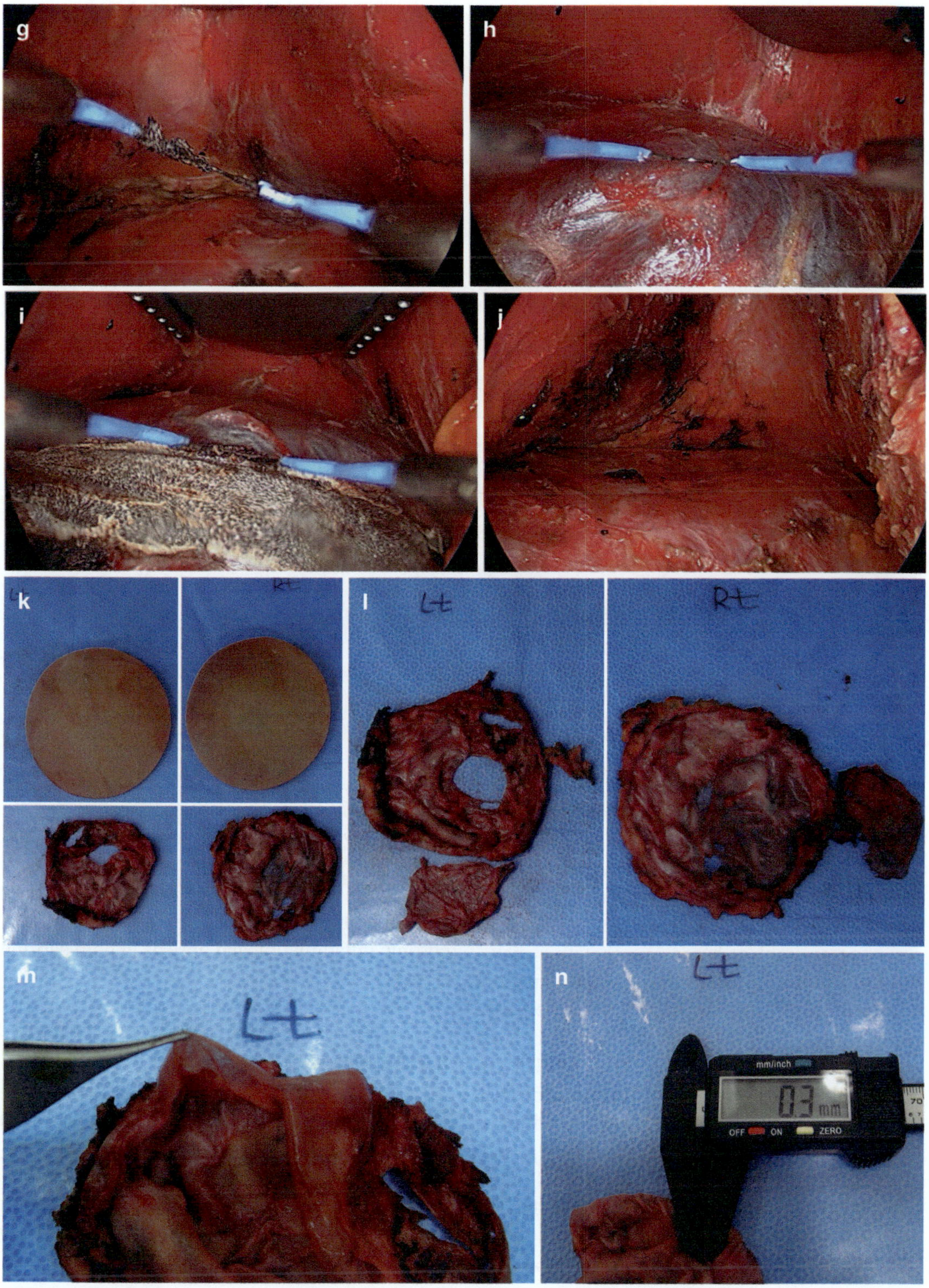

Fig. 8.30 (continued)

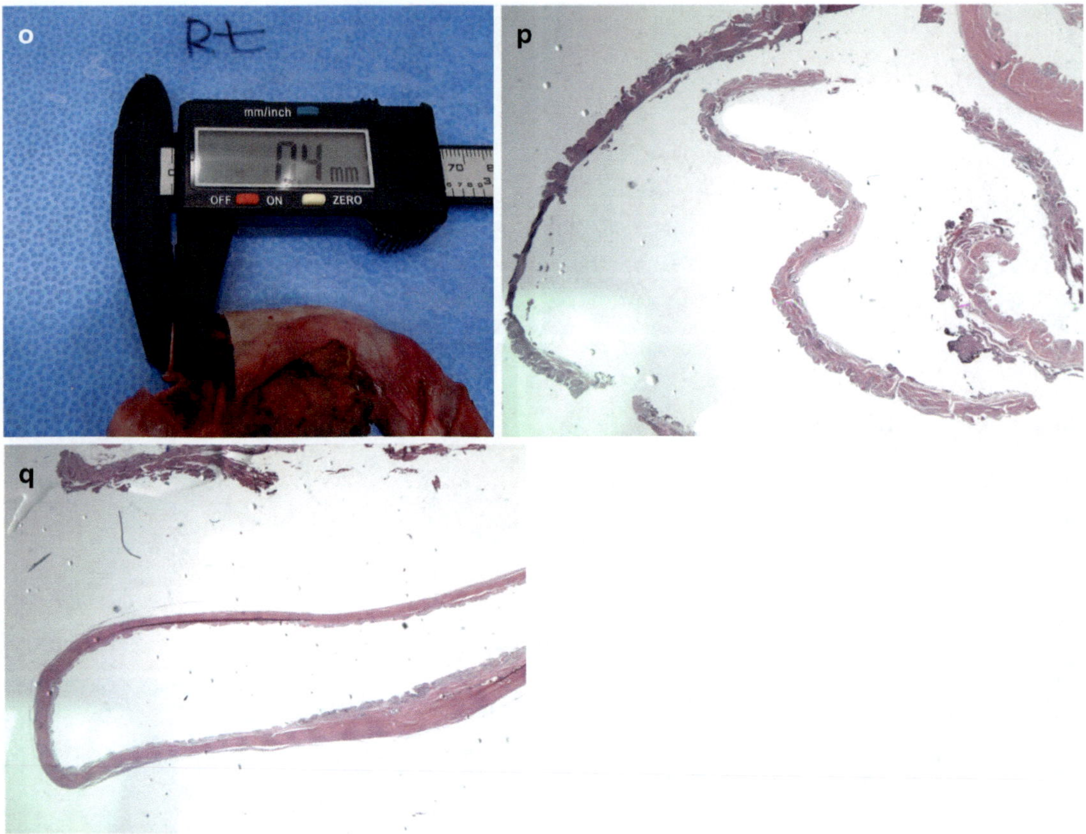

Fig. 8.30 (continued)

8.2.31 Case 31

On physical examination and history taking, a 34-year-old woman had an 8-year history of receiving an implant-based augmentation mammaplasty *via* an axillary incision. The patient wanted to receive explantation, whose chief complaint was concern for breast implant-associated anaplastic large cell lymphoma (BIA-ALCL). On preoperative ultrasonography, the patient was found to have a round textured shell type silicone gel-filled breast implant in the subpectoral pocket (Videos 8.42 and 8.44). The patient had a folding *as well as* an upside-down rotation on the left side. But there were no findings that are suggestive of folding, seroma, thickened capsule, upside-down rotation, rupture, and capsular mass. The patient underwent subtotal capsulectomy with explantation *via* a previous axillary scar on both sides (Video 8.43). There were focal chronic inflammation and fibrosis in both capsule (Fig. 8.31).

8.2.32 Case 32

On physical examination and history taking, a 58-year-old woman complained of breast hardness on both sides. The patient had a 5-year history of receiving an implant-based augmentation mammaplasty *via* an areolar incision.

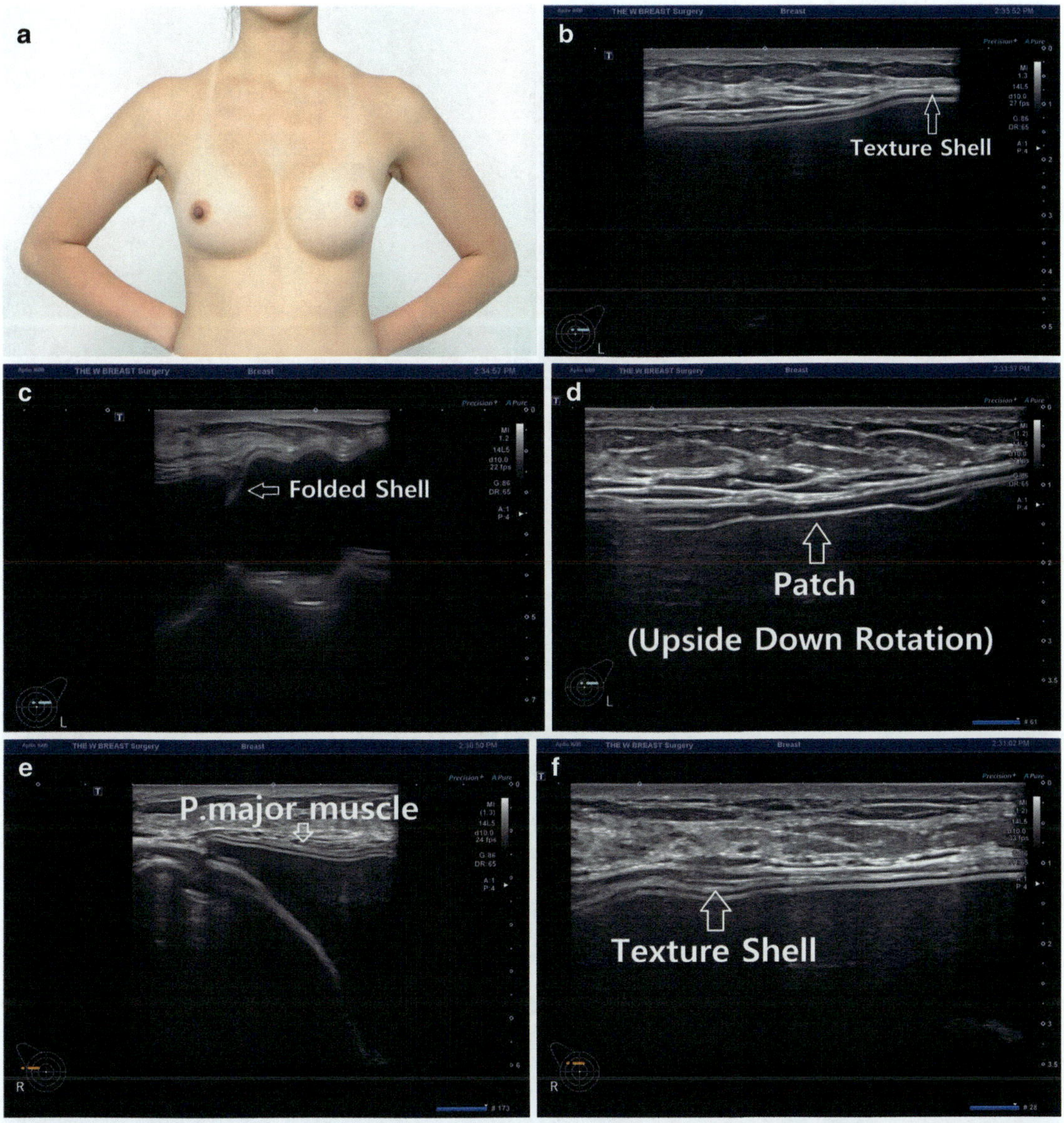

Fig. 8.31 (**a**) A preoperative front view. (**b**) Left textured shell type breast implant in subpectoral pocket is checked in preoperative ultrasonography. (**c**) Left breast implant shell folding is checked in preoperative ultrasonography. (**d**) Left breast implant upside-down rotation is checked in preoperative ultrasonography. (**e, f**) Right textured shell type breast implant in subpectoral pocket is checked in preoperative ultrasonography. (**g, h**) Left intraoperative view of breast implant with periprosthetic capsule. (**i**) Left intraoperative view of breast pocket after subtotal capsulectomy. (**j**) Right intraoperative view of breast implant with periprosthetic capsule. (**k**) Right intraoperative view of texturing between breast implant and capsule. (**l**) Right intraoperative view of breast pocket after subtotal capsulectomy. (**m**) Both removed breast implant Allergan round texture style 115 272 cc. (**n**) Both removed periprosthetic capsule after subtotal capsulectomy. (**o**) Left capsule thickness is measured by digital caliper, 0.3 mm. (**p**) Right capsule thickness is measured by digital caliper, 0.4 mm. (**q**) Microscopic view of the left capsule. (**r**) Microscopic view of the right capsule

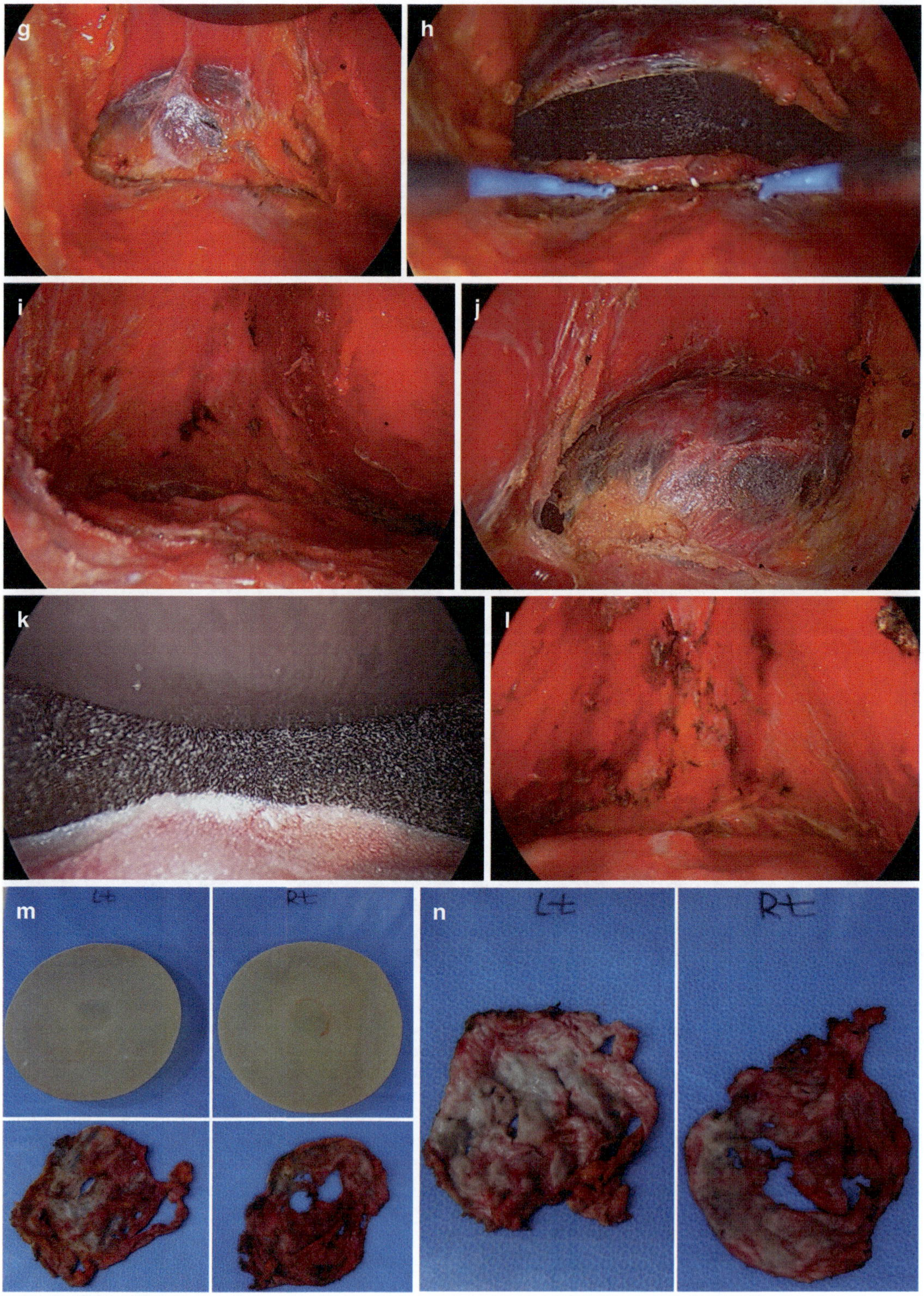

Fig. 8.31 (continued)

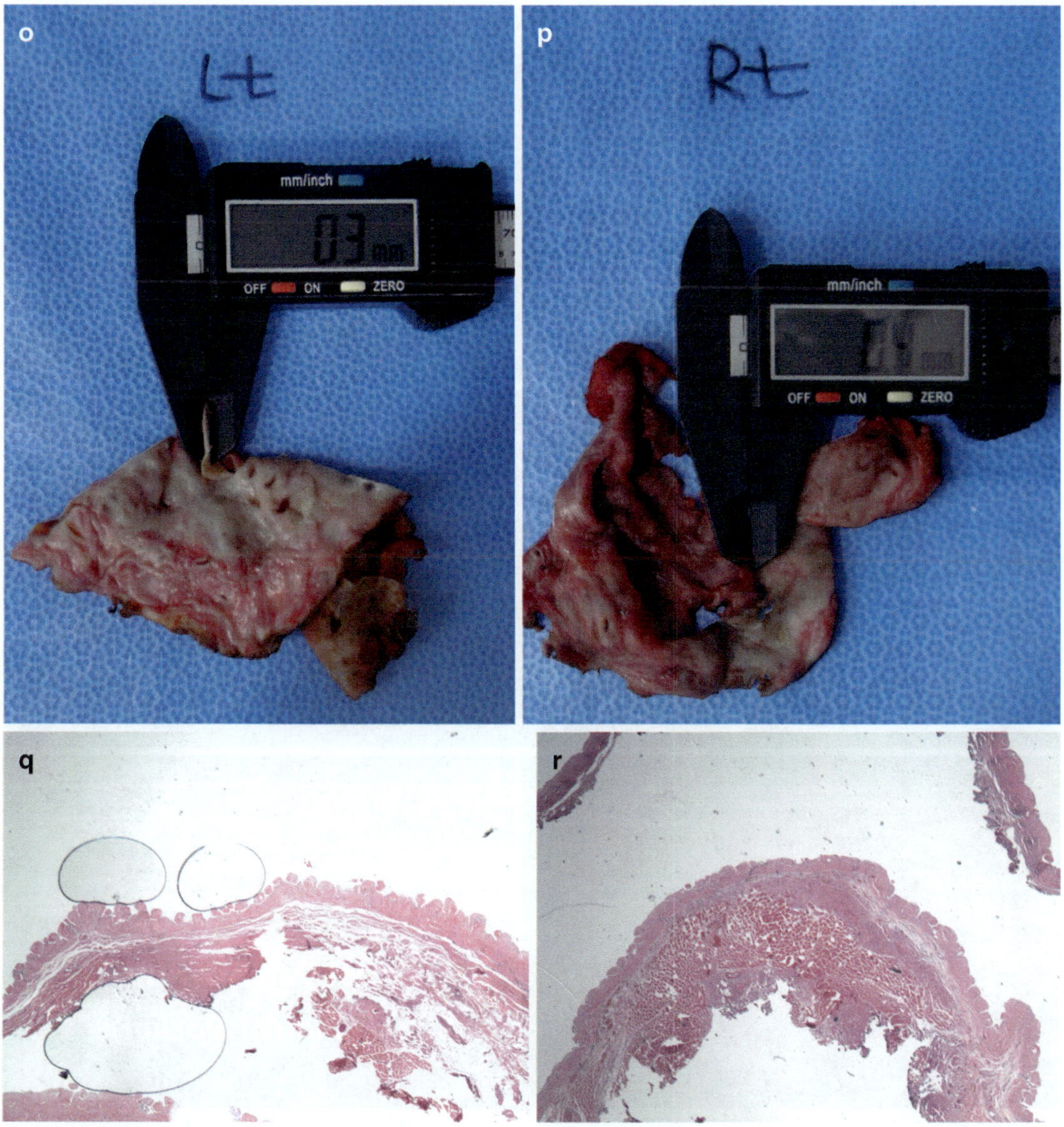

Fig. 8.31 (continued)

On preoperative ultrasonography, the patient was found to have a round smooth shell type silicone gel-filled breast implant on the right side and a round textured shell type one on the left side in the subglandular pocket. The patient had a folding *as well as* a thickened capsule on both sides (Video 8.45). But there were no findings that are suggestive of seroma, upside-down rotation, rupture, and capsular mass.

The patient underwent total capsulectomy with replacement of the device *via* a previous areolar scar on both sides (Video 8.46). There were focal chronic inflammation with fibrosis and multinucleated giant cells, suspicious for foreign body reaction in both capsule (Fig. 8.32).

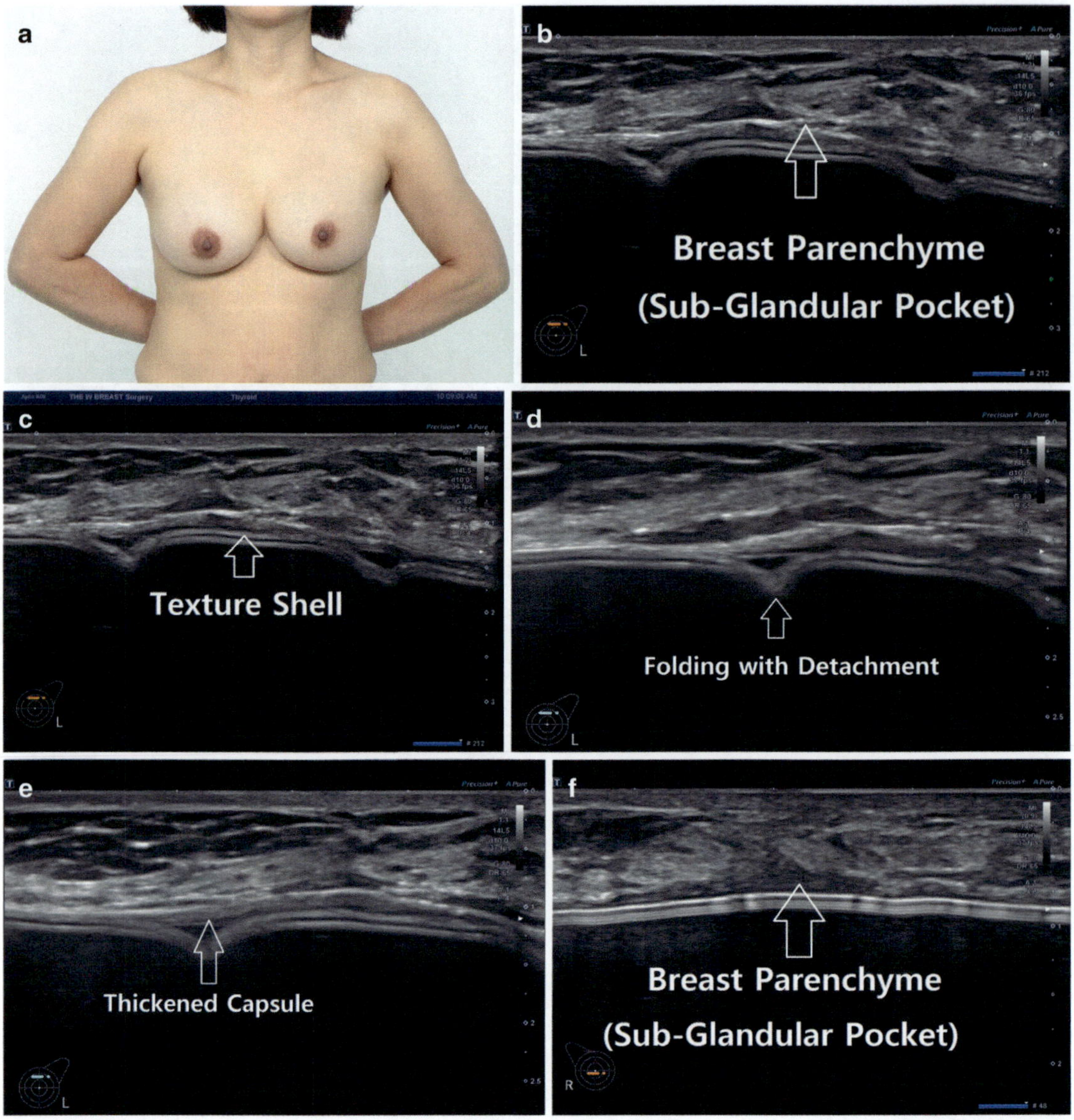

Fig. 8.32 (**a**) A preoperative front view. (**b**, **c**) Left texture type breast implant in subglandular pocket is checked in preoperative ultrasound. (**d**) Left breast implant shell folding is checked in preoperative ultrasound. (**e**) Left periprosthetic thickened capsule is checked in preoperative ultrasound. (**f**) Right breast implant in subglandular pocket is checked in preoperative ultrasound. (**g**) Right smooth type shell is checked in preoperative ultrasound. (**h**) Left intraoperative view of breast implant with periprosthetic capsule. (**i**) Left intraoperative view of breast pocket after total capsulectomy. (**j**, **k**) Right intraoperative view of breast implant with periprosthetic capsule. (**l**) Right intraoperative view of breast pocket after total capsulectomy. (**m**) Both removed breast implant; left Allergan round texture style 115 222 cc, right Sebbin round smooth type breast implant 220 cc. (**n**) Both removed periprosthetic capsule after total capsulectomy. (**o**) Left capsule thickness is measured by digital caliper, 2.1 mm. (**p**) Right capsule thickness is measured by digital caliper, 2.1 & 1.3 mm. (**q**) Microscopic view of the left capsule. (**r**) Microscopic view of the right capsule

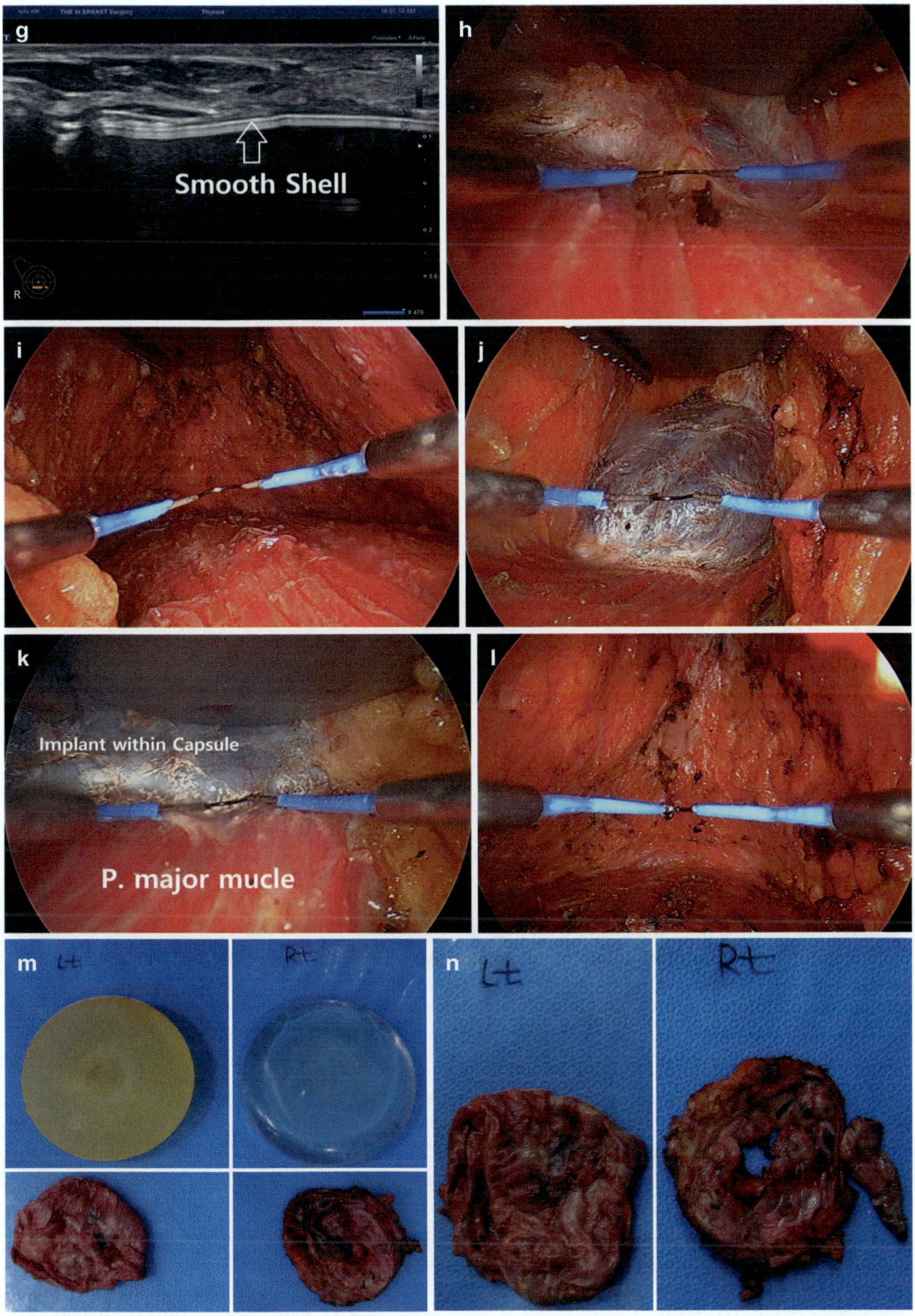

Fig. 8.32 (continued)

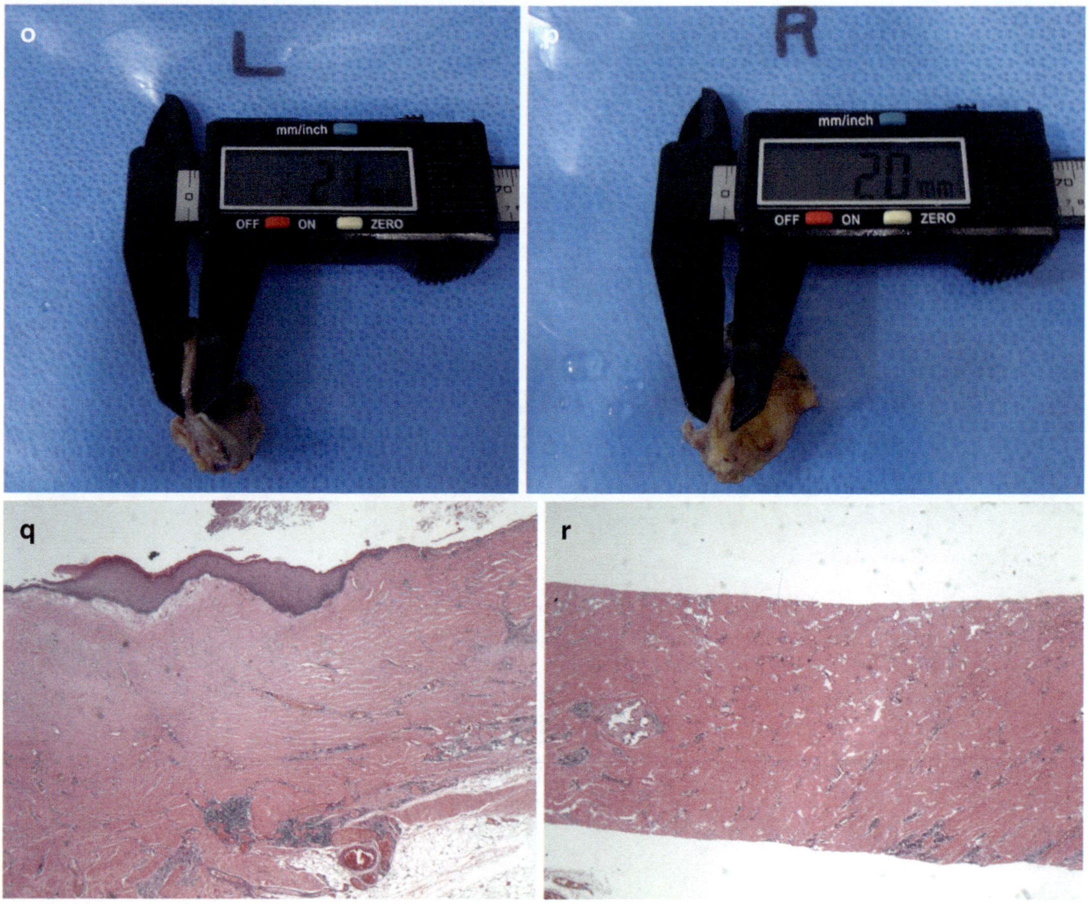

Fig. 8.32 (continued)

8.2.33 Case 33

On physical examination and history taking, a 33-year-old woman complained of breast pain, whose chief complaint was concern for breast implant-associated anaplastic large cell lymphoma (BIA-ALCL). The patient had an 8-year history of receiving an implant-based augmentation mammaplasty *via* an inframammary fold incision.

On preoperative ultrasonography, the patient was found to have an anatomical silicone gel-filled breast implant (Allergan Inc., Irvine, CA) in the subpectoral pocket (Video 8.47). But there were no findings that are suggestive of folding, seroma, thickened capsule, upside-down rotation, rupture, and capsular mass.

The patient underwent subtotal capsulectomy with explantation *via* a previous axillary scar on both sides. There were right chronic inflammation and fibrosis and left focal chronic inflammation and fibrosis (Fig. 8.33).

8.2.34 Case 34

On physical examination and history taking, a 45-year-old woman complained of breast hardness and pain on the right side. The patient had a 6-year-history of receiving an implant-based augmentation mammaplasty *via* an axillary incision.

On preoperative ultrasonography, the patient was found to have an anatomical silicone gel-

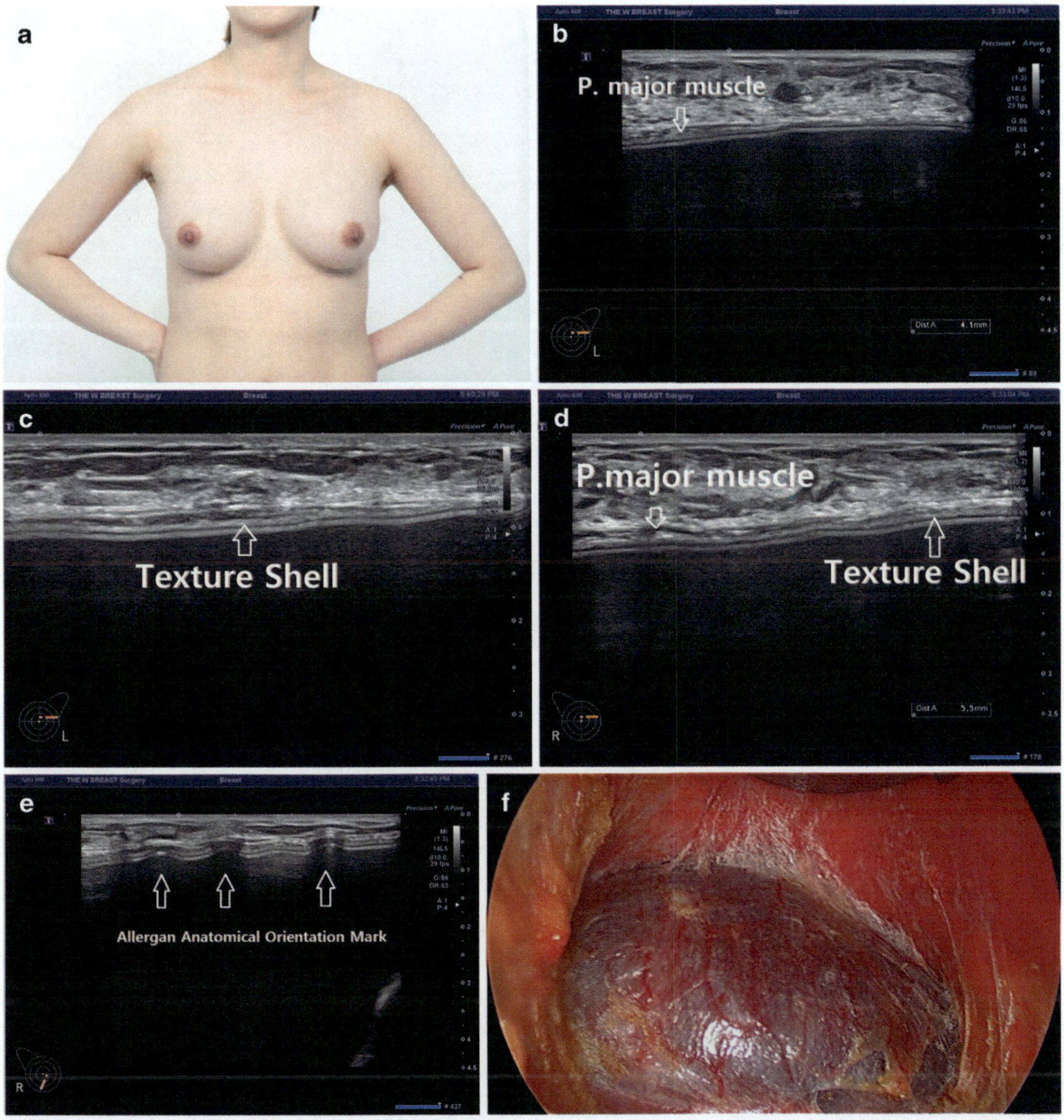

Fig. 8.33 (**a**) A preoperative front view. (**b**) Left breast implant in subpectoral pocket is checked in preoperative ultrasonography. (**c**) Left textured shell type breast implant in subpectoral pocket is checked in preoperative ultrasonography. (**d**) Right textured shell type breast implant in subpectoral pocket is checked in preoperative ultrasonography. (**e**) Right Allergan anatomical type breast implant orientation mark is checked in ultrasonography. (**f**) Left intraoperative view of breast implant with periprosthetic capsule. (**g**) Left intraoperative view of texture type breast implant with periprosthetic capsule. (**h**) Left intraoperative view of breast implant pocket. (**i**) Left intraoperative view of breast pocket after subtotal capsulectomy. (**j**) Right intraoperative view of breast implant with periprosthetic capsule. (**k**) Right intraoperative view of texture type breast implant with capsule. (**l**) Right intraoperative view of periprosthetic capsule after explantation. (**m**) Right intraoperative view of breast implant pocket. (**n**) Right intraoperative view after subtotal capsulectomy. (**o**) Both removed Allergan anatomical type breast implant 410 MF 295 cc. (**p**) Both removed periprosthetic capsule after subtotal capsulectomy. (**q**) Left capsule thickness is measured by digital caliper, 0.2 mm. (**r**) Right capsule thickness is measured by digital caliper, 0.1 mm. (**s**) Microscopic view of the left capsule. (**t**) Microscopic view of the right capsule

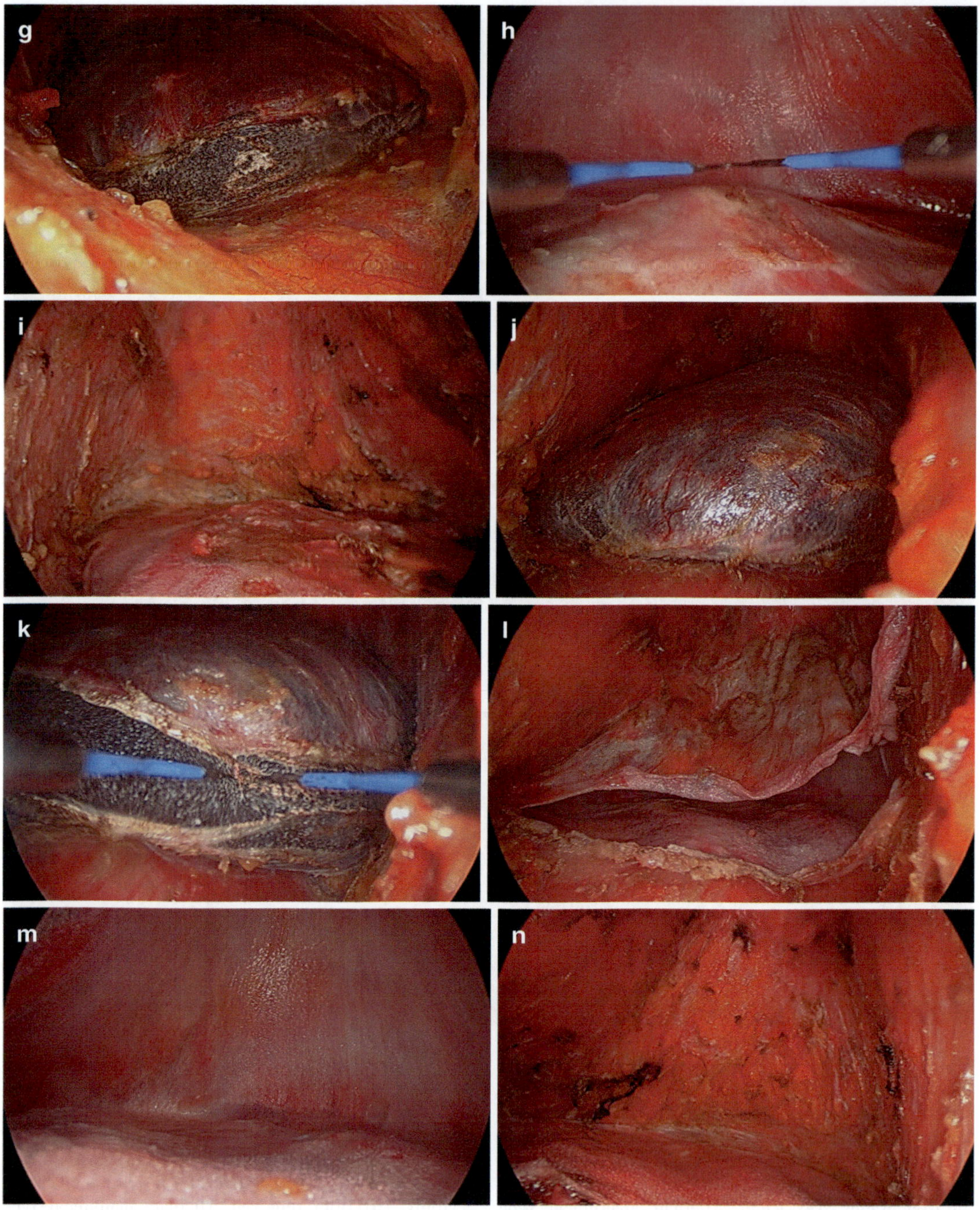

Fig. 8.33 (continued)

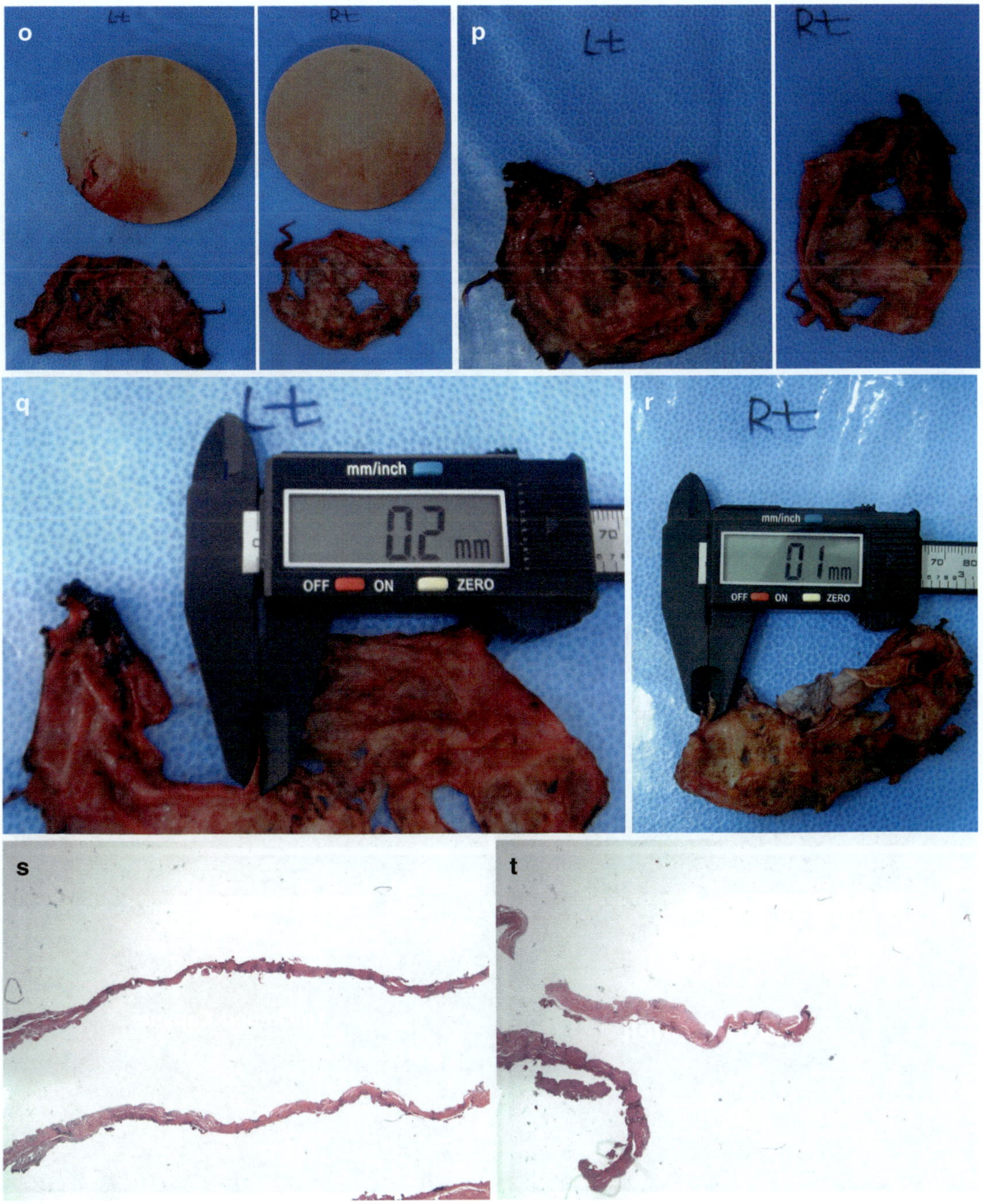

Fig. 8.33 (continued)

filled breast implant (Allergan Inc., Irvine, CA) in the subpectoral pocket. The patient had a rupture (gel bleed) on the left side (Video 8.48). Moreover, the patient also had a double capsule *as well as* a thickened capsule which was measured as 1.1–2.6 mm on the right side. But there were no findings that are suggestive of malrotation, folding, seroma, upside-down rotation, and capsular mass.

The patient underwent total capsulectomy with replacement of the device via a previous axillary scar on both sides. There were right focal chronic inflammation and fibrosis and left chronic inflammation with fibrosis (Fig. 8.34).

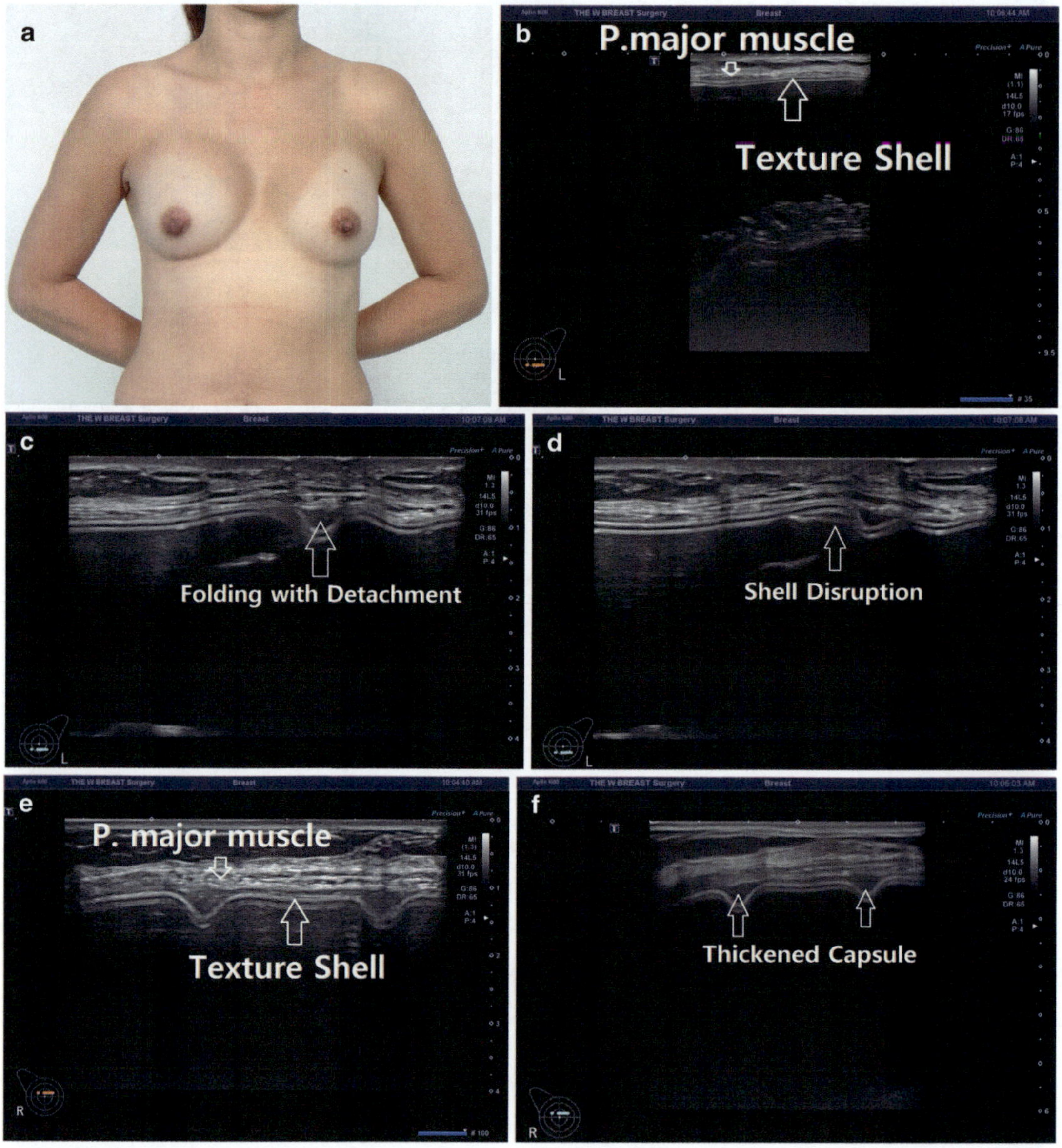

Fig. 8.34 (**a**) A preoperative front view. (**b**) Left textured shell type breast implant in subpectoral pocket is checked in preoperative ultrasonography. (**c**) Left breast implant folded shell with detachment is checked in preoperative ultrasonography. (**d**) Left breast implant shell disruption is checked. (**e**) Right textured shell type breast implant in subpectoral pocket. (**f**) Right periprosthetic thickened capsule is checked in preoperative ultrasonography. (**g**) Left intraoperative view of breast implant with periprosthetic capsule. (**h**) Left Intraoperative view of breast pocket after total capsulectomy. (**i, j**) Right intraoperative view of breast implant with periprosthetic capsule. (**k**) Right intraoperative view of breast pocket after total capsulectomy. (**l**) Both removed Allergan anatomical type breast implant 410 MM 280 cc and periprosthetic capsule after total capsulectomy. (**m**) Right double capsule. (**n**) Left capsule thickness is measured by digital caliper, 0.3 mm. (**o, p**) Right capsule thickness is measured by digital caliper, 0.7 & 1.9 mm. (**q**) Microscopic view of the left capsule with silicone invasion to capsule. (**r**) Microscopic view of the right capsule

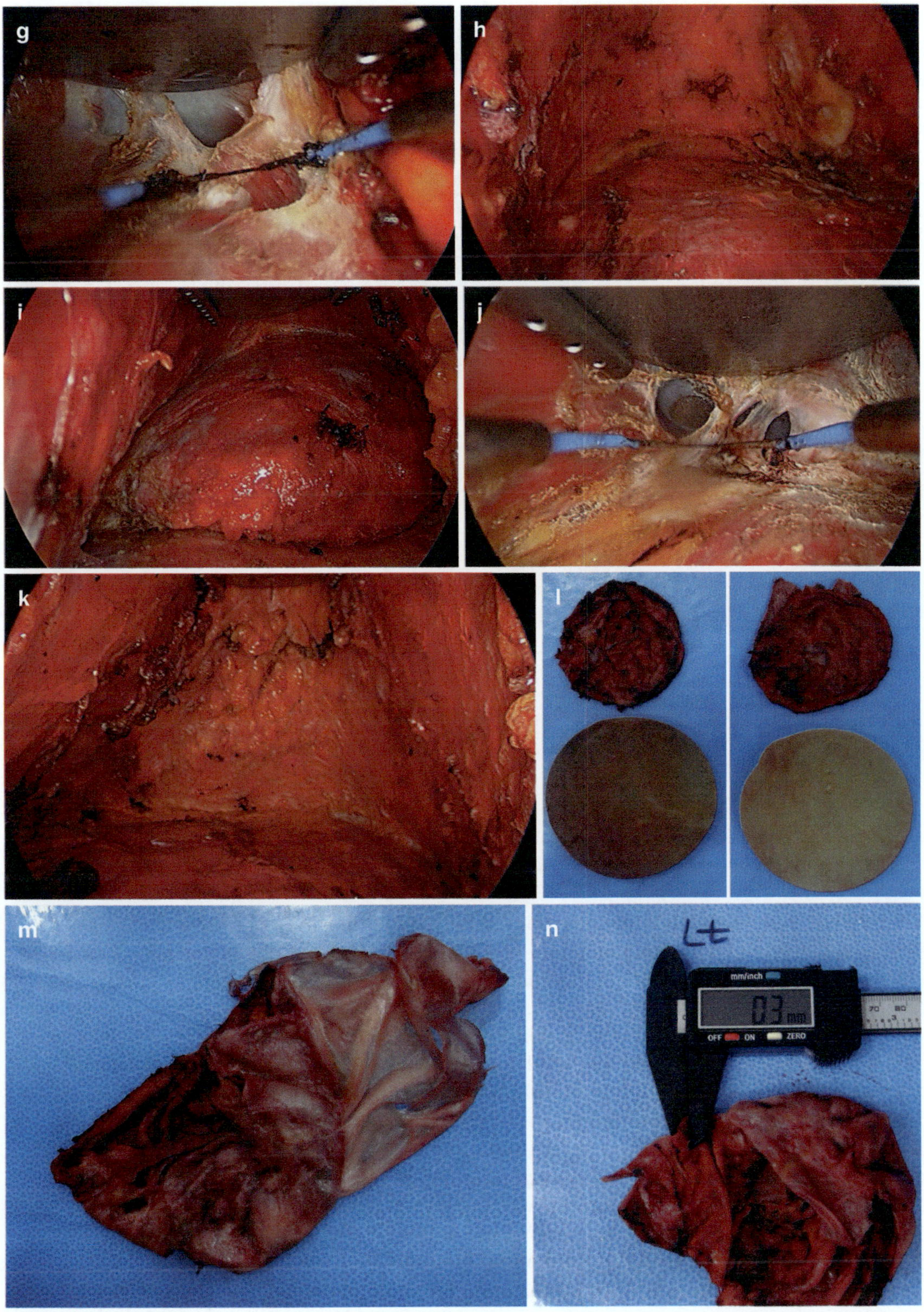

Fig. 8.34 (continued)

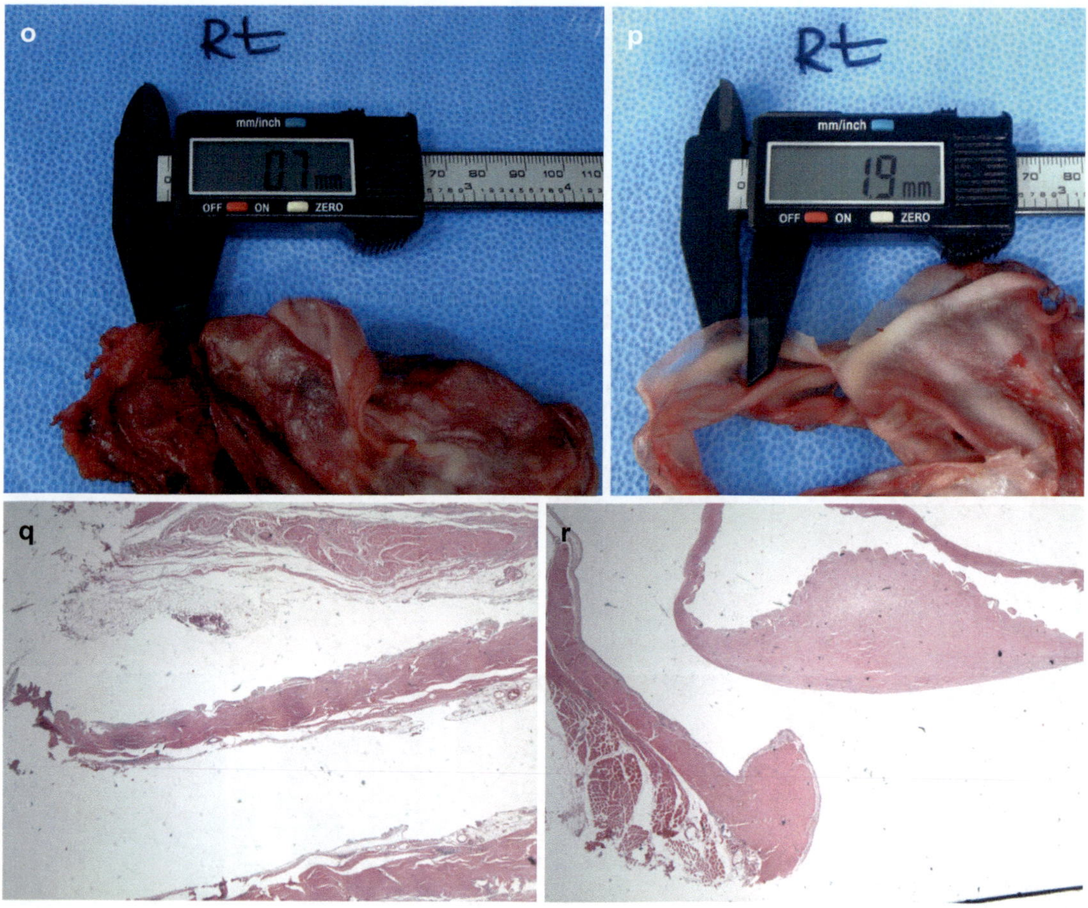

Fig. 8.34 (continued)

8.2.35 Case 35

On physical examination and history taking, a 44-year-old woman complained of breast pain. The patient had an 8-year history of receiving an implant-based augmentation mammaplasty.

On preoperative ultrasonography, the patient was found to have a round textured shell type silicone gel-filled breast implant in the subpectoral pocket and extra-capsular rupture on right side. The patient had a folding on the left side. Moreover, the patient also had an intracapsular rupture *as well as* a thickened capsule which was measured as 1.7 mm on the right side (Video 8.49). But there were no findings that are suggestive of seroma, upside-down rotation, and capsular mass.

The patient underwent total capsulectomy with explantation *via* a previous axillary scar on both sides. There were right chronic inflammation and accumulation of foam cells and left mild fibrosis (Fig. 8.35).

8.2.36 Case 36

On physical examination and history taking, a 32-year-old woman complained of foreign body sensation, whose chief complaint was concern for breast implant-associated anaplastic large cell lymphoma (BIA-ALCL). The patient had a 7-year history of receiving an implant-based augmentation mammaplasty *via* an axillary incision.

On preoperative ultrasonography, the patient was found to have a round textured silicone gel-filled breast implant in the subpectoral pocket (Video 8.50). The patient had a folding with

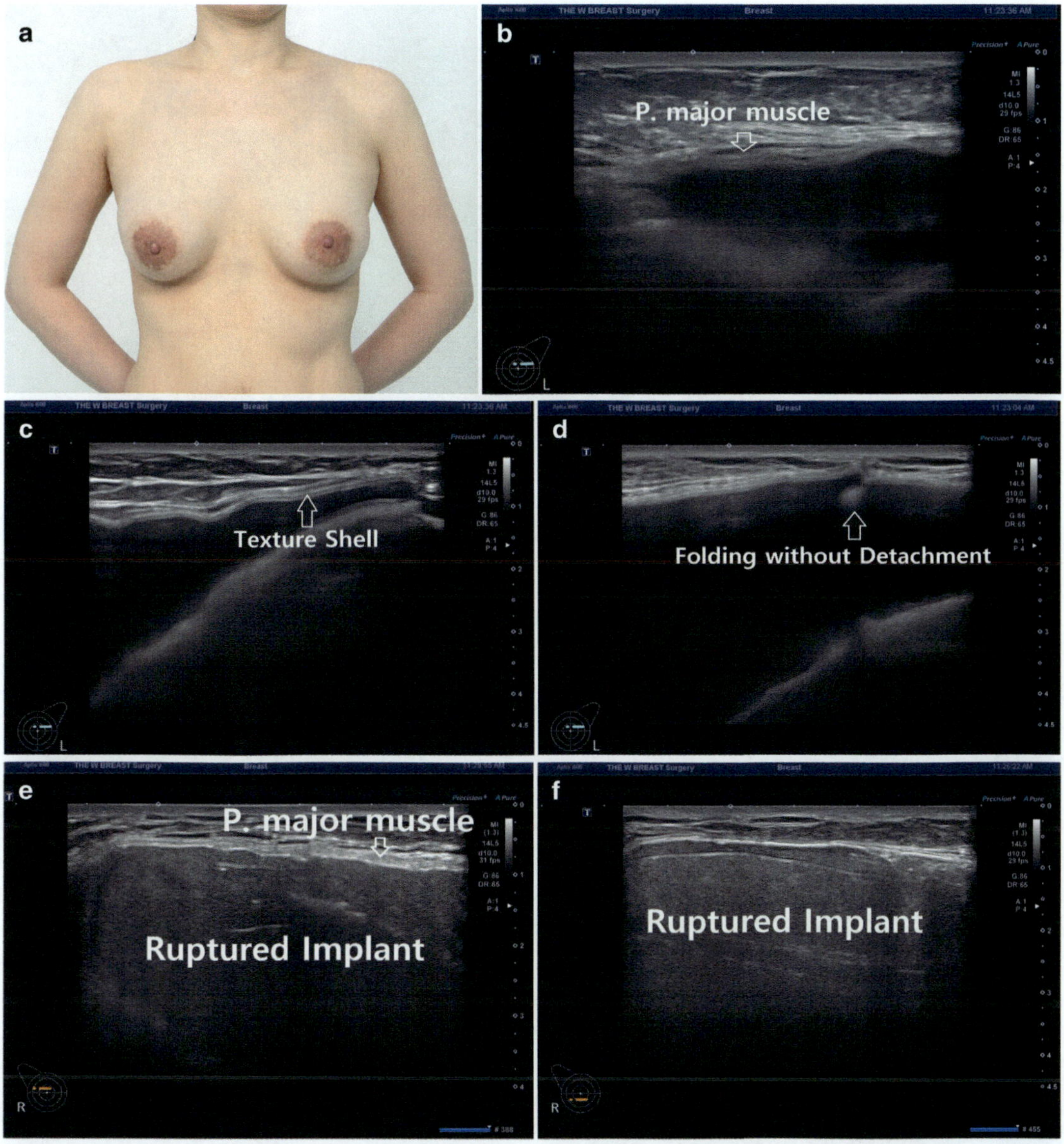

Fig. 8.35 (**a**) A preoperative front view. (**b, c**) Left textured shell type breast implant in subpectoral pocket is checked in preoperative ultrasonography. (**d**) Left breast implant folded shell is checked in preoperative ultrasonography. (**e, f**) Right ruptured silicone breast implant in subpectoral pocket is checked in preoperative ultrasonography. (**g**) Both removed periprosthetic capsule and unknown manufacturer, 240 cc. (**h**) Both removed implant within periprosthetic capsule. (**i**) Both removed periprosthetic capsule after total capsulectomy. (**j**) Left capsule thickness is measured by digital caliper, 0.3 mm. (**k**) Right capsule thickness is measured by digital caliper, 1.7 mm. (**l**) Microscopic view of the left capsule. (**m**) Microscopic view of the right capsule with silicone invasion to capsule

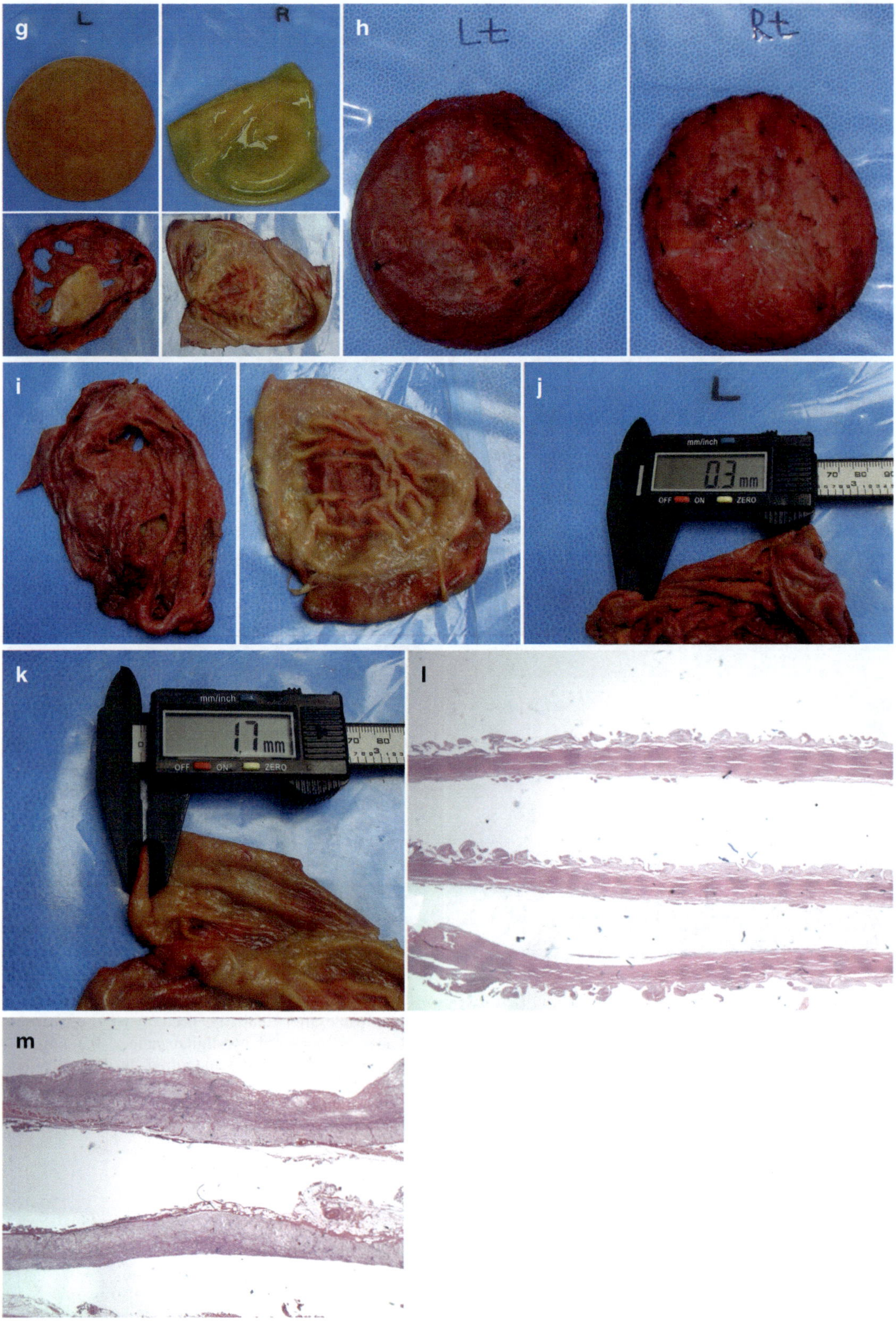

Fig. 8.35 (continued)

detachment on the right side. But there were no findings that are suggestive of seroma, thickened capsule, upside-down rotation, rupture, and capsular mass.

The patient underwent near-total capsulectomy with replacement of the device *via* a previous axillary scar on both sides. There were right focal chronic inflammation and fibrosis and left mild fibrosis (Fig. 8.36).

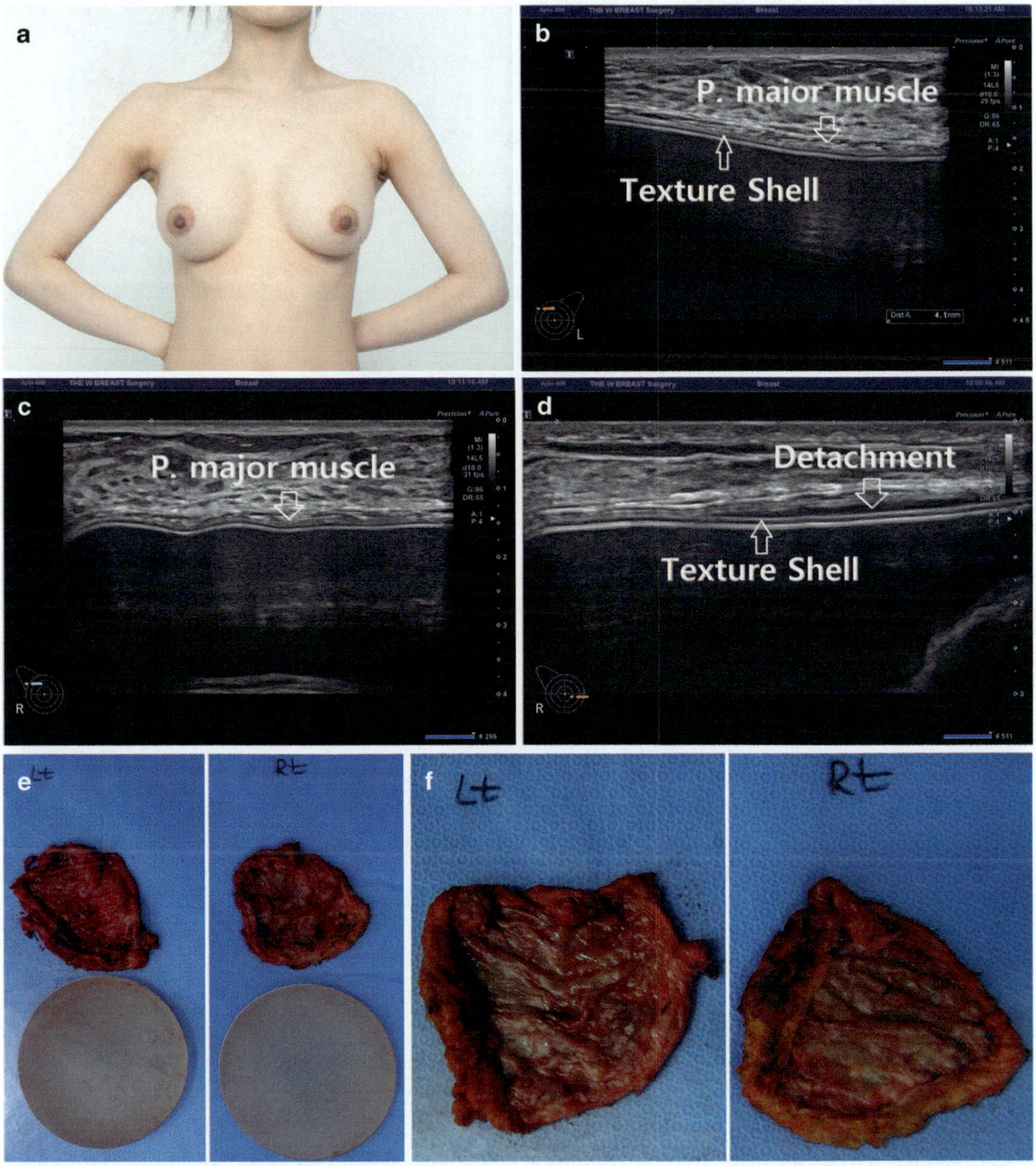

Fig. 8.36 (**a**) A preoperative front view. (**b**) Left textured shell type breast implant in subpectoral pocket is checked in preoperative ultrasonography. (**c**) Right textured shell type breast implant in subpectoral pocket is checked in preoperative ultrasonography. (**d**) Right breast implant detachment is checked in ultrasonography. (**e**) Both removed Mentor round textured shell type breast implant, both 250 cc and periprosthetic capsule. (**f**) Both removed periprosthetic capsule by near-total capsulectomy. (**g**) Left capsule thickness is measured by digital caliper, 0.3 mm. (**h**) Right capsule thickness is measured by digital caliper, 0.3 mm. (**i**) Microscopic view of the left capsule. (**j**) Microscopic view of the right capsule

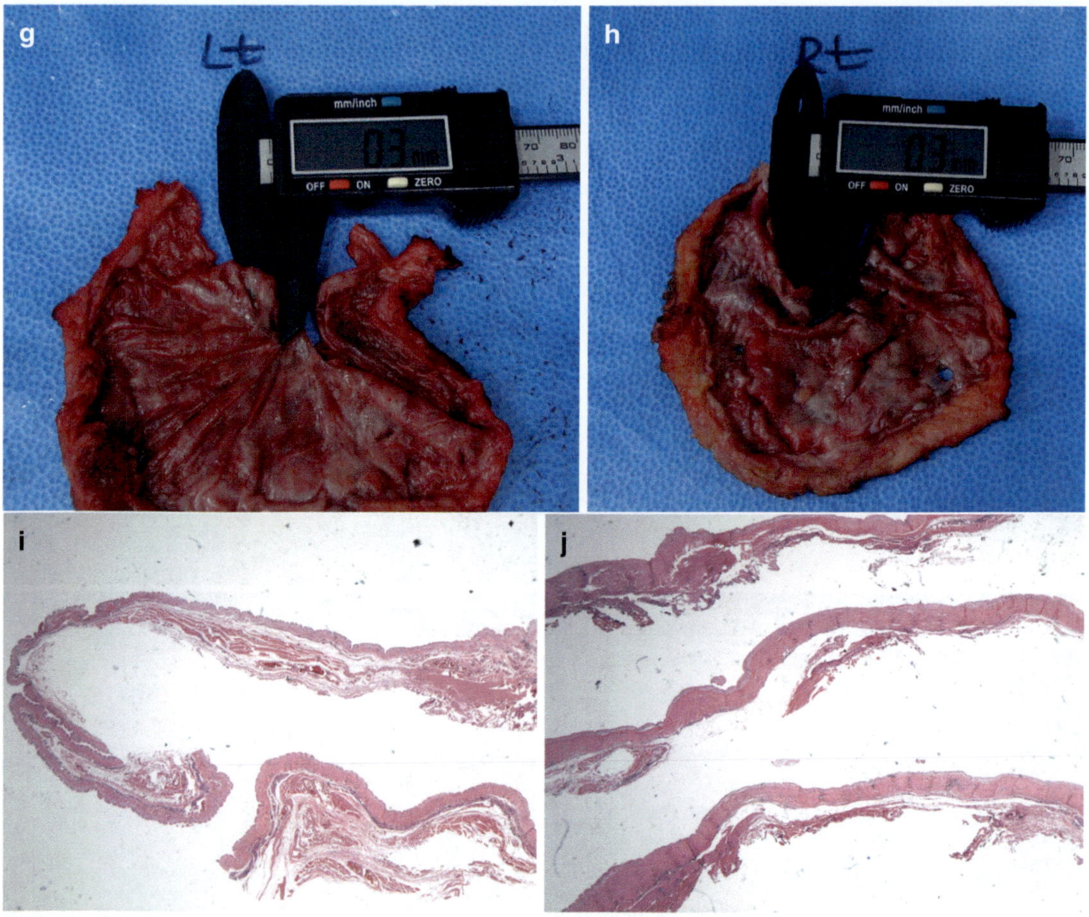

Fig. 8.36 (continued)

8.2.37 Case 37

On physical examination and history taking, a 48-year-old woman complained of dissatisfaction with shape. The patient had a 10-year history of receiving an implant-based augmentation mammaplasty *via* an areolar incision.

On preoperative ultrasonography, the patient was found to have an anatomical textured silicone gel-filled breast implant (Polytech Health & Aesthetics, Dieburg, Germany) in the subpectoral pocket (Video 8.51). But there were no findings that are suggestive of malrotation, folding, seroma, thickened capsule, upside-down rotation, rupture, and capsular mass.

The patient underwent near-total capsulectomy on the right side and subtotal capsulectomy with explantation *via* a previous areolar scar on the left side. There were right mild fibrosis and left focal chronic inflammation and fibrosis (Fig. 8.37).

8.2.38 Case 38

On physical examination and history taking, a 58-year-old woman complained of dissatisfaction with shape and breast pain. The patient had an 8-year history of receiving an implant-based augmentation mammaplasty *via* an inframammary fold incision.

On preoperative ultrasonography, the patient was found to have an anatomical silicone gel-filled breast implant (Groupe Sebbin SAS,

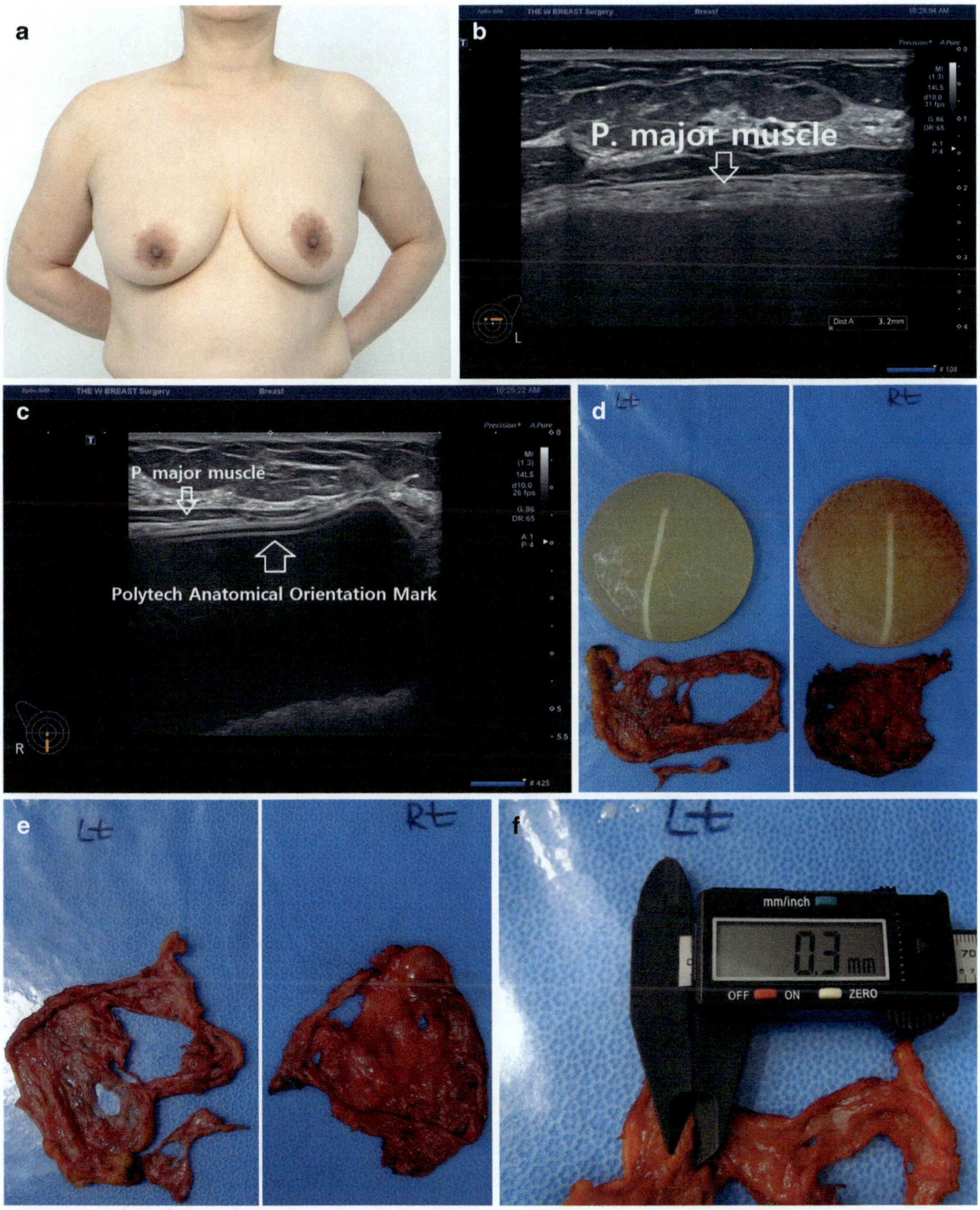

Fig. 8.37 (**a**) A preoperative front view. (**b**) Left textured shell type breast implant in subpectoral pocket is checked in preoperative ultrasonography. (**c**) Right Polytech anatomical breast implant orientation mark in subpectoral pocket is checked in preoperative ultrasonography. (**d**) Both removed Polytech anatomical type breast implant (250 cc) with periprosthetic capsule. (**e**) Both removed periprosthetic capsule by capsulectomy. (**f**) Left capsule thickness is measured by digital caliper, 0.3 mm. (**g**) Right capsule thickness is measured by digital caliper, 0.4 mm. (**h**) Microscopic view of the left capsule. (**i**) Microscopic view of the right capsule

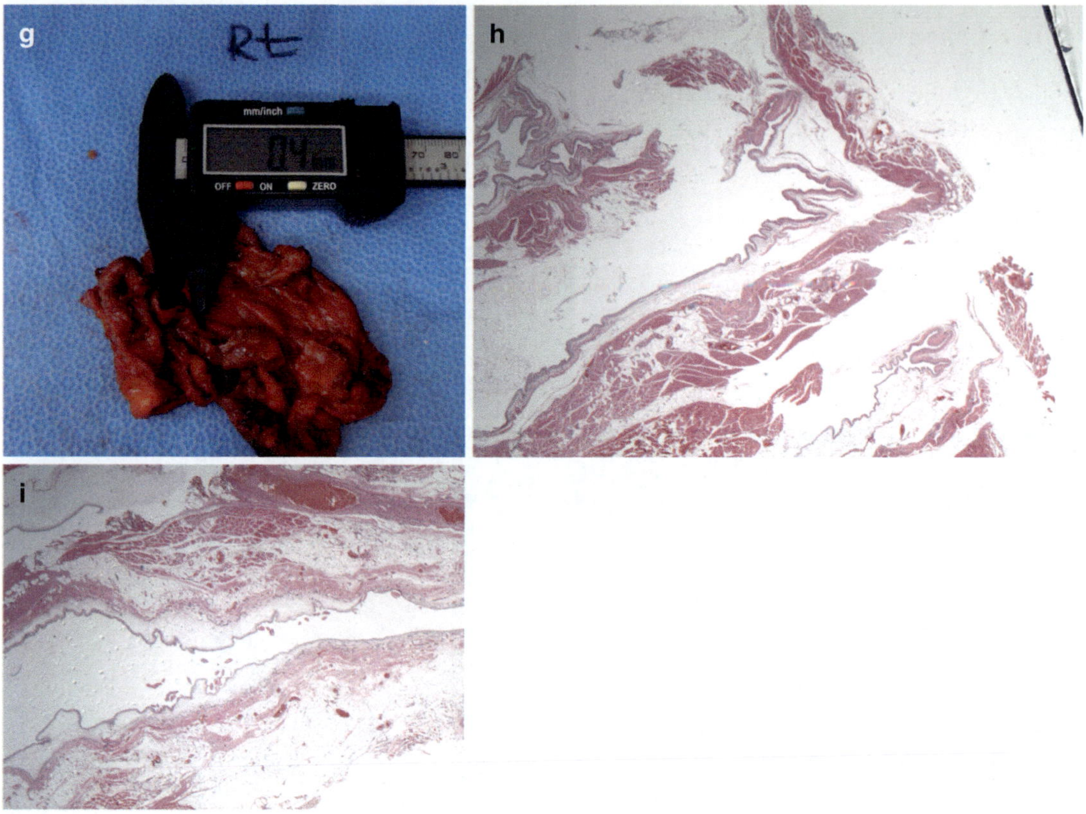

Fig. 8.37 (continued)

Boissy-l' Aillerie, France) in the subpectoral pocket. The patient had a folding on the right side. Moreover, the patient also had an upside-down rotation, double capsule, and a thickened capsule which was measured as 1.1 mm, on the left side (Video 8.52). But there were no findings that are suggestive of malrotation, rupture, and capsular mass.

The patient underwent subtotal capsulectomy with replacement of the device *via* a previous inframammary fold scar on both sides. There were right mild fibrosis and left chronic inflammation with fibrosis (Fig. 8.38).

8.2.39 Case 39

On physical examination and history taking, a 46-year-old woman complained of dissatisfaction with shape. The patient had a 21-year history of receiving an implant-based augmentation mammaplasty *via* an axillary incision.

On preoperative ultrasonography, the patient was found to have a round textured shell type silicone gel-filled breast implant in the subglandular pocket. But there were no findings that are suggestive of folding, seroma, thickened capsule, upside-down rotation, rupture, and capsular mass.

The patient underwent subtotal capsulectomy with replacement of the device *via* a previous axillary scar on both sides. Moreover, the patient received an excision of the left breast using ultrasound-guided vacuum-assisted biopsy. There was mild fibrosis in both capsule (Fig. 8.39).

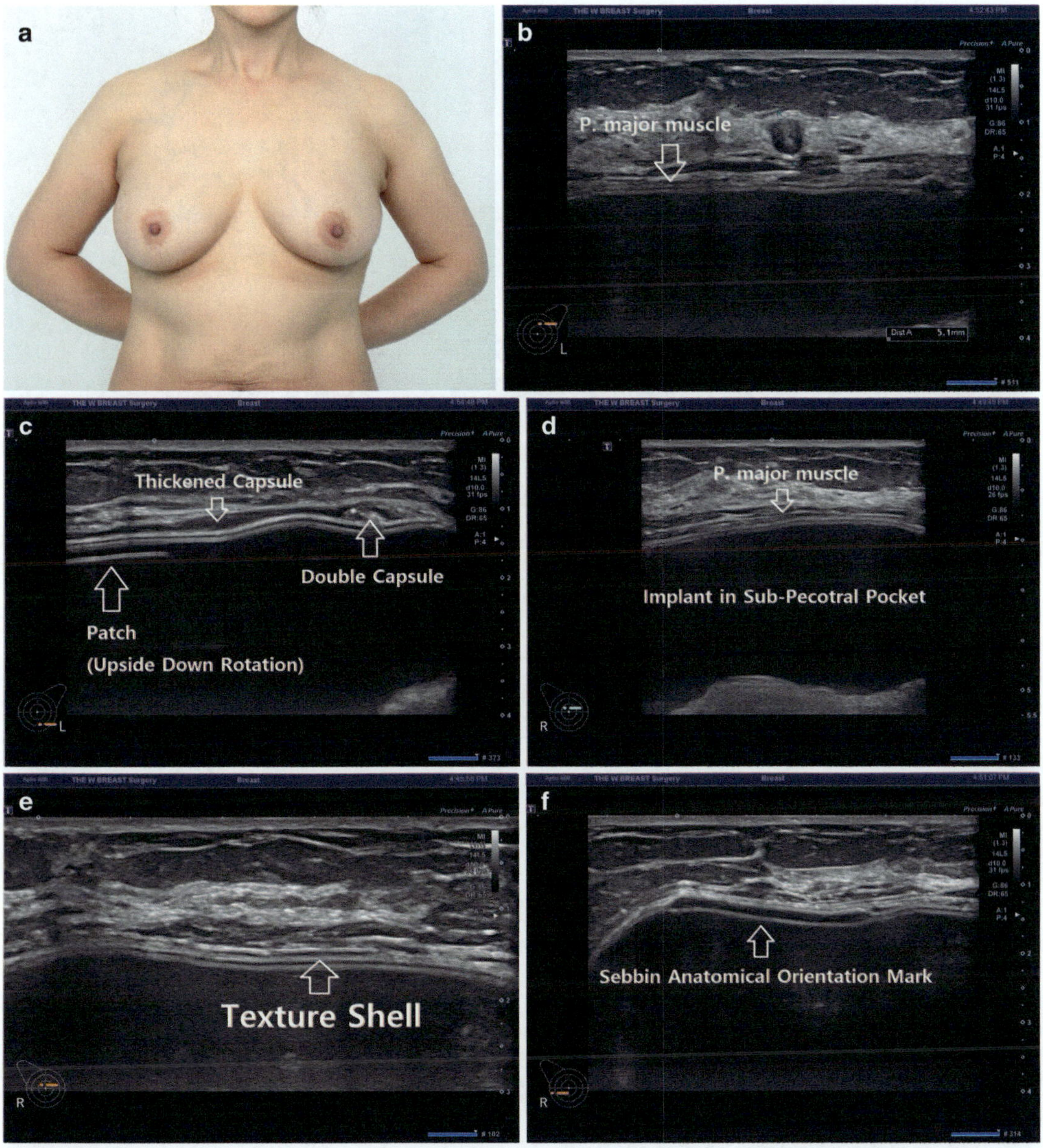

Fig. 8.38 (**a**) A preoperative front view. (**b**) Left textured shell type breast implant in subpectoral pocket is checked in preoperative ultrasonography. (**c**) Left breast implant upside-down rotation, thickened capsule, double capsule is checked in preoperative ultrasonography. (**d**) Right breast implant in subpectoral pocket is checked in preoperative ultrasonography. (**e**) Right textured shell type breast implant is checked in ultrasonography. (**f**) Sebbin anatomical type orientation mark is checked in ultrasonography. (**g**) Both removed Sebbin anatomical type breast implant, 245 cc. (**h**) Both removed periprosthetic capsule by subtotal capsulectomy. (**i**) Left double capsule thickness is measured by digital caliper, 1.8 mm. (**j**) Left periprosthetic capsule thickness is measured by digital caliper, 1.4 mm. (**k**) Right capsule thickness is measured by digital caliper, 0.3 mm. (**l**) Microscopic view of the left capsule. (**m**) Microscopic view of the right capsule

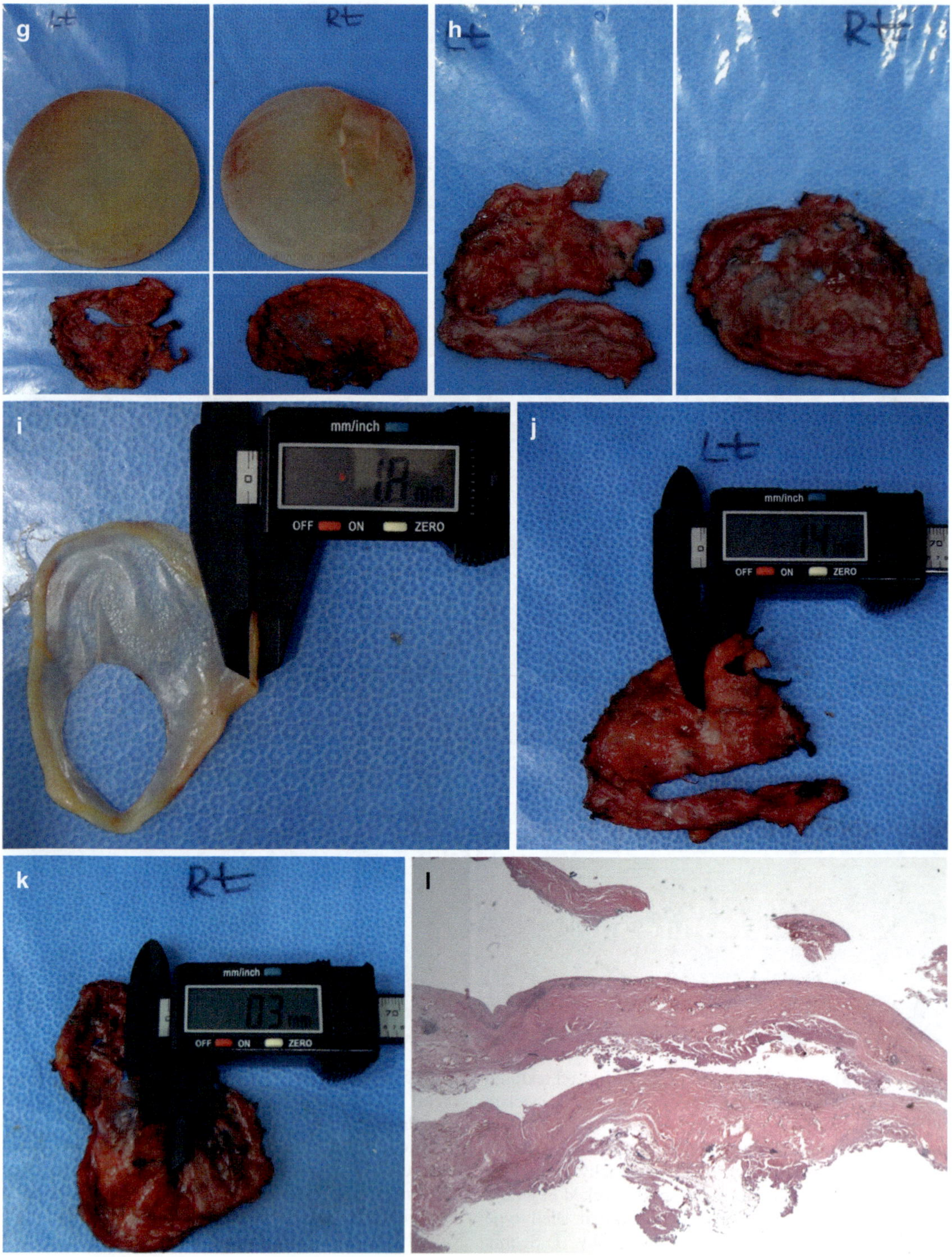

Fig. 8.38 (continued)

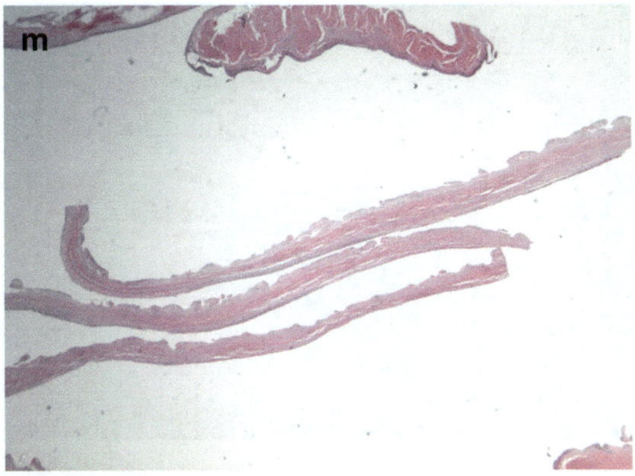

Fig. 8.38 (continued)

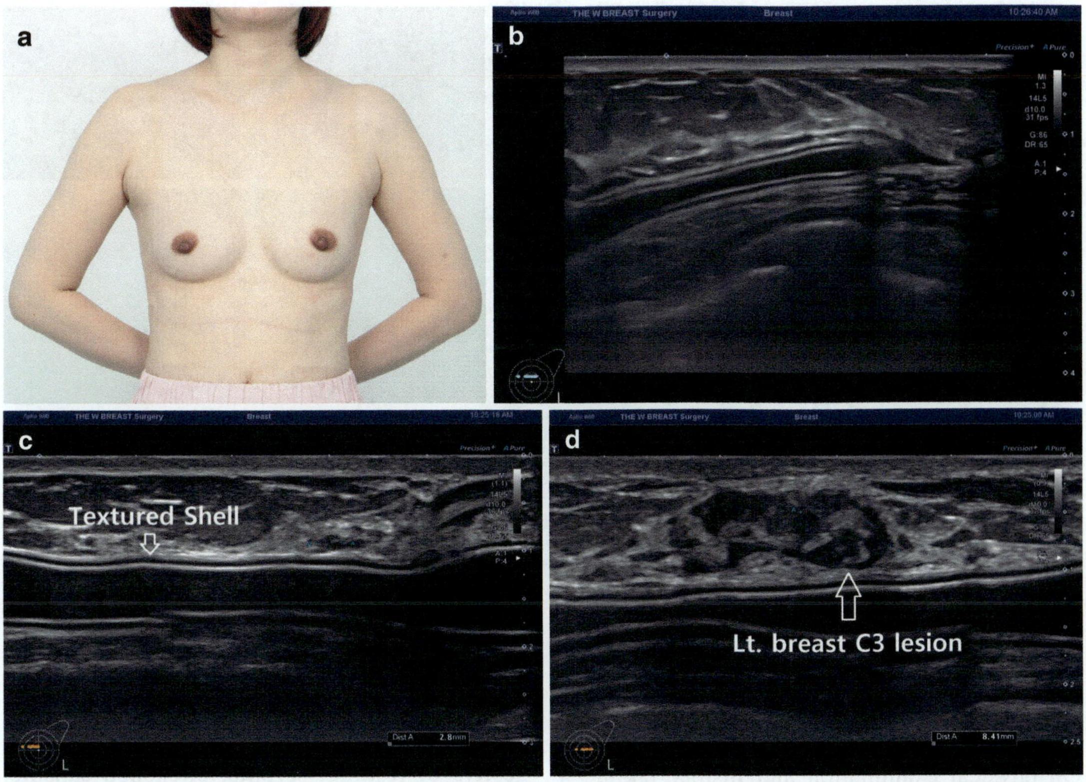

Fig. 8.39 (**a**) A preoperative front view. (**b**) Left breast implant in subglandular pocket is checked in preoperative ultrasonography. (**c**): Left textured shell type breast implant is checked in preoperative ultrasonography. (**d**) Left breast BI-RADs category C3 lesion is checked. (**e**) Right breast implant in subglandular pocket is checked in preoperative ultrasonography. (**f**) Right textured shell type breast implant is checked in preoperative ultrasonography. (**g**) Left intraoperative view of breast pocket, hematoma is seen in upper extracapsular site after vacuum-assisted breast excision. (**h**) Right intraoperative view of breast pocket with periprosthetic capsule. (**i**) Right intraoperative view of breast pocket after subtotal capsulectomy. (**j**) Microscopic view of the left breast benign mass

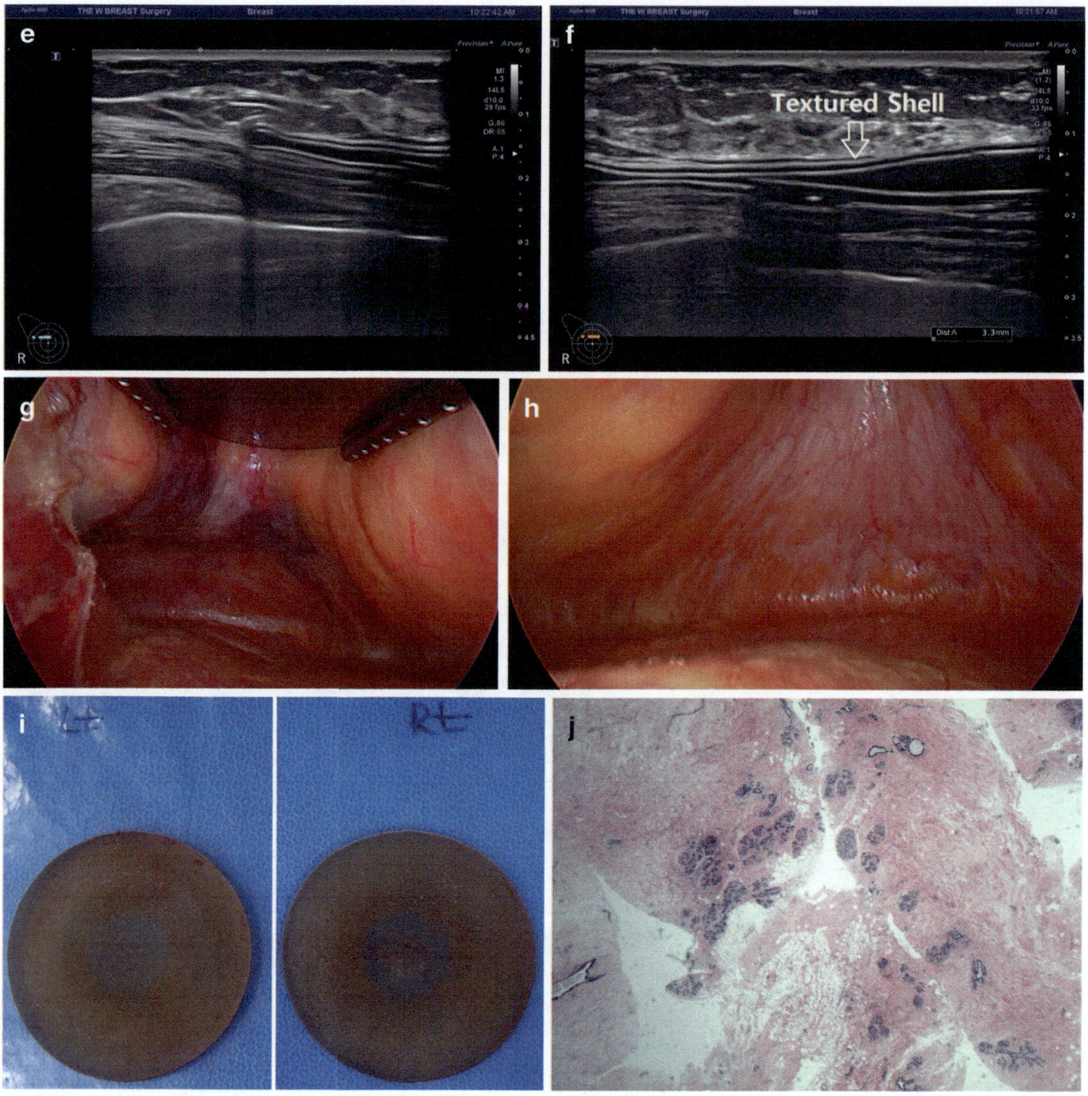

Fig. 8.39 (continued)

8.2.40 Case 40

On physical examination and history taking, a 28-year-old woman complained of breast pain and fear of BIA-ALCL. The patient had a 6-year history of receiving an implant-based augmentation mammaplasty *via* an axillary and inframammary incision.

On preoperative ultrasonography, the patient was found to have a Allergan anatomical silicone gel-filled breast implant and left round smooth type breast implant in the subpectoral pocket. But there were no findings that are suggestive of folding, seroma, thickened capsule, upside-down rotation, rupture, and capsular mass.

The patient underwent subtotal capsulectomy with breast implant pocket change and replacement of the breast implant *via* a previous axillary scar on both sides. There were right focal chronic inflammation and fibrosis and left mild fibrosis in capsule (Fig. 8.40).

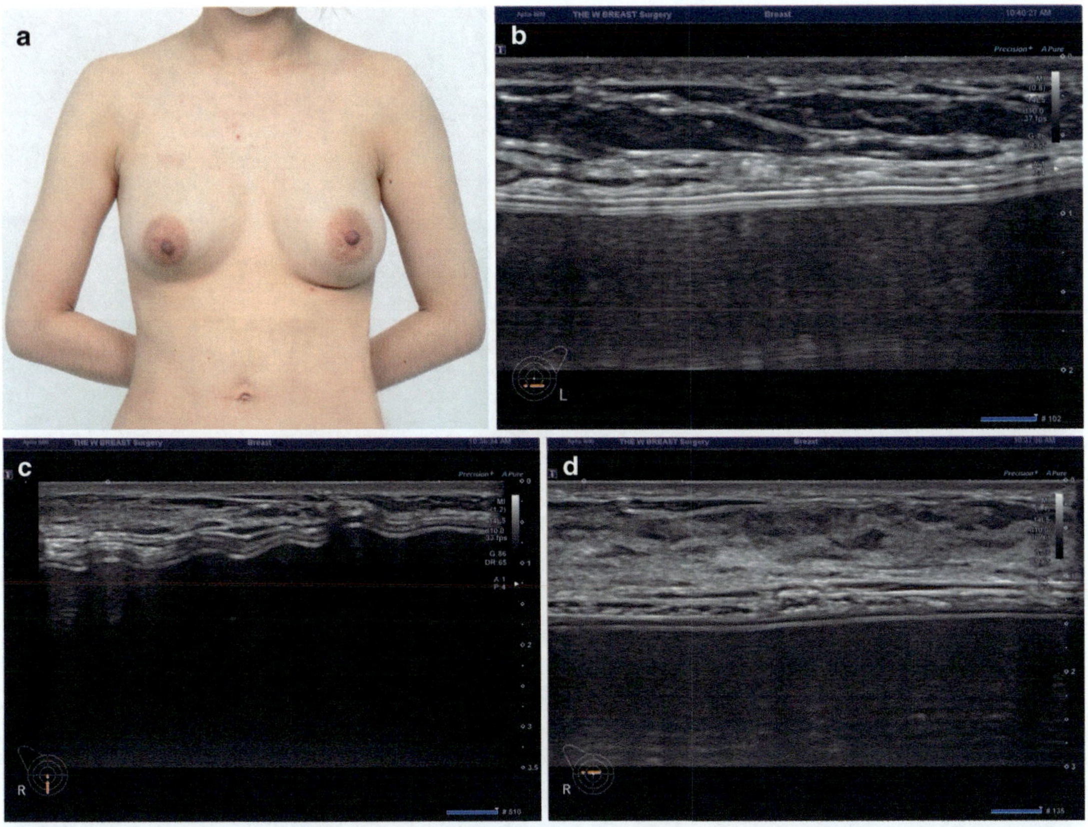

Fig. 8.40 (**a**) A preoperative front view. (**b**) Left smooth shell type breast implant in subglandular pocket is checked in preoperative ultrasonography. (**c**) Right Allergan anatomical type breast implant orientation mark is checked in preoperative ultrasonography. (**d**) Right textured shell type breast implant is checked in ultrasonography. (**e**) Left intraoperative view of breast pocket after subtotal capsulectomy. (**f**, **g**) Right intraoperative view of texture shell type breast implant with periprosthetic capsule. (**h**) Right intraoperative view of periprosthetic capsule after explantation for capsulectomy. (**i**) Removed Allergan style 15 339 cc (left) and Allergan anatomical type 410 MF 335 cc (right). (**j**) Left removed periprosthetic capsule after subtotal capsulectomy. (**k**) Right removed periprosthetic capsule after subtotal capsulectomy. (**l**) Microscopic view of the left capsule. (**m**) Microscopic view of the right capsule

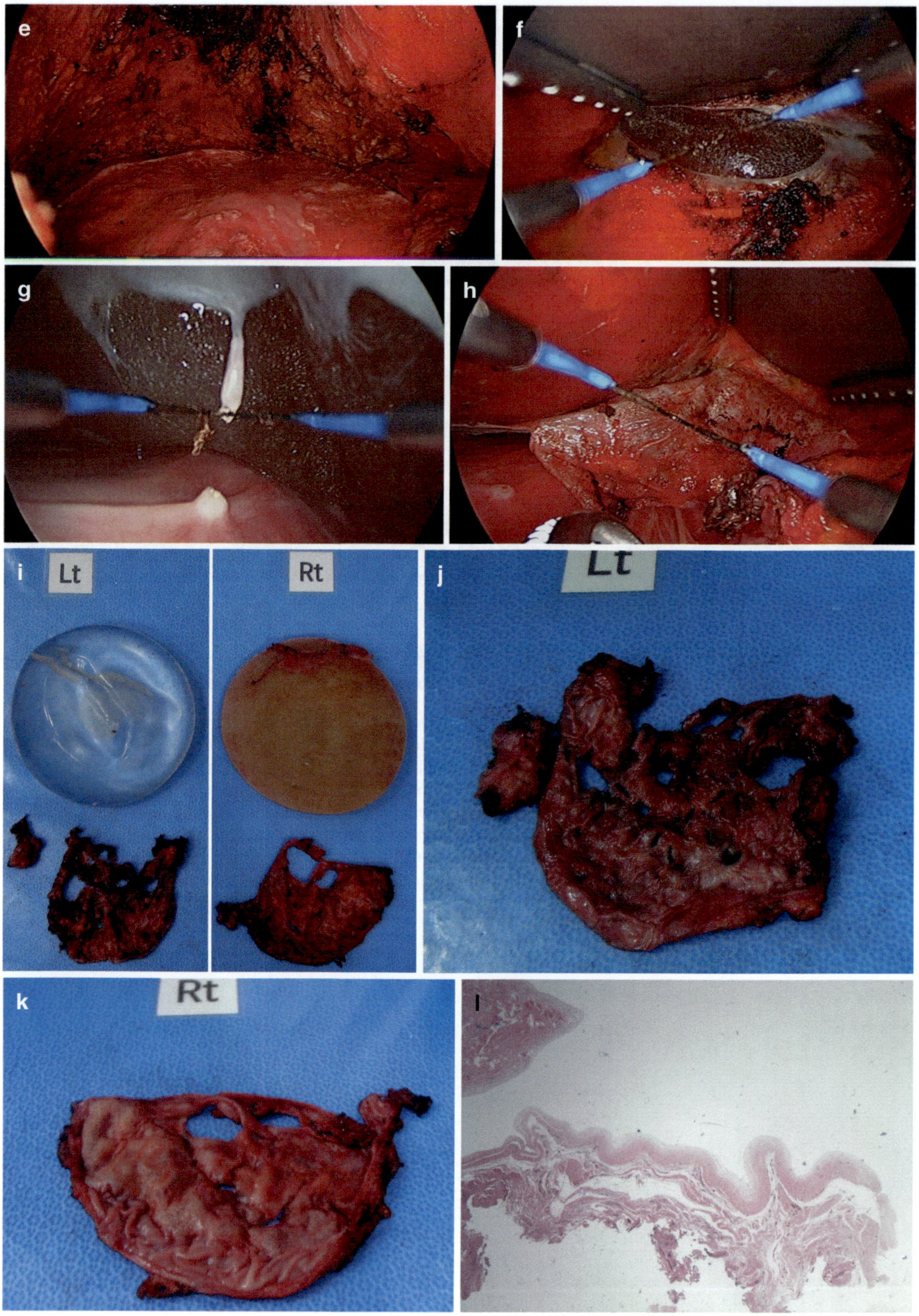

Fig. 8.40 (continued)

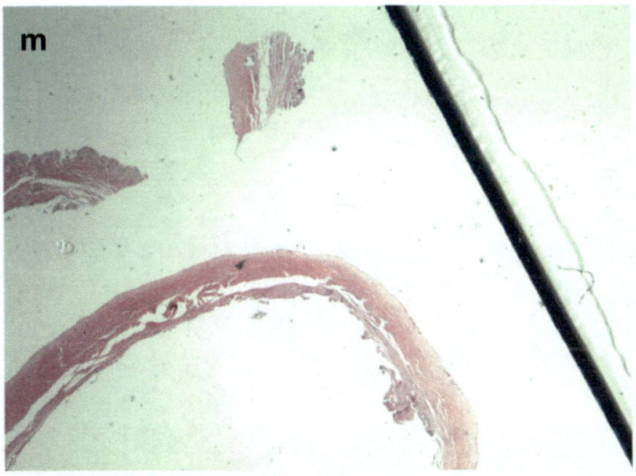

Fig. 8.40 (continued)

8.2.41 Case 41

On physical examination and history taking, a 52-year-old woman complained of dissatisfaction with shape. The patient had a 20-year history of receiving an implant-based augmentation mammaplasty *via* an inframammary incision.

On preoperative ultrasonography, the patient was found to have a round smooth shell type silicone gel-filled breast implant in the subpectoral pocket. There were findings of folding, thickened capsule, and upside-down rotation (Videos 8.53 and 8.54). But there were no findings that are suggestive of seroma, rupture, and capsular mass.

The patient underwent right breast total capsulectomy and left partial capsulectomy with replacement of the breast implant *via* a previous inframammary scar on both sides (Video 8.55). There was mild fibrosis in both capsule (Fig. 8.41).

8.2.42 Case 42

On physical examination and history taking, a 47-year-old woman complained of foreign body sense. The patient had a 13-year history of receiving an implant-based augmentation mammaplasty *via* an axillary incision.

On preoperative ultrasonography, the patient was found to have a round textured shell type silicone gel-filled breast implant in the subpectoral pocket. There was sonographic finding of folded shell and left extracapsular rupture with axillary lymph node silicone invasion (Videos 8.56, 8.57 and 8.58). But there were no findings that are suggestive of seroma, thickened capsule, upside-down rotation, and capsular mass.

The patient underwent right subtotal capsulectomy and left near-total capsulectomy with replacement of the breast implant *via* a previous axillary scar on both sides (Video 8.59). There were focal chronic inflammation and fibrosis in both capsule (Fig. 8.42).

8.2.43 Case 43

On physical examination and history taking, a 53-year-old woman complained of breast pain. The patient had a 12-year history of receiving an implant-based augmentation mammaplasty *via* an areolar incision.

On preoperative ultrasonography, the patient was found to have a round smooth shell type silicone gel-filled breast implant in the subglandular pocket. There was a finding of extra-capsular rupture of right breast implant (Video 8.60). But there were no findings that are suggestive of folding, seroma, thickened capsule, upside-down rotation, and capsular mass.

The patient underwent explantation and both near-total capsulectomy *via* a previous areolar scar on both sides. There were right mild fibrosis and left focal chronic inflammation and fibrosis (Fig. 8.43).

8.2.44 Case 44

On physical examination and history taking, a 35-year-old woman complained of breast pain. The patient had a 4-year history of receiving an implant-based augmentation mammaplasty *via* an axillary incision.

On preoperative ultrasound, the patient was found to have a round textured silicone gel-filled breast implant in the subpectoral pocket. There was a sonographic finding of upside-down rota-

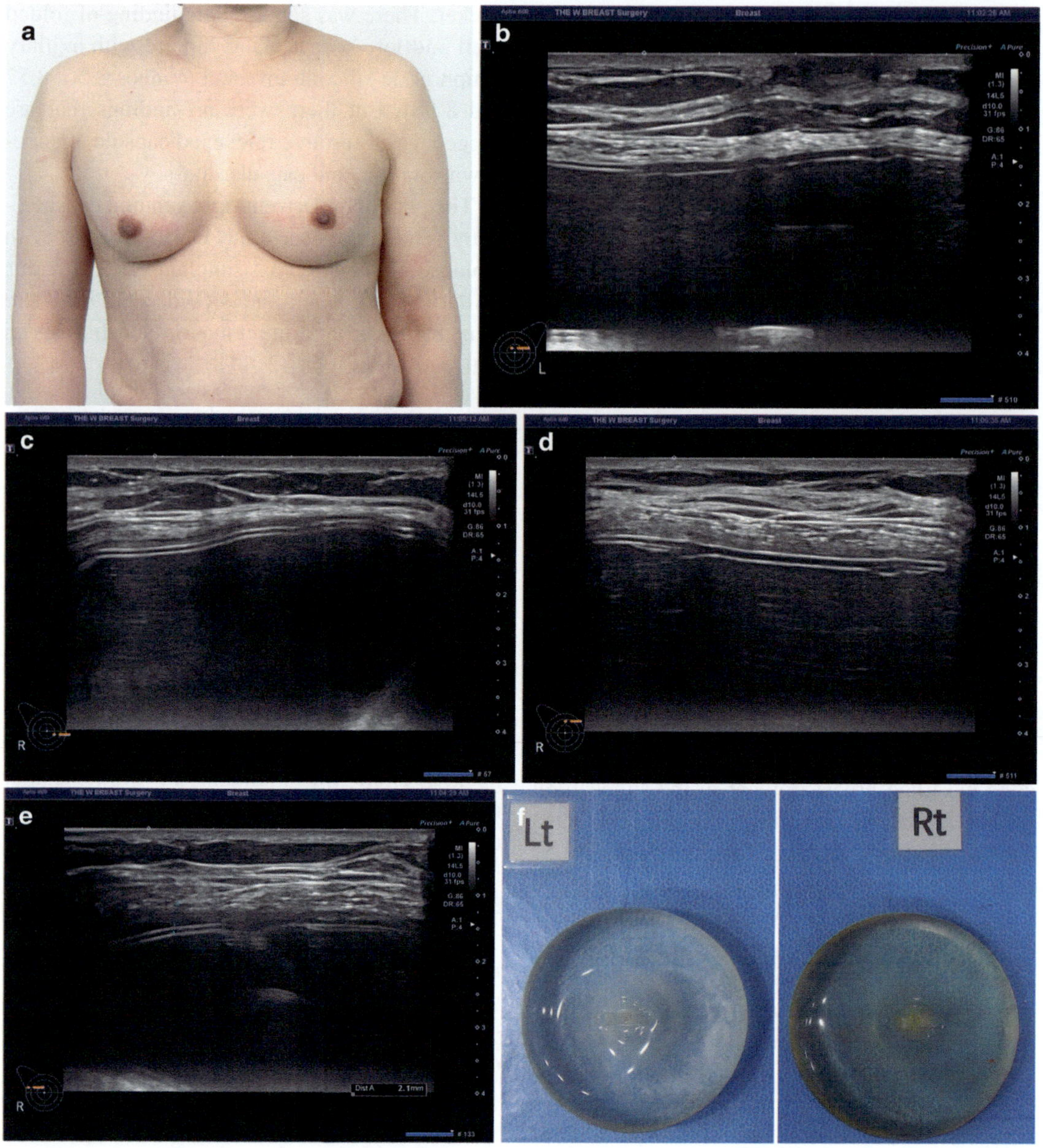

Fig. 8.41 (**a**) A preoperative front view. (**b**) Left smooth shell type breast implant in subpectoral pocket with upside-down rotation is checked in preoperative ultrasonography. (**c**) Right smooth shell type breast implant in subpectoral pocket with thickened periprosthetic capsule is checked in preoperative ultrasonography. (**d**) Right breast implant with upside-down rotation is checked in preoperative ultrasonography. (**e**) Right breast periprosthetic thickened capsule with folded shell is checked in ultrasonography. (**f**) Both removed Allergan smooth type breast implant, 210 cc. (**g**) Right outer surface of removed periprosthetic capsule. (**h**) Right inner surface of removed periprosthetic capsule. (**i**) Right capsule is measured by digital caliper, 2.2 mm. (**j**) Microscopic view of the right capsule

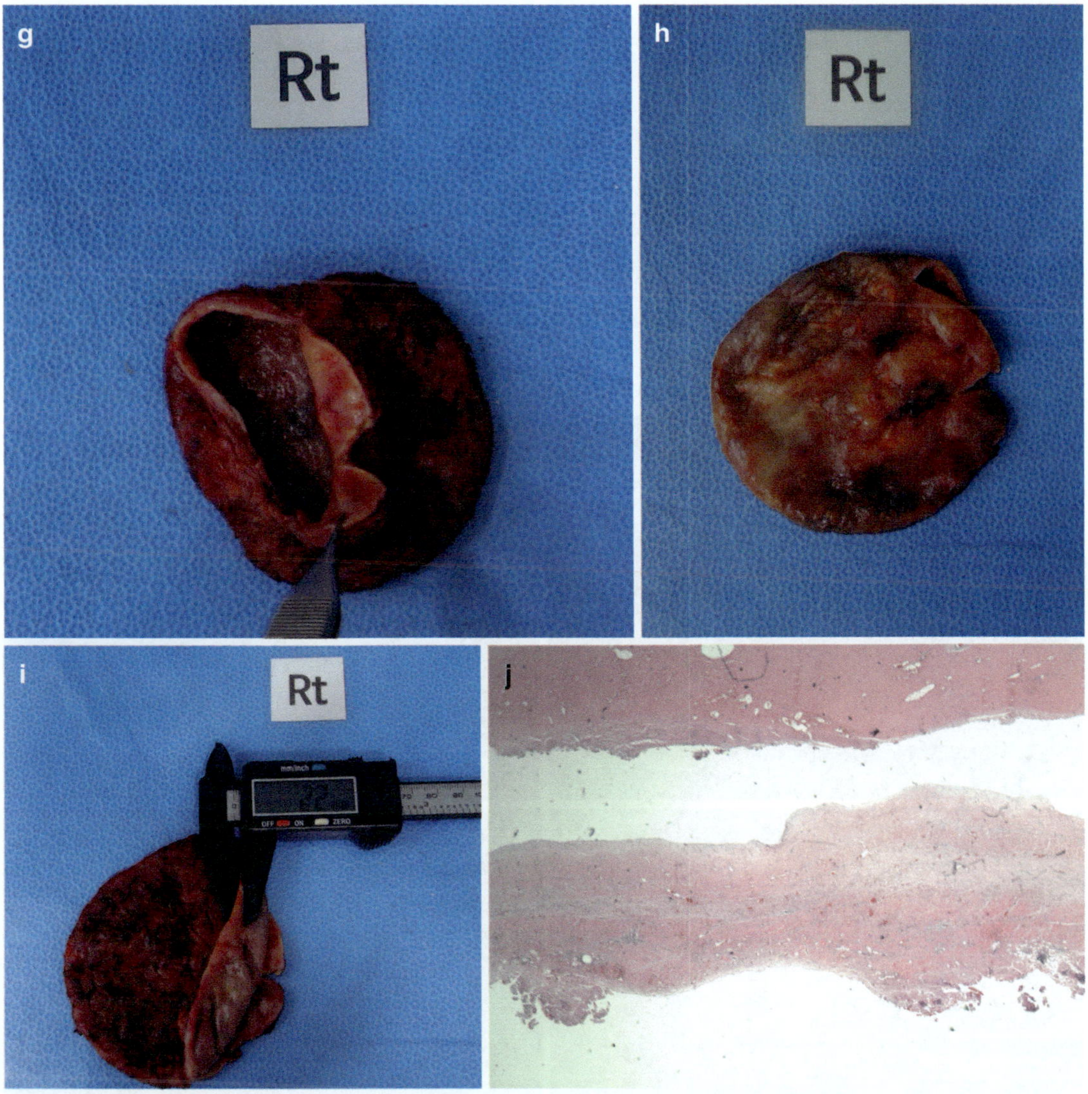

Fig. 8.41 (continued)

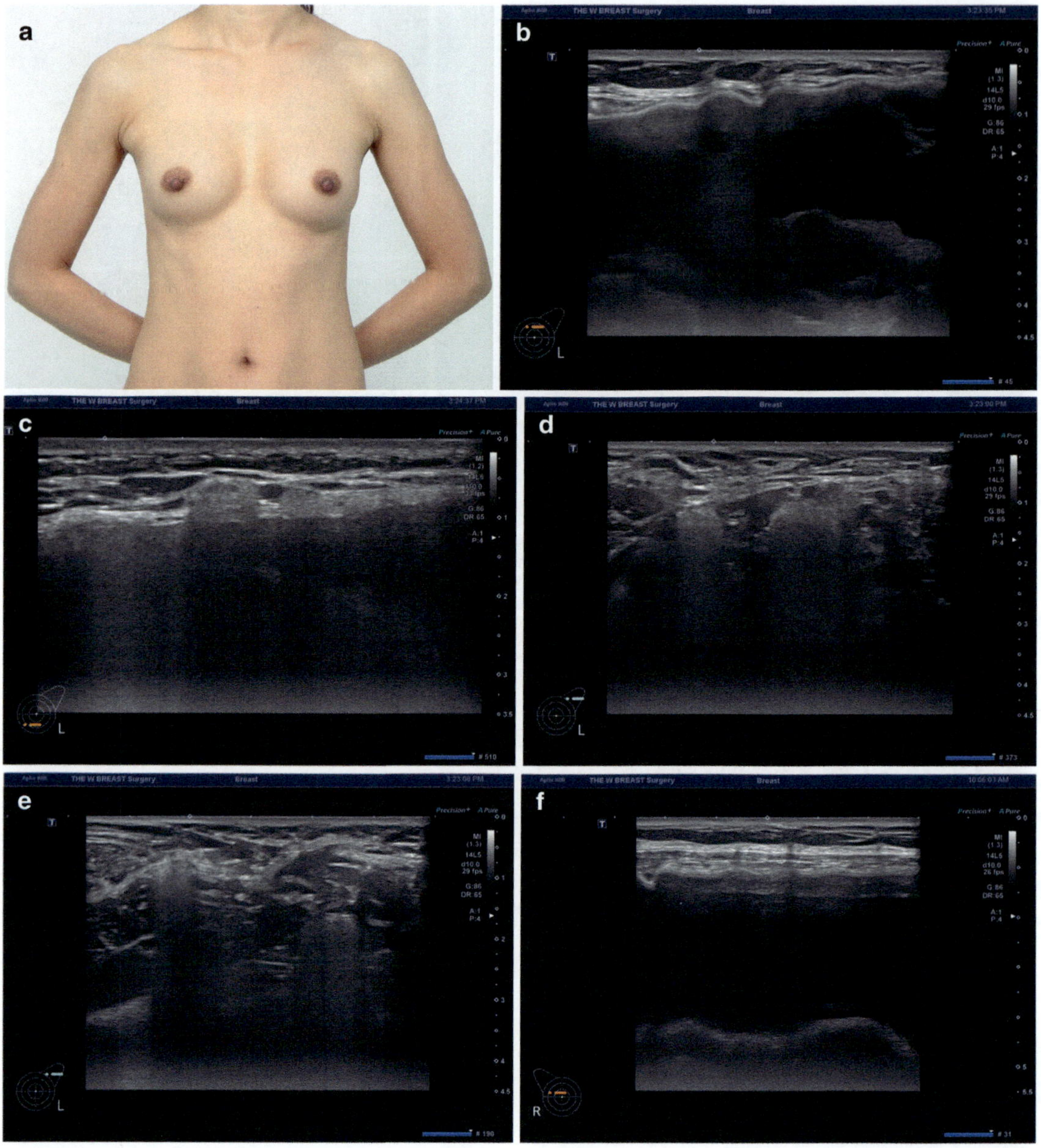

Fig. 8.42 (**a**) A preoperative front view. (**b**) Left textured shell type breast implant in subpectoral pocket is checked in preoperative ultrasonography. (**c**) Left extracapsular silicone invasion is checked in preoperative ultrasonography. (**d**, **e**) Left axillary lymph node silicone invasion in ultrasonography. (**f**) Right textured shell type breast implant in subpectoral pocket is checked in preoperative ultrasonography. (**g**) Left intraoperative view of periprosthetic capsule before capsulectomy. (**h**) Left intraoperative view of ruptured breast implant within capsule. (**i**) Left intraoperative view of breast pocket after near-total capsulectomy. (**j**) Left removed unknown manufacturer breast implant with periprosthetic capsule. (**k**) Left periprosthetic capsule thickness is measured by digital caliper, 0.6 mm. (**l**) Microscopic view of left capsule with silicone invasion to capsule

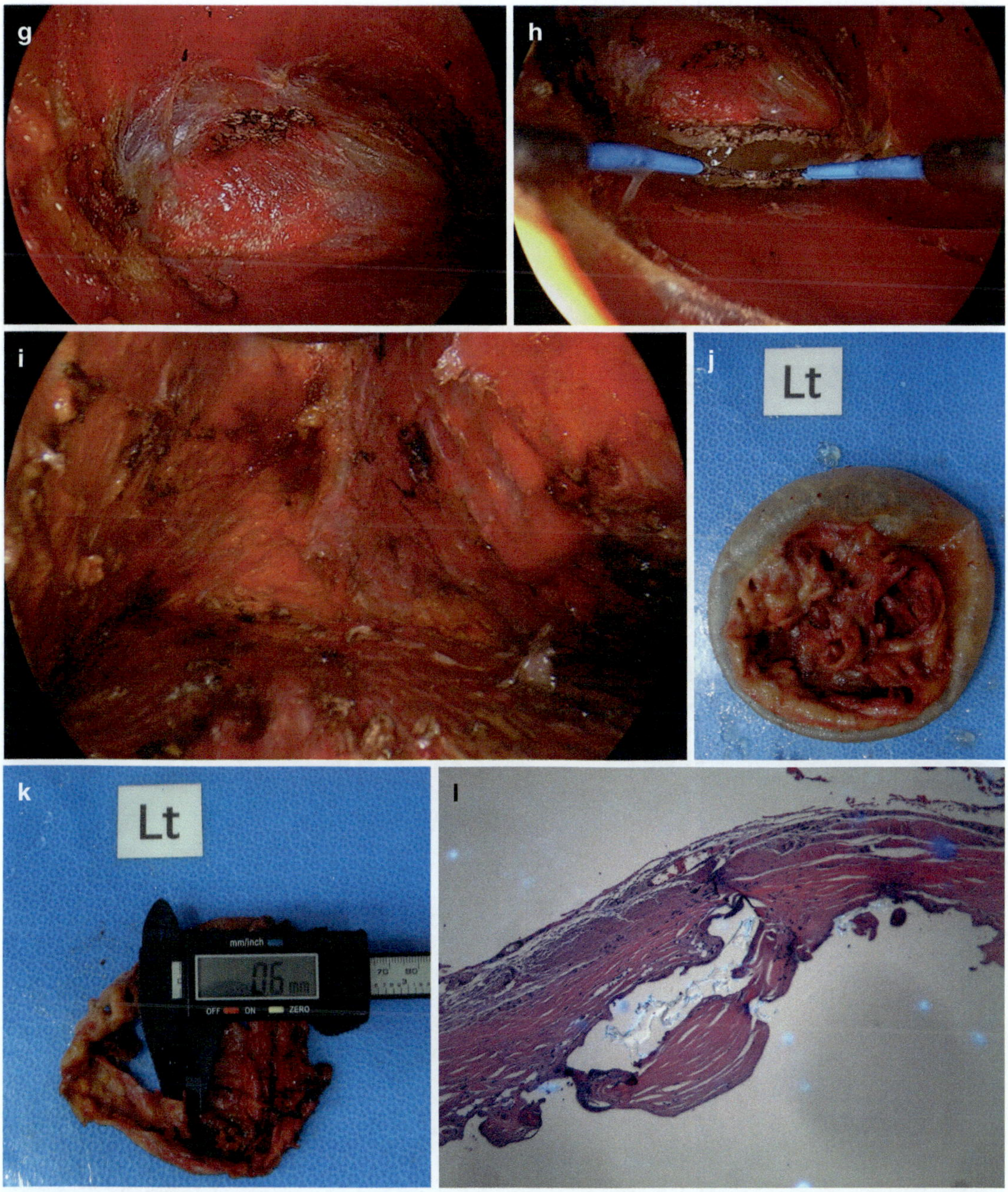

Fig. 8.42 (continued)

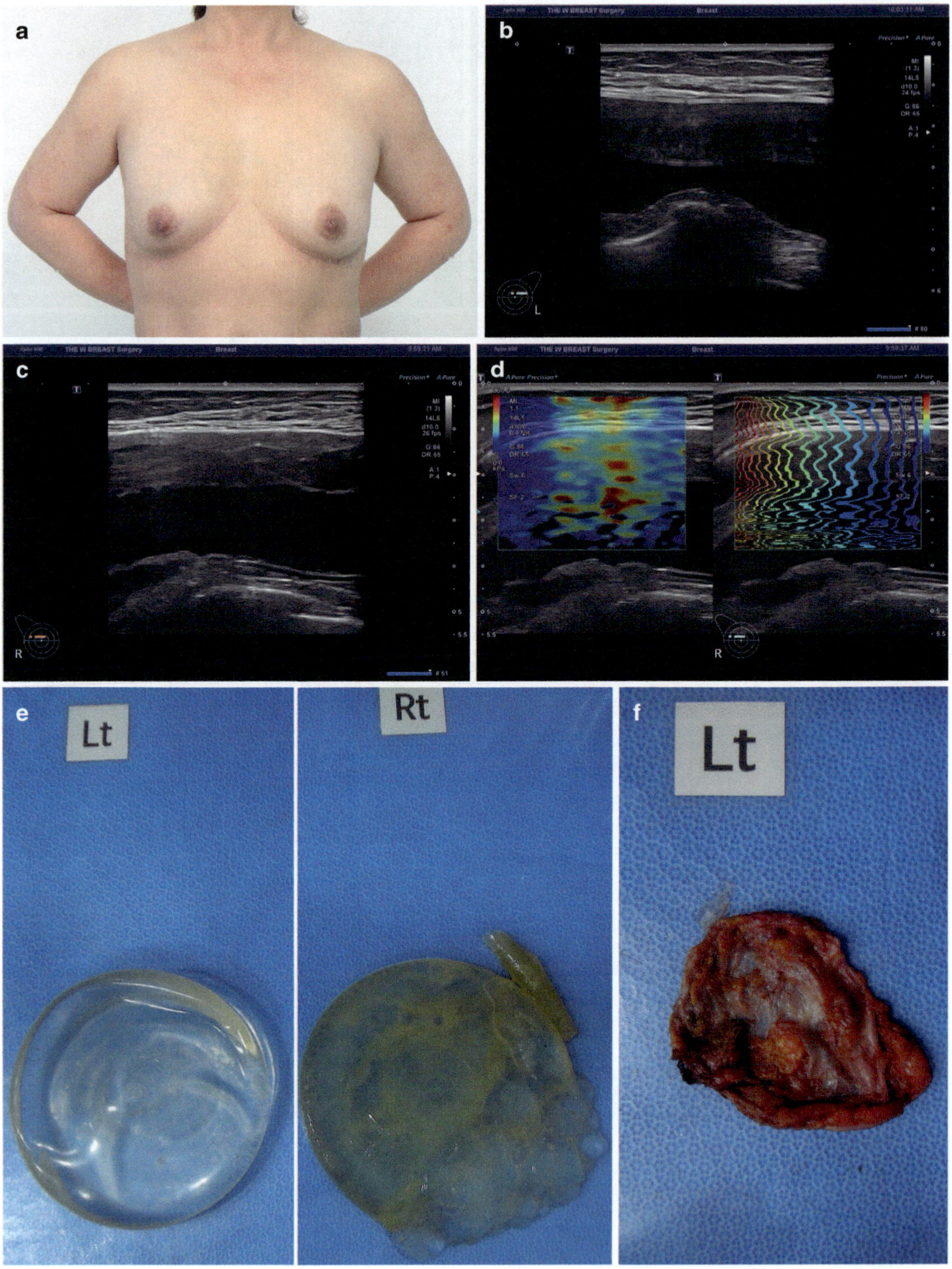

Fig. 8.43 (**a**) A preoperative front view. (**b**) Left smooth shell type breast implant is checked in preoperative ultrasonography. (**c**) Right ruptured breast implant in preoperative ultrasonography. (**d**) Shear wave elastography of right ruptured breast implant. (**e**) Both removed Mentor round smooth shell type breast implant, 200 (left) and 225 cc (right). (**f**) Left removed periprosthetic capsule after near-total capsulectomy. (**g**) Right removed periprosthetic capsule after near-total capsulectomy. (**h**) Left periprosthetic capsule thickness is measured by digital caliper, 0.4 mm. (**i**) Right periprosthetic capsule thickness is measured by digital caliper, 0.4 mm. (**j**) Microscopic view of the left capsule. (**k**) Microscopic view of the right capsule with silicone invasion

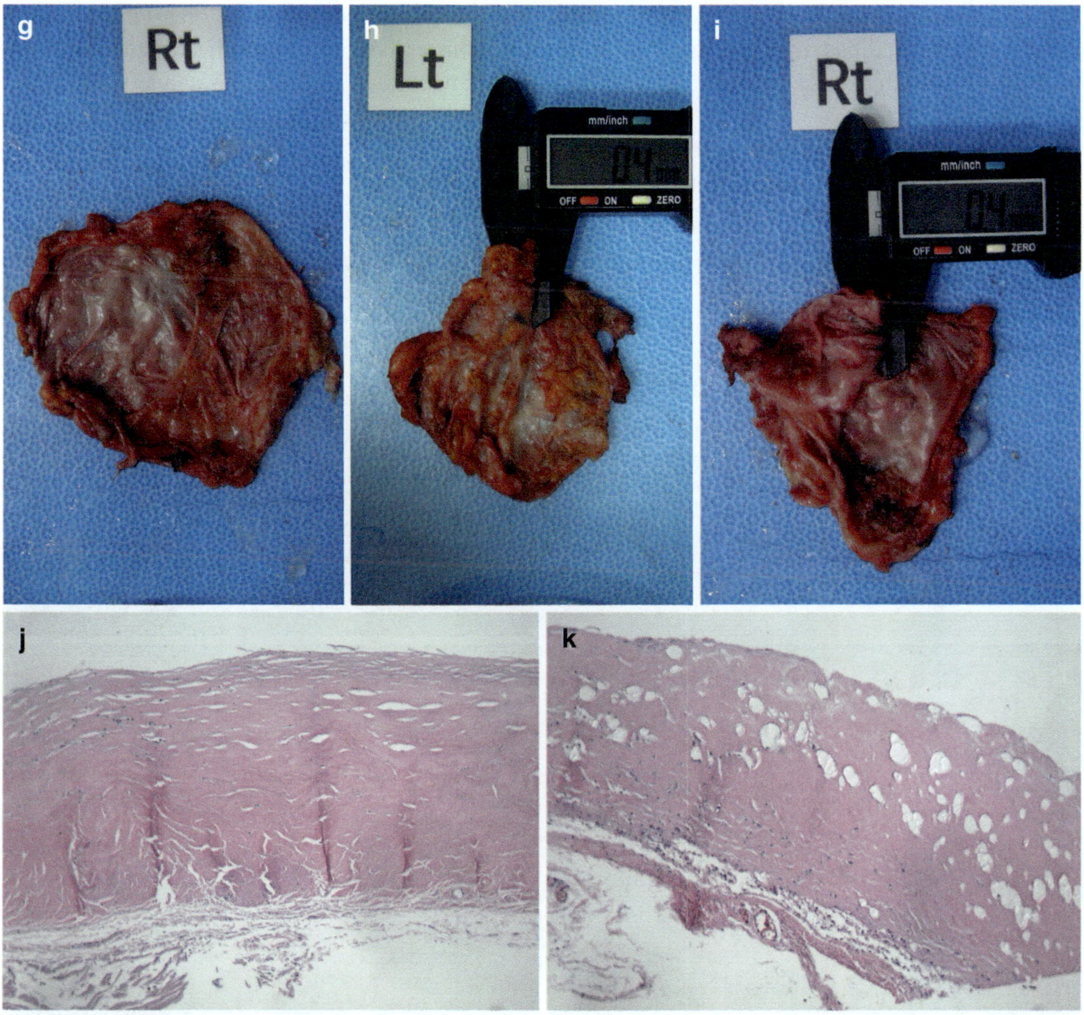

Fig. 8.43 (continued)

tion of right breast implant (Video 8.61). But there were no findings that are suggestive of folding, seroma, thickened capsule, rupture, and capsular mass.

The patient underwent right breast near-total capsulectomy and left breast subtotal capsulectomy with replacement of the breast implant *via* a previous axillary scar on both sides (Video 8.62). There were right mild fibrosis and left mild fibrosis and hemorrhage (Fig. 8.44).

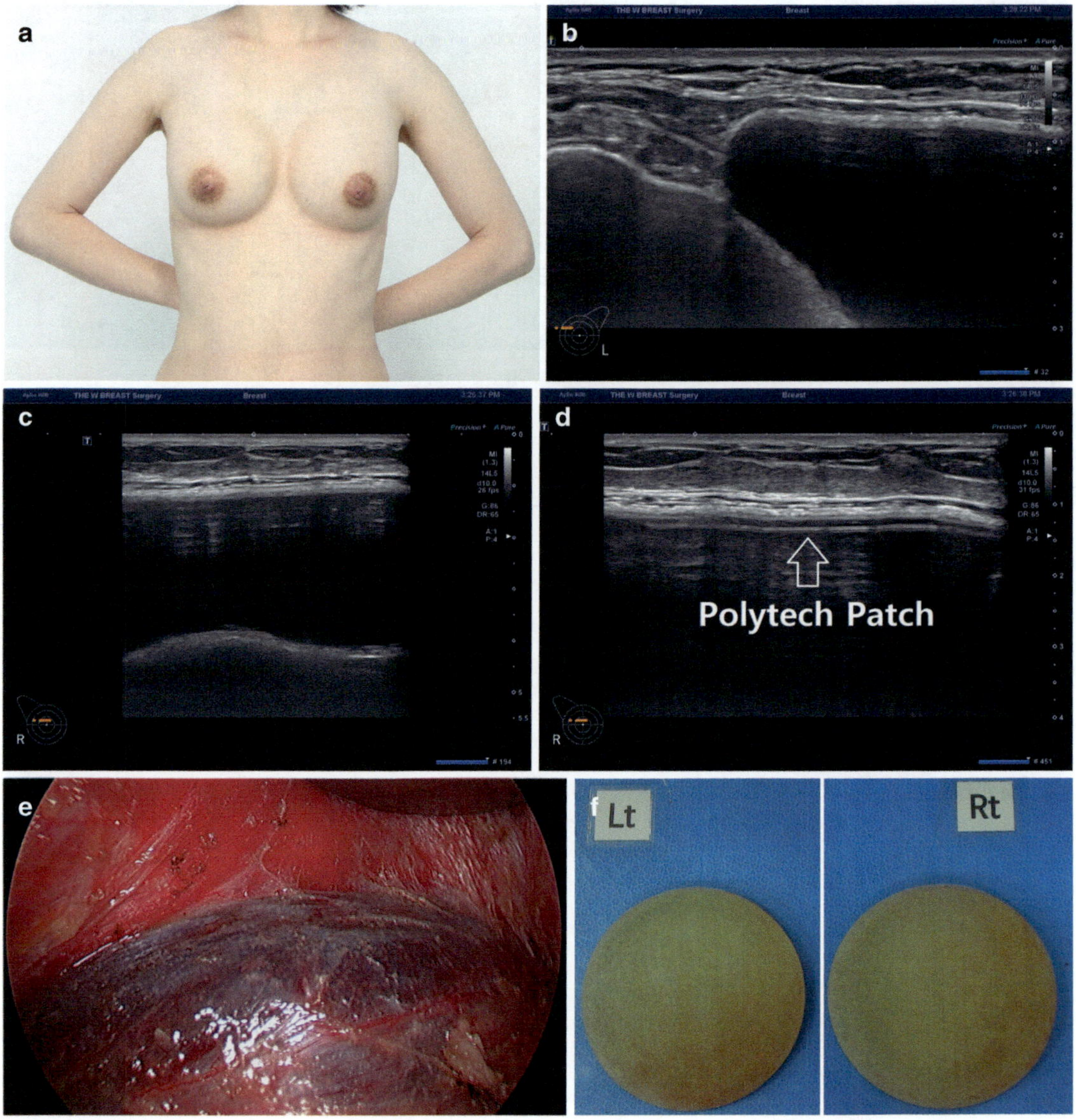

Fig. 8.44 (**a**) A preoperative front view. (**b**) Left textured shell type breast implant in subpectoral pocket is checked in preoperative ultrasonography. (**c**) Right textured shell type breast implant in preoperative ultrasonography. (**d**) Right Polytech round breast implant upside-down rotation is checked in preoperative ultrasonography. (**e**) Right intraoperative view of breast implant with periprosthetic capsule. (**f**) Both removed Polytech round texture type breast implant, 270 cc. (**g**) Left removed periprosthetic capsule after subtotal capsulectomy. (**h**) Right removed periprosthetic capsule after near-total capsulectomy. (**i**) Left periprosthetic capsule thickness is measured by digital caliper, 0.3 mm. (**j**) Right periprosthetic capsule thickness is measured by digital caliper, 0.4 mm. (**k**) Microscopic view of the left capsule. (**l**) Microscopic view of the right capsule

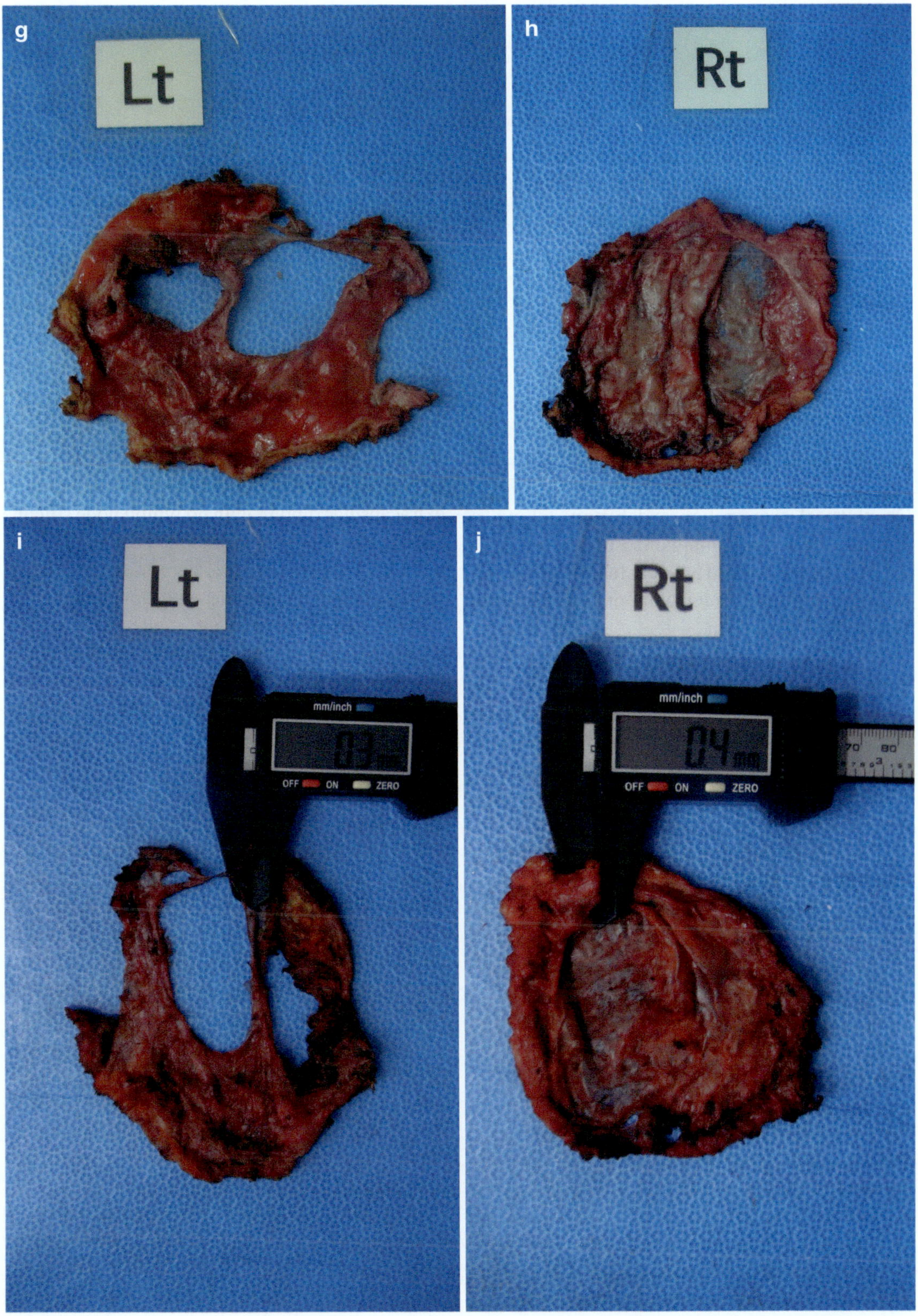

Fig. 8.44 (continued)

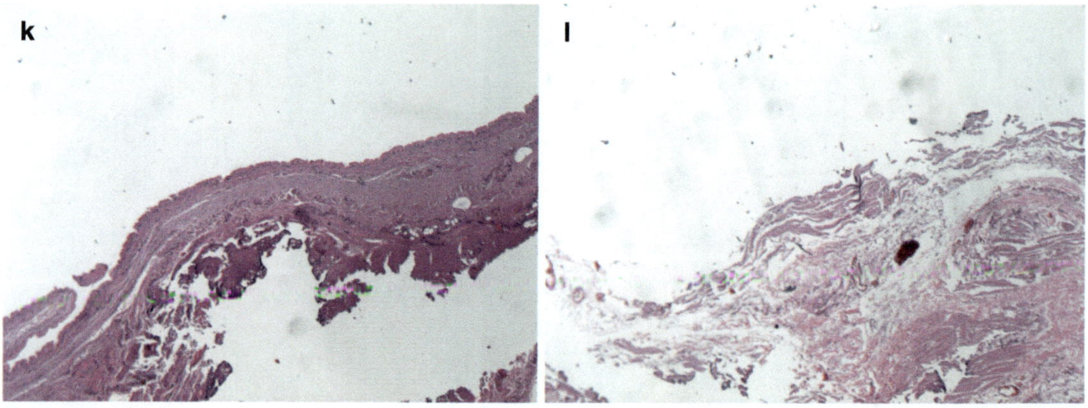

Fig. 8.44 (continued)

8.2.45 Case 45

On physical examination and history taking, a 33-year-old woman complained of fear of BIA-ALCL. The patient had a 8-year history of receiving an implant-based augmentation mammaplasty *via* an axillary incision.

On preoperative ultrasonography, the patient was found to have a round textured shell type silicone gel-filled breast implant in the subpectoral pocket. There was a sonographic finding of partial thickened capsule. But there were no findings that are suggestive of folding, seroma, upside-down rotation, rupture, and capsular mass.

The patient underwent explantation and both subtotal capsulectomy *via* a previous axillary scar on both sides. There were right chronic inflammation with fibrosis and hemorrhage and left focal chronic inflammation and mild fibrosis (Fig. 8.45).

8.2.46 Case 46

On physical examination and history taking, a 61-year-old woman complained of dissatisfaction with size. The patient had a 20-year history of receiving an implant-based augmentation mammaplasty *via* an axillary incision.

On preoperative ultrasonography, the patient was found to have a round smooth shell type silicone gel-filled breast implant in the subglandular pocket. There was a sonographic finding of the left breast implant upside-down rotation and right extracapsular rupture with no lymph node silicone invasion and left gel bleed (Video 8.63). But there were no findings that are suggestive of folding, seroma, thickened capsule, and capsular mass.

The patient underwent total capsulectomy with replacement of the device *via* a previous axillary scar on both sides. There was mild fibrosis in both capsule (Fig. 8.46).

8.2.47 Case 47

On physical examination and history taking, a 39-year-old woman complained of foreign body sensation. The patient had a 13-year history of receiving an implant-based augmentation mammaplasty *via* an axillary incision.

On preoperative ultrasonography, the patient was found to have a round textured shell type silicone gel-filled breast implant in the subglandular pocket. There was a sonographic finding of right extra-capsular rupture. But there were no findings that are suggestive of folding, seroma, thickened capsule, upside-down rotation, rupture, and capsular mass.

The patient underwent explantation with both total capsulectomy *via* a previous axillary scar on both sides. There were right mild fibrosis and left focal chronic inflammation and fibrosis (Fig. 8.47).

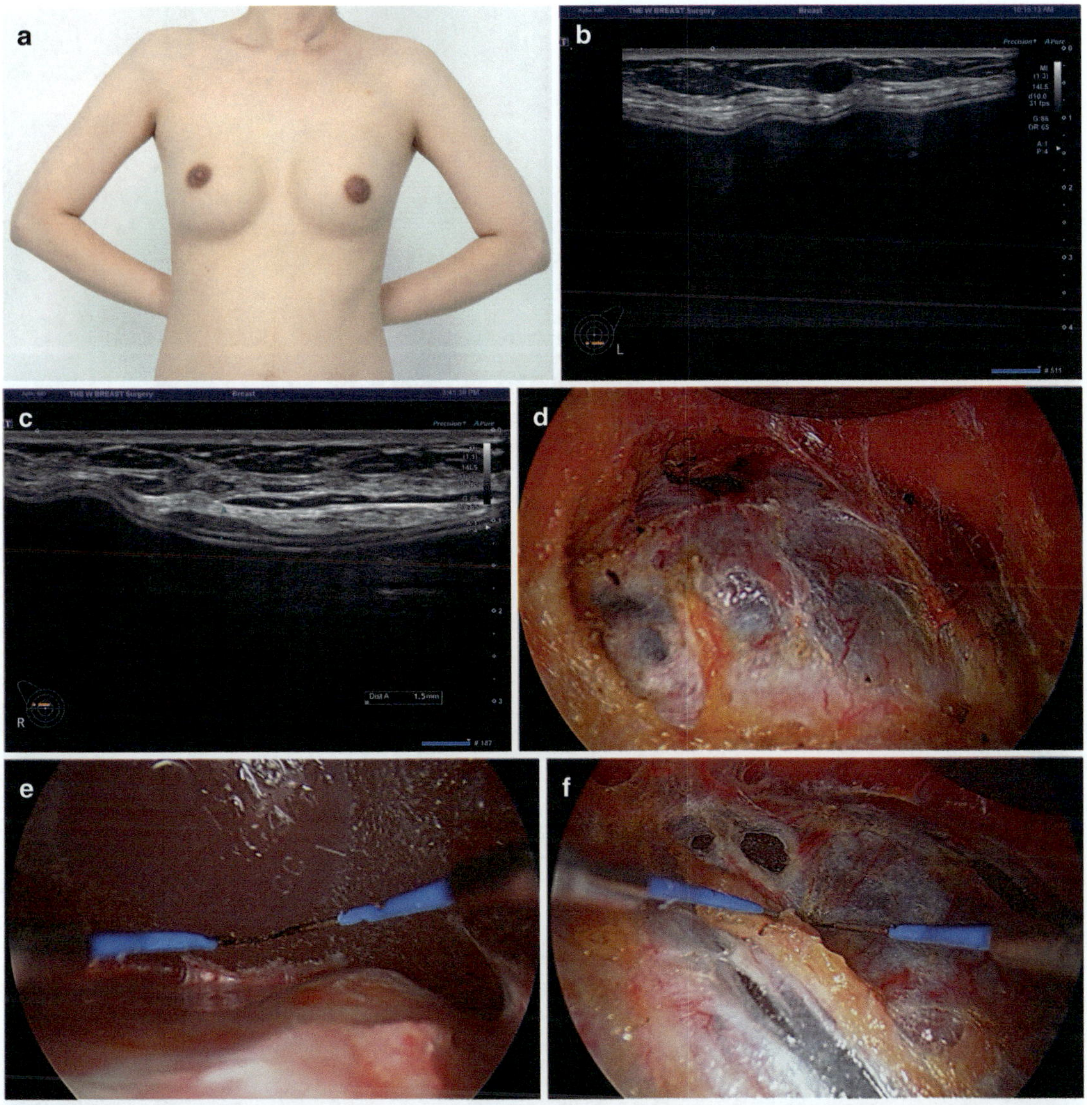

Fig. 8.45 (**a**) A preoperative front view. (**b**) Left textured shell type breast implant in subpectoral pocket is checked in preoperative ultrasonography. (**c**) Right textured shell type breast implant with thickened periprosthetic capsule is checked in preoperative ultrasonography. (**d**) Left intraoperative view of breast implant with periprosthetic capsule. (**e**) Left intraoperative view of Allergan breast implant patch. (**f**) Right intraoperative view of breast implant with periprosthetic capsule. (**g**) Right intraoperative view of Allergan breast implant patch. (**h**) Right intraoperative view of breast pocket with periprosthetic capsule before capsulectomy. (**i**) Right intraoperative view of breast pocket after subtotal capsulectomy. (**j**) Both removed Allergan round texture type breast implant style 120, 220 cc and periprosthetic capsule. (**k**) Both removed periprosthetic capsule after subtotal capsulectomy. (**l**) Left periprosthetic capsule thickness is measured by digital caliper, 0.6 mm. (**m**) Right periprosthetic capsule thickness is measured by digital caliper, 1.5 mm. (**n**) Right periprosthetic capsule thickness is measured by digital caliper, 0.5 mm. (**o**) Microscopic view of the left capsule. (**p**) Microscopic view of the right thickened capsule. (**q**) Microscopic view of the right capsule

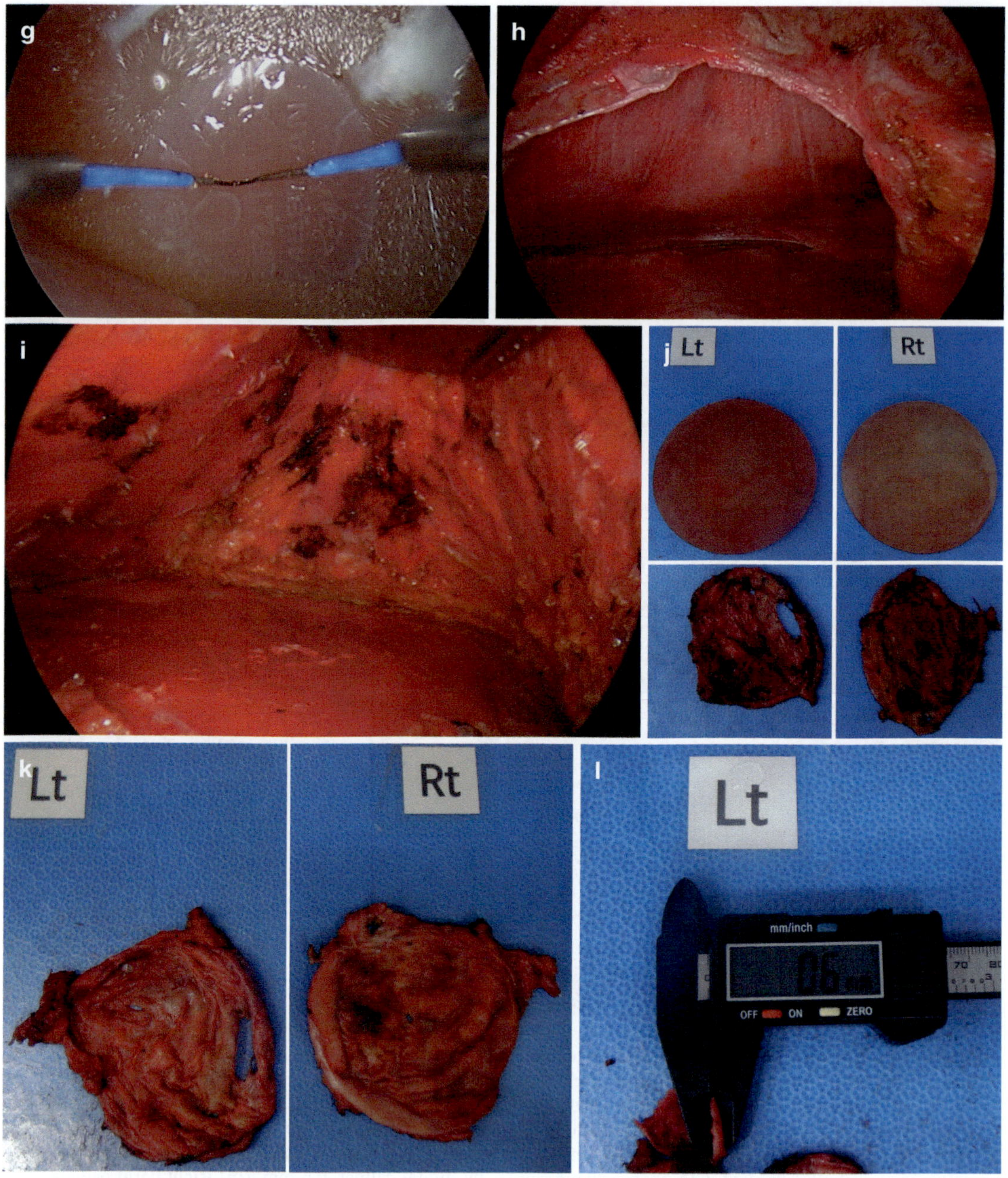

Fig. 8.45 (continued)

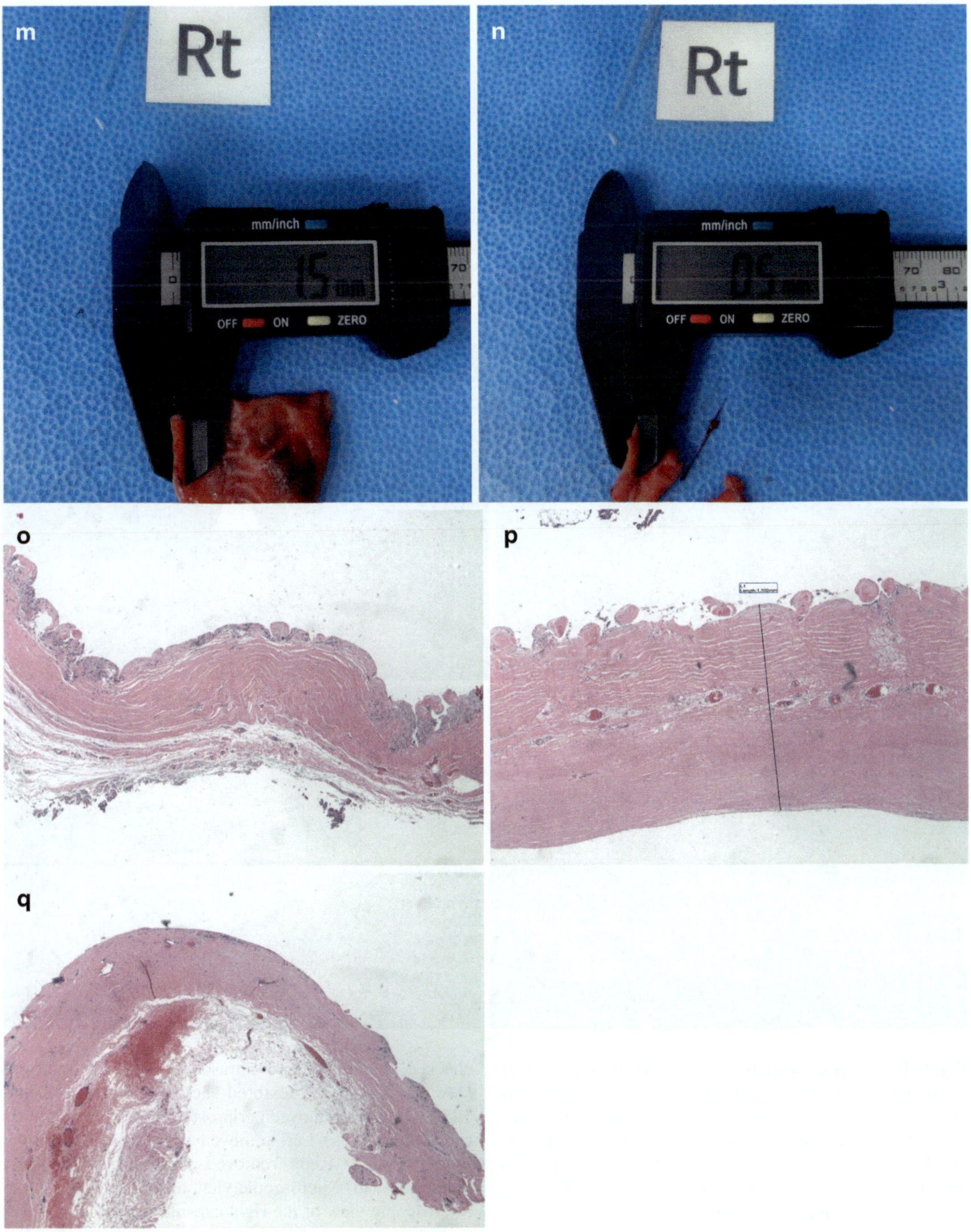

Fig. 8.45 (continued)

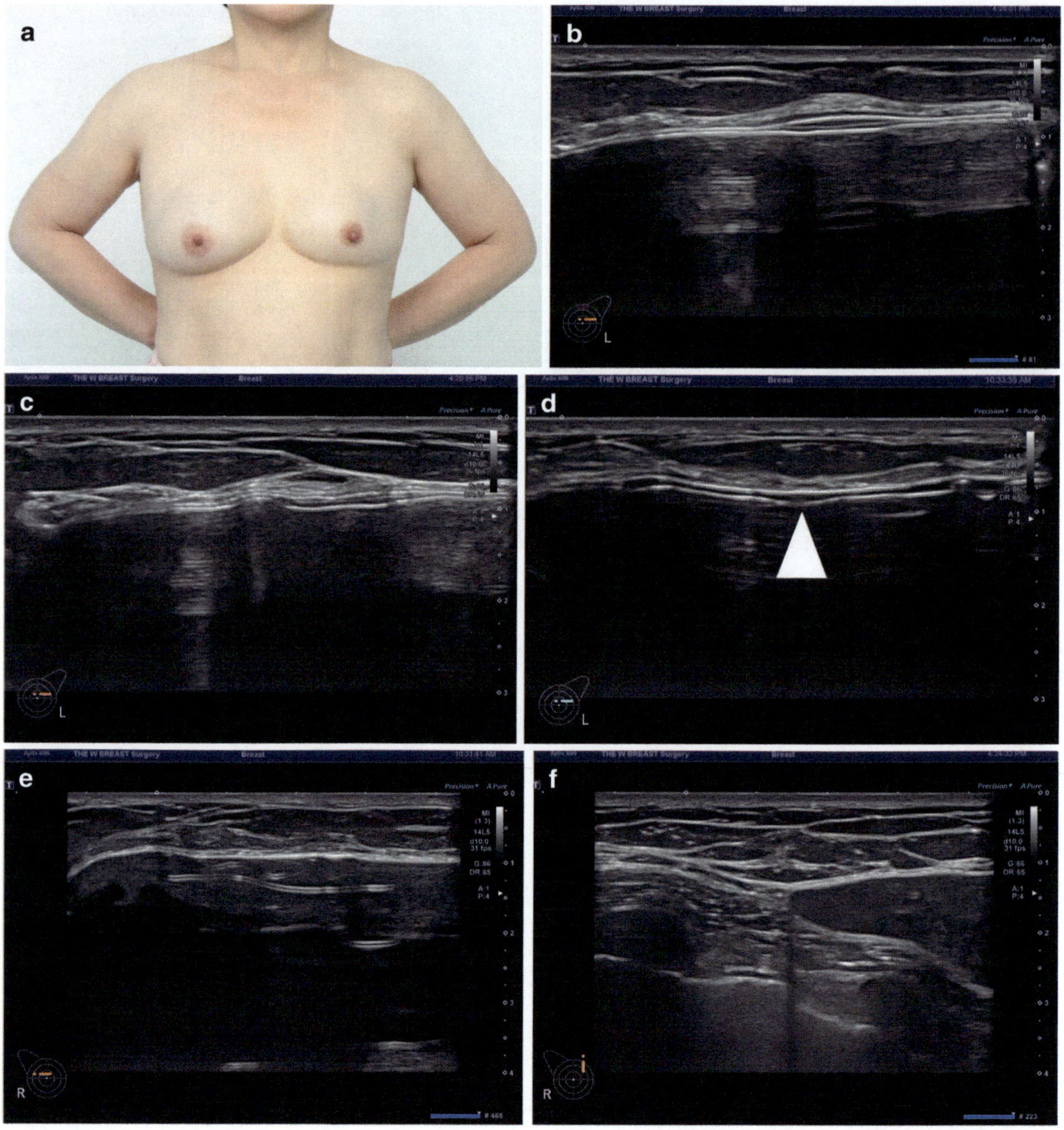

Fig. 8.46 (**a**) A preoperative front view. (**b**, **c**) Left textured shell type breast implant with gel bleeding is checked in preoperative ultrasonography. (**d**) Left breast implant with upside-down rotation (white triangle) is checked in ultrasonography. (**e**) Right breast implant with rupture sign in preoperative ultrasonography. (**f**) Right breast implant rupture with extracapsular silicone invasion is checked in preoperative ultrasonography. (**g**) Right normal axillary lymph node is checked in ultrasonography. (**h**) Right breast implant in subglandular pocket is checked in preoperative ultrasound. (**i**) Both removed Dow Corning round textured shell type breast implant, 125 cc. (**j**) Both removed periprosthetic capsule after total capsulectomy. (**k**) Left removed periprosthetic capsule; inner view. (**l**) Right removed periprosthetic capsule; inner view. (**m**) Microscopic view of the left capsule. (**n**) Microscopic view of the right capsule with silicone invasion to capsule. (**o**) Microscopic view of the right extracapsular mass

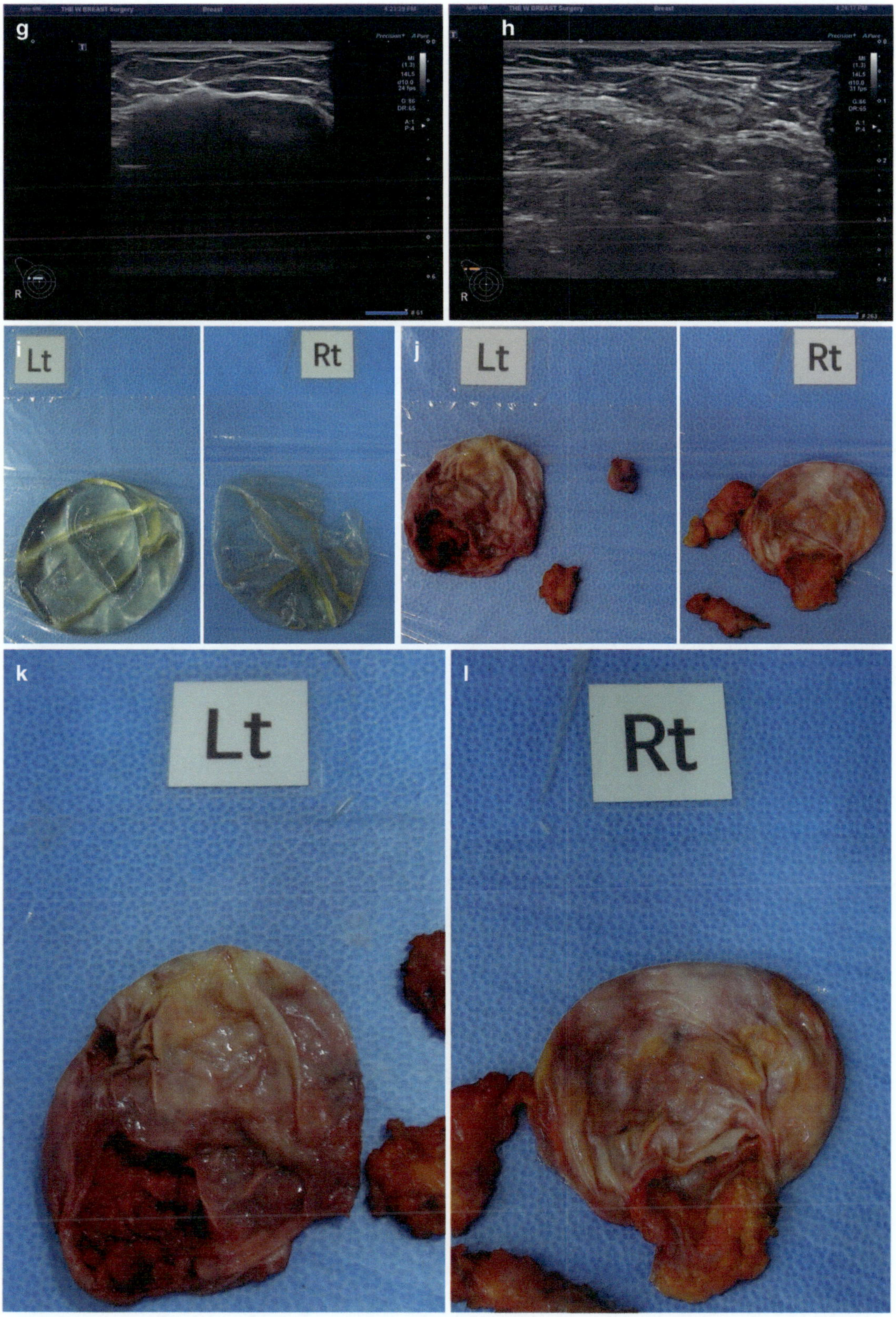

Fig. 8.46 (continued)

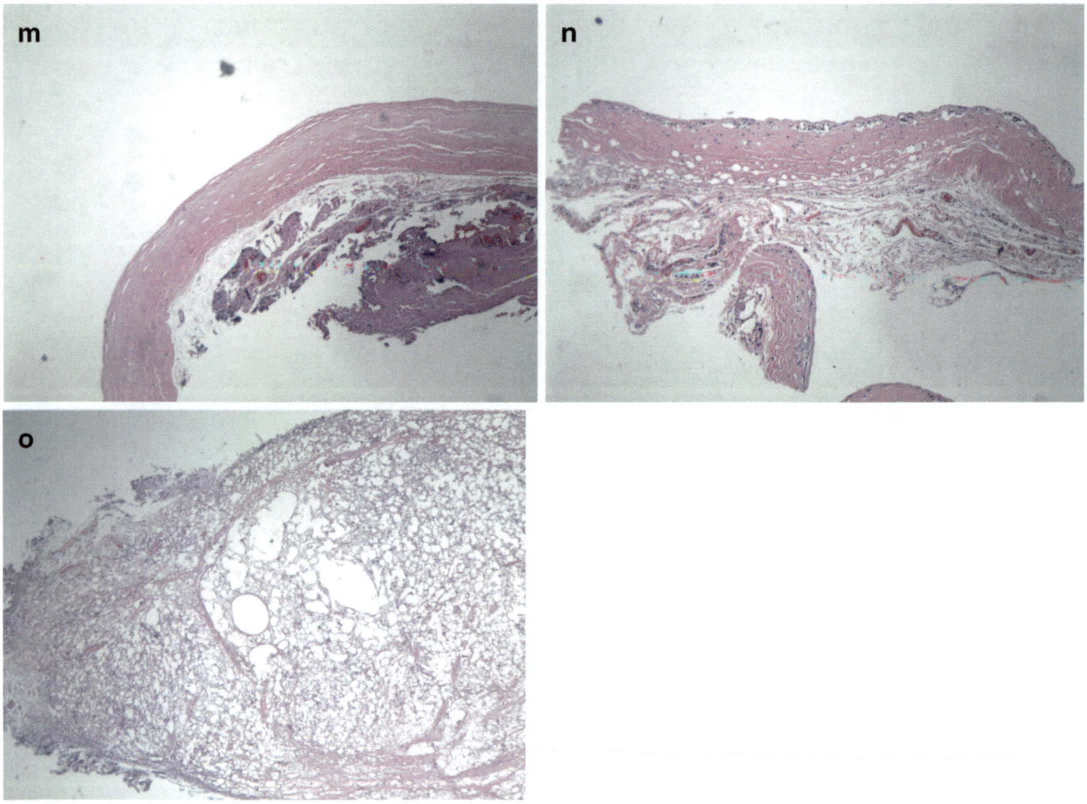

Fig. 8.46 (continued)

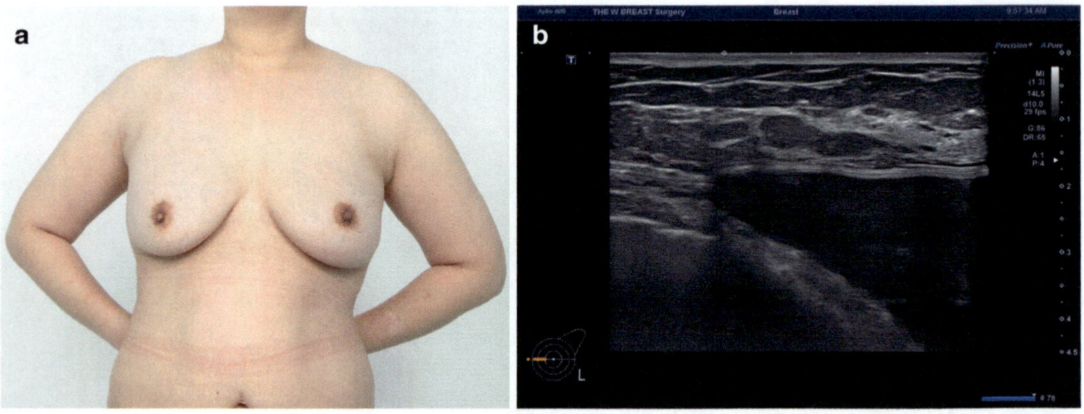

Fig. 8.47 (**a**) A preoperative front view. (**b**) Left smooth shell type breast implant in subglandular pocket is checked in preoperative ultrasonography. (**c**) Right breast implant with intracapsular rupture is checked in preoperative ultrasonography. (**d**) Left intraoperative view of periprosthetic capsule in subglandular pocket. (**e**) Left intraoperative view of intracapsular breast implant pocket. (**f**, **g**) Right intraoperative view of periprosthetic capsule. (**h**) Right intraoperative view of intracapsular breast implant pocket. (**i**) Right intraoperative view of breast pocket after total capsulectomy. (**j**) Both removed Allergan round smooth type breast implant style 40 220 cc. (**k**) Left removed periprosthetic capsule after total capsulectomy. (**l**) Right removed periprosthetic capsule after total capsulectomy. (**m**) Microscopic view of the left capsule. (**n**) Microscopic view of the right capsule with silicone invasion

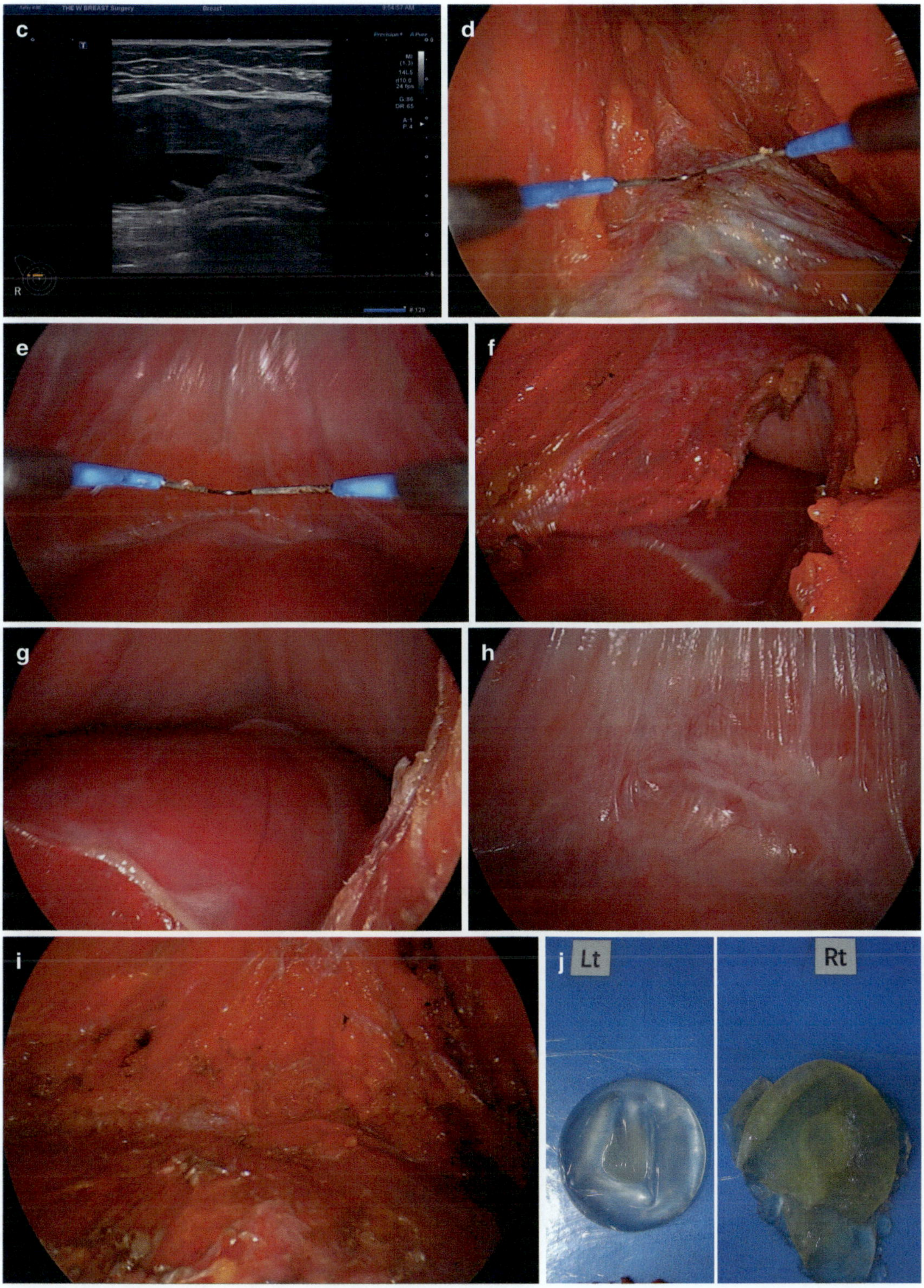

Fig. 8.47 (continued)

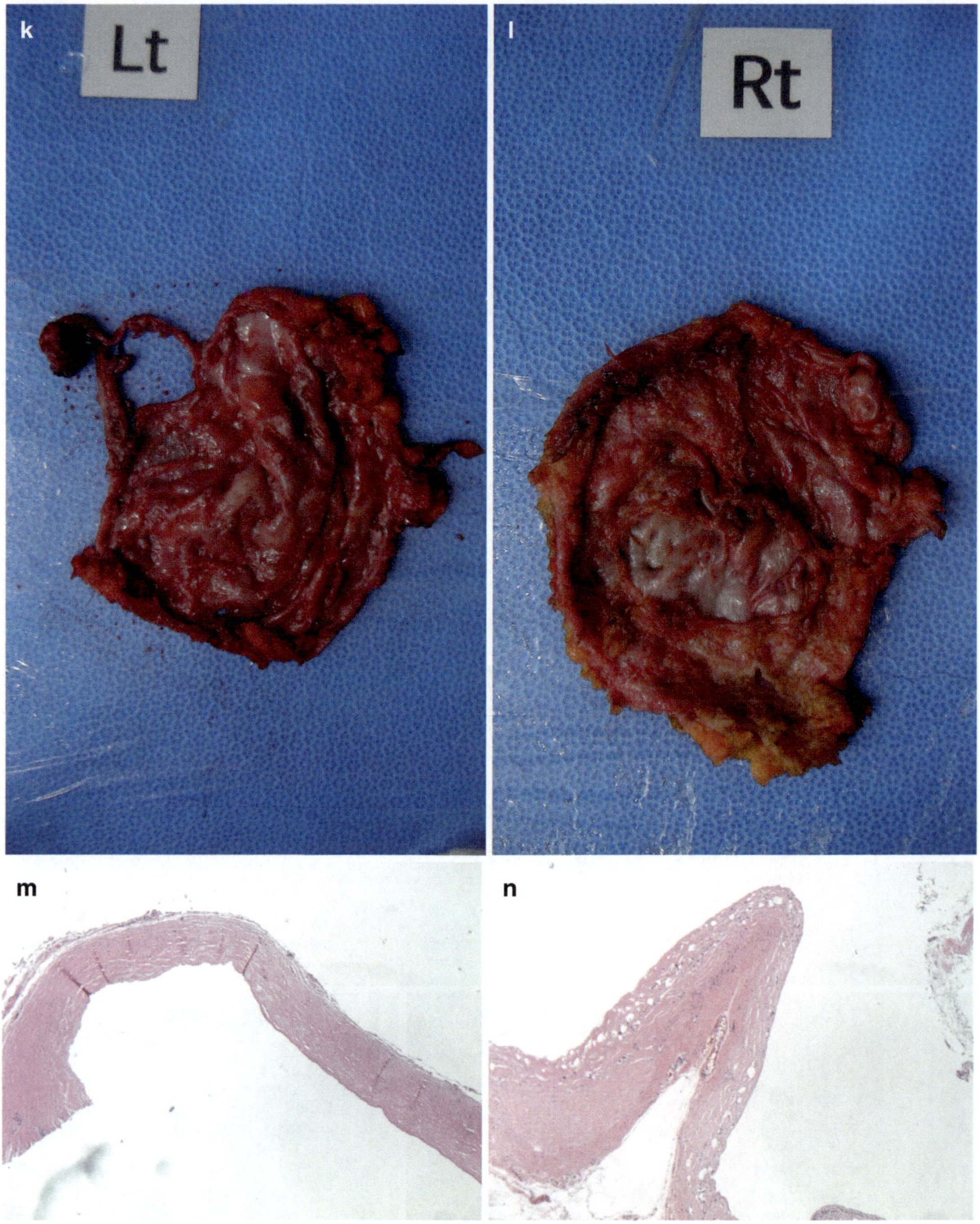

Fig. 8.47 (continued)

8.2.48 Case 48

On physical examination and history taking, a 53-year-old woman complained of change of breast softness. The patient had a 18-year history of receiving an implant-based augmentation mammaplasty *via* an inframammary incision.

On preoperative ultrasonography, the patient was found to have a round textured shell type silicone gel-filled breast implant in the subpectoral pocket. There was a sonographic finding of the right extracapsular rupture with axillary lymph node silicone invasion and folded shell, thickened capsule (Videos 8.64 and 8.65). But there were no findings that are suggestive of seroma, upside-down rotation, and capsular mass.

The patient underwent subtotal capsulectomy with replacement of the breast implant *via* a previous inframammary scar on both sides (Video 8.66). There were chronic inflammation and fibrosis in both capsule (Fig. 8.48).

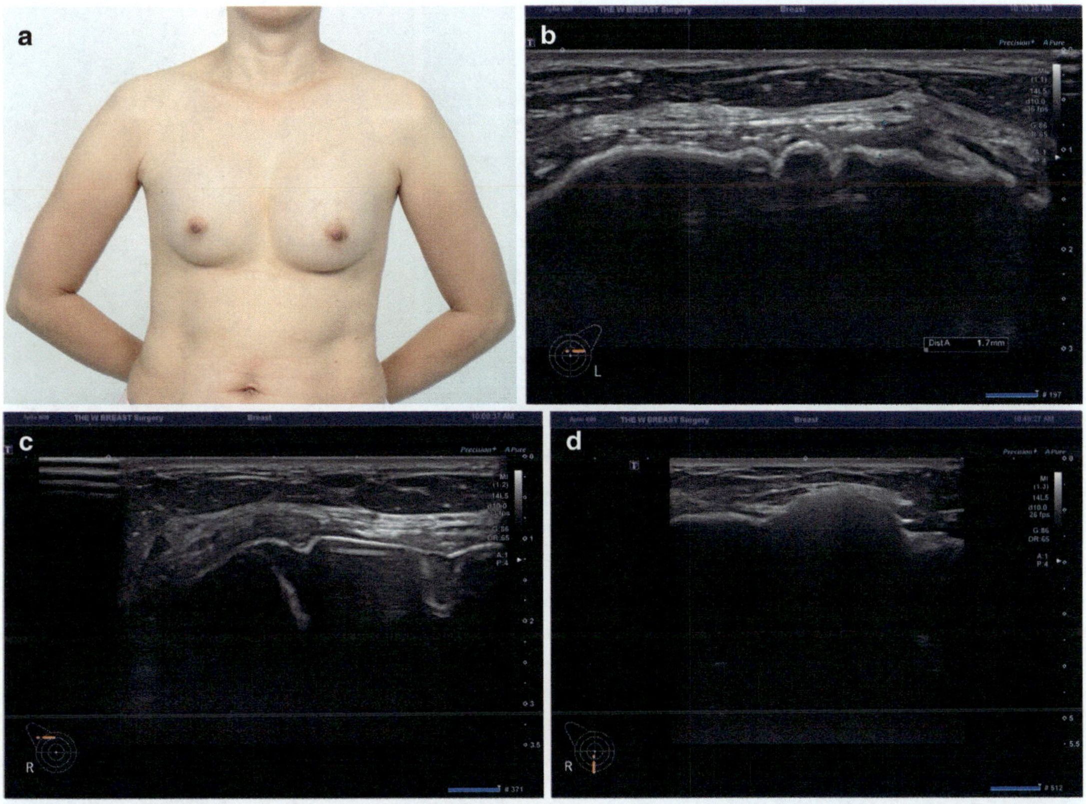

Fig. 8.48 (**a**) A preoperative front view. (**b**) Left textured shell type breast implant in subpectoral pocket is checked in preoperative ultra sonography. (**c**) Right textured shell type breast implant with rupture is checked in preoperative ultrasonography. (**d**) Right extracapsular rupture is checked in preoperative ultrasonography. (**e**) Right breast implant rupture with thickened capsule is checked in preoperative ultrasonography. (**f**) Right axillary lymph node silicone invasion is checked in preoperative ultrasonography. (**g**) Both removed periprosthetic capsule and unknown manufacturer round textured shell type implant, 200 cc. (**h**) Left removed periprosthetic capsule after subtotal capsulectomy. (**i**) Right removed periprosthetic capsule and extracapsular mass after subtotal capsulectomy. (**j**) Right removed periprosthetic capsule. (**k**) Right removed extracapsular mass. (**l**) Microscopic view of the left capsule. (**m**) Microscopic view of the right capsule. (**n**) Microscopic view of right extracapsular silicone granuloma

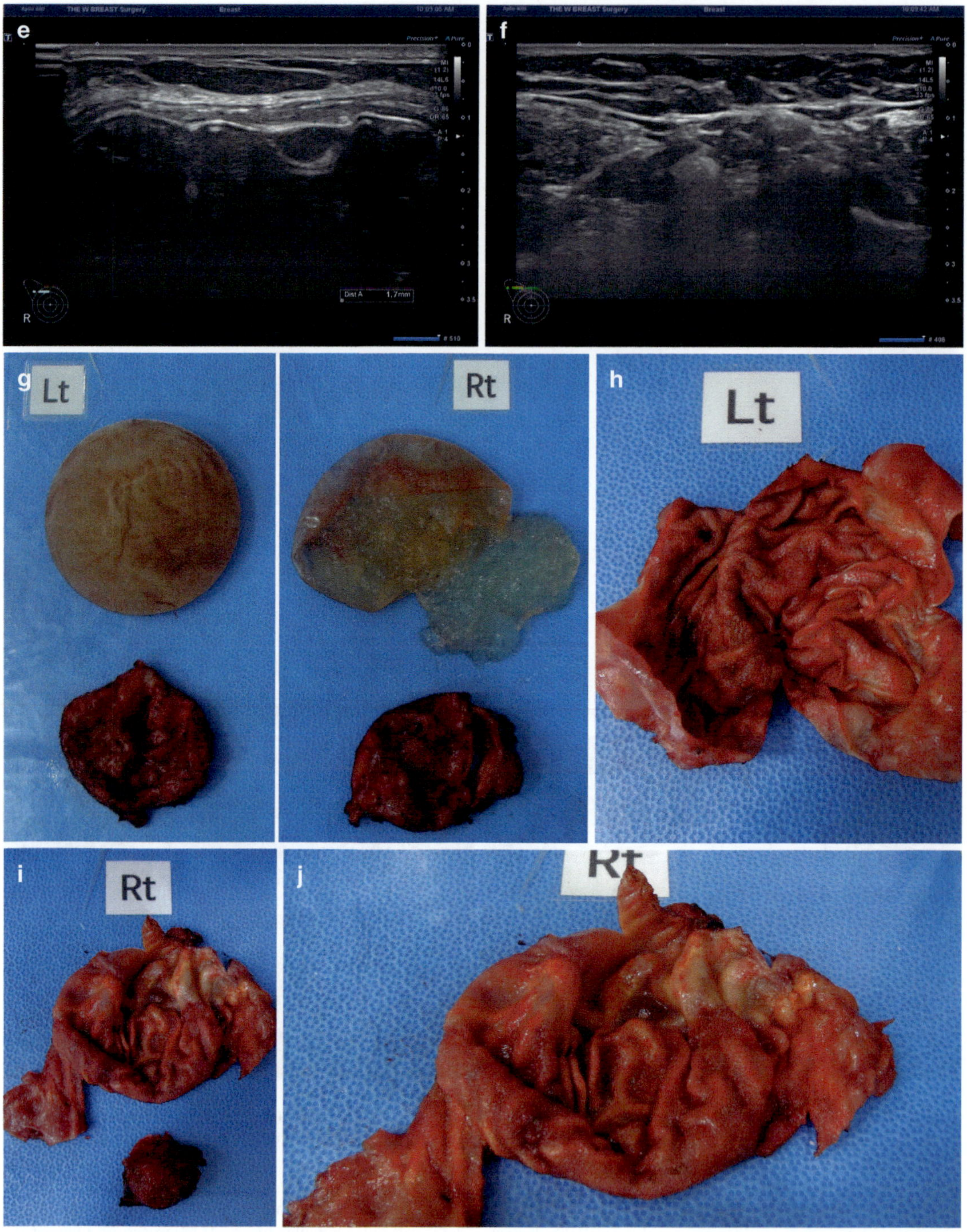

Fig. 8.48 (continued)

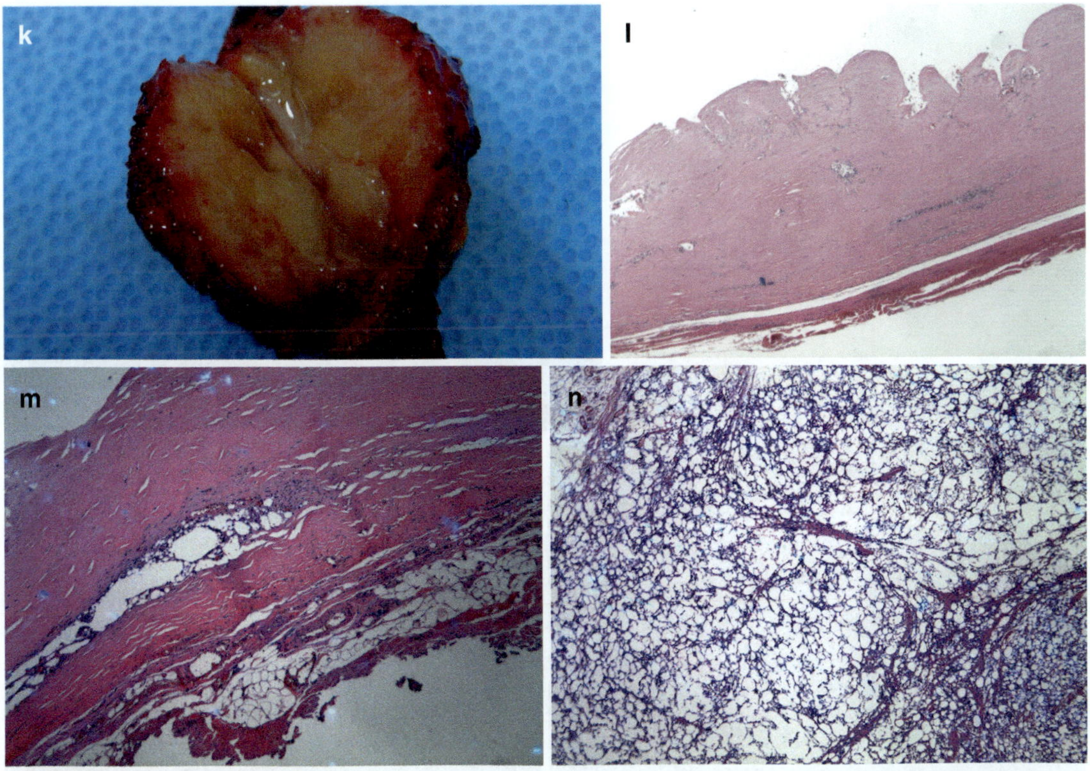

Fig. 8.48 (continued)

8.2.49 Case 49

On physical examination and history taking, a 44-year-old woman complained of breast pain. The patient had a 7-year history of receiving an implant-based augmentation mammaplasty *via* an areolar incision.

On preoperative ultrasonography, the patient was found to have a Sebbin anatomical type silicone gel-filled breast implant in the subpectoral pocket. There were sonographic findings of both extra-capsular rupture without silicone infiltration to lymph node (Video 8.67). But there were no findings that are suggestive of folding, seroma, thickened capsule, upside-down rotation, and capsular mass.

The patient underwent explantation with both near-total capsulectomy *via* a previous areolar scar on both sides. There were chronic inflammation and fibrosis in both capsule (Fig. 8.49).

8.2.50 Case 50

On physical examination and history taking, a 54-year-old woman complained of both breast hardness. The patient had a 7-year history of receiving an implant-based augmentation mammaplasty *via* an areolar incision.

On preoperative ultrasonography, the patient was found to have a Polytech anatomical silicone gel-filled breast implant in the subglandular pocket (Video 8.68). There were sonographic findings of both folded shell and thickened capsule (Video 8.69). But there were no findings that

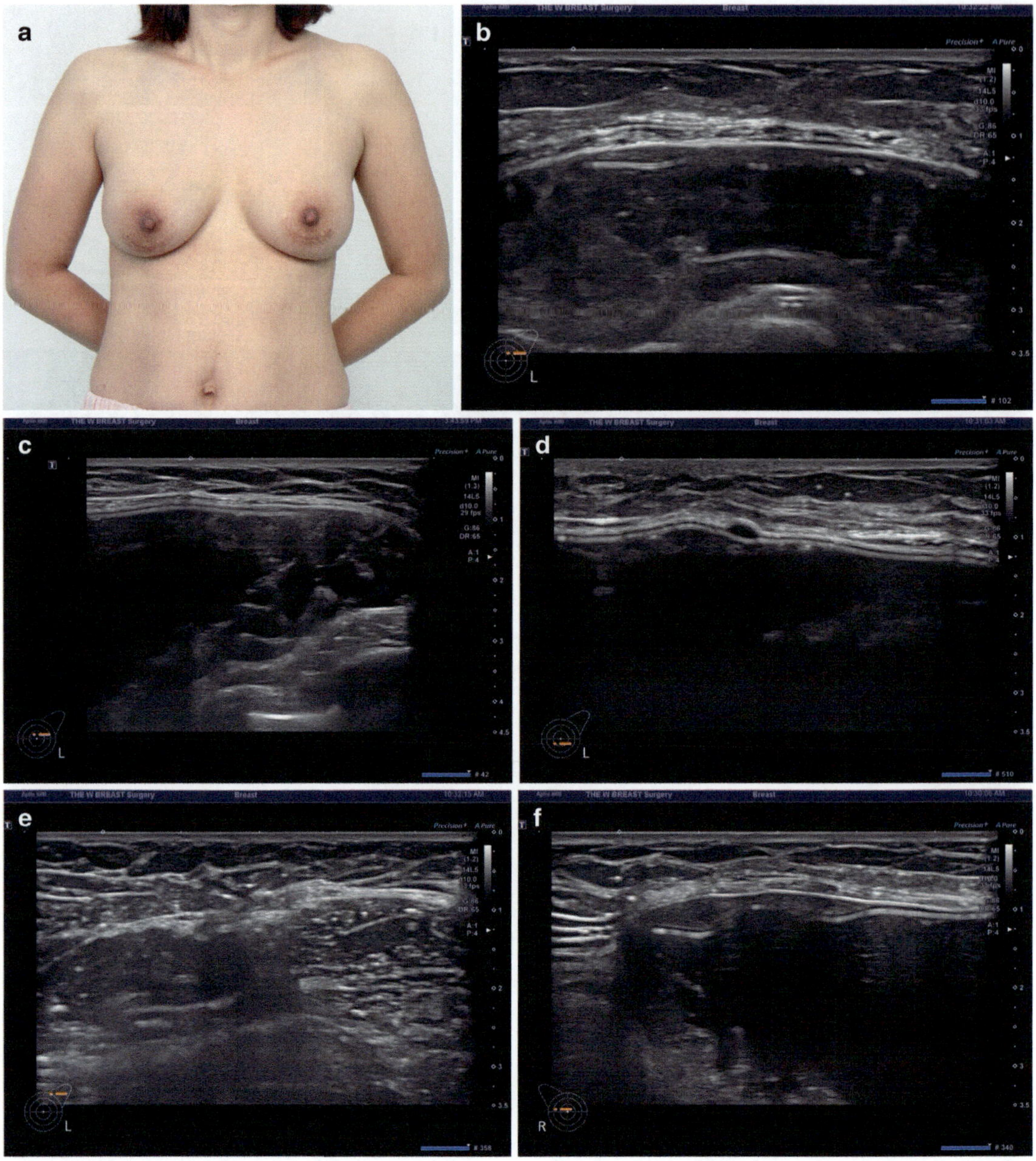

Fig. 8.49 (**a**) A preoperative front view. (**b**, **c**) Left ruptured textured shell type breast implant in subpectoral pocket is checked in preoperative ultrasonography. (**d**) Left Sebbin anatomical type breast implant orientation mark is checked in preoperative ultrasonography. (**e**) Left axillary normal lymph node status is checked in preoperative ultrasonography. No LN silicone invasion. (**f**, **g**) Right ruptured textured shell implant in subpectoral pocket is checked in preoperative ultrasonography. (**h**) Right Sebbin anatomical type breast implant orientation mark is checked in preoperative ultrasonography. (**i**) Right breast implant in subpectoral pocket is checked in preoperative ultrasonography. (**j**) Right axillary lymph node in preoperative ultrasonography. No LN silicone invasion. (**k**) Left ruptured Sebbin anatomical type breast implant and removed periprosthetic capsule after near-total capsulectomy. (**l**) Right ruptured Sebbin anatomical type breast implant and removed periprosthetic capsule after near-total capsulectomy. (**m**) Microscopic view of the left capsule with silicone invasion to capsule. (**n**) Microscopic view of the right capsule with silicone invasion to capsule

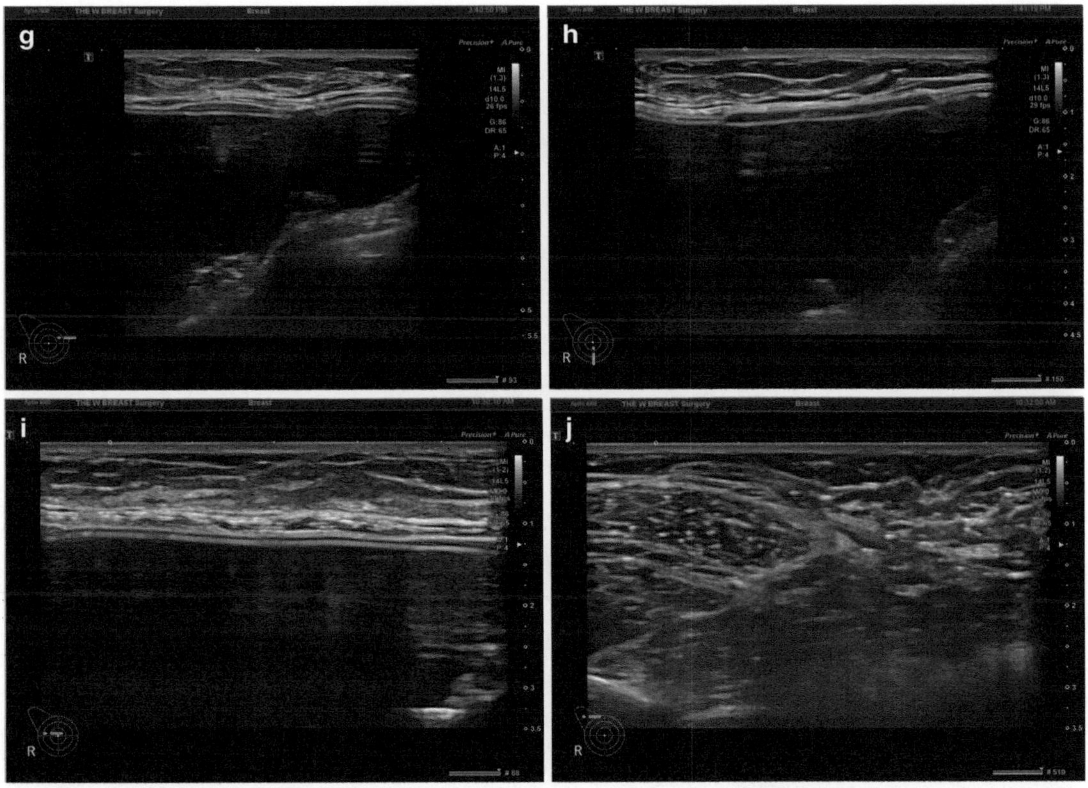

Fig. 8.49 (continued)

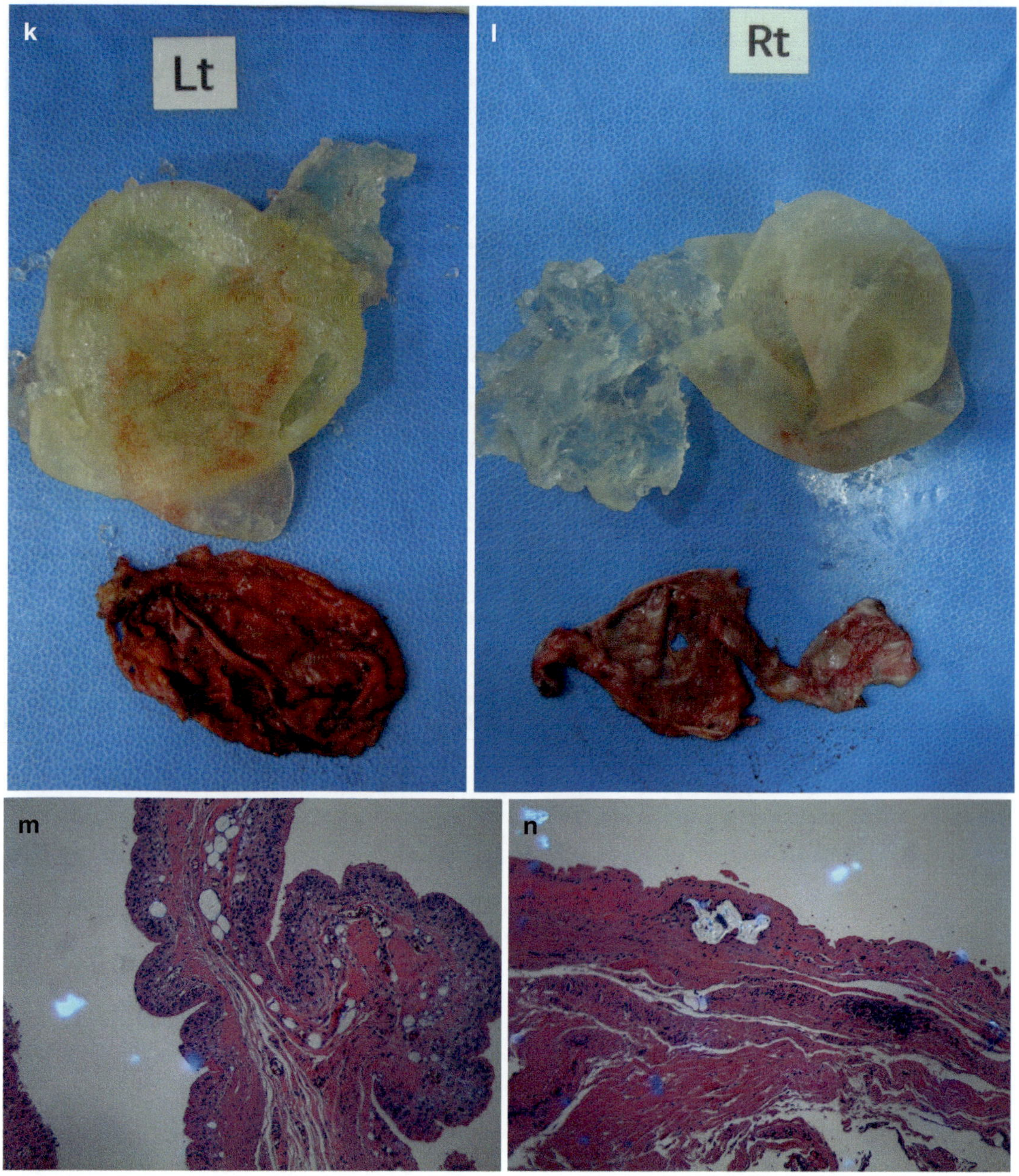

Fig. 8.49 (continued)

are suggestive of seroma, upside-down rotation, rupture, and capsular mass.

The patient underwent explantation with both total capsulectomy *via* a previous areolar scar on both sides. There were chronic inflammation and fibrosis in both capsule (Fig. 8.50).

8.2.51 Case 51

On physical examination and history taking, a 33-year-old woman complained of dissatisfaction of shape and breast pain. The patient had a 7-year history of receiving an implant-based augmentation mammaplasty *via* an areolar incision.

On preoperative ultrasonography, the patient was found to have a round textured shell type silicone gel-filled breast implant in the subpectoral pocket (Video 8.70). There was a sonographic finding of folded shell on both breasts. There was silicone contamination on the right side in preoperative ultrasonography (Video 8.71). But there were no findings that are suggestive of seroma, thickened capsule, upside-down rotation, rupture, and capsular mass.

The patient underwent right subtotal capsulectomy and left partial capsulectomy with replacement of the breast implant *via* a previous areolar scar on both sides. There were chronic inflammation and fibrosis in both capsule (Fig. 8.51).

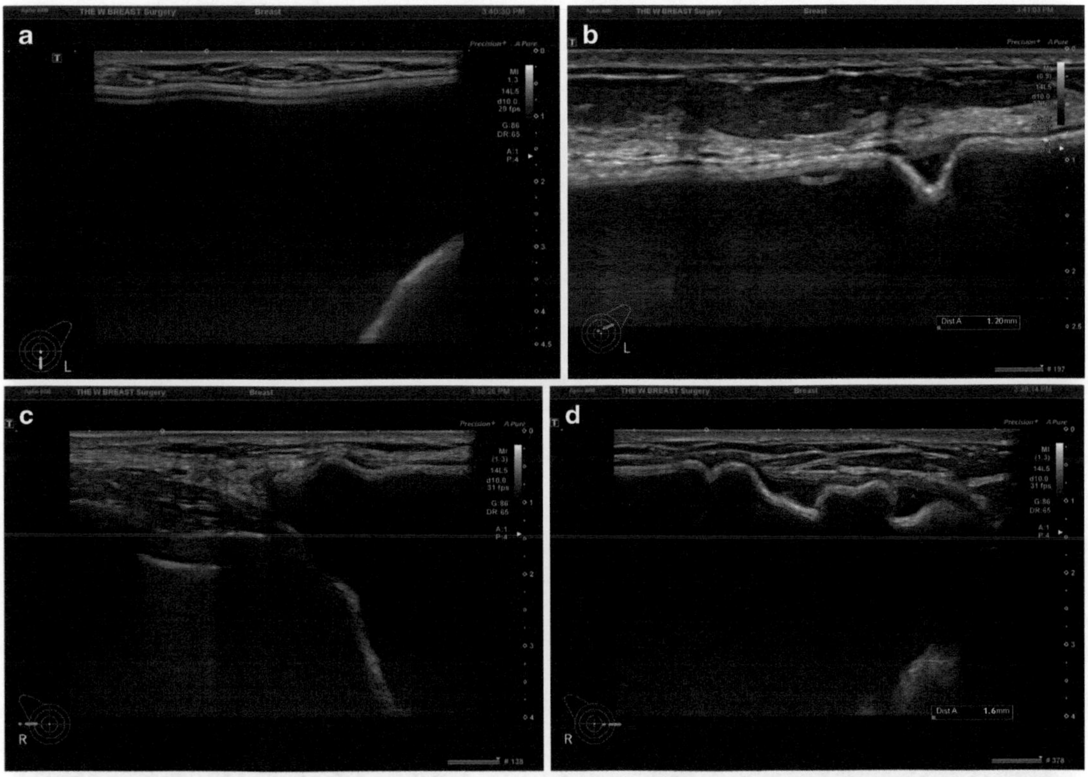

Fig. 8.50 (**a**) Left Polytech anatomical type breast implant orientation mark is checked in preoperative ultrasonography. (**b**) Left periprosthetic thickened capsule with folded shell is checked in preoperative ultrasonography. (**c**) Right texture type breast implant in subglandular pocket is checked in preoperative ultrasonography. (**d**) Right periprosthetic thickened capsule with multiple folded shell is checked in preoperative ultrasonography. (**e**) Left removed periprosthetic capsule and Polytech anatomical type breast implant 280 cc. (**f**) Right removed periprosthetic capsule and Polytech anatomical type breast implant 280 cc. (**g**) Left periprosthetic capsule thickness is measured by digital caliper, 1.3 mm. (**h**) Right periprosthetic capsule thickness is measured by digital caliper, 1.7 mm. (**i**) Microscopic view of the left capsule. (**j**) Microscopic view of the right capsule

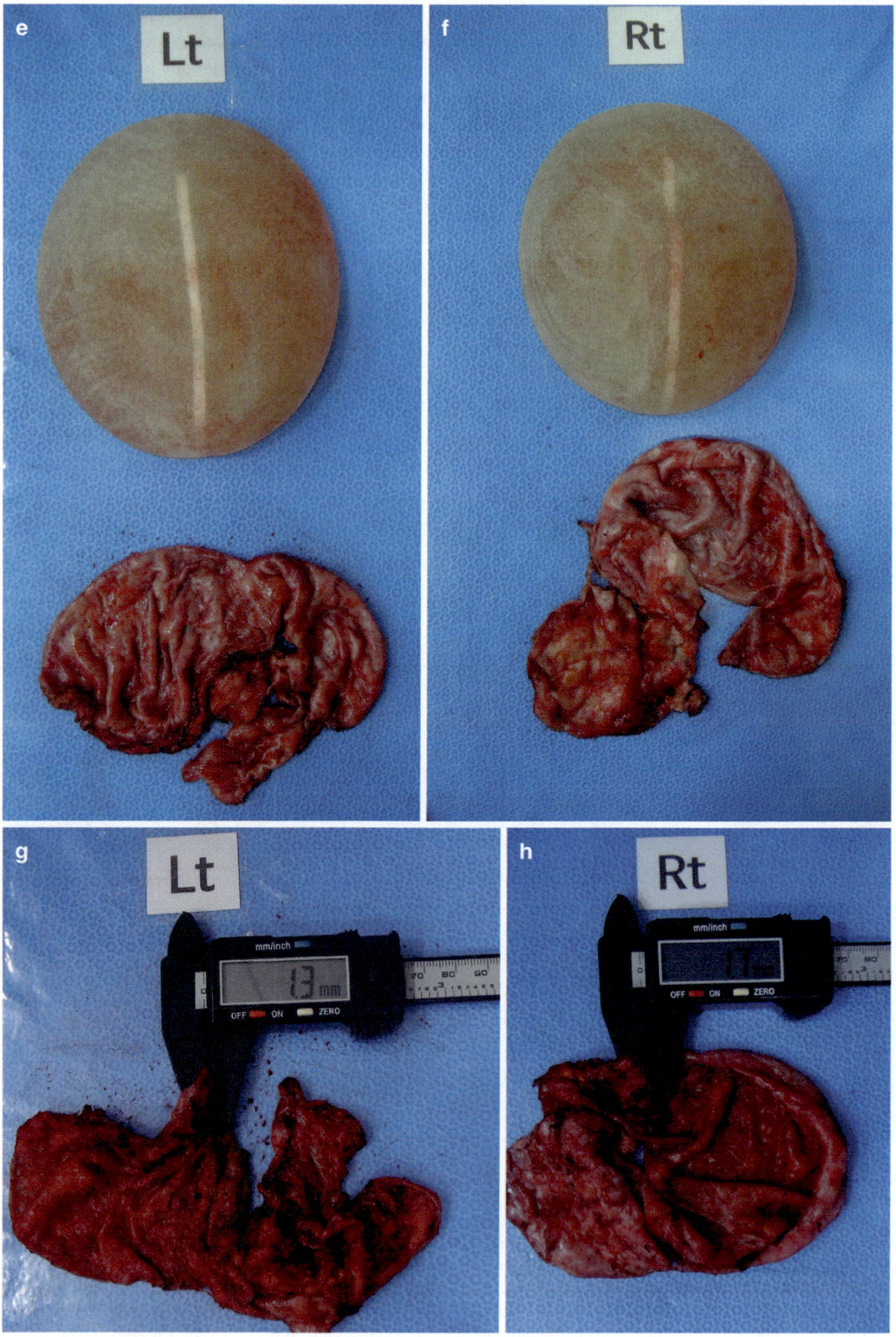

Fig. 8.50 (continued)

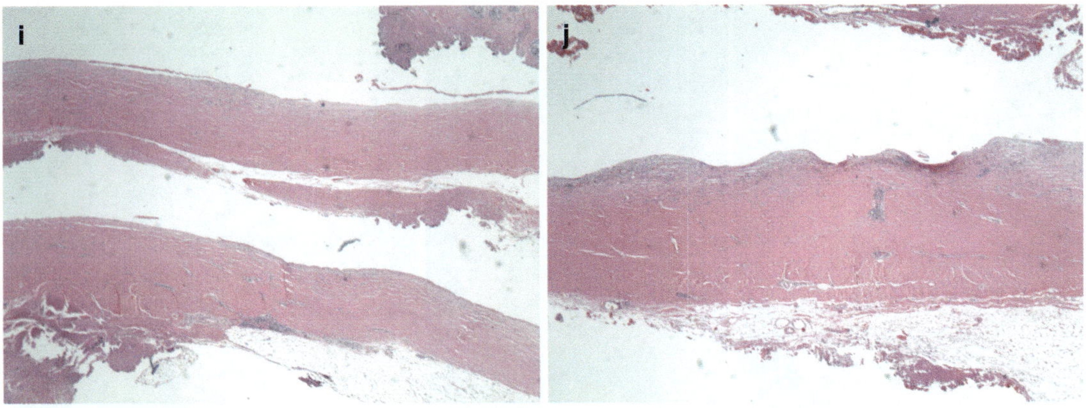

Fig. 8.50 (continued)

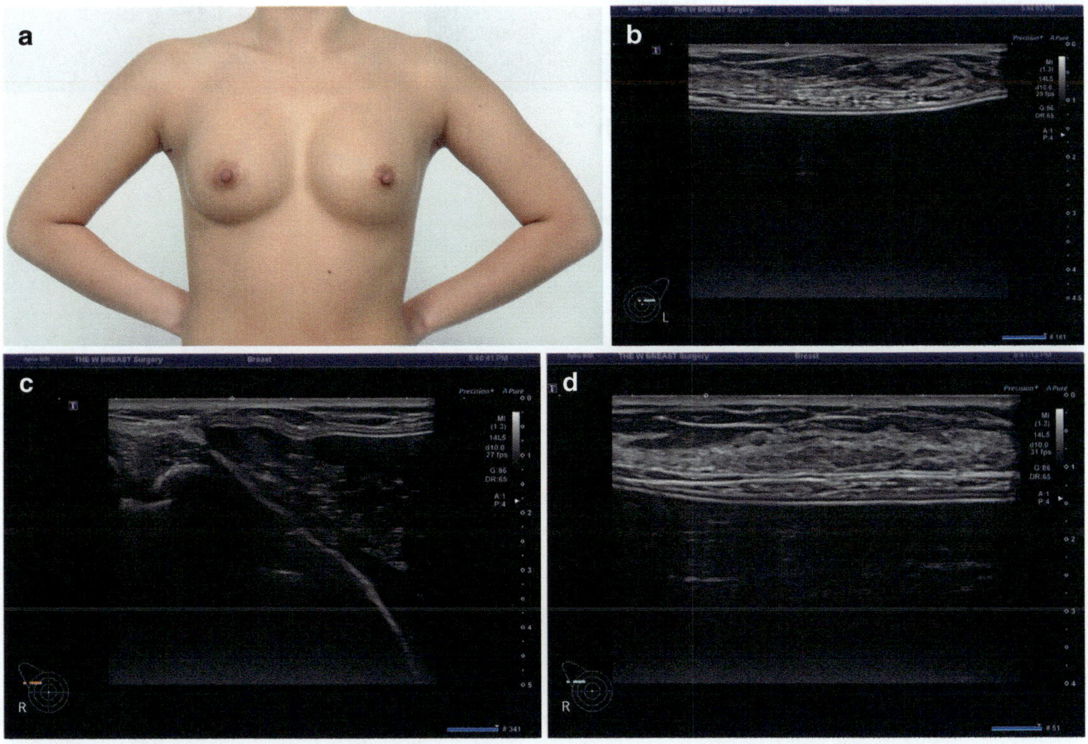

Fig. 8.51 (**a**) A preoperative front view. (**b**) Left textured shell type breast implant in subpectoral pocket is checked in preoperative ultrasonography. (**c**) Abnormal intraluminal silicone finding of right breast implant preoperative ultrasonography but there was not rupture in gross finding. (**d**) Right round textured shell type breast implant is checked in preoperative ultrasonography. (**e**) Both removed periprosthetic capsule and Mentor round texture breast implant, 250 cc. (**f**) Left periprosthetic capsule thickness is measured by digital caliper, 0.4 mm. (**g**) Right periprosthetic capsule thickness is measured by digital caliper, 0.5 mm. (**h**) Microscopic view of the left capsule. (**i**) Microscopic view of the right capsule. (**j**) Gross finding of the right removed breast implant

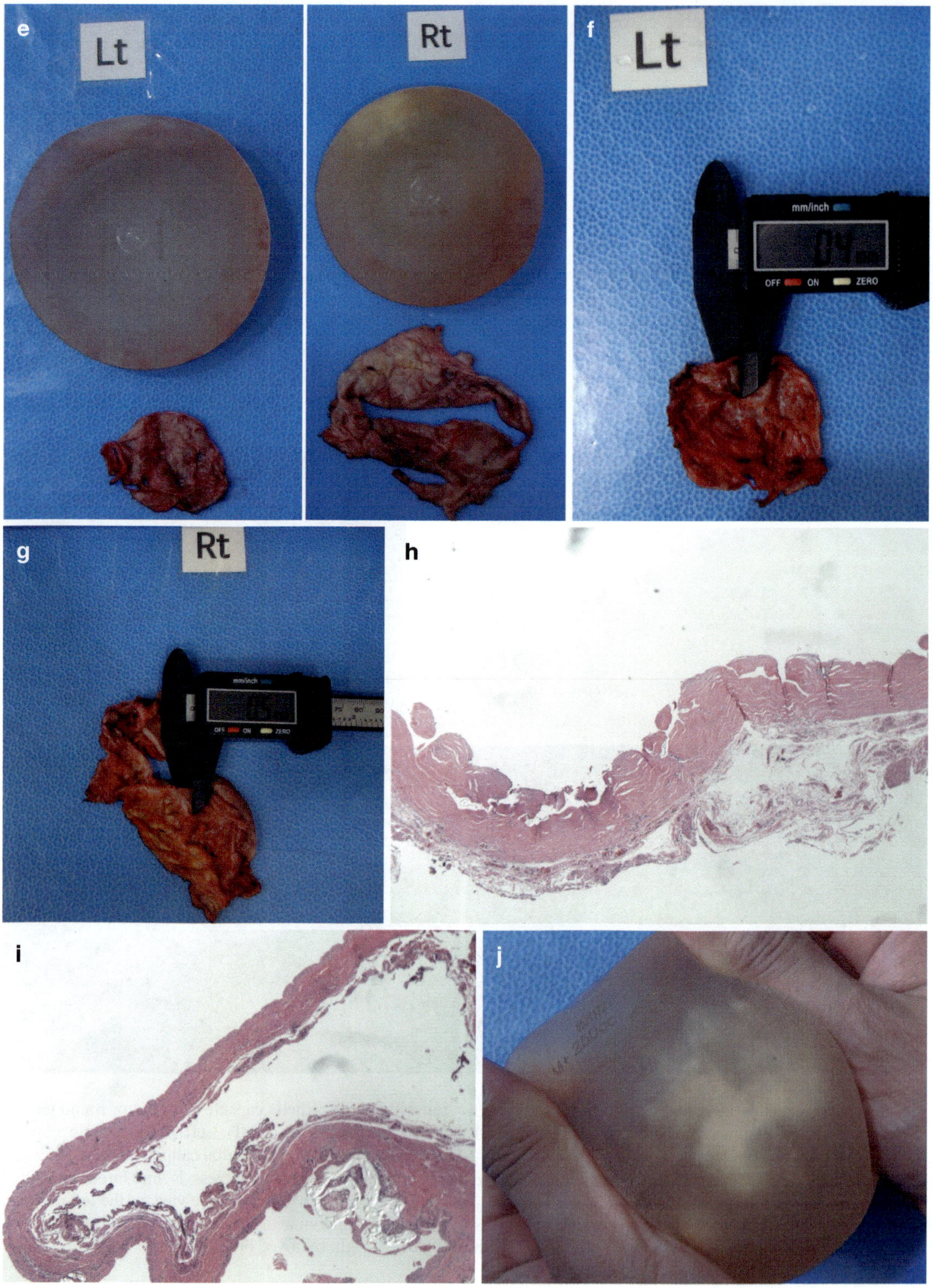

Fig. 8.51 (continued)

8.2.52 Case 52

On physical examination and history taking, a 52-year-old woman complained of breast discomfort. The patient had a 9-year history of receiving an implant-based augmentation mammaplasty *via* an axillary incision.

On preoperative ultrasonography, the patient was found to have a round smooth type silicone gel-filled breast implant in the subpectoral pocket. There was a sonographic finding of post-status of fat graft on both breasts and right intracapsular rupture with hyperechoic capsule and both thickened periprosthetic capsule (Video 8.72). But there were no findings that are suggestive of folding, seroma, upside-down rotation, and capsular mass.

The patient underwent explantation with both total capsulectomy *via* a previous axillary scar on both sides. There were chronic inflammation and fibrosis in both capsule (Fig. 8.52).

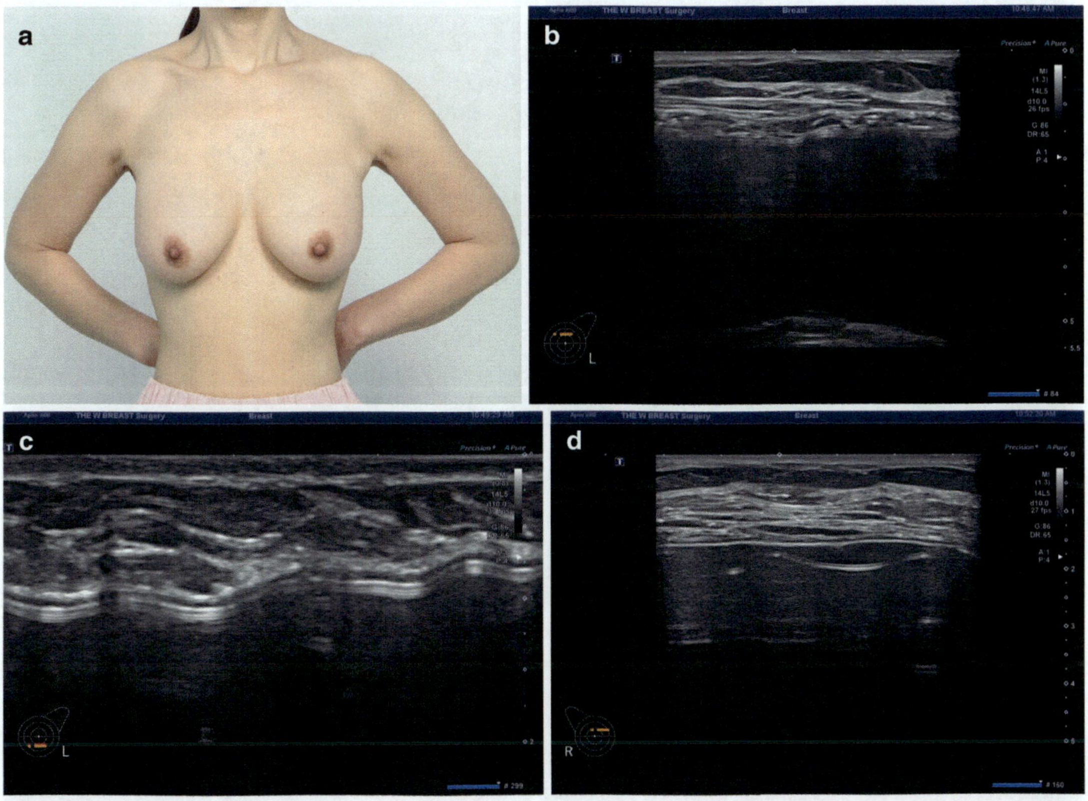

Fig. 8.52 (**a**) A preoperative front view. (**b**) Left smooth shell type breast implant in subpectoral pocket is checked in preoperative ultrasonography. (**c**) Left periprosthetic thickened capsule is checked in preoperative ultrasonography. (**d–h**) Right breast implant with rupture in subpectoral pocket is checked in preoperative ultrasonography. (**i**) Right breast implant with thickened periprosthetic capsule. (**j**) Right normal axillary lymph node. (**k**) Right intraoperative view of breast implant with periprosthetic capsule. (**l**) Right intraoperative view of ruptured breast implant. (**m**) Right intraoperative view of intracapsular breast pocket with free silicone. (**n, o**) Right intraoperative view of breast pocket after total capsulectomy. (**p**) Both removed periprosthetic capsule and Mentor round smooth shell type breast implant 300 cc. (**q**) Both removed periprosthetic capsule after total capsulectomy. (**r**) Microscopic view of the left capsule. (**s**) Microscopic view of the right capsule

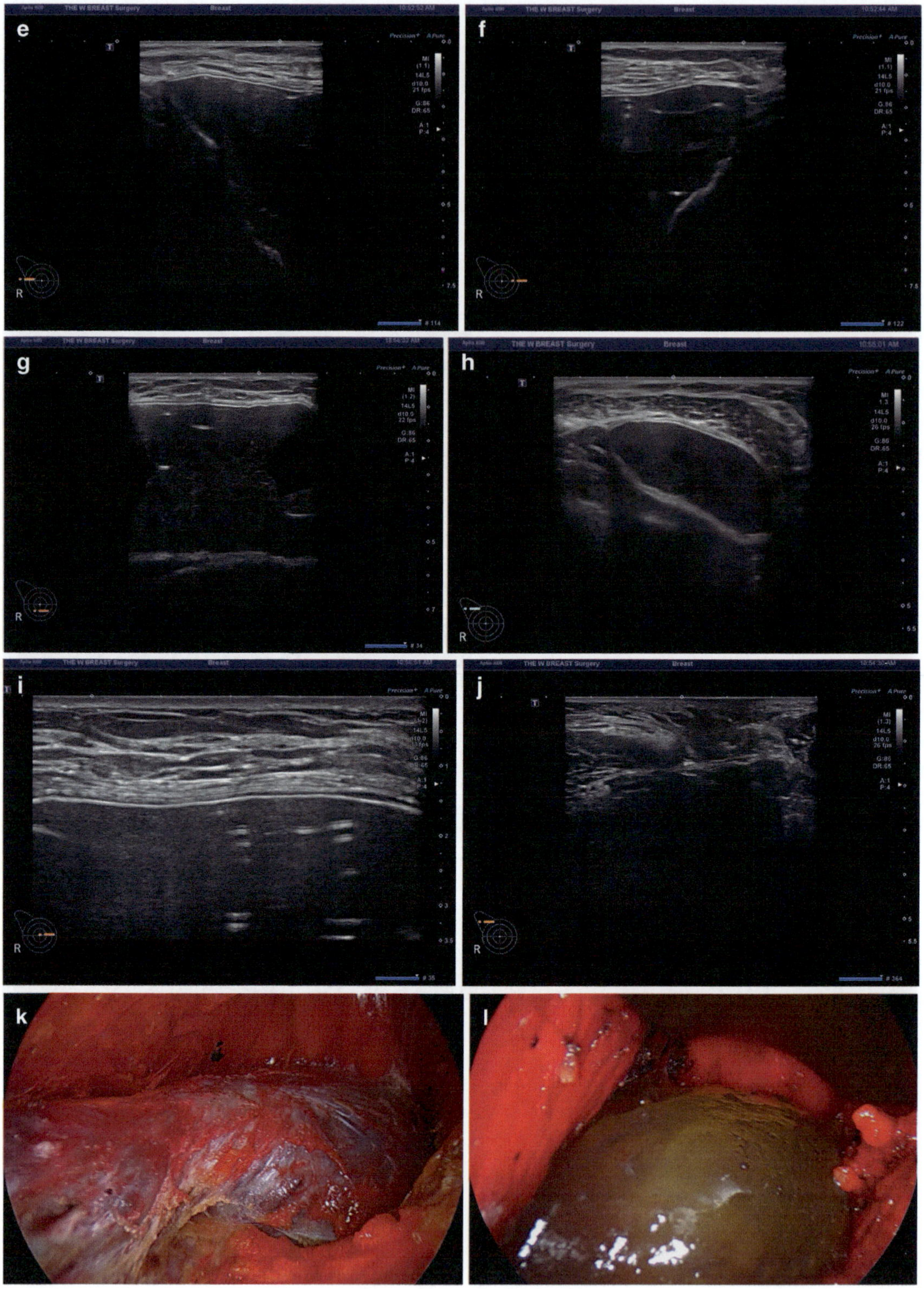

Fig. 8.52 (continued)

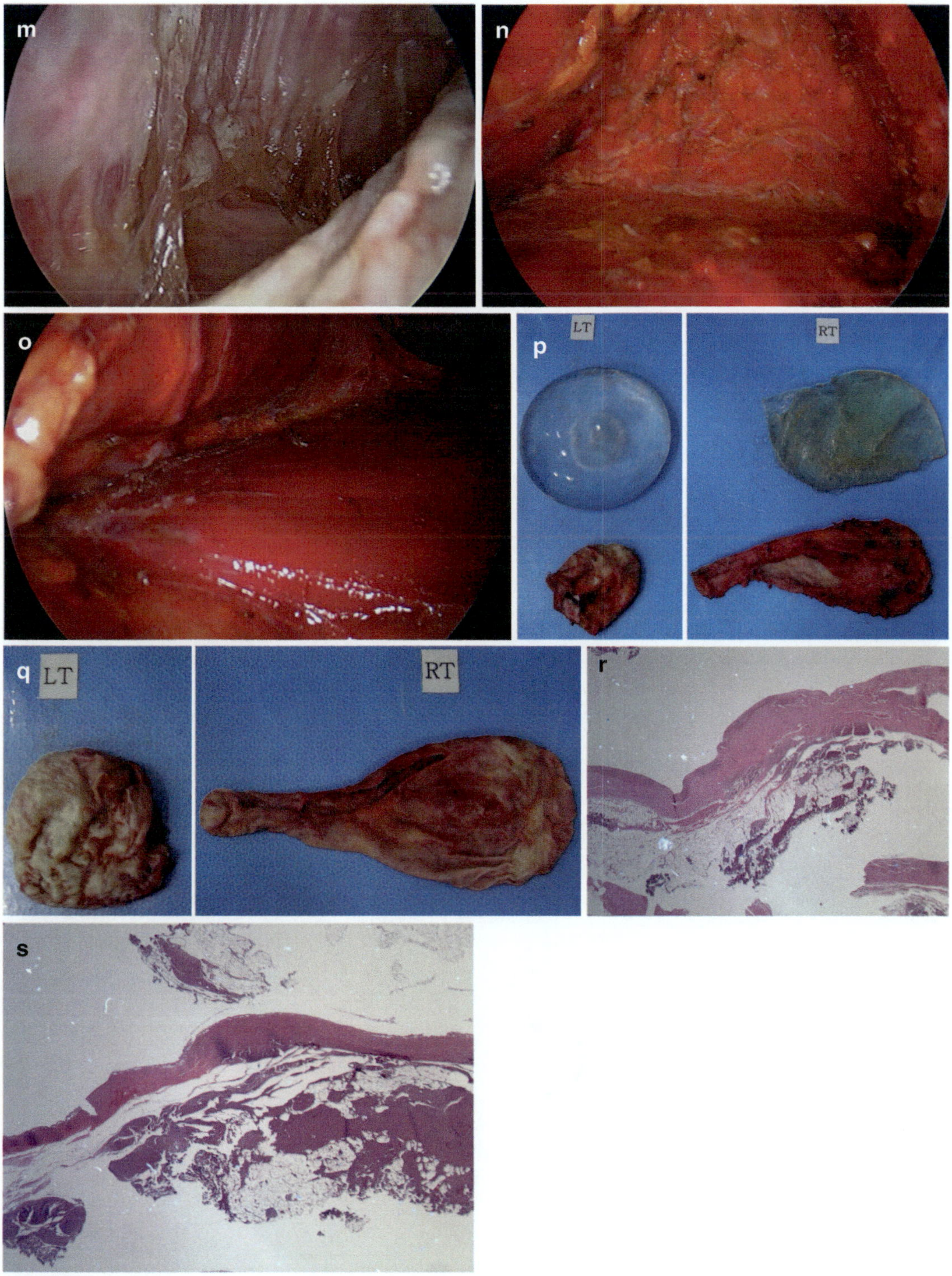

Fig. 8.52 (continued)

References

1. Sung JY, Jeong JP, Moon DS, et al. Short-term safety of augmentation mammaplasty using the BellaGel implants in Korean women. Plast Reconstr Surg Glob Open. 2019;7(12):e2566.
2. Kim JH, Paik NS, Nam SY, Cho Y, Park HK. The emerging crisis of stakeholders in implant-based augmentation mammaplasty in Korea. J Korean Med Sci. 2020;35(15):e103.

9 Conclusions

A silicone gel-filled breast implant was first developed by Cronin and Gerow in 1962 [1]. Subsequently, it became commercially available by the Dow Corning Corporation (Midland, MI) [2]. This initiated the era of the first generation of a silicone gel-filled breast implant, extending from 1962 to 1970, which is composed of a thick outer silicone shell and a dense inner silicone gel [3]. But their unnatural feel and appearance and a high rate of scar tissue formation around the device, i.e., capsular contracture (CC), remained problematic. To resolve this, the second-generation of a silicone gel-filled breast implant was developed and then commercially manufactured during a period between 1970 and 1982; it was characterized by a softer and less viscous inner silicone gel *as well as* a thinner and semi-permeable outer shell [4, 5]. But the second generation of a silicone gel-filled breast implant was disadvantageous in that it caused diffusion of silicone gel through the implant shell [6].

The third generation of a silicone gel-filled breast implant emerged and was circulated in the market between 1982 and 1992, aiming to achieve a balance between the softness and strength of a device. It was equipped with a multi-layered silicone elastomer shell with less permeability *as well as* a slightly more viscous silicone gel [1, 7].

In 1992, the US Food and Drug Administration (FDA) mandated moratorium on a silicone gel-filled breast implant because of a paucity of the safety data and modifications to medical device regulations. Since then until 2006, its clinical use had been strongly prohibited except for clinical trials in the USA [8]. Meanwhile, a saline-filled breast implant had been used alternatively in the USA, while a silicone gel-filled one remained commercially available in the rest of the world [9]. But this is also accompanied by continuous efforts to improve the design of a silicone gel-filled breast implant, thus initiating the era of the fourth and fifth generation of devices that are currently commercially available in the market.

In 2006, the US FDA approved the clinical use of a silicone gel-filled breast implant. The fourth generation of a silicone gel-filled breast implant, also known as a round device, is characterized by a rigorous manufacturing process in compliance with guidelines of the American Society for Testing Methodology (ASTM). Its advantages include diverse types of shape and surface texture [1, 10, 11].

In 2012, the fifth generation of a silicone gel-filled breast implant, also known as a shaped device, emerged in the market. It is characterized by a more cohesive silicone gel forming a tear-drop shape, thus being advantageous in *not only* achieving ideal goals of breast aesthetics *but also* maintaining the breast integrity in response to physiological forces [1, 12, 13]. This explains why the fifth generation of a silicone gel-filled breast implant is also called as a form-stable, highly-cohesive or anatomical device [1, 12, 14].

Currently, a silicone gel-filled breast is manufactured by several companies around the world;

J. H. Kim, *Atlas of Breast Implant Ultrasound*, https://doi.org/10.1007/978-981-16-8282-7_9

these include Allergan Inc. (Irvine, CA), Mentor Worldwide LLC (Santa Barbara, CA), Sientra Inc. (Santa Barbara, CA), Groupe Sebbin SAS (Boissy-l' Aillerie, France), HansBiomed Co. Ltd. (Seoul, Korea), Establishment Labs Holdings Inc. (Alajuela, Costa Rica), GC Aesthetics PLC (Apt Cedex, France), Polytech Health & Aesthetics (Dieburg, Germany), Nagor Ltd. (Glasgow, UK), and Guangzhou Wanhe Plastic Materials Co. Ltd. (Guangzhou, China) [15, 16].

Since breast implants are a medical device that is placed in a human body, their safety should be rigorously assessed. Most of the published studies in this series include those about the safety of breast implants manufactured by Allergan and Mentor.

One of the most common complications of augmentation mammaplasty is CC. This is a pathologic hardening and tightening of the capsule around the implant. Still, little is known about its exact etiologic and pathophysiologic mechanisms, for which various hypotheses have been proposed [17–19].

Previous published studies have shown that the incidence of CC is relatively lower in patients undergoing augmentation mammaplasty using textured implants [20, 21]. But this remains controversial; the use of smooth implants has also been advocated based on reports that there is no significant difference in the incidence of CC between the textured and smooth types [22–25]. Textured implants are characterized by an ability to modify the host response to wound healing. Tissue ingrowth may not only stabilize the interface of implants but also increase compatibility. This leads to an inhibition of the formation of CC [26]. In more detail, irregular surface properties of textured implants promote the growth of fibroblasts into and around their interface. The resulting contact inhibition effect may lead to the formation of a thinner capsule around the implant [27, 28]. By contrast, smooth implants promote the fibrosis characterized by the deposition of collagen fibrils in a capsule composed of the connective tissue around the implant [29, 30].

To date, various types of silicone gel-filled breast implants have become commercially available and then used in a clinical setting. Their safety profiles have been well studied and described in the literature. According to the 10-year follow-up results about Natrelle 410 anatomical form-stable silicone-filled breast implants, CC of Baker grades III and IV occurred at an incidence of 9.2% in patients who underwent breast augmentation. Moreover, other complications include rupture (9.4%), malposition (4.7%), asymmetry (6.9%), and seroma (1.6%). Furthermore, there was a case of breast-implant-associated anaplastic large cell lymphoma (BIA-ALCL) [31]. On the other hand, the 410 Allergan core study has drawn a conclusion that capsular contracture occurred most frequently after breast implant surgery; there was a time-dependent increase in the risk of capsular contracture despite a relatively lower incidence of capsular contracture seen in the Natrelle round gel (fourth generation) core study (56.2%) [32]. In a similar context, according to the 6-year follow-up data about the form-stable Mentor Contour Profile Gel (CPG) implants (Mentor Worldwide LLC, Santa Barbara, CA), the incidence of capsular contracture was lower as compared with smooth-surface round gel breast implants [33, 34]. Of note, the implant rippling or wrinkling occurred at a very low rate of 0.9% in patients undergoing breast augmentation according to the 10-year data [35].

In addition to the formation of CC, patients undergoing augmentation mammaplasty using prosthetic implants are also vulnerable to other complications, such as infection, hematoma, seroma, rupture, malposition, and ripple deformity [36, 37]. Furthermore, BIA-ALCL is the most fatal complication of an implant-based augmentation mammaplasty. It also occurred in Korea. There were a total of three cases of BIA-ALCL; it was reported on August 16 and December 24, 2019 and October 5, 2020. This warns stakeholders in an implant-based augmentation mammaplasty of the importance of evidence-based approach to an early detection of its complications in women receiving augmentation mammaplasty [16].

Breast implant ultrasound is somewhat unfamiliar to readers of this book. Over the past decade, as a surgical practitioner, I have made considerable efforts to broaden the understanding of how it is a useful modality in making a diagnosis of complications of an implant-based augmentation mammaplasty. Then, I have dedicated myself to collecting patients' data in an effort to accumulate evidences demonstrating the feasibility of breast ultrasound in examining the integrity of breast implant *as well as* making an accurate diagnosis of complications of an implant-based augmentation mammaplasty. I strongly believe that this is the best way to perform evidence-based clinical practice for patients receiving it.

Knowledge about a breast implant is an essential factor for surgeons dealing with it and other physicians who are involved in examination of it. Still, however, there is a paucity of publications about it. I have therefore made an effort to innovate methods for examining patients, which will be of interest to readers of this book.

Currently, use of high-resolution ultrasound makes it possible to examine the integrity of a breast implant and to obtain detailed information about it. A surgeon's use of high-resolution ultrasound is useful in detecting postoperative complications at the earliest opportunities possible, taking active measures against patients' discomfort and establishing a good rapport with them. Moreover, it is also useful in accurately confirming the location of breast pocket, which may contribute to developing the surgical technique. Thus, it is an efficient modality in identifying a manufacturer of a breast implant and its types, thus enabling a surgeon to identify a textured implant associated with BIA-ALCL. It would therefore be mandatory for a surgeon to examine whether patients complain of symptoms arising from the breast parenchyma or an implant when receiving an implant-based augmentation mammaplasty. I feel confident that this book will provide healthcare professionals with useful information; a complete understanding of the breast implant ultrasound would be a surprise for them.

In preparation for the future, I'm currently involved in developing a portable high-resolution ultrasound equipment that transmits the data from a patient to healthcare professionals.

In this book, I have described the current and future perspectives of ultrasound-assisted examination of a breast implant. Use of high-resolution breast ultrasound is an operator-dependent modality and therefore requires a long learning curve. I hope that this book will be help readers obtain a sufficient understanding of it.

In the near future, based on the image data accumulated by the author so far, AI software related to implant failure and distinguishing by ultrasonography will be completed. It is expected that this will provide practical help to many plastic surgeons.

www.waibio.co.kr

References

1. Maxwell GP, Gabriel A. Breast implant design. Gland Surg. 2017;6(2):148–53.
2. Cronin TD, Brauer RO. Augmentation mammaplasty. Surg Clin North Am. 1971;51:441–52.
3. Cronin TD, Greenberg RL. Our experiences with the silastic gel breast prosthesis. Plast Reconstr Surg. 1970;46:1–7.
4. Oh JS, Jeong JH, Myung Y, Oh J, Kang SH, Park E, Kim A, Bang SI, Heo CY. BellaGel breast implant: 6-year results of a prospective cohort study. Arch Plast Surg. 2020;47(3):235–41.
5. Headon H, Kasem A, Mokbel K. Capsular contracture after breast augmentation: an update for clinical practice. Arch Plast Surg. 2015;42(5):532–43.
6. Vázquez G, Pellón A. Polyurethane-coated silicone gel breast implants used for 18 years. Aesthet Plast Surg. 2007;31(4):330–6.
7. Maxwell GP, Gabriel A. The evolution of breast implants. Plast Reconstr Surg. 2014 Jul;134(1 Suppl):12S–7S.
8. Young VL, Watson ME. Breast implant research: where we have been, where we are, where we need to go. Clin Plast Surg. 2001;28:451–83.
9. Jewell ML. Silicone gel breast implants at 50: the state of the science. Aesthet Surg J. 2012;32(8):1031–4.
10. Handel N, Garcia ME, Wixtrom R. Breast implant rupture: causes, incidence, clinical impact, and management. Plast Reconstr Surg. 2013;132(5):1128–37.
11. Nava MB, Rancati A, Angrigiani C, Catanuto G, Rocco N. How to prevent complications in breast augmentation. Gland Surg. 2017;6(2):210–7.
12. O'Shaughnessy K. Evolution and update on current devices for prosthetic breast reconstruction. Gland Surg. 2015;4(2):97–110.
13. Hedén P, Jernbeck J, Hober M. Breast augmentation with anatomical cohesive gel implants: the world's largest current experience. Clin Plast Surg. 2001;28(3):531–52.
14. Choi MS, Chang JH, Seul CH. A multi-center, retrospective, preliminary observational study to assess

the safety of BellaGel® after augmentation mammaplasty. Eur J Plast Surg. 2020;43:577–82.
15. Kim JH, Paik NS, Nam SY, Cho Y, Park HK. The emerging crisis of stakeholders in implant-based augmentation mammaplasty in Korea. J Korean Med Sci. 2020;35(15):e103.
16. Chao AH, Garza R 3rd, Povoski SP. A review of the use of silicone implants in breast surgery. Expert Rev Med Devices. 2016;13(2):143–56.
17. Steiert AE, Boyce M, Sorg H. Capsular contracture by silicone breast implants: possible causes, biocompatibility, and prophylactic strategies. Med Devices. 2013;6:211–8.
18. Huang CK, Handel N. Effects of Singulair (montelukast) treatment for capsular contracture. Aesthet Surg J. 2010;30:404–8.
19. Bachour Y, Bargon CA, de Blok CJM, Ket JCF, Ritt MJPF, Niessen FB. Risk factors for developing capsular contracture in women after breast implant surgery: a systematic review of the literature. J Plast Reconstr Aesthet Surg. 2018;71:e29–48.
20. Spear SL, Elmaraghy M, Hess C. Textured-surface saline-filled silicone breast implants for augmentation mammaplasty. Plast Reconstr Surg. 2000;105:1542–52.
21. Pollock H. Breast capsular contracture: a retrospective study of textured versus smooth silicone implants. Plast Reconstr Surg. 1993;91:404–7.
22. Biggs TM, Yarish RS. Augmentation mammaplasty: a comparative analysis. Plast Reconstr Surg. 1990;85:368–72.
23. Handel N, Jensen JA, Black Q, Waisman JR, Silverstein MJ. The fate of breast implants: a critical analysis of complications and outcomes. Plast Reconstr Surg. 1995;96:1521–33.
24. Becker H, Springer R. Prevention of capsular contracture. Plast Reconstr Surg. 1999;103:1766–8.
25. Fagrell D, Berggren A, Tarpila E. Capsular contracture around saline-filled fine textured and smooth mammary implants: a prospective 7.5-year follow-up. Plast Reconstr Surg. 2001;108:2108–12.
26. Bergmann PA, Tamouridis G, Lohmeyer JA, Mauss KL, Becker B, Knobloch J, Mailänder P, Siemers F. The effect of a bacterial contamination on the formation of capsular contracture with polyurethane breast implants in comparison with textured silicone implants: an animal study. J Plast Reconstr Aesthet Surg. 2014;67:1364–70.
27. Lei ZY, Liu T, Li WJ, Shi XH, Fan DL. Biofunctionalization of silicone rubber with microgroove-patterned surface and carbon-ion implantation to enhance biocompatibility and reduce capsule formation. Int J Nanomedicine. 2016;11:5563–72.
28. Minami E, Koh IH, Ferreira JC, Waitzberg AF, Chifferi V, Rosewick TF, Pereira MD, Saldiva PH, de Figueiredo LF. The composition and behavior of capsules around smooth and textured breast implants in pigs. Plast Reconstr Surg. 2006;118:874–84.
29. Moyer KE, Ehrlich HP. Capsular contracture after breast reconstruction: collagen fiber orientation and organization. Plast Reconstr Surg. 2015;131:680–5.
30. Spano A, Palmieri B, Taidelli TP, Nava MB. Reduction of capsular thickness around silicone breast implants by zafirlukast in rats. Eur Surg Res. 2008;41:8–14.
31. Maxwell GP, Van Natta BW, Bengtson BP, Murphy DK. Ten-year results from the Natrelle 410 anatomical form-stable silicone breast implant core study. Aesthet Surg J. 2015;35:145–55.
32. Spear SL, Murphy DK; Allergan Silicone Breast Implant U.S. Core Clinical Study Group. Natrelle round silicone breast implants: Core Study results at 10 years. Plast Reconstr Surg. 2014;133:1354–61.
33. Hammond DC, Migliori MM, Caplin DA, Garcia ME, Phillips CA. Mentor Contour Profile Gel implants: clinical outcomes at 6 years. Plast Reconstr Surg. 2012;129:1381–91.
34. Cunningham B, McCue J. Safety and effectiveness of Mentor's MemoryGel implants at 6 years. Aesthet Plast Surg. 2009;33:440–4.
35. Hammond DC, Canady JW, Love TR, Wixtrom RN, Caplin DA. Mentor contour profile gel implants: clinical outcomes at 10 years. Plast Reconstr Surg. 2017;140:1142–50.
36. Ballard TNS, Hill S, Nghiem BT, Lysikowski JR, Brandt K, Cederna PS, Kenkel JM. Current trends in breast augmentation: analysis of 2011-2015 maintenance of certification (MOC) tracer data. Aesthet Surg J. 2019;39:615–23.
37. McGuire P, Reisman NR, Murphy DK. Risk factor analysis for capsular contracture, malposition, and late seroma in subjects receiving natrelle 410 form-stable silicone breast implants. Plast Reconstr Surg. 2017;139:1–9.

GPSR Compliance

The European Union's (EU) General Product Safety Regulation (GPSR) is a set of rules that requires consumer products to be safe and our obligations to ensure this.

If you have any concerns about our products, you can contact us on ProductSafety@springernature.com

In case Publisher is established outside the EU, the EU authorized representative is:

Springer Nature Customer Service Center GmbH
Europaplatz 3
69115 Heidelberg, Germany

Batch number: 10732801

Printed by Printforce, the Netherlands